Craig **IMPORTANT!** Maley

Confined Space and Structural Rope Rescue

It is critical that the following changes and corrections are noted.

Page Number	Figure Number	Corrections
50	3.11	Horizontal axis is the Minor Axis. Vertical axis is the Major Axis.
76	(A)	Line with arrow should indicate that the rope continues to wrap around the anchor.
77	(middle)	Line with arrow should pass underneath the loop (as shown in last figure).
84	(C)	Line with arrow should pass behind the red webbing.
92	5.1	Example of an extended anchor rather than a load-sharing bridle.
93	(B)	Example of a screw-link attachment rather than a butterfly knot in rope.
115	6.14	Excessive rope wraps are shown.
132	(3rd figure)	Line is incomplete; 4th figure shows the completed lock-off.
166	9.23	Shows BTLS strapping technique rather than a Figure-8 weave.
186	10.25	Incorrect photo. Long spineboard in Sked is shown in Figure 10.28.
221	11.28	Illustration should show the attendant's feet slightly below the litter.
277	15.6	Warning: Not Recommended! Procedure violates manufacturer's recommendations and therefore violates OSHA regulations.
298	17.6	This system is called CSR System 5.

Confined Space and Structural Rope Rescue

Confined Space and Structural Rope Rescue

Michael Roop

Tom Vines

Richard Wright

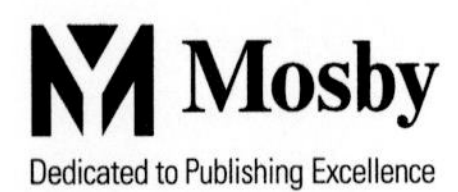

A Times Mirror
Company

Publisher: Don Ladig
Acquisitions Editor: Jennifer Roche
Editorial Assistant: Jeanne Murphy
Senior Production Editors: Nadine Fitzwilliam, Shannon Bates
Art Director: Max Brinkmann
Design: Frank Loose Design, Portland, OR
Manufacturing Manager: Betty Mueller
Photography: Camille Gerace, Cam-Works
Line Art: Beverly Ransom

FIRST EDITION

Printed in the United States of America.

Composition by: GGS Information Services
Printing/Binding by: Von Hoffman Press

Mosby-Year Book, Inc.
11830 Westline Industrial Drive
St. Louis, MIssouri 63146

Library of Congress Cataloging-in-Publication Data

Roop, Michael.
Confined space and industrial rescue / Michael Roop, Tom Vines, Richard Wright.
p. cm.
Includes index.
ISBN 0-8151-7383-0 (pbk.)
1. Industrial safety--Handbooks, manuals, etc. 2. Rescue work--Handbooks, manuals, etc. 3. Industrial accidents--Handbooks, manuals, etc. I. Wright, Richard. II. Vines, Tom. III. Title.
T55.R63 1997
628.9'2--dc21 97-22071
CIP

98 99 00 01 02 / 9 8 7 6 5 4 3 2 1

Dedication

This book is dedicated to the people who have made the conscious decision to put themselves at some risk to save another person's life. The National Association for Search and Rescue's motto is *"So that others may live"* . . . obviously, a rescuer is a unique sort of person. While the general public may consider rescuers heroes because of what they do, we believe rescuers are special just because they voluntarily put themselves in a position to be called upon. Then respond without hesitation. The true measure of rescuers (and maybe, heroes) is how they prepare themselves to respond with the greatest possibility for success. We intend this book to better prepare these very special people.

Introduction

This book is a collaboration of three individuals whose backgrounds have little in common other than rescue. A retired law enforcement officer, a former firefighter/paramedic, and a writer/rural rescuer have all been drawn to the rescue field, a field in which they all currently make their living. While their combined experience of over seventy years in the rescue field might seem impressive, **it is not**, particularly, if experience only equates to survival. Hopefully, the authors' experience and training has resulted in knowledge that eventually has evolved into wisdom.

Practitioners in the field of rescue should focus on the safest and most efficient rescue method or piece of rescue equipment. This search for better techniques and technology requires an open and questioning mind. So the authors' combined wisdom has enabled them to compile this book of techniques, strategies, and, yes, philosophies about industrial/structural rope rescue.

The authors offer this book as "battle-proven" ideas. However, the offerings here are not the only way to approach structural rope rescue. The one perfect technique or perfect piece of equipment simply does not exist. There is no one magical way to approach, package, and move a victim from a hazardous location to a safe location. There are numerous "right" methodologies and, more importantly, **numerous wrong ones**. Rather than attempting to write a generic text that addresses a multitude of rescue approaches using a variety of techniques and equipment types, the authors have limited the content to specifics they use, teach, and recommend. This book is not intended as **the** answer for the rescuer, but rather a compilation of answers that have been used successfully time and again.

Acknowledgments

The authors gratefully acknowledge the many rescuers, students, instructors, and manufacturers who have contributed to the concepts and ideas presented in this book. We are especially appreciative to our friends and family members who endured countless hours of aggravation and separation, yet continued to support us, as we developed this text. While it is impossible to thank everyone individually, we would like to acknowledge the following individuals:

Robert Aguiluz, Roco Rescue
Capt. Mark Baker, Wichita Fire Department
Dan Bestwick, Roco Rescue Adjunct Instructor
Don Cooper, Cuyahoga Falls Fire Department
Chief Leonard Deonarine, Refinery Terminal Fire Company
Capt. Tim Gallagher, Phoenix Fire Department
Jim Gillingham, Weyerhauser-Kamloops, British Columbia
Lynn Harp, Amoco-Evanston, Wyoming
Steve Hudson, PMI-Petzl
Andy Ibbestson, Con-Space Communications
Kenny Moore, Shell Oil DPMC-Deer Park, Texas
Michael Reimer, South Technical Education Center
Kay Roop, Roco Rescue
Capt. Bob Salo, North Vancouver Fire Department
Capt. Jimmy Sibley, Baton Rouge Fire Department
Norma Sibley, Chevron Chemical-St. James, Louisiana
Chaplin Durrell Tuberville, Shreveport Fire Department

THE AUTHORS WOULD ALSO LIKE TO ESPECIALLY THANK THE FOLLOWING ORGANIZATIONS:

CMC Rescue; PMI-Petzl; and Roco Rescue (Staff & Instructors).

PHOTOGRAPHY:

Bob Davis, Photography; Don Allen, Photography; and John Voinche' of Roco Rescue.

GRAPHIC ILLUSTRATIONS:

2121 Graphics (Baton Rouge, Louisiana) and Jeff Forrest of Roco Rescue.

Preface

Confined Space and Structural Rope Rescue is directed at the industrial rescuer, but the techniques are applicable to all fields of rescue that include confined spaces or elevated environments. The urban or rural fire-rescue team will find this book invaluable for their applications. This book is, however, limited to **structural** rescue; meaning man-made structures. Wilderness, vehicle, and water rescue disciplines are not addressed in this text.

The authors have designed this book as detailed reference material that can be used as a textbook by a qualified rescue teacher that chooses to teach these specific techniques. Rescue instruction can only be safely accomplished by an experienced professional because the field work required to learn rescue encompasses some risk to the student's health and safety. The calm application of accumulated knowledge to deal with those risks, when they evolve from possibilities into realities, cannot come only out of a book, video, or classroom training. A professional rescue instructor can, however, utilize this well organized, step-by-step instructional text as the basis of a complete lesson plan to achieve the students' dual goals of preparedness and compliance.

Contents

CHAPTER 1

Team Development

This chapter will cover the following topics:

- Developing objectives
- Management's Committment
- Creating the Team
- Training the Team
- Selecting Rescue Equipment
- Creating Standard Operating Procedures
- Marketing the Team
- Performance Evaluation
- Effective Communication

Introduction

Federal regulations require that an industrial site have rescue capabilities. Of course, the biggest reason for creating a rescue team is to provide the final cornerstone in a complete emergency response (ER) structure. The other three vital components are fire, hazardous materials (HazMat), and medical. Without a rescue capability, you cannot have a comprehensive program. Most important, a comprehensive ER program provides workers the protection they deserve.

You can achieve this rescue capability by establishing a team from within your facility. However, the U.S. Occupational Safety and Health Administration (OSHA), does allow the use of an off-site rescue service for an employer's permit required confined spaces (PRCS). Any employer who chooses an off-site rescue service must evaluate it and verify that the service is capable of a timely response. The employer must verify that the service is properly equipped and its personnel are properly trained to function appropriately for rescue within the employer's facility. Specific issues of confined space rescue (CSR) will be addressed in later chapters.

Developing Objectives

Once you decide to establish a rescue team, you must create a clear strategy for developing the team. A coherent strategy is essential in creating an effective and viable rescue service. It is important to document all major elements of team development. Putting the major elements in writing will:

1. help transform ideas into concrete team goals.
2. help develop standardized operational guidelines.
3. provide a legal record to deal with issues of compliance and liability.
4. develop a historical reference that remains through changes of management and other personnel.

Assuming you have decided to create an on-site rescue team, what steps should you take, and in what order? You must first establish objectives and goals.

Needs Assessment

One effective way to develop objectives is to make a complete analysis of your needs (see Figure 1.1). This Needs Assessment should answer three important questions:

1. What is the current status of rescue response on site?

Text continued on p. 9

Needs Assessment: The following information will be used in establishing goals and objectives for the rescue program. Surveyor to review questions and check yes or no, along with target date for completion. Notes & Recommendations are included in the Comments section and are to be reviewed. Surveyor to fill in any additional information or comments regarding goals and objectives for the rescue team.

QUESTION	Yes	No	Target Date	Comments / Suggestions:
1. Have you evaluated the current readiness of emergency response personnel to handle a "rescue" incident?				▯ This report is being used as a means to evaluate current readiness.
2. Do you have management's support for the development (or further development) of a rescue team?				▯ Management's Support ▯ Study-phase only at this time.
3. Has funding been approved for the development of a rescue team?				If not, when is funding expected?
4. Have you established an Action Plan for the step-by-step development of a rescue team?				▯ Will use this document as a guideline.
5. Will you develop a Mission Statement for your Rescue Team?				▯ To develop Mission Statement ▯ To use the following example... **Example:** "In order to provide complete emergency response services for our facility, the Rescue Team of (Company Name) is to be capable of competently performing technical rescue operations (both elevated and confined space rescue) in a safe, timely, and effective manner while avoiding further harm to the patient or compromising the safety of the rescuer(s).
6. Would existing Emergency Response Procedures be applicable to a rescue incident if it happened today?				Briefly describe existing procedures:
7. What "confined space" procedures are in place at this time? ▯ Permitting ▯ Entry ▯ Rescue				Describe:
8. Are Emergency Response Personnel comprised of "volunteers" or are personnel assigned to specific duties?				**Note:** Using "voluntary" participation is highly recommended in that volunteers are normally more enthusiastic and motivated to learn new skills and then devote sufficient time for practice drills. The learning process for volunteers is enhanced dramatically, and team members are usually very committed to the program. It is also recommended that "Day Shift" and "Supervisors" not be excluded from team participation.
9. Are current Emergency Response Personnel eager to learn and further develop their skills?				**Note:** Enthusiastic personnel can be your greatest asset!

Figure 1.1 Needs Assessment Form

QUESTION	Y e s	N o	Target Date	Comments / Suggestions:
10. Will you establish membership criteria for the Rescue Team? (considering physical health, shift assignment, interest, etc.)				**Note:** Guidelines established for other emergency response team members can be used and adapted for rescue team membership.
11. Will your Rescue Team be given adequate authority (via company policy) to perform its duties in an emergency?				**Note:** A clearly established command structure and written policy is critical. Supervisors must be advised of such policy and procedures.
12. Will "rescue coverage" be provided for all hours of operation? Will 24-hour coverage be needed? What about during industrial "turnarounds"?				**Recommendations:** A minimum of two (2) trained rescuers be on-duty at all times. Plant coverage area, type of operations, and number of employees on site are significant factors when determining adequate rescue coverage.
13. Will written SOP's (Standard Operating Procedures) be developed for your Rescue Team?				**Recommendation:** It is recommended that SOP's include items such as: team structure, leadership responsibilities, response policies, and other safety rules and guidelines.
14. Will detailed site Preplans* be developed for each area of the facility, including all confined space areas? *Preplans to include detailed diagrams with anchor placement, technique strategy, equipment needed, egress routes, safety-line positioning, etc.				**Note:** The Site Specific problem areas noted in this report plus any others on site need to be carefully examined... it is recommended that "extensive" preplanning and regular practice drills be conducted at these sites in particular. **Reference: ANSI Z117.1-1989** 3.1 Confined Space Survey - A survey shall be conducted of the premises, or operations, or both to identify confined spaces... This survey shall be conducted by a qualified person. **ANSI Note:** The purpose of the survey is to develop an inventory of those locations or equipment, or both, which meet the definition of a confined space so that personnel may be made aware of them and appropriate procedures developed for each prior to entry.

Figure 1.1, Cont'd Needs Assessment Form

Continued

QUESTION	Yes	No	Target Date	Comments / Suggestions:
15. Once preplans (surveys) are completed, will a detailed Emergency Response /Rescue Plan* be completed? *Plan should include detailed information and specific procedures for all problem areas and confined spaces identified in the inventory process.				**Note: OSHA requires that rescue procedures be listed on the entry permit.** ANSI specifically requires plans for confined spaces; however, **Recommendation:** develop preplans for all potential problem areas in which a rescue may be performed. **Reference: ANSI Standard Z117.1-1989** **14.1 Emergency Response Plan** - "A plan of action shall be written with provisions to conduct a timely rescue for individuals in a confined space should an emergency arise." **ANSI Note:** These rescue provisions will normally be present in the form of emergency response procedures. Included in these provisions shall be: "determination of what methods of rescue must be implemented to retrieve individuals." A review should be conducted of all the different types of confined spaces which will be entered and what steps/equipment it will take to get someone out. Consideration should be given to the size and configuration of the confined space and the body size of entering personnel.
16. Will sufficient equipment be acquired for your rescue team... for training purposes and for actual rescues? Will all team members be outfitted with their own personal gear? Will necessary rescue equipment be provided in amounts adequate for practice or training drills and actual rescue operations? Will a "history" be maintained on all rescue equipment and will equipment be replaced as needed?				**Note:** Standardized equipment that meets the guidelines of NFPA, ANSI, ASTM, or OSHA and SPRAT is recommended. Sufficient equipment is needed for training applications as well as for actual rescue operations. **Recommendation:** All rescue equipment be acquired prior to the training so that rescue team members can use their own equipment during the training.

Figure 1.1, Cont'd Needs Assessment Form

Continued

QUESTION	Yes	No	Target Date	Comments / Suggestions:
17. What rescue training will be provided for your team members? ☐ On-site Training ☐ Off-site Training ☐ Basic Rescue (40 hrs) ☐ Advanced Rescue (40 hrs) ☐ Other: When will the training be conducted? <u>QUESTIONS:</u> • How many rescue personnel will need to be trained? • Will 24-hour rescue coverage be required? • How many rescuers are to be on-duty per shift? • Number of training sessions? • Number of students per session? • Will support personnel be trained in basic rescue techniques?				**<u>RESCUE TRAINING RECOMMENDATIONS</u>:** It is important to note that most "confined space" rescues also involve lowering or raising personnel to ground level. Therefore, structural rescue techniques are critical to any confined space training program. **Description of basic Rescue Program:** The program begins with the basics of knots, rigging, equipment technology, and safety precautions in rope rescue. Secondary back-up safety lines are used in all evolutions as well as secondary anchors. Patient management and packaging techniques (including spinal immobilization, litter lashings, and patient harnessing) are demonstrated and practiced repeatedly. Mechanical advantage theory, hauling systems, tripod deployment, and litter management are also included. Rappelling and other lowering systems are also taught during field evolutions. OSHA requirements and ANSI standards pertaining to Confined Space Rescue are thoroughly covered.
18. What medical training will team members receive? Will <u>all</u> team members at least be trained in First Aid and CPR?				**Recommendation:** Certain rescue team members (if not all) should be trained to the EMT (Emergency Medical Technician) level or at least to the First Responder level. **OSHA Note:** OSHA states that <u>all</u> rescue team members be trained in first aid and CPR and, at a minimum, one rescue team member be currently certified in first aid and CPR.
19. Once initial rescue training is completed, will regular drill times be established for rescue personnel to practice the techniques learned?				**Note:** As with all emergency response operations, skills must be regularly practiced and reinforced to maintain proficiency levels. The authors recommend 16-to-24 hours per quarter in structured, prescribed drill time.

Figure 1.1, Cont'd Needs Assessment Form

Continued

QUESTION	Yes	No	Target Date	Comments / Suggestions:
20. Will a yearly rescue team maintenance plan be developed to include a prescribed methodology of refresher training and practice drills that encompasses "elevated" as well as "confined space" techniques?				**OSHA Note:** OSHA finds that "refresher or on-going safety instruction has invariably been an important component of training programs." OSHA believes that paragraphs (g)(2)(ii), (g)(2)(iii), and (g)(2)(iv) of the Confined Space Regulation (1910.146), which addresses the issue of refresher training, will ensure that employers provide on-going training to their employees, including "refresher" or "follow-up" training... **Note:** A documented training schedule is needed to maintain the team's skill level in all areas of technical rescue. Topics need to be prescribed specifically in order to prevent the team from de-emphasizing any technique that may not be as "exciting" as another. Problem-solving drills are extremely beneficial for focusing learned techniques. **Recommendation:** A minimum of 16-to-24 hours per quarter for practice drills, etc.
21. Will all training be documented and records maintained for the team as well as individual team members?				**Recommendation:** All rescue training sessions should be documented with signed, daily roster sheets describing training evolutions and a reference or source material sited for each technique taught. **OSHA Note:** "OSHA strongly believes that certification of employee training provides a valuable record to employers, employees, and OSHA in determining whether or not required training has been accomplished." **Note:** All training sessions should be documented with a signed, daily roster sheet, which includes specific topics taught and reference material sited.
22. Will your team be provided rescue reference manuals which include modern, industrial rescue technique schematics and performance criteria?				**Note:** Rescue manuals or study guides should include detailed schematics of rescue techniques as well as performance criteria information. This reference material should be directed specifically towards industrial situations using modern rescue equipment and techniques. **Reference:** Confined Space and Structural Rope Rescue

Figure 1.1, Cont'd Needs Assessment Form

Continued

QUESTION	Yes	No	Target Date	Comments / Suggestions:
23. Do you plan to educate and equip rescue personnel with breathing air systems specifically designed for confined space rescue operations?				**Recommendation:** Use Supplied Air Systems (SAR) for confined space operations; SAR provides the rescue with virually an unlimited supply of air as well as the advantage of a lowprofile apparatus. **ANSI Reference:** (Z117.1-1989 - 14.2 Breathing Equipment - "All rescue personnel must use self-contained breathing apparatus (SCBA), or Combination Type C Airline/SCBA breathing apparatus, when entering the confined space to rescue victims. If it is established that the cause of the emergency is not a hazardous atmosphere, rescue breathing apparatus is not required." **ANSI Note:** In some instances the entrance to the confined space may be such that an SCBA unit on the rescuer will not fit through the opening of the confined space. This should have been pre-determined in hazard identification and evaluation or drills. In this event, the rescuer may be required to use Combination Type C Airline/SCBA-type breathing equipment.
24. Will you provide more advanced training for your rescue team or at least for key team members?				**Description of typical advanced training (40 hours):** This program teaches more advanced rigging and mechanical advantage techniques as well as more complex confined space extrication methodology. Entry permits, MSDS, and atmospheric monitoring are discussed in reference to rescue operations. Other confined space rescue considerations, such as PPE and breathing air management are also addressed. Third-man rescue, line transfers, and traverse operations are also included in this program.
25. Will a "Resource Library" be established for Rescue Team Members?				**Recommendation:** A Resource Library should be established for Rescue Team Members which includes rescue-related books, periodicals, newsletters, video tapes, etc.

Figure 1.1, Cont'd Needs Assessment Form

Continued

QUESTION	Yes	No	Target Date	Comments / Suggestions:
26. Will annual "team" and "individual" performance evaluations be conducted?				**OSHA Note:** OSHA believes that a **periodic demonstration** of the on-site rescue service's ability to extract authorized entrants from permit spaces will provide the necessary feedback regarding the **adequacy** of the rescue equipment, the rescue procedures, and the training provided for performance of rescue from permit spaces." **Reference: ANSI Standard 15.5.1** - "Periodic assessment of the effectiveness of employee training shall be conducted by a qualified person." **Note:** Training effectiveness may be evaluated by several techniques. Written, as well as practical testing is recommended..."
27. Do you have (or have you considered) a "Mutual Aid" agreement with a nearby neighbor who has technical industrial rescue capabilities?				**Recommendation:** Include local emergency agencies and/or neighboring plants in their rescue training programs. Consistency in training could be invaluable in a major disaster in which additional manpower is required. **Note:** Often, local emergency response agencies do not have the funds for rescue training (or equipment). Including them in company rescue training provides a valuable service to the community and affords the opportunity to build a good working relationship prior to an emergency.
28. Do you plan to educate management as well as company personnel of the specialized capabilities of the Rescue Team? ☐ company newsletters ☐ rescue demonstrations ☐ other means:				**Note:** This promotes a sense of pride in the rescue team as well as an added sense of security for employees.
29. Do you plan to educate the public, area industries, public agencies, etc. about the capabilities of your Rescue Team? ☐ news releases ☐ rescue demonstrations ☐ mutual aid meetings				**Note:** This is an excellent way to provide support to local emergency agencies and the community.
30.				
31.				

Figure 1.1, Cont'd Needs Assessment Form

2. Considering management's desires and compliance with the law, what does the site need?
3. How will the site establish an action plan to get from its current state to its desired state?

In other words, where are we now? Where do we want to be? How are we going to get there? The ideas are simple, but they might be difficult to carry out.

Managers can choose to conduct their own needs assessment or hire outside expertise. They can also consult managers of other industrial sites with established teams or private consultants who are knowledgeable and experienced in developing rescue teams.

One critical step in a needs assessment is establishing what the site wants to accomplish with its rescue team. Since both elevated and confined space rescue are usually needed in industry, the rescue team should be capable of handling both. Many confined space rescues also require elevated techniques. So, a well-prepared team is one that can complete a safe, efficient rescue from any location in the facility.

Legal Compliance

What about compliance with the law? Many safety managers mistakenly believe that CFR 1910.146 is the only OSHA regulation requiring trained, equipped rescuers (see Chapter 18). The OSHA Fall Protection, Respiratory, and HAZWOPER regulations all require specific rescue capabilities. Additionally, the rescue team is going to have to function according to all of OSHA's laws such as those dealing with lockout-tagout, personal protective equipment (PPE), and process safety. It is vital that the needs assessor know the regulations and use them to establish the ultimate objectives of the rescue team.

Current Readiness

As stated earlier, the first step is to establish exactly where the facility stands as far as current readiness. Start by looking at the big picture. What are the general capabilities of the site in relation to ER? Most facilities possess fire brigades and some medical capabilities, and since the appearance of HAZWOPER, HAZCOM, and SARAH Title III, most sites have added capabilities to handle emergencies involving hazardous materials. By requiring a rescue service for permit spaces, the confined space regulation has helped to emphasize the need for rescue teams in industry.

Although helpful, the CSR regulations do not address the total need for industrial rescue. In fact, most of the facilities in the United States are not in complete compliance with those basic requirements. The assessor should look at what the facility is currently doing to be prepared for rescue and whether that service actually meets the goals of management and the requirements of federal law.

It is apparent that the needs assessment is a valuable tool for sites that already have a rescue team as well as for those just starting one. The needs assessment is an excellent tool to measure the status of all rescue teams, no matter what their stage of development.

The Mission Statement

Once the status of the site's rescue response has been determined, you must decide where the facility wants to go. This direction must be clear to everyone involved in this process. A written mission statement is a concise summation of what a group is ultimately trying to accomplish. At the beginning of any new endeavor it is a logical focal point for planners, and eventually for team members, as well as managers. Later it is helpful as a reference to evaluate progress.

A good, generic mission statement might read:

> In order to provide complete emergency response capabilities, the Acme rescue team will be able to competently perform technical rescue from both elevated structures as well as confined spaces. The team will carry out these rescues safely and efficiently while avoiding further injury to the patient or harming the rescuer.

Authority

After approving the mission statement, management must decide under whose authority the rescue team will operate. In most cases, the team should fall under the emergency response manager. The ER manager may function in the Safety or Industrial Hygiene Departments, or as the fire brigade chief.

Of the other three cornerstones of ER, rescue is most closely associated with medical emergencies. Often the rescue involves an injured or sick worker. Rescue can also require the team to work in locations containing a hazardous substance. Therefore, HazMat response has an important role.

If the fire chief is responsible for all emergency response, then he or she might also be rescue manager. In this case, however, it is important that the chief is not already overwhelmed with other responsibilities such as fire training, maintaining fire equipment, overseeing water supply systems, obtaining permits, monitoring regulations, and record keeping. If the chief is heavily committed to other activities, then the responsibility for rescue should be delegated to a deputy.

Management's Commitment

As mentioned earlier, compliance with OSHA regulations such as the Confined Space Final Rule is often inadequate (see chapter 18: *Confined Space Rescue: Compliance Issues*). Of course, management's priority must be to produce product for the company to sell. All legitimate companies are dedicated to cost-efficiency and safety while producing a quality product.

While this fact is often frustrating to the team that needs more of the company's resources, each member must realize that his or her job depends on accomplishing management's goals. Managers, on the other hand, must realize that rescue requires competent team members who are confident in their training and equipment. Although it is possible to be too confident, it is impossible for rescuers to be competent if they are not confident in themselves and their fellow team members.

While assessing needs and writing the needs assessment, management must declare its support for the rescue team. To become well-trained and capable, the team must have management's clear commitment. In addition to the financial obligation for equipment, management must support the long-term time commitment to training. Its commitment, or lack of it, to adequate training time for all personnel is often the cause of great conflict. The facility must commit resources for overtime, compensation time, and replacements for members while they train.

Creating the Team

To comply with OSHA's requirements a competent rescue team must be properly trained, adequately equipped, and capable of functioning appropriately in specific situations. Management's support should go beyond the requirements. Although initial training and equipping of a fully capable rescue team can be expensive, the real investment comes in precious work-hours. The least anticipated expense of an on-site rescue team is ongoing training. Unless practice time is scheduled during regular shifts, the overtime bill can mount quickly.

Rescuers are not fully prepared after initial training. To become proficient in new skills takes hours of practice and drills. Follow-up practice, according to OSHA, is absolutely necessary in any type of safety training. Many new teams, although once highly motivated, have fallen by the wayside due to a lack of practice. Those teams were unfortunate because their management only supported the *idea* of a rescue team, but not the reality of what is required to become capable and to maintain team competency. Management must make the commitment to train and maintain the team or outsource the rescue function.

Initial training of a fully capable rescue team may take from 40 to 160 hours. This initial phase must be reinforced by regularly scheduled practice sessions.

Within the first year following initial training, at least 24 hours of practice time is recommended every three months for the team to develop competency. For best results, these quarterly training hours should be grouped into one session (usually three days). Dividing the hours into shorter monthly sessions usually does not provide the same quality of training. This is due to the need for review each time a session begins. By the time the team has finished reviewing what it previously learned, the training session is almost over. Longer sessions can provide complete review and still allow plenty of time to practice and become more proficient.

After this year of follow-up training, many industrial teams find it possible to maintain their level of skill with only 12 to 16 hours of practice per quarter. It may be possible to *maintain* skills with these limited practice sessions; it certainly is not possible to *improve* them. Every time the team is introduced to new techniques and technology, the more practice time it needs to assimilate the new knowledge. Of course, each team is different. The amount and type of rescue training required to reach and maintain competency varies. General recommendations will be discussed later in this chapter, however, a few key issues must be considered when organizing a rescue team.

Team Size

Before choosing team members you must decide how many you need. The team size depends on the following facts.

1. **The team's mission, or responsibility.** If the team is responsible for contractors' employees and mutual aid response, a larger team is needed.
2. **The size of the facility.** A large plant with many employees requires a sizeable team. More people plus more places to get hurt equals more opportunities for accidents.
3. **The number of work shifts.** Every shift should have a minimum of four to six trained rescuers on the site. This allows rapid response by rescuers to an incident.
4. **The frequency and times of PRCS entries.** Are PRCS entries made 24 hours a day or only during day shifts? Confined spaces are a priority with OSHA. Coverage of possible incidents requires a larger team if entries are made on a 24-hour basis instead of an 8-hour basis.
5. **The location of off-site employees.** Off-duty help can be either a few minutes away or 30 to 45 minutes away. Longer response time requires a larger on-duty team.
6. **The number and training of rescue response personnel.** Many plants train the entire emergency response team in basic rescue. This can speed response and assist a smaller, more highly trained core group of rescuers.
7. **The availability of outside rescue response agencies.** According to OSHA, for CSR, a combination of on-site and off-site rescuers is an employer's option. This option is not limited to teams that provide only confined space rescue. It also works for full-function industrial rescue teams. If trained off-site responders are used, the on-site team can be smaller.

It's also necessary to consider maintenance shutdowns. Many plants use outside rescuers as an on-site standby service to work night shifts during maintenance and the in-plant team covers the day shift. This standby team is capable of functioning as a first response team. It can detect and possibly mitigate hazards, establish and monitor conditions of the accident victim(s) including the mechanism of injury, and begin rigging.

The team's size also depends on the nature of the incidents to which it will respond. It depends on how complicated potential injuries are and, most important, how hazardous the rescue environment may be. A situation involving hazardous materials, for example, increases the need for specially trained team members. When rescuers work in these environments, there is always the potential for injury. This possibility requires still other personnel to back up the primary rescuers in case of a problem.

There must be adequate coverage for each shift. If shift patterns change seasonally or with turnarounds (scheduled maintenance), the number of team personnel must be altered accordingly. Coverage must also compensate for vacations, comp time, sick leave, and other situations when team members will be away.

All of the above factors should be considered when trying to arrive at the right number of team members for a particular facility. The average-sized industrial rescue team is approximately sixteen members. There are plants that actually have a different rescue team for each shift (usually four), each team consisting of about eight members. Most sites lean toward training several persons on each shift, all of whom (on-duty and off-duty) combine to make one team.

Membership Criteria

Whom should you invite to be part of the rescue team? Why not anybody in the plant? While most sites automatically gravitate toward asking for volunteers from the current emergency response team, there is really no reason that a secretary in the administration building or a 50-year-old plant operator could not be valuable team members. The biggest asset a prospective team member can bring to the team is a good attitude and a true desire to help others. The only people who might be discouraged from joining the rescue team are fire brigade members because of the amount of training required for both types of emergency response assignments. An employee's supervisor can become very impatient with an employee who is constantly leaving his or her primary job to go do some type of emergency training.

The primary consideration for rescue team membership should be the candidate's attitude toward the job. It is highly recommended that the team be composed mostly, if not entirely, of volunteers. Elevated and confined space rescue involves overcoming fears such as acrophobia and claustrophobia. These feelings can be strong and very difficult to overcome, even for a willing rescuer. In addition, rescue team members might be asked to voluntarily place themselves in harm's way. A "captive" rescuer is less likely to offer a positive response. Finally, team members have to make a personal commitment to learn new skills that can be applied automatically during a crisis, almost without thinking. Team members soon realize that they have to dedicate themselves to learning if they are to be successful. For all of these reasons, it is easy to imagine the lack of confidence the team will have in a member who obviously does not want to be on the team.

Sometimes even willing participants are not suited for the job. A hidden agenda may be behind their desire to be on the team. Thoughts of glory and overtime have no place in the motivation of a true rescuer. Ideas about screening applicants will be discussed later in this chapter.

Routine job assignments cannot be ignored when considering potential team members. A less desirable candidate would be the person with a job function so critical that he or she could not leave it, especially in an emergency, to go to a rescue call. It is good to have team members representing the Safety Department, since that department's support and guidance is crucial to a successful rescue team.

Qualification for team membership should not be limited by age, gender, or physical ability. Rescue operations can at times be physically taxing, but anybody in sound health can make a valuable contribution. A person with a disability such as extreme obesity, an unhealthy heart, or only having one lung or kidney would probably have a tough time coping with the demands of the job. However, it does not take an extraordinary athlete to perform rescue. In fact, the participation of an older, perhaps less physically adept, more experienced team member often proves vital to the success of the rescue.

A solicitation letter for volunteers should be straightforward about the personal commitment. Applicants must understand they will need to commit personal time for studying techniques, understanding law, and attending practice and drills. Team members often make the mistake of thinking that their personal development as a rescuer is the sole responsibility of the employer. This might be technically accurate; it is far from realistic. A team member must have a personal responsibility to his or her betterment as a rescuer. There is no reason individuals cannot practice certain rescue skills, study technical information, or otherwise work to improve themselves independently of scheduled drill time.

The Applicant's Motivation

Ask prospective members during interviews or in writing why they want to join the team. This can be an early indicator of the applicant's attitude and true motivation for membership. Answers that suggest the "right stuff" include:

- "I like to help people." This is a truly great answer. After all, it is the ultimate reason for rescue. But be cautious. The applicant may have contrived the answer, thinking it is what you want to hear.
- "I have First Responder EMS training, and need a way to use it." This applicant could be a great asset and a motivator of other team members.
- "It seems like fun." Potential team members must have an interest in the activities to continue the necessary training.

Identify the volunteer's motivation. Be certain the person is not volunteering because he or she sees only the glory of doing rescue or seeks the position only to get overtime pay or time off from the regular job to train.

Health and Fitness

Rescue activities generally do not employ brute strength but use technique and finesse to achieve their ends. However, rescue activities can be physically demanding and stressful. Rescue team members should be in good health and physical condition. They need physical stamina and flexibility, which automatically screens out applicants with medical problems that might physically limit them or endanger their health when they are physically stressed. It is good practice to require an initial physical examination during the application process and then repeat it annually. Results of the physical exam also establish a baseline for monitoring the rescuer's physical condition. In addition, most rescuers operate in confined spaces and other situations where they have to wear breathing apparatus. To comply with OSHA's respiratory regulation, the wearer must be able to use and perform in a respirator. This generally requires good physical health.

Psychological Considerations

The challenge of rescue work is often mental, not physical. The psychological aspects of dealing with one's fears and the fears of others can be daunting. Among the extreme fears are acrophobia (fear of heights), and claustrophobia (fear of confined spaces). Other psychological aspects will be having to deal with co-workers who are severely injured and panicky or, even worse, deceased. The prospect of using practiced rescue skills to recover a body requires a psychological review process. A healthy attitude toward life and people, as well as mental and emotional strength and stability are essential ingredients.

Training the Team

Once the team is organized, the next step is to train it. Selecting the method of training and the people to conduct the training is critical to the ultimate established goal of the rescue team. The mission statement, approved by management, defines the team's capabilities—to be able to perform industrial rescue *safely and efficiently*. These two elements, safety and efficiency, are the equal legs that every rescue has to stand on. Therefore, the training should be planned and structured to accomplish those goals.

Training Regulations

Of course, the training cannot just concentrate on confined spaces. There are other types of rescue and other requirements to consider. Specifically, OSHA has rescue regulations for HAZWOPER, Respiratory Protection, and Fall Protection. Additionally, rescuers have to be familiar with Lockout-Tagout, Personal Protective Equipment, Process Safety, and other OSHA regulations. Rescuers should also be schooled on standards for rescue equipment set by the American National Standards Institute (ANSI) and the National Fire Protection Association (NFPA). The team's training must include all regulations that

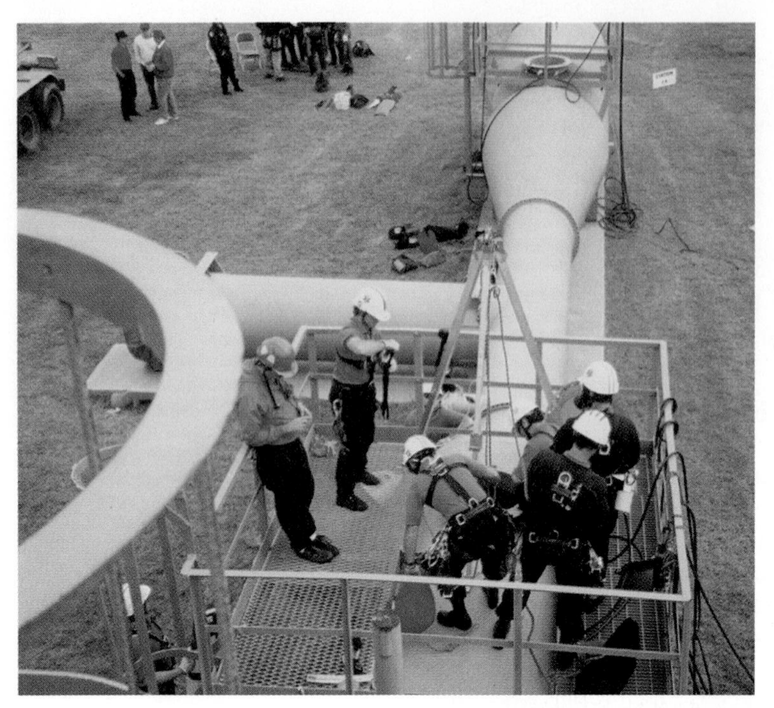

Figure 1.2 Rescuers practicing in-plant

apply to the particular facility and a working knowledge of elevated and confined space rescue.

Training Methods

Training methods must include classroom instruction and extensive fieldwork. Besides regulations and standards, the team has to learn rescue equipment technology and practice the techniques to use the equipment in both confined spaces and elevated structures. It is important to keep in mind that no single rescue class can by itself produce a competent rescuer. Competence comes from practice that produces confidence.

The initial training should cover safety rules and guidelines, rescue/retrieval equipment and its uses and limitations, and some simple methods of extraction from confined space as well as basic lowering techniques. Upon completion of the initial training, the team should be able to *safely* make the rescues for which it was trained. The trainees will not be capable of performing all rescues *efficiently* without additional training and many hours of structured practice sessions. Competent rescuers, according to OSHA, can accomplish the task successfully by incorporating both attributes into their practices.

The most important test of the team will be its ability to build and maintain competence with continual practice. There should be more than the minimum required by regulations. Minimum training results in minimum performance. Regular training develops not only competence, but confidence.

Rescue activities involve specific skills that must be done automatically and in proper sequence. This can only be achieved with regular training. Rescue practice must occur in realistic situations representative of plant conditions (see Figure 1.2). Realistic rescue training cannot be only in a place team members find clean and convenient. For instance, OSHA's Confined Space Regulation requires the rescue service to practice in actual or representative spaces with respect to opening size, configuration, and accessibility. The team must do this for every type of permit required confined space in the plant. This is based on OSHA requirements and the need to know the problems unique to each space configuration and hazard. How can rescuers achieve this when they continue to train in the same place with the same scenario time after time? They cannot.

The team should instead design a structured drill plan. These drills should be based on rescue objectives. They should also be balanced, written, and scheduled in advance. Doing this can avoid the trap of practicing only those activities (such as rappelling) that may be attractive to the members, but do not contribute significantly to rescue capabilities.

The Trainer

When published in 1993, OSHA's Confined Space Regulation implied that "Confined space training will be the HazMat of the 90s." This prediction has come true. The number of CSR trainers has grown from a handful in the 1980s to hundreds currently. The good news is that this exponential growth of trainers brings new ideas and competition. The bad news is that there are currently no national standards or criteria for rescue trainers. So, many well-intentioned teaching programs are not offering what industrial rescuers need. Competition among training providers is good, but it is wise for the buyer to beware.

General industry regulations published by OSHA are mostly oriented to performance rather than based on specifications. Rather than specify what kind or how much training is required, OSHA instead requires compliance to rules that state what the employer has to accomplish.

Since OSHA leaves it to the employer to get the rescue team where it needs to be, most employers simply throw that ball to the trainer. There really is no problem with using a consultant to help the manager lay out the training action plan, if the consultant/trainer is knowledgeable and experienced. It may be beneficial to bring in a professional rescue trainer at the onset of the needs assessment to provide valuable insight. The trainer would then have an intimate knowledge of the goals and philosophies of management. This would make it easier for him or her to develop and carry out the appropriate training program to meet the organization's needs.

Select a trainer who can put the team in a position to save lives and possibly save the employer money by avoiding fines, legal fees, and civil settlements.

A trainer's competence is indicated by credentials and references, but also by background and experience. Whom has the trainer taught? There are many who can "talk the talk"; there are fewer who can "walk the walk." If the instructors do not have a background in emergency response, the employer should question competency. How can an instructor express what it feels like to perform under pressure-packed and dangerous conditions when he or she has never experienced it?

Another key element in the qualification of prospective trainers involves speaking to their former students. Did the trainer teach a philosophy of safety along with the rescue skills? Were the classes structured and organized? Was the material covered with detailed printed references backed by field learning and practice? Did the trainer bully his or her way through the course without regard for quality of instruction and safety? Does the team now have a complete understanding of what is required to comply with federal mandates? Is the team properly equipped? Can it respond in a timely manner? Is each member trained to act in a safe and responsible manner? How or what measuring device has the employer used to decide the above? Has the team been evaluated in realistic training scenarios to determine its level of competency?

Another excellent method for assessing the qualifications of a trainer is to ask for written training specifications (specs). The specs should give the student/instructor ratio. Based on the average span of control, it should never be more than 7:1 for hands-on training. There should be printed reference material specific to the course content (not just a manual written by somebody else and used as a partial reference), training equipment, instructors' biographies, insurance coverage, waivers of liability, and accessible references for contact. The trainer should have no trouble providing copies of his or her manual, certificates, insurance coverage, written tests, and course outlines. The trainer should be able to customize courses to meet the site's specific needs. It is usually inappropriate to request lesson plans from the trainer because of the competitive nature of the rescue training field. These lesson plans are usually considered highly protected proprietary information.

The trainer should also be able to provide a written plan of action to accomplish the site's goals. The plan should contain realistic, measurable objectives, complete with time lines. Recommendations for follow-up training are crucial if the team is to become proficient. The trainer should outline a prescribed method for the team to learn, practice, and demonstrate its new skills. In addition, a good trainer must be knowledgeable of and helpful in team motivation. This is important to managers because they bear the burden of keeping a team interested, which can be very difficult for teams that have few actual rescue calls.

Finally, the trainer should generally be a full-time, professional rescue specialist. There are many part-timers who work for somebody else and say they have training expertise in many areas of emergency response. Beware of the "Jack of all trades and master of none." Trainers with broad expertise are full-time trainers. Whatever their employment status, experienced professionals have excellent reputations and sound credentials. They also have a multitude of satisfied customers who will be glad to discuss their performance.

How Much Is Enough?

Realistically, in the ER arena, there is no such thing as too much training. All ER training should be planned, structured, and documented to make the best of available resources. Training should be planned because there is a vast amount of information to be learned in a prescribed time. It should be structured to make sure all appropriate areas are covered initially and each area is practiced. It should be documented not only because documentation is required, but a history will help in planning structured practices.

Most competent trainers can produce a 40-hour course that will give rescuers the bare necessities of confined space and elevated rescue. This level of training should enable a rescue team to manage most of the basic incidents faced in an average industrial facility. This is a minimum recommendation only. A rescue team should pursue more advanced training if it wants to expand capabilities beyond the minimum. It is highly recommended that a team be trained to a level that will allow it to handle most of the possible incidents in its facility. Competent trainers can usually provide an intermediate-level course to meet this goal. Although the number of hours varies with the trainer, at least 40 additional hours are recommended.

Many trainers offer additional courses to provide students with advanced skills appropriate for more complex elevated and confined space rescues. Even with all this training, there may still be incidents beyond the rescue capability of the team. Examples include atmospheres that require fully encapsulated protective (Level A) suits and respiratory protection because of highly toxic or enclosed explosive atmospheres. There will be rescues a team cannot perform safely, whatever its level of training. Good training includes understanding limitations.

Be cautious of the quick fix. A course lasting two or three days may teach only enough to get a rescuer in trouble. Unless the rescue team has a highly unusual situation requiring only one or two types of rescue, a brief course is sure to be a problem. Workshops and seminars cannot substitute for hands-on field exercises.

Documentation and records of all training should include the specific training performed, when it took place, which members were present, the hours, and the trainers. Other sections of this text that will prove helpful in developing the right approach to training discuss the required and recommended training for confined space rescue, the regulations, and how to manage the rescue incident.

Selecting Rescue Equipment

Select equipment specifically designed for rescuing live persons (see Figure 1.3 A, B). Industrial equipment designed for moving equipment may be too bulky or not have sufficient safety margins for rescue activities. Rope and hardware designed for sporting activities, such as rock climbing or caving, may not have appropriate properties or safety margins for rescue. Most equipment designed for rescue carries the manufacturer's certification that it was designed for carrying human loads.

Government regulations mention "rescue and retrieval equipment," but do not specify which equipment to use. The team's equipment must be appropriate for the most difficult rescue operation it can safely accomplish in its facility. For example, a simple tripod and winch cannot provide confined space retrieval/rescue in all situations. This system might work in a simple vertical extraction but, because of entanglement problems, it is not appropriate for vessels with internal obstacles.

A rescue from an internal confined space may involve moving a patient along various levels and through interior obstructions such as trays and pipes. The rescue would most likely require lowering or raising the patient through this difficult configuration. The team may need specialized equipment for rope anchoring and rigging, for litter hauling and lowering systems, and for securing the patient (or patient packaging).

Federal rules require the employer to properly equip the rescue team member. The requirements include rescue, retrieval, communication, ventilation, air monitoring, personal protective, lighting, barrier, and egress equipment. The law says that the team must also be trained in the proper use of the equipment. The problem arises when a site's management decides to purchase equipment to be in compliance rather than equipment that it actually needs.

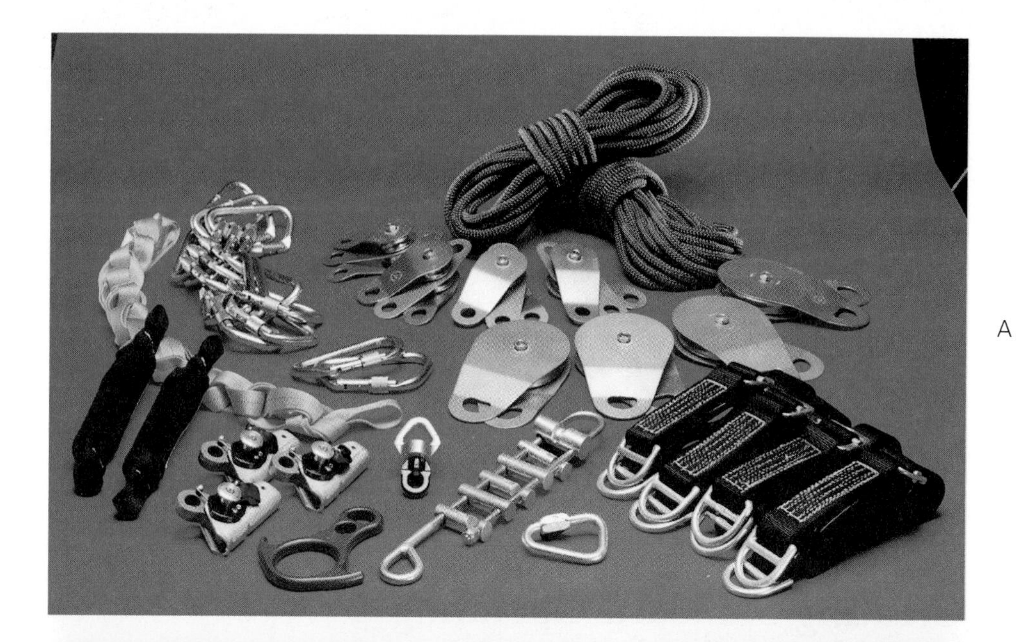

A

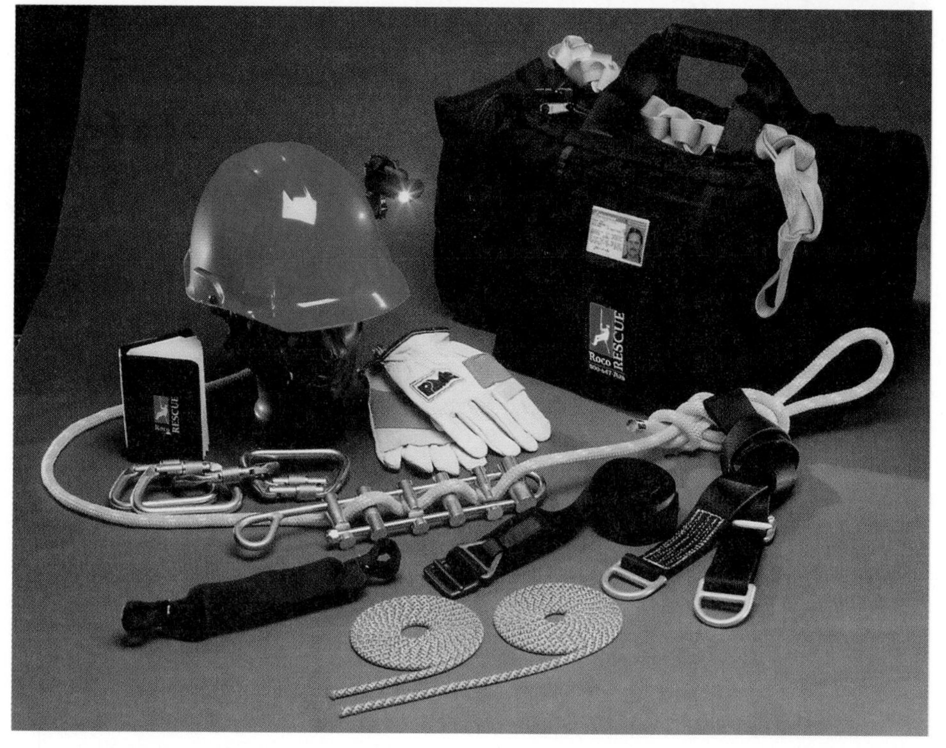

B

Figure 1.3 **A, B Rescue equipment**

All rope rescue equipment should meet or exceed national standards and regulations (see Chapters 2 and 3). The equipment should be purchased only after a trainer has been selected. An enormous variety of equipment is available, most of it expensive. The trainer can recommend equipment that will be used in training and subsequent operations.

OSHA regulations consider timeliness of response an important attribute of a capable team. Therefore, it is a good idea to equip each team member with gear for which he or she is responsible. This allows team members to start the rescue effort no matter who arrives first on the scene. A complete rescue cache should be maintained on the response vehicle to provide the primary equipment for the team's operation (see Figure 1.4). Equipment that will be used in actual rescues should be separate from practice rescue equipment. This ensures that the equipment used in an actual rescue has not been compromised by the rigors of constant use in drill sessions. The team should maintain a history of use on all rope rescue equipment.

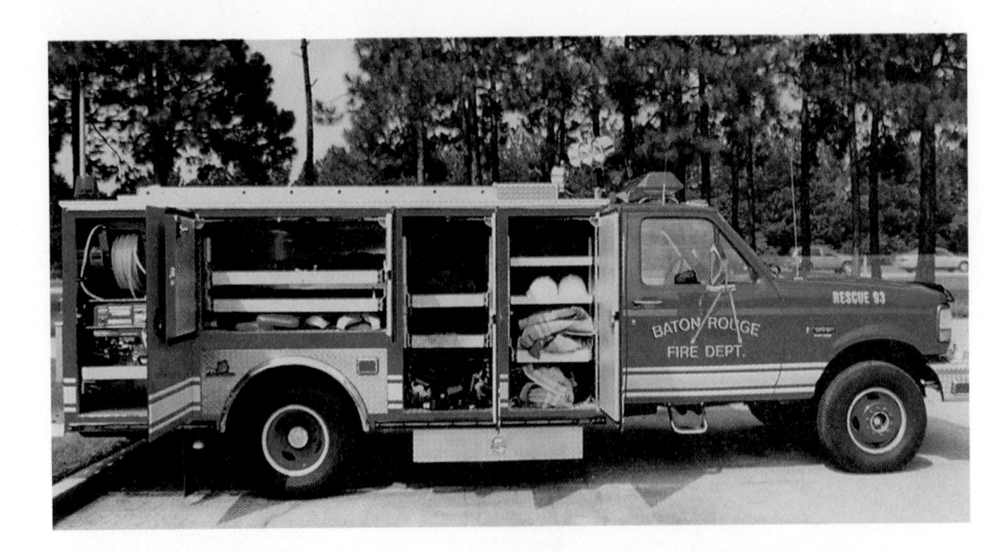

Figure 1.4 Rescue equipment on emergency response vehicle

Creating Standard Operating Procedures/Guidelines

It is important to establish standard operating procedures (SOPs) for the rescue team. A more recent approach applies the term "suggested operating guidelines (SOGs)" rather than SOPs. The very name suggests that these operational procedures are simply guidelines designed to eliminate much of the guesswork associated with the decision-making processes in emergency operations. Guidelines should not be so specific as to limit latitude for independent judgment based on the circumstances of the incident. However, latitude for independent judgment brings individual responsibility to the person who makes the call. A rescuer who strays from the standard bears the responsibility for such a decision. The following are advantages that SOGs provide to emergency response organizations.

1. They allow many decisions commonly associated with the emergency to be made automatically. This will allow the incident commander (or manager) to devote attention to the more complex aspects of the incident.
2. They help provide uniformity in the operations of the emergency response agency. All rescuers are familiar with the way the operation should go and understand their individual roles.
3. They provide the scope of authority for all personnel, who know their rights and limitations.
4. They assign responsibility to all personnel, who understand their functions and their responsibilities to carry them out. Each person is responsible for something and to someone. This is a very important concept in incident command (incident management).

Suggested operating guidelines should always be written to avoid misinterpretation and confusion. In general, they help the team in terms of response, safety, and communications. They can also help in terms of liability and legality.

Examples of rescue team SOGs include:

- Team Structure
- Membership/Leadership Selection
- Communications
- Notification and Response
- Confined Space Rescue
- Incident Management System (IMS), also known as an Incident Command System (ICS)

Every team member must have access to SOGs and understand them. Team members must know what they can and cannot do.

Supporting the Team

Management, security, and personnel in other interested units must understand the activities of the rescue team. Poor communication and failure to keep them involved will cause problems with managers faster than anything else. One way to gain their support is to include them early in the game, perhaps by selling them on the necessity of the team in view of regulations and the site's needs. Management should be heavily involved in the initial phases of team development. This includes the needs assessment and generation of goals.

Another method for gaining the support of management is a demonstration. It can also be used to grab the attention of the plant's employees and even the general public. It provides an opportunity for established teams to show off their capabilities in a way that will instill confidence and respect for their ability. A successful demonstration can also be a big source of pride and motivation for the team itself.

Successful Demonstrations

Demonstrations (demos) should be planned carefully (see Figure 1.5). The attention span of most people is short, so keep demos brief, 20 minutes at maximum. Make certain that all team members look sharp, are dressed uniformly, and are neatly groomed. Keep the demonstration fast-paced, with multiple evolutions, to avoid lulls in the action. Here are some suggestions:

1. **Plan the stations.** A station is the demonstration area where different evolutions will be performed. A large demonstration would involve three or four stations where elements of rescue are performed in rapid succession from one to the other. Each station may require as many as seven people. Plan stations that have good visual appeal. Some examples include litter lowers with attendants, pick-offs from significant heights, and traverse systems.
2. **Keep it moving.** All stations must be prerigged and ready to go before the demo begins. Most people do not want to watch you rig your stations. It takes too long. Keep it fast-paced. As one station begins its demonstration, the next station is made ready. When the first is almost done, attention is diverted to the second demo, which is already in progress. This cycle continues from one station to the next. Each station should be reset as quickly as possible following its demo. Using lightweight manikins in litter demos can speed this process. The litter can be left rigged and simply pulled back up to start the evolution again. Once reset, a station's personnel should prepare to repeat the demo. This demonstration cycle should continue for approximately 15 minutes, or as long as most of the observers remain. Never run a demonstration longer than 20 minutes unless dictated by unusual circumstances.
3. **Practice, practice, practice!** The team should rehearse the entire demonstration in detail either on the day before or on the day of the scheduled event. Without rehearsals, embarrassing errors can occur. The team should practice until the demonstration is polished. Schedule at least 4 hours of practice time for three or four stations. This will allow plenty of time for setup, practice, problem solving, and breakdown. Be prepared for mistakes that could occur in the operation. If problems occur, shift immediately to the next evolution and keep going. Each team member should be aware of what to do in case of a glitch.
4. **Use a narrator.** It is important to use a narrator with a written script for the demonstration. The narrator should have a thorough understanding of the operation, be aware of problems that could occur, and understand his or her role in adapting to any problems. The narrator, using a public address system, should describe what is occurring in detail and in understandable language. The narrator should help the audience relate to the demonstration by describing situations in the plant where the evolution they are watching might occur. In character with the demonstration, the narration should be brief, concise, and to the point.
5. **Consider inviting the media.** Publicity about your demonstrations can promote the team. Be sure to assign a person such as a public information officer to escort the media and keep them informed.

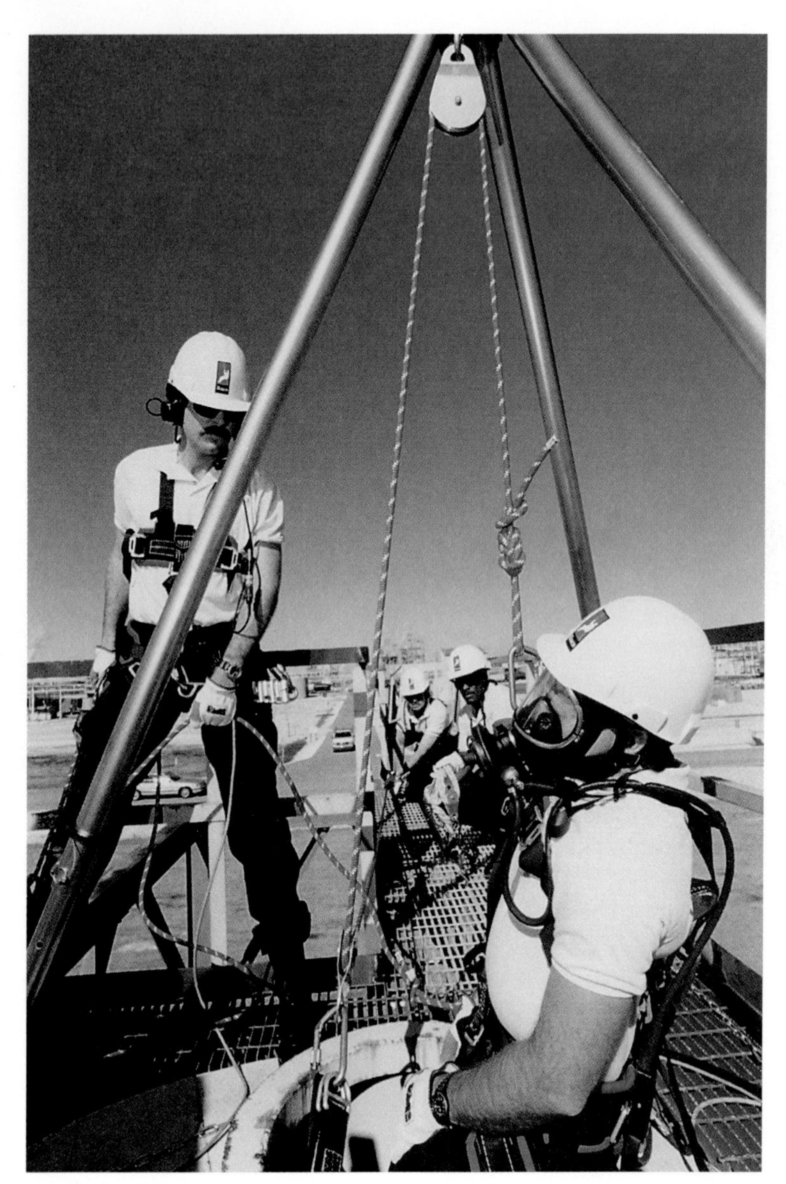

Figure 1.5 **Rescuers performing a demonstration**

Demonstrations can be performed for plant family gatherings and picnics. They can even be used as a great public relations tool for the surrounding community. It is most important, however, that every employee and manager know that there is a competent rescue team on-site. This is the best way to ensure rapid notification when an incident occurs. If personnel do not know about or believe in the rescue team, they will not be quick to call for them.

Video Production

Another effective educational tool involves producing an in-plant videotape describing the rescue team and showing them in action. These videos should be about 5 minutes long. You can send them to unit safety meetings in the facility to help employees understand the capability of the team. The better the distribution, the better plant personnel will understand its capability. The better they understand, the quicker they will call the ER team in an emergency.

Supporting Management

Remember to give credit where credit is due. Rescue teams often receive the credit for their successful rescues. One of the most honorable gestures when discussing a success is to give credit to the management for its support. If management does not give strong support to the rescue team's efforts, public attention can strengthen management's support.

Performance Evaluation

Demonstration of the team's competence is extremely important. The in-plant team should be evaluated annually to make certain that it remains capable (see Figure 1.6). These team performance evaluations (TPEs) should evaluate the group in relation to preset performance objectives or competencies. This method of evaluation should take the form of a simulated, but realistic, rescue scenario. A qualified person should evaluate and rate the team's performance. This can be done by independent training agencies or even other rescue teams with similar environments and goals. The evaluations should be well documented so management can show that the team has been trained and has performed adequately. Performance evaluations are also a good way to establish team competency in addressing issues of legal compliance.

Team members have to rely on and be confident in one another's abilities. This confidence promotes teamwork and communication—attributes that develop efficiency. Consequently, individual team members' skills should also be tested at least biannually. An individual performance evaluation (IPE) should rate each individual against an established set of competencies or performance objectives. Besides maintaining team quality, it provides incentives for members to maintain their skills.

What happens to team members who do not score well? Individuals who score below the designated standard should be given additional training and assistance to return them to the desired level of proficiency. This helps to reestablish an individual's competency. The SOGs should establish recommendations for handling individuals who do not meet the standards. Although it may be easier to simply dismiss a substandard member, it is better by far to try to salvage him or her. The team member

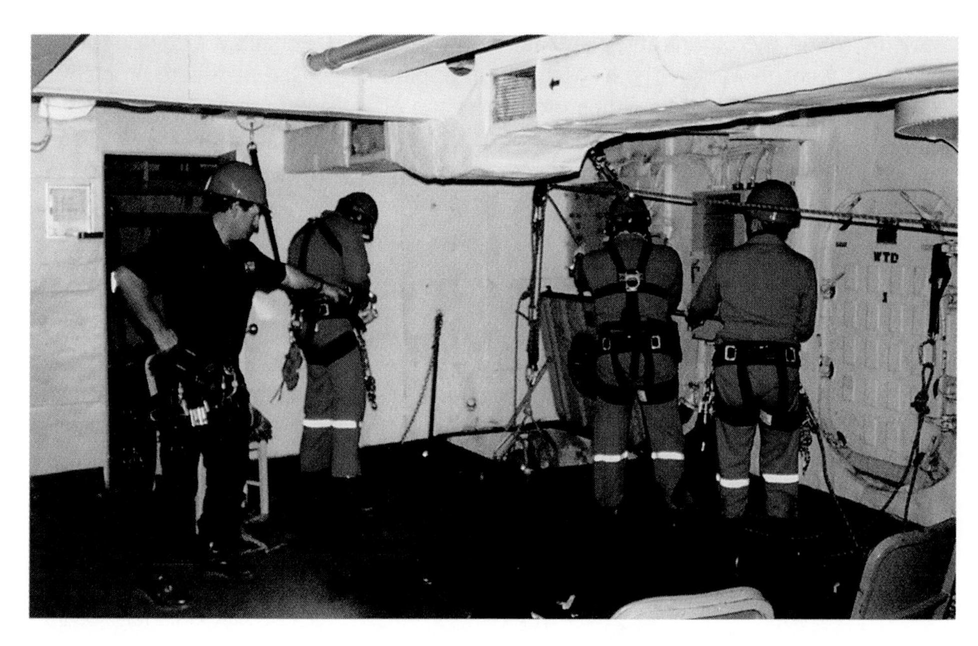

Figure 1.6 Team Performance Evaluation

should be placed on probation during this period. Guidelines should restrict him or her from response to actual rescues until satisfactorily completing an IPE. Given additional training to get up to speed with the rest of the team, the poorly performing team member often responds by exceeding all expectations the next time he or she is tested.

Effective Communication

Intergroup communications include interpersonal relationships and group dynamics. A team is made up of individuals with different thoughts and attitudes. It is important that a team include people who get along well and work together toward the same goals.

Goals can be set that will mesh individual goals with the goals of the team and management, so that everyone will strive for the same objectives. Personality conflicts that interfere with the operation of the rescue team must be avoided. Even with the best of teams, this is not always possible.

There will be differences in opinions on rigging, techniques, or equipment to be used. Argument on the scene is detrimental to the rescue. Training and the SOGs can help reduce potential conflict before it starts. One way to resolve conflicts is to establish strong leadership.

The good news is that different people bring different abilities and skills to the industrial rescue team. A person skilled at knots and rigging, for example, may not be good at caring for injured people. Or a person skilled in operating in confined spaces may not be a good leader. The object is to develop a team of individuals whose various skills and abilities complement each other for the betterment of the entire group. Often a person's greatest attribute is not apparent until after several training sessions or real operations. All team members should be trained and practiced in every part of a rescue operation. This is particularly important when team members respond at different times. Anyone could be needed anywhere.

A team is a group of individuals with particular skills who come together to operate as a single unit. Placing the right person in the right position is crucial for the best effect. In an actual rescue, when possible, place members where you know they can excel.

One of the most important ingredients in a successful rescue team is a good leader. The team leader is not necessarily the one who is best in all areas of skill. The team leader, instead, should have the right balance of technical and perceptual skills. Perceptual skills allow the team leader to see things as they really are and mitigate problems within the organization. A team leader must lead. To lead effectively, the team must want to follow. The leader must anticipate needs and negotiate problems while considering the individual team members. An effective leader seeks input and feedback from all team members. Differences of opinion are normal and healthy, but the team leader must not allow arguments to jeopardize anyone's life or safety. The leader can make or break a successful rescue team.

Summary

The development of an effective rescue team starts with a vision, a vision that often includes many hopes and dreams. It requires much planning and effort to realize the goals set forth because of these ideas. But it should not end there. A team must continually set new goals for itself to keep the effort strong. Satisfaction with current status precludes growth. A rescue team's growth and development should be a never-ending process.

CHAPTER 2

Rescue Rope

The information in this chapter is provided as a basis for continued training. Each rescuer should consult with his or her own team leader for the correct SOGs for the team. The NFPA Standard 1983, ANSI and ASTM guidelines will be referred to throughout this chapter.

Topics covered in this chapter include:

- Standard Governing Rope Rescue Equipment
- Rope Composition
- Rope Construction
- Fall Factors
- Choosing Rope
- Rope Care, Maintenance, and Storage
- Deploying Rope

Introduction

In rescue, each piece of equipment is a critical link in a very important chain. All links must work together safely to build systems to move persons from a hazardous place to a safe area. If any link fails, it threatens the entire system. Therefore, you, the rescuer, must thoroughly train yourself to identify, select, and safely use each piece of rescue equipment.

You have to know what equipment you need for a rescue task, and the things equipment can do and cannot do. You must know how to check equipment and maintain it after the job is done. It may sound like a lot of work. But consider that the only thing between you and death or injury may be a single component of a rescue system.

Standards Governing Rescue Rope

Many years ago an accident in a large city claimed the lives of two firefighters. The incident involved an attempt by a firefighter to rescue another. During the rescue attempt, the rope failed and both firefighters fell to their deaths. The only good that comes from such tragedy is that rescuers take notice of safety, or lack of it, in operating guidelines.

The International Association of Firefighters (IAFF) did just that. The IAFF took a hard look at rope handling practices and developed new guidelines concerning rescue rope and equipment. They called their recommendation "Line to Safety." It was the predecessor to the present equipment standard created by the National Fire Protection Association (NFPA).

Guidelines versus Law

Certain recommendations by agencies such as the NFPA, the ANSI, and the ASTM specify minimum standards for much of the equipment used for structural rope rescue. Unless adopted by a governmental agency, however, these recommendations do not carry the weight of law.

Some industrial and municipal organizations ignore such recommendations. These organizations fail to realize that recommendations such as those developed by the NFPA make up nationally recognized "safe practices." They could be used as a basis for prosecution for an incident leading to litigation. Although not bound legally by such a recommendation, rescuers are obviously bound ethically and morally.

Consider this disturbing scenario: You are called to testify during litigation involving an accident that occurred in your facility during practice rappelling. The incident involved failure of a rope that did not meet NFPA standards for construction and strength of life safety rope. The plaintiff's lawyer asks if you are familiar with this nationally recognized recommendation. You are familiar with it through your rescue training. The problem is, you and your team decided a few months before the incident not to adopt NFPA rope standards. Everyone on the team thought that these recommendations were for municipal fire departments and did not apply to industry. So you answer the attorney, "Yes, I know the standard exists."

He then asks, "Why would you want to ignore recommendations designed to ensure the safety of your team members in hazardous practice?"

All rescuers and the agencies they work for have the responsibility to make their practice as safe as possible. National standards can help make this happen.

The National Fire Protection Association's Standard 1983 provides recommendations concerning life safety ropes, harnesses, and other items of equipment designed for rescue. This standard establishes some stringent safety guidelines designed to help compensate for the harsh realities of the structural rescue environment.

Rope Condition

The previous NFPA 1983 standard on life safety rope (1990 edition) recommended that rope employed in rescue be unused. Ropes used in an actual rescue, despite their conditions, were to be rendered unusable to avoid accidentally returning the rope to life safety service.

However, according to the NFPA 1983 standard (1995 edition), "Life safety rope used for rescue at fires or other emergency incidents or for training can be reused if all of the following conditions are met:"

"(A) Rope has not been visibly damaged." This means the naked eye with 20/20 visual acuity cannot see signs of damage.

"(B) Rope has not been exposed to heat, direct flame impingement, or abrasion." This requirement might eliminate most rescues performed during working fires. Exposure to abrasion virtually eliminates every rope used over an edge (even a padded one) for lowering or hauling.

"(C) Rope has not been subjected to any impact load." This does not say "severe" or "significant" impact loads. It means all impact loads. Any drop on a rope creates an impact load.

"(D) Rope has not been exposed to liquids, solids, gases, mists, or vapors of any chemical or other material known to deteriorate rope." This requires a study of chemistry and keeping the telephone number of the rope manufacturer in a convenient place.

"(E) Rope passes inspection when inspected according to the manufacturer's inspection procedure by a qualified person both before and after each use." This inspection procedure obviously depends on the manufacturer of the rope. The statement also implies that the "qualified person" received qualifications through the manufacturer or according to manufacturers' guidelines.

The NFPA standard suggests rope should be virtually new when you use it as a single line for rescues or training. Also, the standard is directed toward personnel who may not have adequate training in rope inspection. By making it nearly impossible to qualify a rope for reuse, the NFPA has made it difficult to accidentally place a damaged rope into service for life safety.

This requirement applies to ropes for training as well as ropes for actual incidents. So, to the NFPA, safety in training is just as important as safety in actual rescues. There is also the need for common sense when it comes to the reuse of rope for training. If teams follow the standard verbatim, they will find themselves replacing some rope after every training session. Unfortunately, the replaced rope may have nothing more wrong with it than slight surface abrasion. By the standard, this is enough to retire the rope, but trained rescuers recognize it as a normal process of use.

The NFPA focuses on all users, whatever their level of training. Trained rescuers educated in the proper care and maintenance of rescue rope should have a superior knowledge of what constitutes damage and what does not. However, for the less experienced rope user, it may be more difficult to reconcile common sense and all recommendations of the standard.

Many training agencies recommend that life safety ropes used in single-line rescue techniques (where only one rope will support the entire load) meet the specific recommendations of the NFPA 1983 standard. Some ropes may no longer meet the standard. But through the process of proper care, maintenance, and inspection, trained rescuers recognize the lines as safe for use. The authors recommend that these ropes be used only in training and that a "backup line," or safety line, always be employed. This second line gives an added margin of safety to training operations using good ropes that technically no longer meet standards.

With this method of use comes great responsibility and liability. Even with additional safety lines in training, the rescuers must properly maintain and inspect the rope constantly. This helps eliminate the chance of placing a damaged rope in a life safety situation.

The rescue team must thoroughly assess its used ropes to decide whether to retire or destroy them. The team may use the information found in the NFPA standard and the information in this chapter to help establish proper assessment procedures. The 1983 edition of the 1993 NFPA Standard requires rescue rope be inspected by a qualified person. The most important phrase to remember when any article of rescue equipment has been compromised is: WHEN IN DOUBT, THROW IT OUT!

Rope Strength

In developing recommendations for life safety rope, the NFPA had to decide the average weight of a firefighter in full turnout gear with self-contained breathing apparatus (SCBA). They decided to designate the weight of this one-person load as 300 pounds.

The NFPA then established a safety margin of 15:1 for rope strength. This safety margin is expressed as a ratio of rope strength to weight of the load. In other words, according to the recommendation, a one-person load (300 pounds) will need a rope 15 times stronger than that, or 4,500 pounds minimum breaking strength. A rope strength of 4,500 pounds for a load of only 300 pounds will provide a significant margin of safety. This will help the rope hold up better to abusive surroundings and practices. Most $\frac{3}{8}$-inch life safety ropes exceed this requirement.

Sometimes in rescue it is necessary to place the weight of two persons on a rope. The NFPA recognized this and wanted strength standards that would allow up to two persons to be suspended on a single rope. They used the same safety margin (15:1) used for one-person loads. The NFPA decided that a two-person load, for purposes of the standard, would be 600 pounds. Using a rope 15 times stronger than this requires a rope with a minimum breaking strength of 9,000 pounds. Again, this will provide a significant margin for error should the rope meet with extreme conditions. Most manufacturers produce a $\frac{1}{2}$-inch rescue rope that meets or exceeds this requirement.

The NFPA does not advocate suspending more than two persons from a single rope for any reason. Many ropes are strong enough by the safety ratio, but it is not a recommended practice.

There are many contributing standards for construction, workmanship, and testing of rescue equipment such as those of the ANSI and the ASTM. The NFPA refers to most of the relevant standards in its 1983 standard. A review of this and other relevant standards provides a more thorough knowledge of the process requirements for rescue equipment.

Rope Composition

Rescue rope is a synthetic, flexible cordage designed specifically to support human loads during rescue and training. Because it is often the only thing between the rescuer and injury or death, it is important to learn everything possible about the rope in use. Rope analysis will help rescuers choose the right rope for the job and use it properly.

Most rescue rope is 100% nylon. However, nylon is not the only type of rope on the market, nor is it the best material for every situation. But nylon does seem to meet the general needs for rope rescue most of the time. Looking at several materials for rope and reviewing the good and bad points of each will allow a more educated decision on which type of rope will work best in a particular situation.

Natural Fiber Ropes

For many years the fire service used rope constructed of natural fibers from such plants as hemp, sisal, or manila. There are several serious problems with natural fiber ropes. One is that they are not as strong as synthetic fiber ropes. Consequently, a good-quality manila rope would need a very large diameter to meet the strength requirements of the NFPA. This means that the rope would be very heavy and cumbersome. It also means most of the hardware and accessory equipment would be bulky and very expensive. More important, there are safety concerns with natural fiber ropes.

Desirable Properties of Natural Fiber Ropes for Rescue

- None.

Undesirable Properties

- Low shock absorption
- Loses strength over time, even under ideal circumstances
- Lower breaking strengths than synthetic ropes of the same diameter
- Short fibers twisted and held together by friction, in contrast to continuous running fibers in most synthetic ropes
- Permanent degradation (as much as 50%) of strength when wet
- High absorption of moisture (Manila rope can absorb 100% of its weight in water.)
- Poor resistance to damaging chemicals
- Visible effects at temperatures between 250° and 300° Fahrenheit

TECHNOLOGY NOTE

The technology in fiber development is constantly changing. Consequently, much technical literature about rope is outdated. Technical information varies due to differences in testing procedures. The "materials" section of this chapter does not include all available rope materials, but concentrates on those materials most often seen and used.

National organizations such as the NFPA, the IAFF, and the ISFSI (International Society of Fire Service Instructors) have condemned natural fiber ropes in life safety applications. Natural fibers are still used in certain other applications, although most fire departments now also use synthetic materials for utility ropes. In summary, DO NOT USE NATURAL FIBER ROPES FOR RESCUE.

Synthetic Fiber Ropes

There are many synthetic fiber ropes now available. Many of these materials have qualities desirable for specific types of rescue. These desirable qualities may be outweighed by drawbacks associated with the specific material. There is still no one rope that works for all rescue situations. However, at this time, it appears that nylon has the best ratio of desirable to undesirable characteristics for general-purpose rope rescue. Until science creates rescues without rope, rescuers must continue to analyze rescue needs and hazards to decide what ropes best meet their requirements.

Nylon Ropes

Specific Rescue Uses: At this time, nylon rope is considered most suitable for most rope rescue applications. The two major types of nylon used to manufacture rescue rope are (1) Type 6, also known as "Perlon" and found in many European ropes and (2) Type 6,6 found in many ropes in North America. The major differences are that type 6,6 has a slightly higher melting point and a slightly higher breaking strength than type 6.

Desirable Properties of Nylon for Rescue Rope

- Good shock absorption
- Melting point of approximately 480° Fahrenheit (type 6,6)
- Good resistance to abrasion
- Resistant to many chemicals
- Low surface friction
- About 10% stronger than polyester in ropes of comparable diameter

Undesirable Properties of Nylon for Rescue Rope

- Both nylon 6 and 6,6 can lose up to 15% of their strength when wet (but regain full strength when they dry).
- Nylon fiber can be damaged seriously by certain corrosives such as battery acid.

Polyolefins

Specific Rescue Uses: Because they float, polyolefins such as polypropylene and polythylene are often used in water rescue rope. Polyolefins are not very strong and cannot absorb shock well. So most water rescue ropes combine polyolefins and nylon to provide strength.

Desirable Properties

- Highly resistant to water (they float)
- Good resistance to mildew
- Highly resistant to acids

Undesirable Properties

- Low tensile strength (compared to nylon)
- Poor resistance to abrasion
- Poor resistance to sunlight (ultraviolet degradation)
- Heat damage at relatively low temperatures (melts at approximately 235° Fahrenheit)
- Poor shock absorption

Polyesters

Specific Rescue Uses: Polyester fibers such as Dacron and Seran have many properties comparable to those of nylon but have low shock-absorption capability. Because of this characteristic, polyesters are generally not used in rope that might be subjected to shock loading from long falls (i.e., mountain climbing and wilderness applications). Polyesters are, however, found in many life safety applications.

Desirable Properties

- High tensile strength even when wet, relatively water resistant
- Good resistance to abrasion
- High melting point (about 480° Fahrenheit)
- Resistant to damage from acids and organic compounds

Undesirable Properties

- Poor resistance to shock, compared to nylon
- May be damaged by alkalis

Kevlar

Specific Rescue Uses: Kevlar, DuPont's trade name for a type of aramid fiber, cannot tolerate small-radius bending such as in knot tying. This causes the fiber to fail under relatively small loads. It is widely recognized that Kevlar is unsuitable for rappelling, ascending, belaying, and rescue lowering and hauling systems.

Desirable Properties

- ✚ Resistant to high temperatures
- ✚ High tensile strength

Undesirable Properties

- ✖ Poor resistance to abrasion
- ✖ Easily damaged by continued, small-radius flexing
- ✖ Poor shock absorption

Other Synthetic Fibers

There are many other synthetic fibers available that might be used alone or in combination with other fibers for specific rescue purposes. It is up to the rescuer to ensure that the chosen rope fibers will meet the needs of the rescue environment, and that it meets national standards that apply.

Rope Construction

A rope's capabilities are the result of fiber combined with method of construction. Different combinations of fiber and construction make a rope more suitable for one use than another. As with rope fibers, each type of construction has its own set of desirable and undesirable properties. Remember, ropes for life safety applications should not be constructed from natural fibers.

Laid Rope

Construction Characteristics: To make a laid rope (see Figure 2.1), fibers are twisted into yarns. The yarns are twisted into strands. The strands are twisted into finished rope. Fibers in hard-laid rope are twisted much more tightly than those in soft-laid or common-laid rope. This provides better resistance to abrasion, but weakens the rope and makes it much more difficult to tie knots in.

Desirable Properties

- ✚ Every part of the rope can be inspected visually for damage by untwisting the strands. While this may seem desirable, it can prove difficult and extremely time consuming. Also, depending on the rope fiber, certain chemical degradation may not be evident from a visual inspection.
- ✚ This type of rope produces high surface friction (it is not slick). This might be considered desirable when rescuers must use their hands to grasp or pull on the rope.

Undesirable Properties

- ✖ All load-supporting strands are subject to abrasion at some point in the rope. Each fiber is exposed to the surface about every 2 inches along the length of the rope.
- ✖ This type of rope tends to untwist under tension, causing a free-hanging object or person to spin.
- ✖ This type of rope tends to kink easily.

Eight-Strand Plaited

Construction Characteristics: A solid woven rope using eight strands (see Figure 2.1) is typically made of white cotton or nylon. Hardware stores often sell it as general-purpose rope.

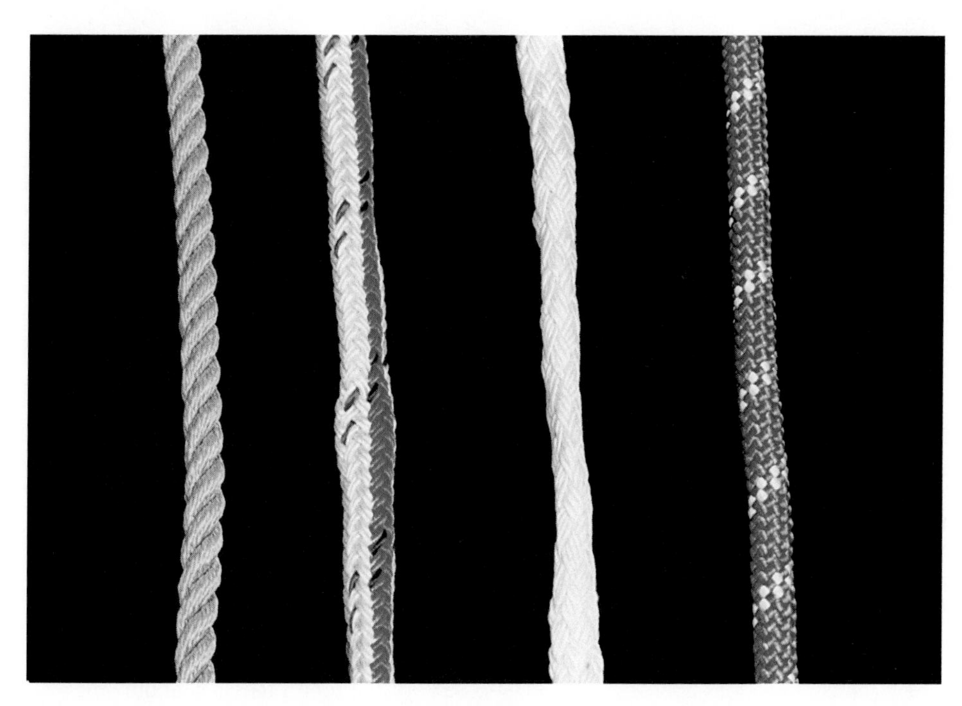

Figure 2.1 Laid Rope, Eight-Strand Plaited Rope, Braid-on-Braid Rope, Kernmantle Rope

Desirable Properties (depending on material used)
- Good resistance to abrasion
- Good tensile strength

Undesirable Properties
- As with laid construction, all fibers are exposed at frequent intervals along the plaited rope's length.
- This type of rope is very susceptible to picking (snagging). This is similar to what happens when threads are snagged and pulled from clothing.

Braid on Braid

Construction Characteristics: This rope is constructed of two braided strands, one encased in the other (see Figure 2.1). In one design, the inside solid-braided strand has about 60% of the tensile strength of the rope. This leaves the outside sheath with approximately 40% of the strength. Braid on braid ropes are usually constructed of synthetic fibers.

Desirable Properties
- Good tensile strength (depending on material used)
- Very pliable if loosely woven
- Resistance to surface abrasion (outside braid helps protect the inside braid)

Undesirable Properties
- Under normal working loads, abrasion resistance is very poor.
- This type of construction has very high stretch under load.

Kernmantle

Construction Characteristics: This rope, low-stretch or dynamic, (see Figure 2.1) is constructed of an internal core (kern) surrounded by a woven sheath (mantle). In most rescue ropes, the core accounts for approximately 80% to 85% of the tensile strength. The sheath provides around 15% to 20% of the tensile strength. It also helps protect the core from surface abrasion and contamination. Kernmantle ropes are always constructed of synthetic fibers.

The core of a low-stretch (static) kernmantle rope is constructed of continuous fibers running parallel to each other and taut throughout the length of the rope. There is generally no twist in the fibers, which allows very little stretch. This makes low-stretch rope ideal for rescue systems requiring control (i.e., hauling systems). Low-stretch kernmantle ropes for rescue stretch between 1.25% and 10% under the weight of a one-person load. They should elongate no more than 45% at 75% of breaking strength.

Dynamic kernmantle rope is designed to absorb shock from falls such as in rock climbing. The specific style of construction varies among manufacturers. The core of one design of dynamic rope is made up of two bundles of fibers twisted in opposite directions to reduce spin. The twisted cores give the rope its stretch by untwisting under load to absorb shock. Most dynamic ropes provide somewhere around 25% stretch under the weight of a one-person load. They will elongate as much as 40% to 60% at failure. The NFPA standard 1983 does not apply to ropes used for dynamic loading.

Desirable Properties

- Good tensile strength (depending on the material)
- Core fibers run continuously throughout the length of the rope (Block creel construction).
- The core provides approximately 80% to 85% of the rope's tensile strength. The outer sheath protects the core from dirt and abrasion.
- Low spin under load
- Does not kink easily

Undesirable Properties

- Core fibers cannot be inspected visually for damage when sheath is intact.

Rescue Rope Recommendations

For most needs, low-stretch kernmantle rope made of 100% nylon that meet the requirements of the NFPA 1983 standard should be used in rescues. The following summary highlights the advantages and disadvantages of this combination of materials and construction rescue rope.

Advantages

- Low stretch for maximum control when hauling or lowering injured people.
- Nylon has a very high tensile strength compared to many materials.
- Nylon kernmantle is very strong. The minimum breaking strength of most manufacturers' $\frac{3}{8}$-inch lifeline is around 5,000 force pounds. The minimum breaking strength for $\frac{1}{2}$-inch is usually over 9,000 force pounds, and for $\frac{5}{8}$-inch is generally over 13,000 force pounds.
- Nylon static kernmantle rope has excellent resistance to abrasion.
- Nylon will not dry-rot.
- Nylon is resistant to extreme heat and extreme cold.
- Nylon melts at temperatures between 480°F and 500°F (depending on the type of nylon). If it remains dry, nylon can withstand temperatures much colder than minus 40°F. However, at this temperature, any ice crystals that form are so hard they can cut the nylon.
- Nylon is resistant to many common chemicals such as most alkalis, antifreeze, alcohols, and hydrocarbons with no additives (most processed hydrocarbons contain additives harmful to nylon).
- Nylon kernmantle rope is lightweight. For example, one manufacturer's $\frac{1}{2}$-inch rescue rope weighs approximately 7 pounds per 100 feet and its $\frac{5}{8}$-inch rope weighs only 10 pounds per 100 feet.

Disadvantages

- Nylon temporarily loses 10% to 15% of its strength when wet. It will return to its original strength after drying.
- Nylon can be damaged by certain chemicals. Acids specifically should be avoided. These will be covered later in this chapter.

Fall Factors

There may be situations in rescue where significant falls are possible. For example, when a rescuer has to climb a tower or antenna. If low-stretch rope is used, the rescuer could be seriously injured by the fall. In these cases, rescuers should use dynamic ropes because they absorb shock rather than transfer it to the rescuer. When planning rescues of this type, consider the fall factor before deciding whether to use low-stretch or dynamic rope.

The "fall factor" is an estimate of the force of a potential fall. It is calculated by dividing the distance the person attached to the rope is expected to fall by the length of the rope between him or her and the rope's anchor attachment. Therefore, a 3-foot fall on a 10-foot rope would have a .3 fall factor. A 3-foot fall on a 3-foot rope would have a 1.0 fall factor. And a 3-foot fall on a 100-ft rope would have a .03 fall factor. This formula assumes the fall takes place in free air without rope drag across a rough surface or through intermediate equipment.

In most situations with fall factors of less than .25 (a $2\frac{1}{2}$-foot fall on a 10-foot rope), static rope is satisfactory. If fall factors greater than .25 could occur, the rescuer should not use static rope alone. With fall factors greater than .25, dynamic ropes or shock absorbers (also known as load limiters) incorporated into the low-stretch system create a dynamic effect. As a rule of thumb, a dynamic rope (or a low-stretch rope with a shock absorber for dynamic effect) is used any time a person is working above the rope's anchor attachment. In industrial rescue, this should seldom happen.

Choosing Rope Size

A rescuer could encounter additional problems by confusing different sized ropes during an emergency. If the rope is poorly marked, it may be difficult to tell the difference between one-person and two-person ropes.

Most manufacturers' $\frac{1}{2}$-inch low-stretch kernmantle rescue ropes meet the NFPA strength requirements for two-person loads. All of the main load lines in a rope rescue system, whether one- or two-person loads, should meet this strength requirement.

Some manufacturers make a smaller-diameter rope that meets the NFPA strength requirements for a one-person load. However, it is always possible that the rescue situation could change. The change could require a two-person load on a single rope. If the rescuer has set up with the one-person rope and must suddenly load it with two people, it could be a dangerous situation. Always plan for a two-person load on your rescue system.

There are some applications for smaller one-person lifelines in rope rescue systems. For example, many industrial rescue teams advocate using short (50 to 75 feet) sections of $\frac{3}{8}$- or $\frac{7}{16}$-inch lifeline for building mechanical advantage systems designed to be attached to a main load line (rated for two-person loads) for hauling. Rescuers can build these piggyback hauling systems and prebag them for rapid deployment. The smaller rope diameter helps reduce friction in the system's pulleys while making the haul easier for the rescue team. They still maintain system strength through the load distribution characteristics of mechanical advantage (see Chapter 12, "Confined Space Rescue: Hauling Techniques," for more information).

Some rescuers advocate the exclusive use of $\frac{5}{8}$-inch rescue rope. The idea of stronger equipment prevails here since most rope manufacturers have a $\frac{5}{8}$-inch rescue rope in excess of 13,000 pounds tensile strength. If bigger is better, shouldn't rescuers all go to $\frac{5}{8}$-inch rope? Is bigger always better? There are pros and cons.

The pro is obvious: $\frac{5}{8}$-inch rescue rope is much stronger than $\frac{1}{2}$-inch rescue rope, although both meet the minimum requirement of the NFPA standard for two-person loads. The cons may not be so obvious: bigger, stronger rope is heavier, bulkier, more expensive and requires larger hardware accessories. Bigger isn't always better.

The final decision on rope size rests with the rescue team. It is important to meet the NFPA standards. The ideal is to do so for both one- and two-person loads while keeping the weight, bulk, and expense to a minimum.

Choosing the Rope Length

Analyzing average and worst-case rescue scenarios helps rescuers make a more informed decision on rope length. The following is an example.

The team knows from its history of rescues that it accomplishes most rope rescues within an average vertical height of 50 feet. The team factors in that a hauling system might be needed and in training they usually use a 4:1 simple mechanical advantage system. This system requires enough rope to reach the full height of the drop four times. Based on these factors the team calculates that it needs rope lengths of 200 feet (50 feet depth × 4) for most rescues in their facility. In reality, this length seems to work well as the standard for most industrial rescue teams. The number of rope sections needed depends on the rescue systems a team commonly builds.

WARNING

Do not mark ropes with phenol-based markers or use any process that will cause nylon to degrade.

What about the worst-case scenario? Suppose that the same team has in its response area a digester unit 250 feet high. Maintenance personnel occasionally work atop the unit and would require rescue in case of illness or injury. The team realizes from training drills that it cannot conveniently use the 200-foot rope sections to perform this rescue. The team decides to purchase a few longer ropes to handle this problem should it ever arise. These rescuers have planned and will be prepared for a worst-case rescue.

Training can also help answer the question of rope length. During training a team plans for and practices rescue scenarios it is most likely to experience and those that might be considered worst case. If the rope lengths are not working well in training, they will not work well in actual rescues.

Rope Care and Maintenance

Marking Rope

Every rope should be labeled with identifying markings. This identification (ID) allows a rescue team to maintain a complete history of the rope and its use by keeping a log corresponding to the ID. Many nondestructive methods of marking ropes are available. Identification numbers can be marked with permanent markers or affixed to the ends of the rope with adhesive labels (see Figure 2.2). The identification markings can then be sealed with commercial products to prevent them from wearing off. Rope marking and sealant products are available from most suppliers of rope rescue equipment.

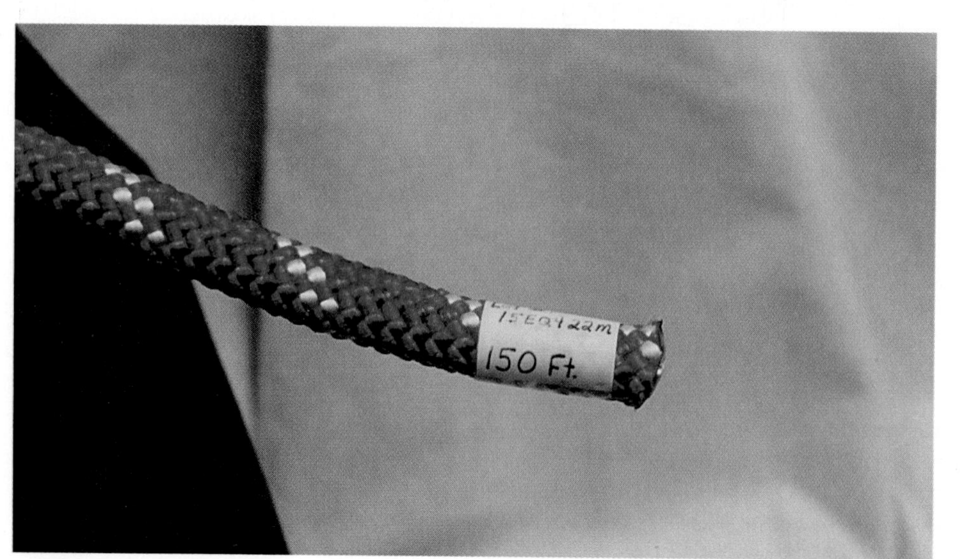

Figure 2.2 Using rope marker to identify rope

Rope History

A team should maintain a history of use on all ropes and rope rescue equipment. A rope log such as the one provided by the rope manufacturer (see Figure 2.3) is very useful. There should be a rope log for every rope. Each time a rescuer returns the rope to storage, he or she should record such information as the date of use, the type of use, and the maintenance performed. Rope intended for single-line use in actual rescues and training should be logged and designated as such.

Storing Rope

Rescue ropes must be protected while in storage. As noted earlier, damage can occur in many ways. Some things to avoid when storing nylon rescue rope are:

- Excessive exposure to direct sunlight (ultraviolet radiation). Store rope in the shade.
- Exposure to certain chemicals such as acids (i.e., battery acid, bleaching agents, and acid vapors), hydrocarbons with acidic additives, and hydrogen-dissolving solvents (i.e., methylene chloride, phenol, benzene, and xylene). Do not store rescue rope in the same compartment with batteries or gas-fueled equipment. Keep the rope out of areas containing grease or exhaust fumes. Do not let it contact any chemical known to harm nylon. If uncertain of the effect of a substance on rope, call the manufacturer of the rope.
- Exposure to dirt and grit. This can damage rope from the inside out. Keep the rope clean and dry.
- Exposure to high temperatures. Keep the rope away from sources of heat such as direct flame, apparatus mufflers, and exhaust pipes.

Some rescue teams store their ropes in airtight cases for maximum protection, which may provide the best storage environment. However, these often heavy, bulky boxes may not be the most practical means of deployment. Most rescue teams choose

Figure 2.3 Rope log

ROPE HISTORY & USAGE

User's ID #	ID Marking	Mfg Lot #
Date of Mfg	Issue Date	Date in Service
Length	Diameter	Color

IMPORTANT: Inspect rope for damage or excessive wear each time it is deployed and again after each use. Retire all suspect ropes immediately!

Date Used	Location Used	Type of Use	Rope Exposure	Date Cked	Inspector	Rope Conditions/Comments

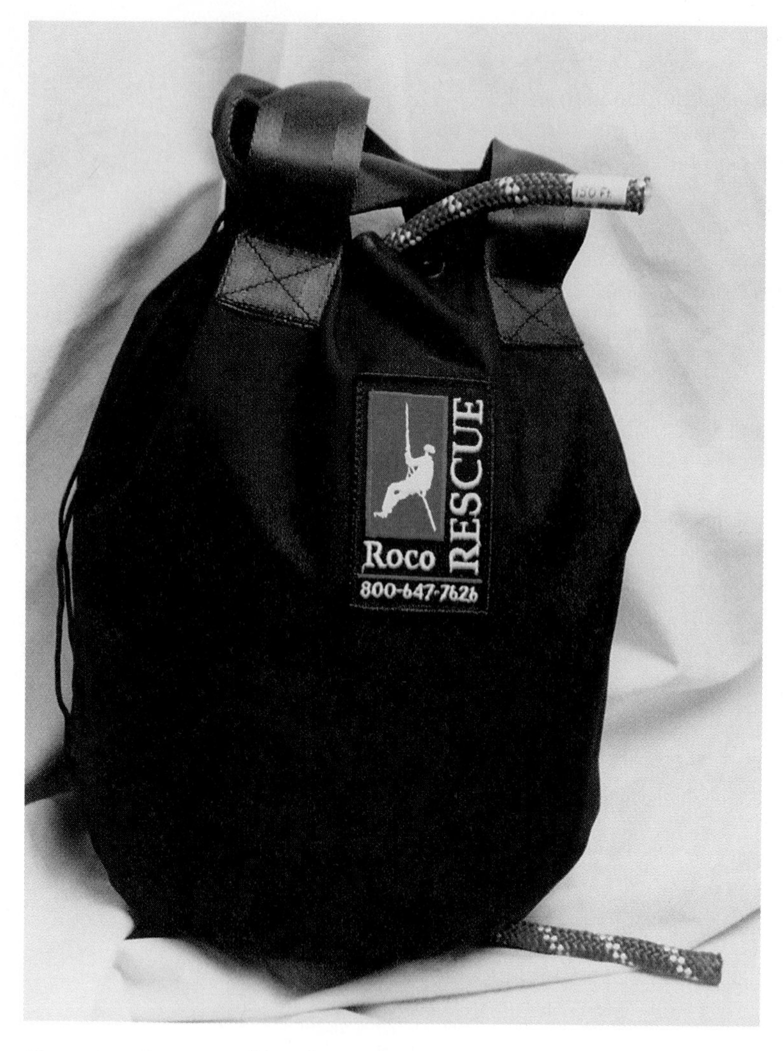

Figure 2.4 Rope stored in a bag

to store their ropes in bags made of nylon and other materials (see Figure 2.4). Bags provide some protection from common hazards while allowing more rapid deployment. Keep them stored in an area shaded, clean, and dry. Avoid caustic or otherwise damaging ambient conditions.

Inspecting Rope

The manufacturers of life safety rope or system components certified as in compliance with the NFPA 1983 standard are required to furnish the purchaser with inspection procedures, maintenance procedures, and retirement criteria. Rescuers should always follow the manufacturer's recommendations concerning these procedures.

A rescue team should inspect its ropes before and after each use. Inspection of kernmantle rope can be simpler than inspection requirements of laid rope. When inspecting rope you should note the following:

1. As with all rescue equipment, inspect ropes by sight and by touch.
2. Run every inch of the rope through your *bare hands.* Visually inspect the sheath for damage and feel for deformities in the core that might suggest damage.
3. If you find visible sheath damage, inspect the area carefully to decide if it should be discarded. One method of inspection involves bending the rope acutely at the damaged area and inspecting the sheath. Most rescue ropes have a core of solid white fibers. If you can see white core fibers through the sheath, "sheath penetration" has occurred. Cut out that area of the rope and discard it.
4. If you find inconsistencies in the feel of the rope's core, suggested by soft, hard, lumpy, or mushy spots, inspect the core for permanent damage. Inconsistencies in feel often result from the core fibers becoming bunched up inside the sheath. This may constitute no real damage to the core. "Popping" the rope often restores the core fibers to their normal state of alignment in the sheath. You can do this by grasping the rope several inches away from the suspect area on either side and popping it several times (see Figure 2.5). After popping, reinspect the rope by running the suspect area through your bare hands. If the inconsistency remains, assume the core is damaged. Cut out and discard that area of the rope.

These procedures are quick and easy to follow and should provide a practical means of inspecting kernmantle rope. There are many other methods of rope inspection, however, the principle method of inspection should be based on manufacturers' recommendations.

Washing Rope

Only used rope needs to be washed. One leading contributor of damage to rope is dirt. Dirt can infiltrate the fibers and damage them. Dirt often contains sand. Sand is silica, a primary component of glass. Rope that remains dirty can, bit by bit, be cut and damaged. A commercial rope washing device can remove big chunks of mud and similar dirt from the rope's surface, but these rope washers are not adequate for a thorough cleaning. Again, consider the manufacturer's recommendations for cleaning. Here are some general guidelines for washing nylon kernmantle ropes:

A

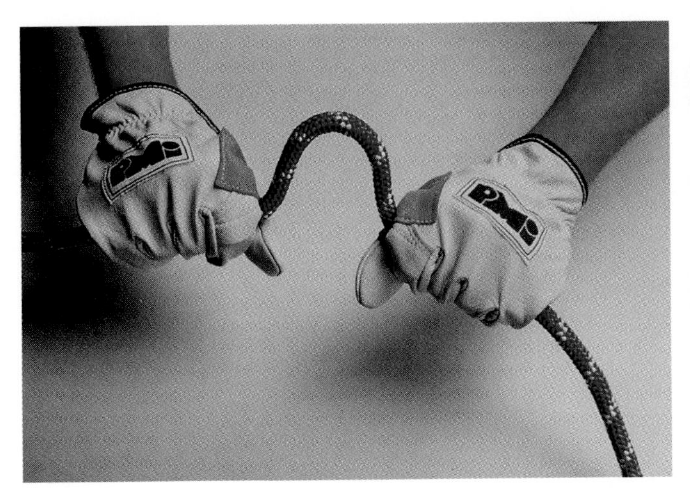

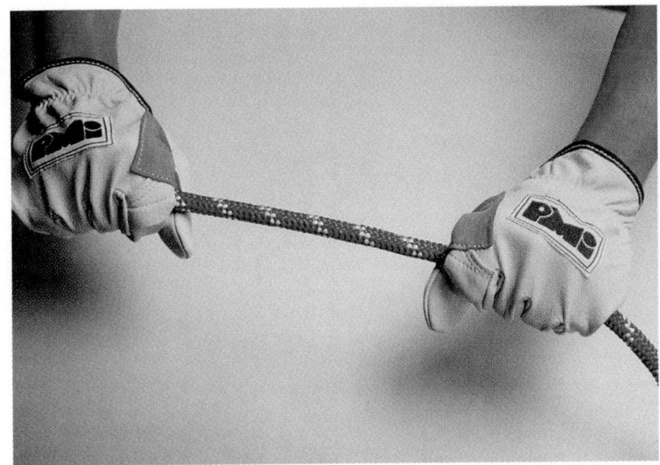

B

Figure 2.5 A, B Popping rope

1. Consider using a clothes washing machine. Many trainers recommend a front-loading washer. A top-loading washer is acceptable if the agitator can be removed. The agitator tends to tangle rope. It can also cause heat damage due to friction between the nylon and the synthetic material of the agitator.
2. If you decide to use a front-loading machine, be sure the view port on the door is glass and not plastic. The plastic door may cause heat damage (glazing of rope sheath). This is caused by friction between the plasic window and the nylon surface of the rope while it is tumbling in the drum.
3. 'Daisy chain' the rope (see Figure 2.6) to prevent tangling while it is tumbling in the wash cycle. You may wish to place the rope in net-type dive gear bags before loading it in the machine.
4. Wash and rinse in cool water. If the rope is very dirty, it may need a warm-water wash, warm-water rinse. To test for temperature, stick your hand in the wash water. If it is too hot for your hand, it is too hot for your rope.
5. Use a gentle detergent. Do not use detergents containing bleaching agents, often advertised as containing "whiteners and brighteners." Bleaching agents can cause deterioration and compromise the rope's integrity.
6. During the rinse cycle, add one capful of fabric softener to the wash load to replace the natural lubricant in nylon rope that is lost through repeated washing. This helps the rope retain its original suppleness. Use fabric softener in moderation and in strict adherence to manufacturers' recommendations. Use regular strength, not concentrated, fabric softener.
7. Remove the rope from the washer and dry before storing. Rescuers should wash rope on a scheduled basis, at least twice a year, and as needed. Every time the rope is cleaned, it should be recorded on the rope log.

Figure 2.6 Rope daisy-chained for washing

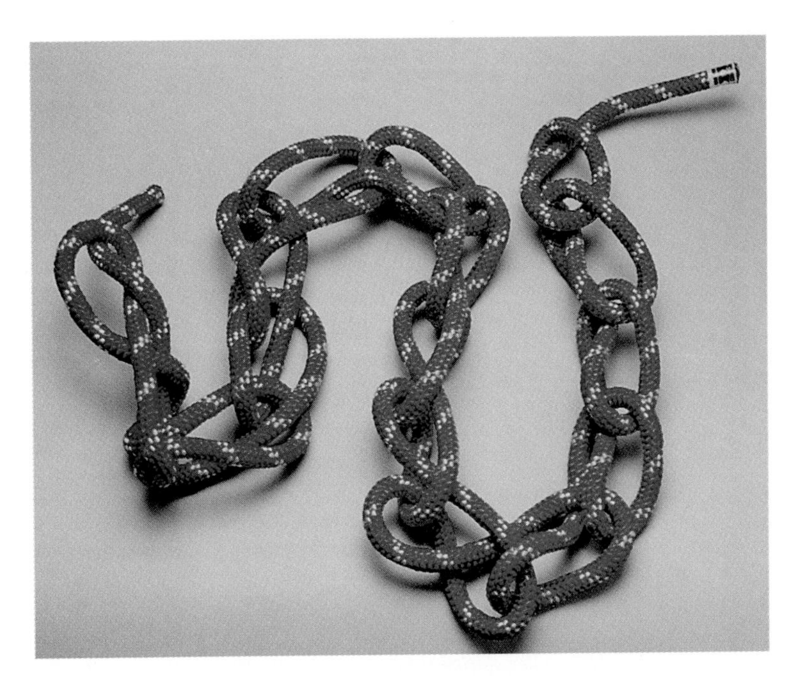

Drying Rope

Nylon rope loses approximately 15% of its strength when wet (saturated) due to the effect of water on its hydrogen bond. This is not a lasting problem because nylon rope completely regains its strength when it is dry. Although nylon kernmantle rope may be used wet, it should be allowed to dry completely before storing it. Follow manufacturers' recommendations.

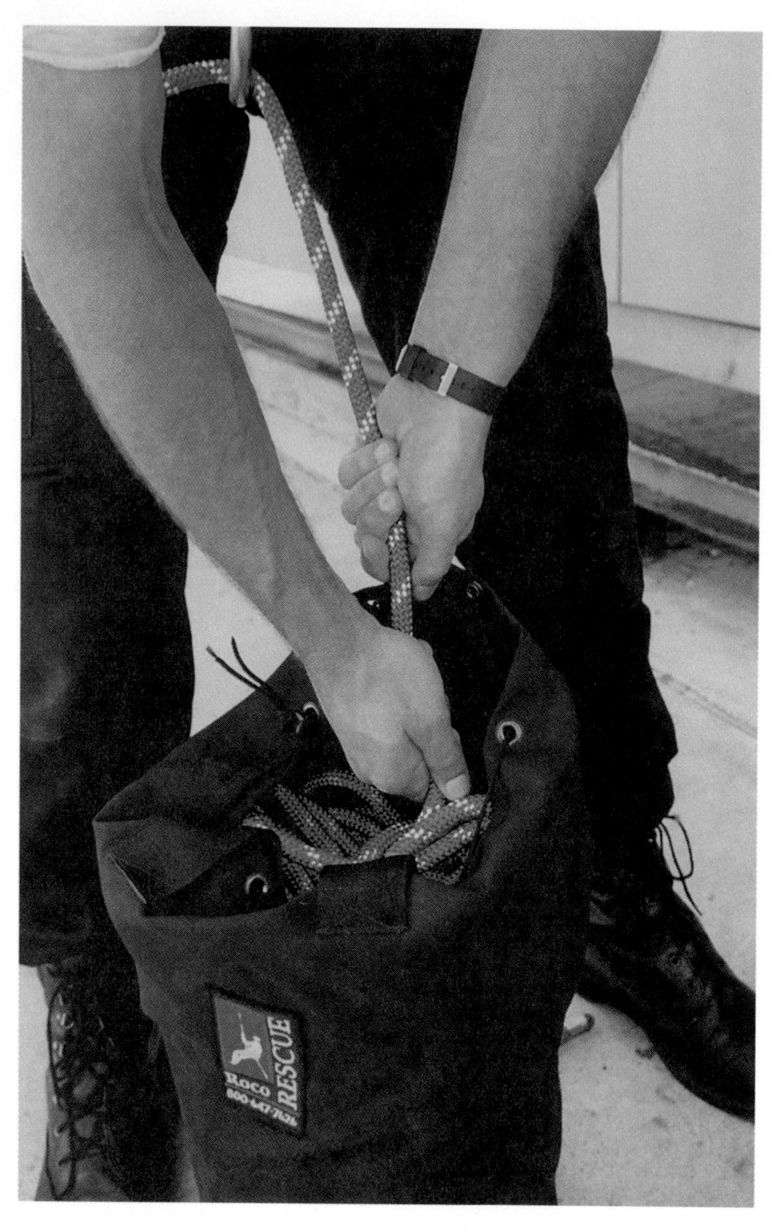

Figure 2.7 Bagging rope

Rope should not be dried in a commercial dryer because temperatures often exceed 180°F. This temperature can cause shrinkage and can damage the rope fibers. The following recommendations provide a general guideline for drying nylon kernmantle rescue rope:

1. Air dry nylon rope but do not dry in direct sunlight. Ropes can be placed in loose coils and left overnight to dry, if outside humidity is not high.
2. Do not lay the rope on a concrete floor. Concrete may contain substances damaging to nylon rope, particularly wet nylon rope.
3. Once thoroughly dry, return rope to storage container.

Retiring Rope

According to NFPA 1983 (1995 edition), the manufacturer of rescue rope must supply the purchaser with retirement criteria. However, many easily recognized conditions render a rope unsafe. Several of these conditions are:

1. Sheath penetration is present.
2. Severe shock loading. NFPA standards suggest that fall factors greater than .25 are unacceptable. This equates to a 2$\frac{1}{2}$-foot fall on a 10-foot rope.
3. The rope has been severely overloaded or used for unapproved procedures such as towing vehicles.
4. The rope has been contaminated by harmful chemicals such as acids, chlorine, or bleach.
5. Soft, mushy or hard spots are not recoverable by popping.
6. The rope has reached a certain age and may have degraded due to use or storage conditions.

According to the manufacturers of nylon, a brand new static kernmantle rescue rope of 100% nylon with a breaking strength of 9,000 force pounds that has been in a perfect storage environment for 100 years can be taken out and, on a break test, theoretically it will break at 9,000 force pounds. The words *perfect* and *theoretically* imply that nylon does not degrade if everything is just right. Unfortunately, most rescue teams cannot store their ropes in ideal environments. It is doubtful these environments even exist outside a laboratory. Although there has been no definitive testing, some rescue trainers suggest that industrial facilities cycle their ropes every 3 to 5 years. This is due to adverse ambient atmospheres frequently associated with industrial processes and training an average of 8 hours per month. For municipalities, the recommendation is usually greater (up to 10 years). Their ropes are not as likely to be exposed to the harsh environments of industrial facilities.

Any time there is a loss of confidence for any reason, the key phrase for retirement of life safety rope is WHEN IN DOUBT, THROW IT OUT!

Bagging Rope

As discussed, there are advantages to placing rescue rope in bags for storage. The following method is one way to rebag rope after use (see Figure 2.7):

1. Tie a loose figure-8 stopper or similar knot in the loose end of the rope. This knot will prevent the rope from sliding through the descent control device if the rope is too short for the operation.

2. Stuff the rope into the bag while running it through your hands, feeling and visually inspecting it. There is no rule concerning how kernmantle rope should be put into the bag. Do not worry about trying to coil the rope into the bag. It does not have to be wound clockwise or counterclockwise. Just stuff it, hand over hand (not in a lump) into the bag.
3. To make it easier to stuff the rope into the bag, try clipping the rope through a carabiner or snap link attached to your belt while you stand directly over the rope bag. This is an excellent method of directing the rope's path over the opening of the bag for easier bagging.

Deploying Rope

The good thing about using a rope bag for storage is how easy it is to deploy in an emergency. If bagged as described in the previous section, it almost never tangles when deployed. To deploy it, simply feed the rope out. Avoid dropping the rope bag to the ground from heights. Drops from elevations higher than 100 feet onto a hard surface can damage rope.

Summary

This chapter discussed the rescue rope needs of the rescue team. Many other important equipment items are needed to complete the rope rescue system. A rescuer must have a thorough knowledge of rope rescue equipment before he or she can construct rope rescue systems. The next chapter discusses these related components. Remember that all rescuers should seek proper hands-on training from a competent trainer before attempting any of the techniques shown in this book.

CHAPTER 3

Related Rope Rescue Equipment

The NFPA Standard 1983, ANSI and ASTM guidelines will be referred to throughout the chapter. The information in this chapter is provided as a basis for continued training. Each rescuer should consult with his or her own team leader for the correct SOGs for the team. Topics covered in this chapter include:

- Equipment Strength Guidelines
- Software
- Hardware

Introduction

In the last chapter, we discussed the importance of rope in the rescue system chain. This chapter will review several hardware (rigid nonflexible) and software (flexible) components of rope rescue systems. We will review items of equipment that have specific application in industrial rescue.

Products useful for industrial and structural rescue are in ample supply. Before you choose a piece of equipment, remember that it must be designed and manufactured to the rigid specifications required for rope rescue. If the manufacturer does not endorse the product for rope rescue purposes, DO NOT use it for rope rescue. For example, slings designed for rigging steel beams to a crane for lifting may be very strong indeed, but the manufacturer does not give approval for lifting human loads. A rescuer who uses it for that purpose has a serious liability. Rescue equipment must be built with a great deal of quality assurance for its intended use in mind. Just as, for example, there is a difference between a ladder designed for painting a house and a ladder designed for fighting fires, there is a lot of difference among items of rescue equipment. This is the reason for national standards such as those developed by the National Fire Protection Association, to help rescuers decide on the safest equipment for rescue.

Equipment Strength Guidelines

Some environments are often more unfriendly to rescue equipment than the others. Therefore, the need for stringent requirements may be even greater. The strength recommendations discussed in the previous chapter involved life safety rope only. The recommendations for hardware and other items of life safety equipment that might also be required to hold the weight of a two-person load are generally less than that required for rope.

Because of this, many trainers recommend that industrial rescuers apply to all equipment the same two-person load standards as for rope. For example, a 9,000 pound rescue rope being used to lower two persons is attached to a lowering device rated at only 6,000 pounds minimum tensile strength. Thus the safety margin has been reduced by a weak link (the lowering device) in the chain. This 9,000 pound strength in rescue with the potential for two-person loads should be carefully considered by industrial rescue teams before purchasing equipment.

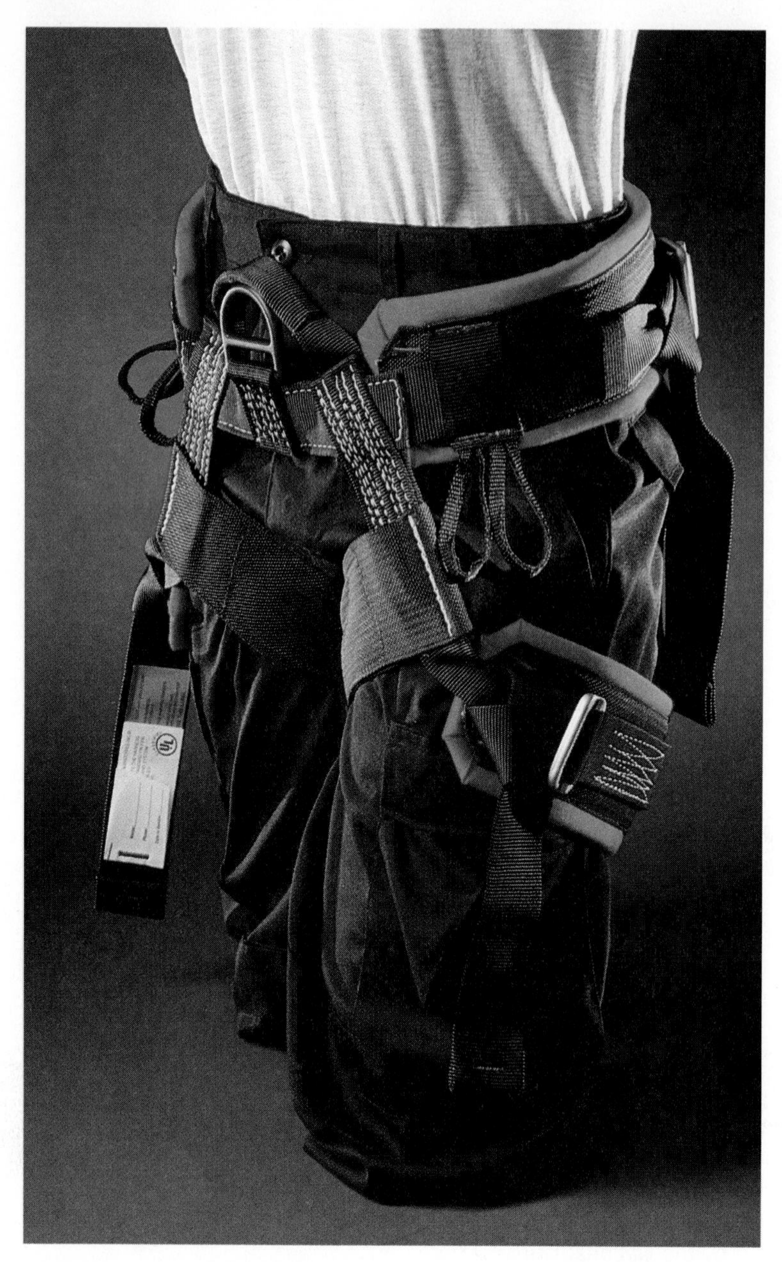

Figure 3.1 Class II safety harness

Software

In addition to rope, the NFPA 1983 standard addresses many types of equipment used for rope rescue. Among them are harnesses and auxiliary software and hardware. Where standards exist, it is important to adhere to criteria relating to construction, inspection, maintenance, and retirement. The manufacturer's recommendations play a big part in this process.

Life Safety Harnesses

The NFPA standard has strict specifications for life safety harnesses worn by rescue personnel. Many types of prefabricated harnesses meet NFPA standards. Most harnesses designed for wilderness use do not meet the stringent requirements of this standard and may not hold up in harsh environments.

Safety Harness Classification

The NFPA lists three basic classifications of life safety harnesses. There are additional specifications for escape and ladder belts, which are not classified as harnesses. The NFPA's description of each harness type follows.

- **Class I life safety harnesses** fasten around waist and around thighs or under buttocks and are designed to be used for emergency escape with one-person loads.
- **Class II life safety harnesses** fasten around waist and around thighs or under buttocks and are designed for rescue with two-person loads (see Figure 3.1).
- **Class III life safety harnesses** fasten around waist, around thighs, or under buttocks, and over shoulders, and designed for rescue where two-person loads can be encountered and inverting might occur (see Figure 3.2). Class III harnesses shall be permitted to consist of one or more parts.

According to these descriptions, only Class II and Class III harnesses should be used for rescuers intending to rescue others. According to NFPA, a Class III harness should be used any time inverting may occur. Inverting while suspended on rope is often done in an effort to extend one's downward reach.

For industrial rescuers, the additional consideration of confined space rescue often dictates the use of a Class III harness. This is due to the frequent need to extract someone vertically through a narrow opening (manway). If attached to a waist connection, an unconscious worker or rescuer will maintain a somewhat horizontal attitude. This is not good for retrieving the fallen rescuer through a 20-inch manway.

Using a Class III harness, connection can be made to a high point (usually the chest area in the front of or between the shoulder blades) on the harness, allowing the stricken rescuer to be retrieved in a somewhat vertical position (see Figure 3.3). This will make it much easier to get them through the narrow opening.

Whatever harness a rescue team chooses, it should meet NFPA 1983 standards. A Class III or combination Class II and III is strongly recommended for industrial rescue.

Construction

The harness in Figure 3.4 is an example of an NFPA 1983 compliant Class II and III combination harness. This is a two-piece unit consisting of a seat harness and a chest harness. The chest harness alone does not meet standards and should not be used without the seat. The seat harness alone meets all of the requirements for NFPA 1983 Class II. In combination, the harness meets the NFPA requirement for a Class III harness.

D-rings

D-rings (not to be confused with carabiners) and buckles on harnesses are load-bearing hardware and are usually rated by "proof load." A proof load is an amount of force the hardware can withstand without permanent distortion. This term should not be confused with "breaking strength," which is the tensile strength that can be applied without failure of the item. The NFPA 1983 standards apply the requirement of "minimum" to these terms. The minimum strength is generally based on a number of standard deviations subtracted from the mean or average strength of a group of these items. In very rough terms, the lowest strength among a group of hardware items tested is the minimum strength. Rescuers should always ask for minimum strengths when inquiring about the proof load and breaking strengths of rescue equipment. These items of equipment should meet NFPA 1983 standards.

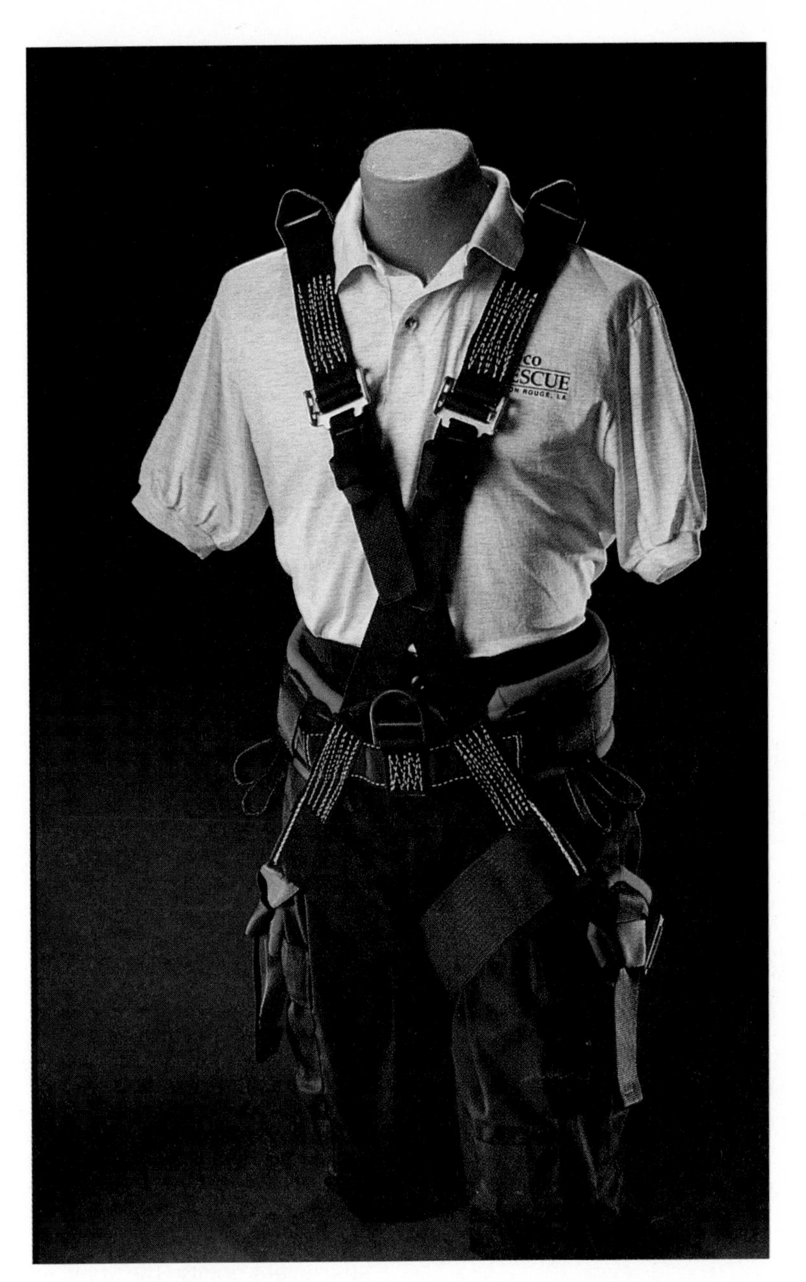

Figure 3.2 Class III safety harness

Attachment Points

The D-rings pictured on the harness in Figure 3.4 are the primary load-bearing attachment points. The D-rings on this harness are located both front and back at the waist area and front and back at the level of the chest. Multiattachment points give the rescuer versatility. This type of harness can be attached to a rope or rope system at the waist to allow the rescuer to invert and maneuver easily, or it can be attached at the chest to allow for vertical retrieval in a confined space.

Most often, primary attachments to a class II seat harness are made at a front D-ring. However, a rear D-ring allows an excellent point of attachment for secondary safety lines if used in training. Chest-level D-rings are used primarily for confined space retrieval systems although they have other applications. Front or back chest-level D-rings may be used interchangeably as dictated by the type of opening through which the rescuer must be retrieved. On this particular harness (see Figure 3.4), maximum comfort is attained through attachment to front D-rings at the waist or the chest level (see Figure 3.4).

Some harnesses incorporate structural loops as attachment points (see Figure 3.5a). These act as the primary attachment point or as a backup to another attachment point.

Structural Webbing

The webbing used to create the soft structural members of most harnesses is a type of flat-weave webbing of various widths made of 100% nylon, similar to the straps used for seat belts. The minimum breaking strength of this type webbing usually has a breaking strength of at least 6,000 force pounds.

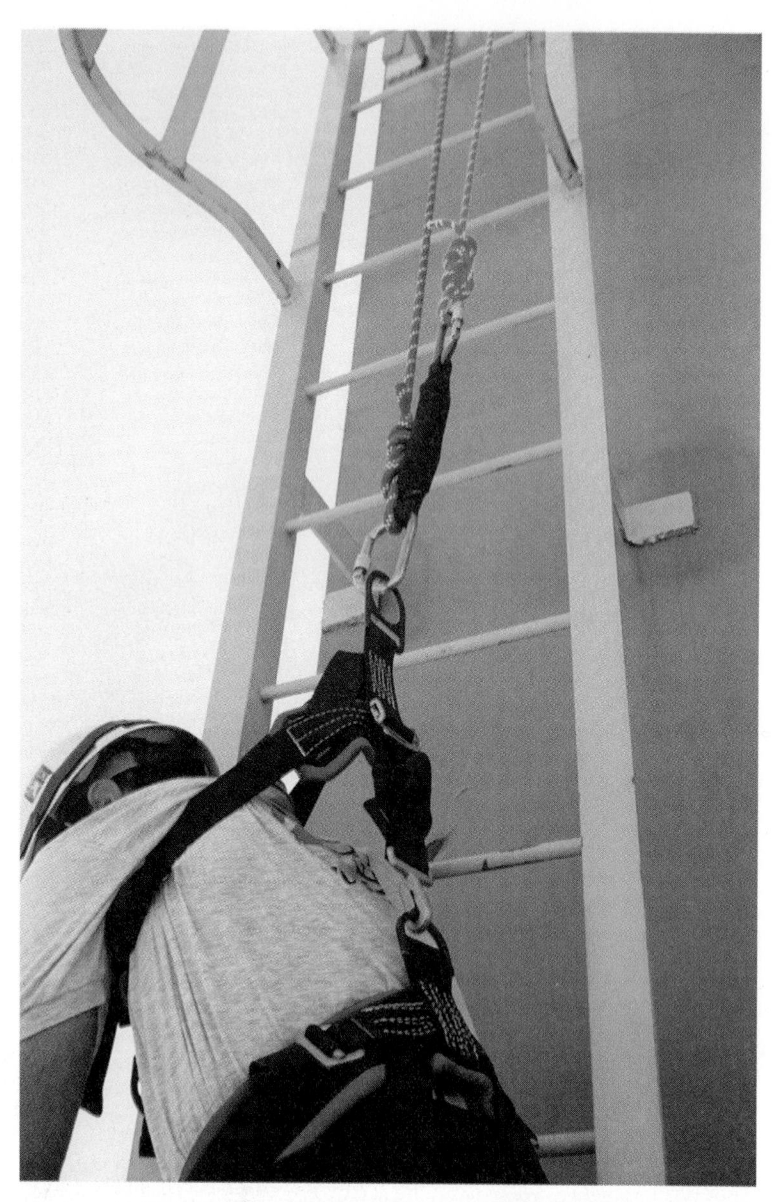

Figure 3.3 Connection to high point on Class III harness

Utility Loops

Many harnesses have small cordage or webbing loops attached to a seat harness designed for carrying auxiliary rescue equipment (see Figure 3.5b). This is convenient and prevents rescue equipment from being kicked or dropped from a height. Utility loops are not designed to be load-bearing items. DO NOT mistakenly attach utility loops to live loads!

Comfort

Many rescue harnesses have padding and design features that promote comfort for the wearer. Comfort during rescue operations is not only desirable, it is vital. A badly designed or poorly fitted harness will apply undue pressure to the wearer's chest, waist, or legs during an extended rescue operation. The rescuer might experience pain or other physiological consequences to the point of incapacitation. The rescuer could become a victim.

Before purchasing a harness, try it out if possible. Ask the manufacturer for a test unit or contact trainers for assistance. Work and hang in the harness in various positions from each attachment point for a length of time. The time to find out that your harness is not suitable for your rescues is *before* the rescue.

Testing Requirements

Although each component maintains its own strength rating, the combination of components makes the harness. For this reason, NFPA 1983 (1995 edition) requires a series of static pull and drop tests to determine the structural integrity of the harness. During the static pull tests, forces between 2,250 and 3,600 pounds are applied to a weighted, harnessed test manikin according to its positioning (upright, horizontal, head down). These specifications require testing from all load-bearing attachment points. The static tests must be successful without destroying or rendering nonfunctional any component of the harness. Drop tests are also specified and require a certain number and height of drops without the test load contacting the ground or adjustment buckles slipping significantly. For maximum safety and minimum liability, harnesses used by industrial rescuers should meet all applicable requirements of the NFPA 1983 standard for life safety harnesses. This testing is the responsibility of the manufacturer and must be conducted by a third party.

Care and Maintenance

A manufacturer certified as compliant with NFPA 1983 (1995 edition) must supply inspection procedures, maintenance procedures, and retirement criteria for the product. It is important to acquire and follow this information for a particular harness, and to pay attention to the manufacturer's donning procedures. Improper application is the leading cause of discomfort and poor performance.

Patient Harnesses

Harnesses meeting NFPA 1983 standards are designed to be worn by rescuers performing rescue work. These harnesses are seldom made for rapid application to subjects being rescued. The method of packaging a patient (patient packaging) must be appropriate for his or her medical condition. For example, if a patient has a suspected spinal injury, it would be much better to immobilize the spine and place him or her in a litter for rescue rather than into a harness and further complicate the injury. Because regulations governing victim packaging differ from state to state, the procedure should be performed according to your rescue team's specific protocols. These decisions, and the priorities surrounding them, are discussed in a later chapter.

Full-Body Harnesses Full-body harnesses with high points of attachment are always the preferred type of harness for victims. It is sometimes desirable for a rescuer to invert, but it is certainly undesirable for the person being rescued, particularly if it is unintentional. Seat harnesses may allow the subject (especially those with greater-than-average upper body weight) to turn upside down or horizontal while suspended. This can cause panic quicker than any other action, except a fall. Attaching the subject to a high attachment point near the chest or middle of the back will keep him or her upright despite a tendency to invert. Some harnesses have D-rings at the shoulder straps for vertical extraction of the patient (see Figure 3.6). DO NOT use these D-rings for extraction without the bridle manufactured for this application. The bridle has a "spreader bar," which prevents the webbing or rope attached to the D-rings from placing lateral-to-lateral pressure on the patient's head during lifting.

Prefabricated Harnesses As a rule, prefabricated full-body harnesses such as the one shown in Figure 3.4 should be used for rescue subjects. Prefabricated harnesses cannot easily come untied, which makes them safer than improvised harnesses. Certain standards pertain to harnesses for employees working from heights, to be worn in conjunction with fall protection equipment (OSHA 1910.126, subpart M). It is recommended that these harness standards be applied to the rescue subject's harness whenever possible.

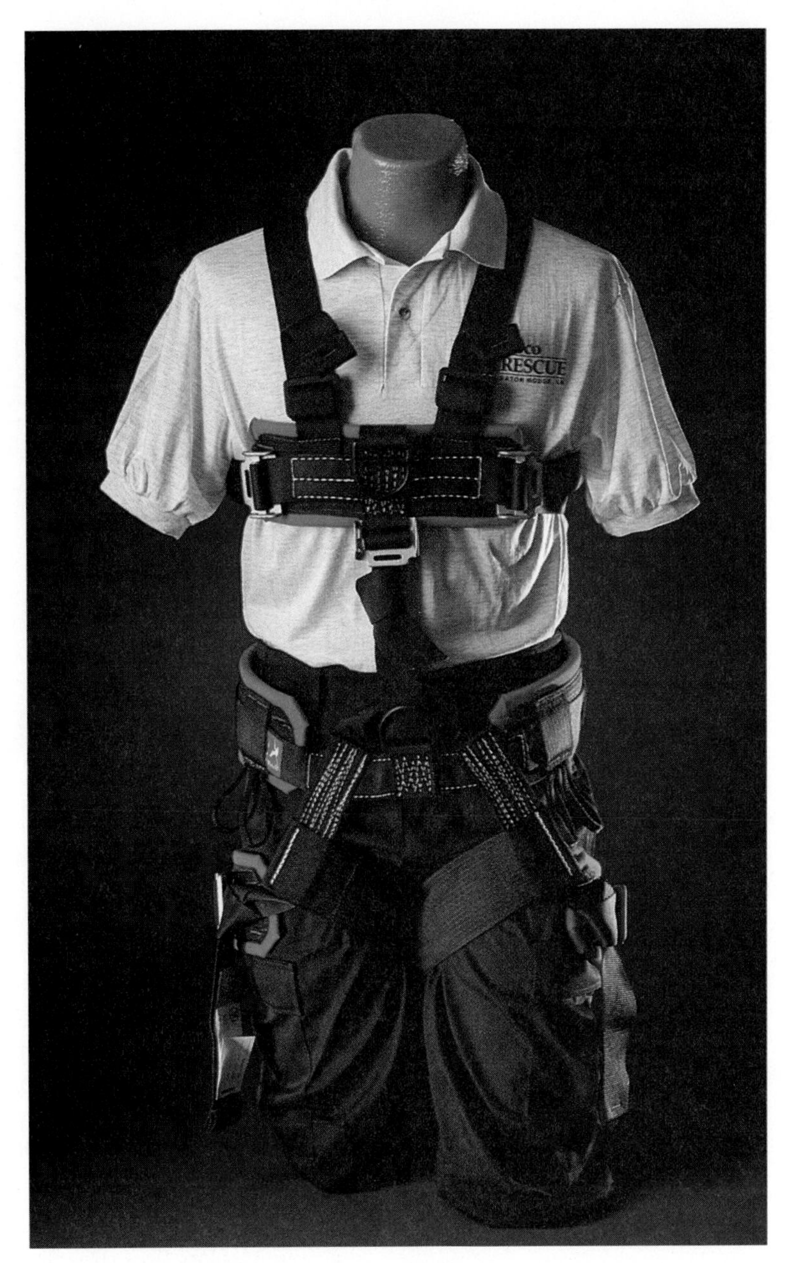

Figure 3.4 Seat/chest harness combo meeting Class III

Improvised Harnesses There may be times when a prefabricated harness is not available or is impractical. It may be that the patient's condition requires immediate removal, which calls for speed in application that is not possible with a prefabricated harness. Many ways to improvise harnesses are being taught by rescue trainers. These harnesses are usually designed for emergency rescue and not for comfort. However, the comfort of the patient should be a consideration whenever possible. A few of the improvised harnesses known to rescuers are presented later in this text.

These harnesses are not ideal for all situations. It is the rescuer's responsibility to seek appropriate training from competent individuals in an effort to make informed decisions on safe and efficient practices during rescue operations.

Webbing

Webbing has many uses in rescue. Webbing is more efficient than rope when passed over squared edges such as beams because the load is distributed over a majority of

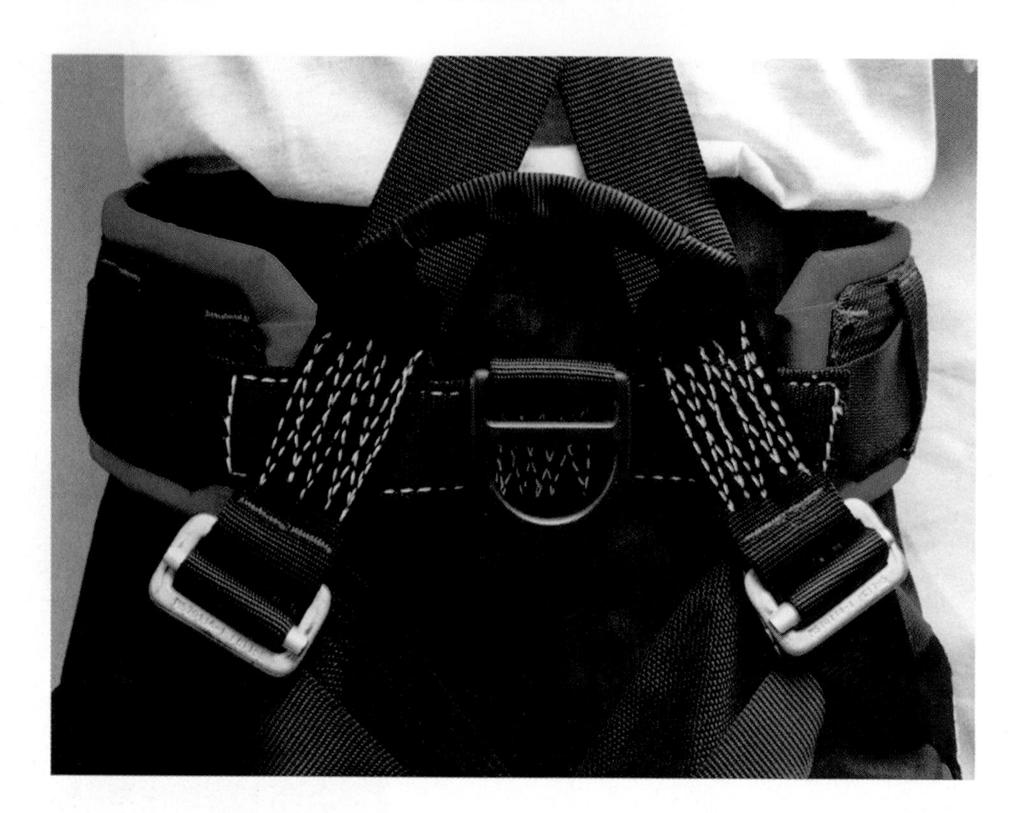

Figure 3.5a Harness with webbing attachment point as safety backup loop.

the fibers. This makes it ideal for anchor slings in industrial environments. It can also be used to lash patients into litters and tie improvised full-body harnesses. It can even be used to create bridles and other components of rescue systems.

All webbing has a very poor tolerance for shock because it stretches even less than low-stretch kernmantle rope. For this reason, webbing should be used with some accompanying means of shock absorption in a rescue system where falls are likely. Webbing must be inspected carefully and replaced frequently. If significant abrasion or other visible damage is noted, get rid of it!

As with rope, a team's webbing should be properly marked and a history kept. Most trainers recommend that webbing used for rescue, regardless of the type, be constructed of 100% virgin nylon continuous-filament fiber.

Flat-Weave Webbing

Flat-weave webbing, of various widths and types, is woven as a flat strip. Seat belt webbing is an example of flat-weave webbing. There are high grades of flat webbing available that exceed 9,000 pounds minimum breaking strength. This high strength webbing is recommended for rescue and is often used in prefabricated harnesses, anchor slings, and pick-off straps. Although fairly expensive, adjustable prefabricated webbing straps like the adjustible Utility Belt in see Figure 3.7 have many uses and may help streamline industrial rescue operations. Webbing in these auxiliary rescue components should meet all requirements specified in NFPA 1983 (1995 edition).

Tubular Webbing

Tubular webbing is sewn as a tube and flattened into straps of various widths. One-half, one-, two-, and three-inch widths are available although one- and two-inch widths are the most popular for rescue. This type of webbing is soft and flexible, making it ideal for tied harnesses, tied anchor slings, and patient lashing. One-inch tubular webbing has a breaking strength of 4,000 pounds, and two-inch around 7,000 pounds. There are two types of construction for tubular webbing (see Figure 3.8):

1. Spiral-stitched (shuttle-loom construction) webbing is sewn as a tube and is considered most desirable for rescue applications.
2. Chain-stitched (needle-loom construction) webbing is actually flat webbing folded over or placed on top of another piece of flat webbing and sewn at the edge(s).

Some types of chain-stitched webbing can unravel if picked or cut, so it is not recommended for industrial rescue use.

To tell the difference between the two types, simply roll the webbing so the flattened edge is easily visible. If the edge is seamless, it is spiral-stitched webbing. If the edge shows a sewn seam, it is chain-stitched webbing. Bright color combinations in tubular webbing should also signal caution since this is common in chain-stitched webbing.

Most authorities recommend that webbing be used in a way that will meet the strength requirements for auxiliary equipment as specified by NFPA 1983. This equates to 4,500 pounds minimum breaking strength for personal use (one-person loads) and 8,000 pounds minimum breaking strength for general use (two-person loads). Many webbing products have much lower strengths than this, so they must often be tied in a loop, perhaps even doubled to attain the strength necessary for a two-person load. Note that the knot used to tie the webbing in a loop will cause some loss of efficiency due to acute bending. This can be compensated for easily.

For example, a rescue team uses one-inch tubular webbing, one of the most common types. The one-inch webbing is rated at 4,000 pounds when pulled end to end. The rescuers have chosen to use the webbing for a sling to attach a rope system to the anchor point. They build the system to support a two-person load but realize the webbing, stretched end to end, is not strong enough. One rescuer figures that if the webbing is tied in a loop, it should have 8,000 pounds breaking strength because the force is now distributed between two pieces of 4,000-pound webbing instead of one. Wrong! The reason the webbing's breaking strength isn't 8,000 pounds is because a knot has been tied in it. The water knot is the knot recommended for webbing and some previously performed break tests show

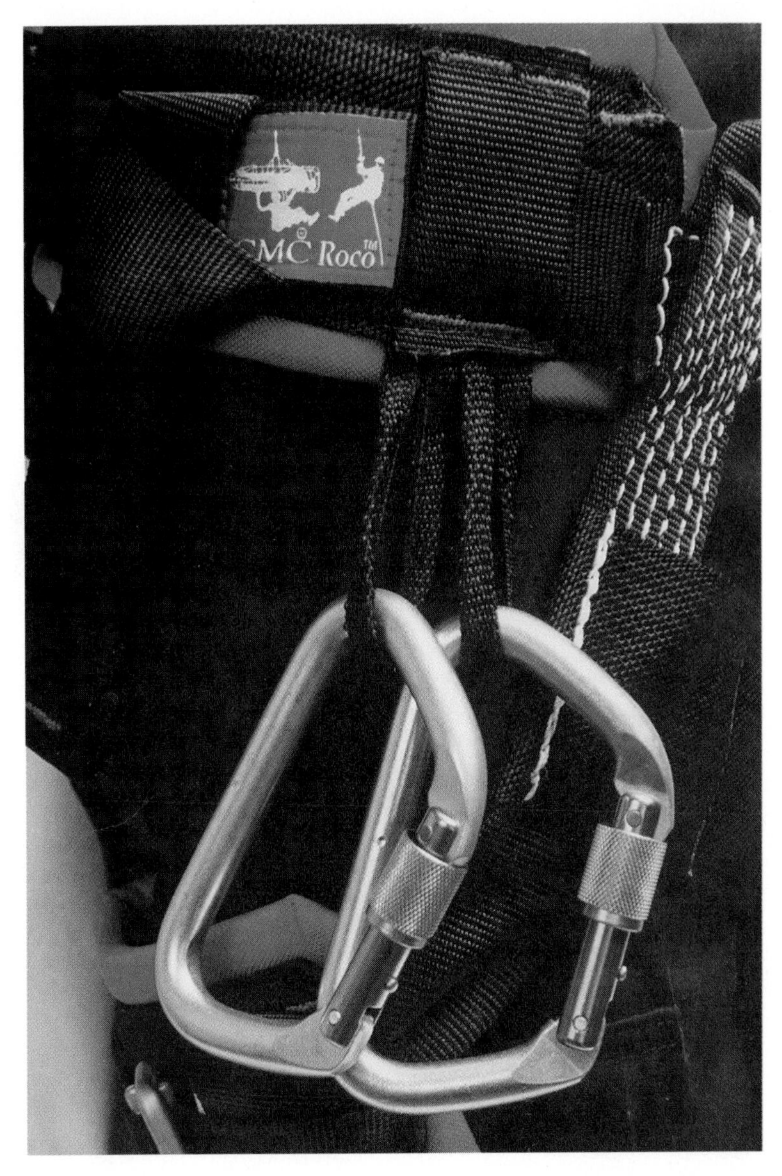

Figure 3.5b **Utility loop on side of seat harness**

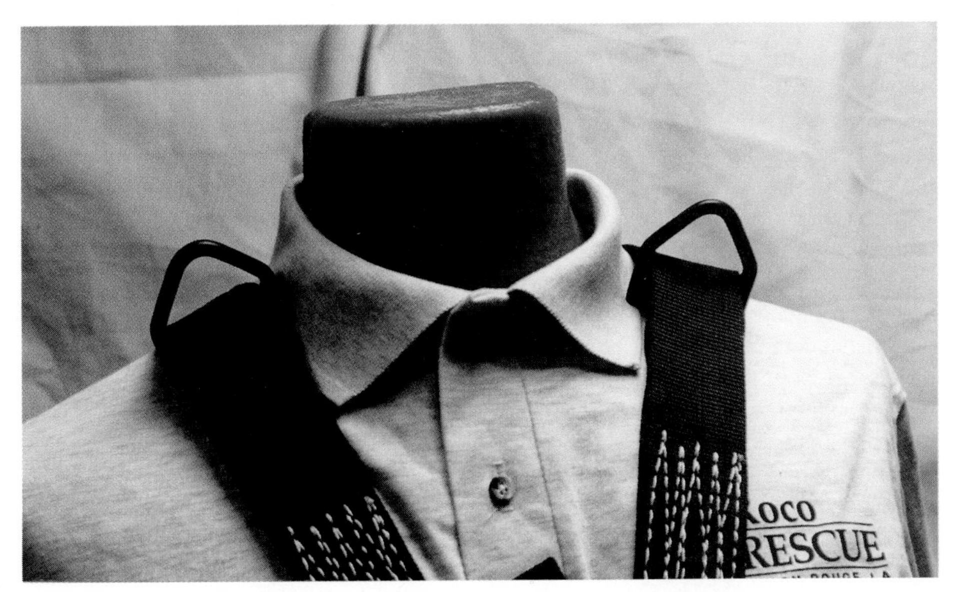

Figure 3.6 **D-rings at shoulder straps**

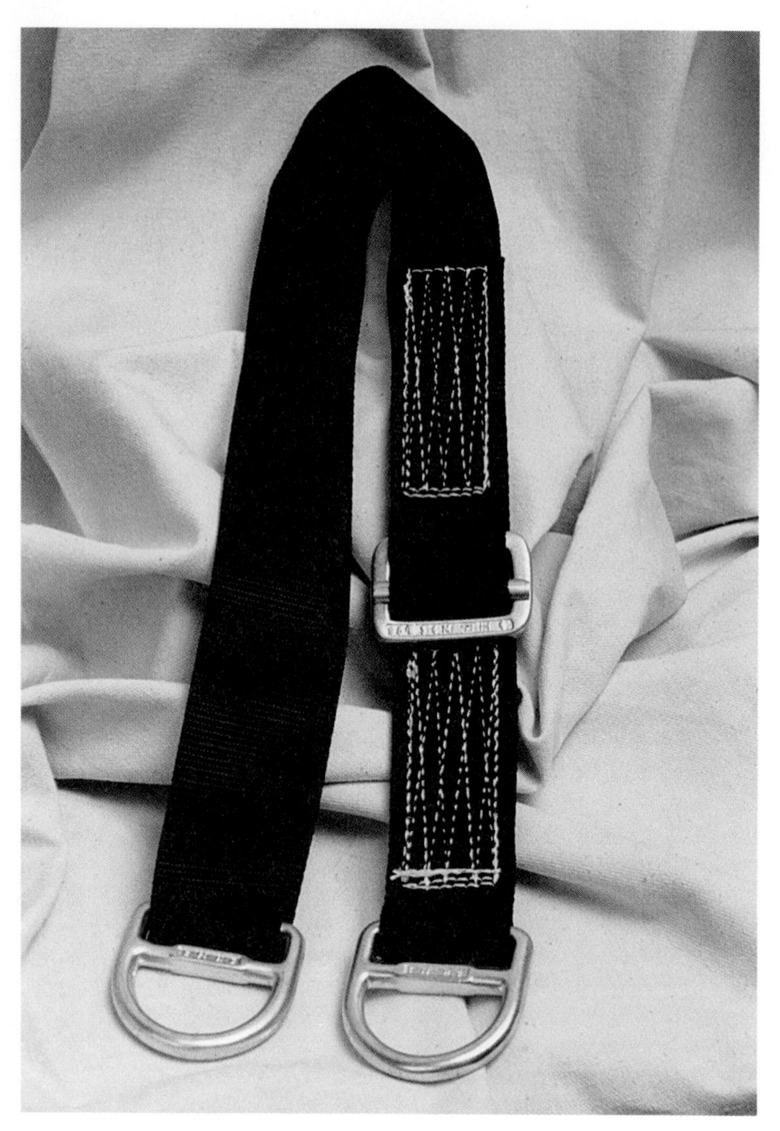

Figure 3.7 Adjustable utility belt

that the webbing loop tied with this knot is reduced to approximately 6,000 pounds breaking strength. This loss occurs only once. Even if four different knots were tied in a rope, the reduction in strength would result from the one knot that is least efficient. It is not a cumulative process.

With this in mind, the tied loop of one-inch webbing is approximately 6,000 pounds breaking strength, still not strong enough for a two-person load. The rescuers can double the loop of webbing by wrapping it around their anchor. Because of the physics of load distribution and since they already deducted once for the knot, the webbing should have a breaking strength of approximately 12,000 pounds. This is well in excess of the NFPA requirement for auxiliary equipment. In short, one-inch tubular webbing should be at least tied in a loop and doubled once to support two-person loads.

Some commercial webbing slings are presewn in a loop. If presewn, the webbing sling should meet the minimum strength requirements of the NFPA Standard and should be certified by the manufacturer. If this is the case, there will be no loss of strength due to a knot.

Accessory Cord

Accessory cord is a small-diameter rope designed for use with relatively small loads (see Figure 3.9). Accessory cord is generally made of 100% nylon and should be of kernmantle construction for rescue. Most authorities recommend 6- to 7-foot long pieces of 6- or 7-millimeter accessory cord, tied in a loop (referred to as a Prusik loop) for general use with $\frac{1}{2}$-inch kernmantle rescue rope. This type of Prusik loop can be attached to a rope with a special knot (double-wrap Prusik) and used for ascending, for self-rescue, or as a simple attachment point for temporarily hanging equipment. Eight-millimeter accessory cord with certain specifications should be used to make Prusik loops for rope grabs in hauling systems or belay systems using $\frac{1}{2}$-inch rescue rope.

WARNING

Accessory cords should be used with relatively small loads and in such a manner as to avoid severe shock loading.

Shock Absorbers

A shock absorber (also known as a load limiter, force limiter, and fall arrestor) is a prefabricated device usually constructed with webbing in a configuration designed to absorb a shock load created by a fall (see Figure 3.10). It is designed to prevent injury of the person to which it is attached. Shock absorbers are used primarily with safety line systems, which are intended to catch the load should the primary rope system fail. If the primary system fails, tremendous force can be generated as the load falls onto the safety line system. If no shock absorber is in place, much of the force will be transmitted to the person on the end of the safety line. Most manufacturers recommend that their shock absorbers be attached directly between the load and the rope system. All of these units have sewn loops on either side of the absorbing mechanism so they can be attached between the load to be protected and the rope system. In advanced applications, shock absorbers may also be useful as stress indicators in mechanical advantage systems.

The mechanism used to absorb the shock varies significantly among commercially manufactured devices but most begin to activate with impact loads between 400 and 600 pounds. Some units use webbing loops sewn with successive rows of stitching, known as bar tacks, engineered to break under a certain amount of force. Each bar

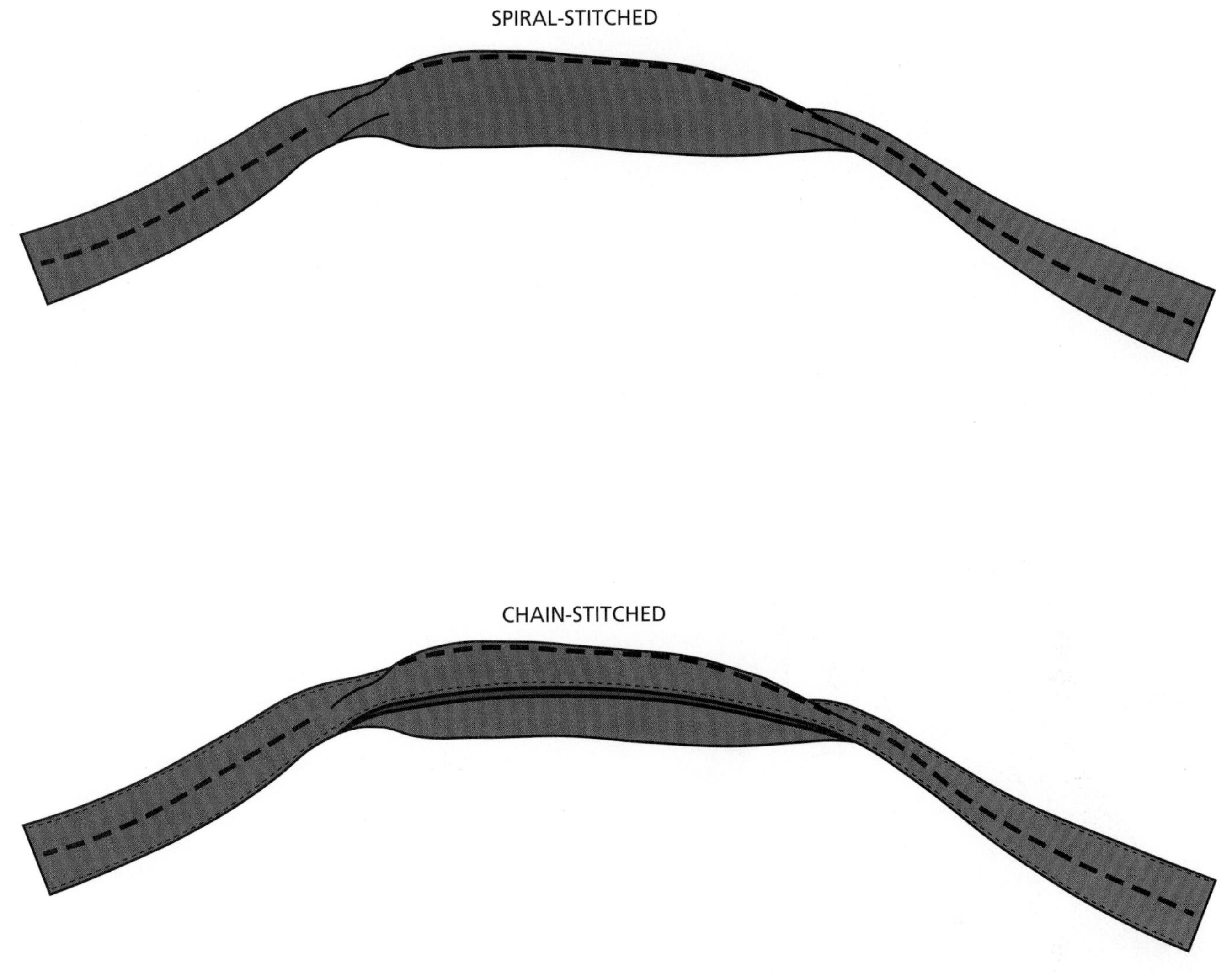

Figure 3.8 Spiral-stitched webbing vs. chain-stitched webbing

tack broken absorbs some of the shock that would otherwise be transferred to the load. This device is often referred to as a "screamer" due to the loud popping sounds created by the breaking of the bar tacks.

Another type of shock absorber uses a coil of heavy-gauge copper wire positioned near a rolled-up piece of flat webbing with sewn loops on each end for attachment. As the webbing begins to unroll, the wire penetrates the middle of the webbing, ripping the latitudinal fibers of the webbing as it unrolls. The longitudinal fibers, which are the strength of the webbing, are left intact while the force of the fall is effectively absorbed.

Yet another type of shock absorber has a compression ring attached to a portion of a sewn loop of flat webbing. As the attachment points are pulled apart, the compression ring allows the loop to which it is attached to slip through, absorbing the shock of the fall.

Although all of these devices help absorb shock, some are much more effective than others. Most of the industrial-grade fall-protection devices effectively reduce shock for falls with one-person loads. However, most do not absorb shock well with two-person loads. Tests have been conducted to see if two shock absorbers, parallel to each other, would absorb shock generated by a two-person load. While the readings varied significantly, it appeared that reduction of force at the load was minimal using this technique. The absorbers either did not activate or activated unevenly. When falls are expected with two-person loads on a single rope, it is best to place a separate shock absorber in-line for each person attached to the rope.

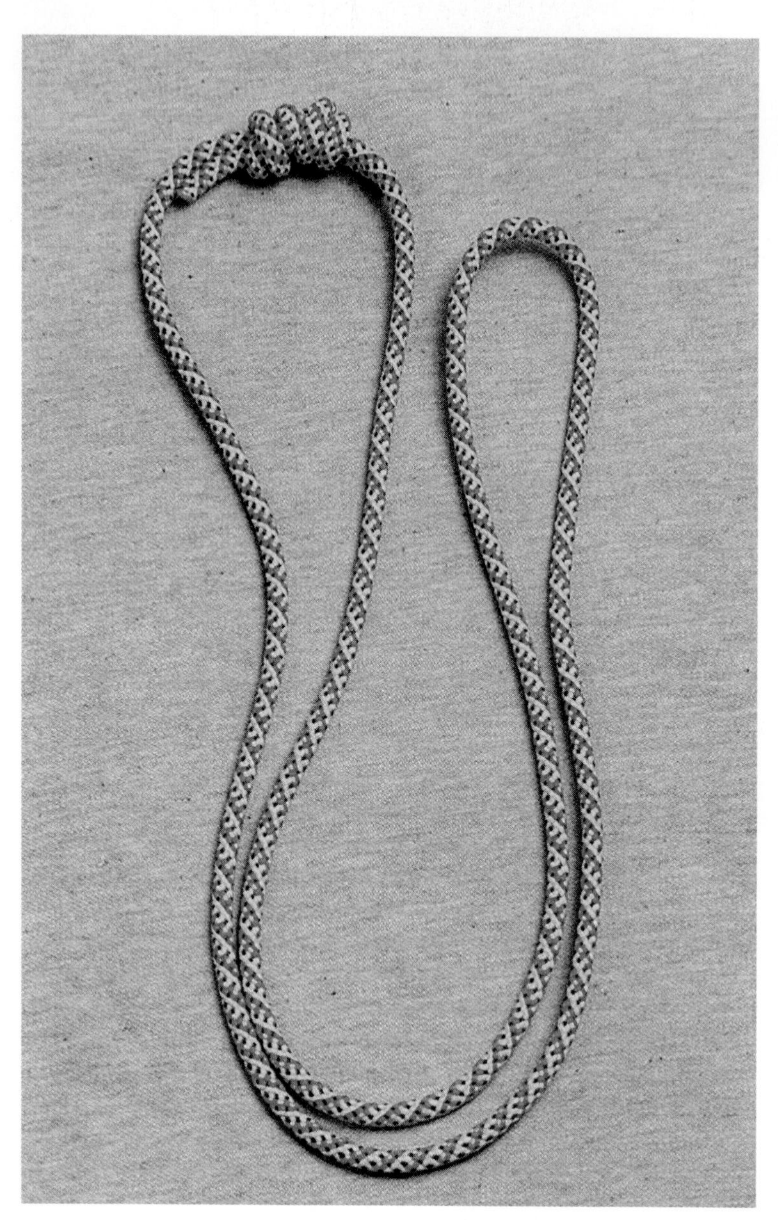

Figure 3.9 Tied loop of accessory cord

Most shock absorbers meet the auxiliary equipment strength requirements of the NFPA 1983 (1995 edition) standard for personal use (one-person loads) but not for general use (two-person loads). For this reason, a single shock absorber should not be the only link between the rope system and a two-person load.

Hardware

Hardware for rescue should be of the highest and strongest quality available and should meet all recommendations of NFPA 1983 (1995 edition).

The NFPA 1983 has recommendations for hardware, referred to as auxiliary equipment, as well as for life safety rope and harnesses. Many items of equipment have specific requirements for certification, product labeling and information, design and construction, and testing. Such items include carabiners and snap links, ascending and rope grab devices, and descent control devices. Other items not specifically addressed are generally covered in a section titled Other Auxiliary Equipment.

Most of the items have requirements for both personal use (one-person load) and general use (two-person load) because they might be used in either capacity. Some have the same requirement regardless of use. It should be reemphasized that the rescuer must make decisions about equipment for the team that will provide the greatest safety and the least margin for error with the least amount of confusion.

If a team has a mixed bag of personal and general-use equipment, members must know how to pull the right equipment out of the kit for the application at hand even under high pressure and in the dark. If they cannot easily do this, they should stick with the recommendation of purchasing only general-use equipment (when that designation applies). Although this may be a more expensive proposition, it certainly increases safety by reducing the margin for error and eliminating a lot of confusion.

Inspection, Maintenance, and Retirement

Procedures for inspection, maintenance, and retirement of auxiliary rescue equipment should be supplied by the manufacturer of the product, although there are some general guidelines that might prove helpful.

- Keep a history of the equipment. Use identification markings that are acceptable to the manufacturer. Some rescuers use markers, some use tape, others use metal stamps, and still others engrave. Call the manufacturers and see what they say, but make sure you know where your equipment has been and how it has been used.
- Keep the equipment clean and dry in storage. Dirty, wet equipment does not help preserve its integrity.
- Inspect the equipment constantly for wear or impaired operation. Before you pack it up, check it out thoroughly! Log its use on the history card.
- Only make alterations and minor repairs to equipment in accordance with the manufacturer's recommendations. If the manufacturer doesn't allow it, don't do

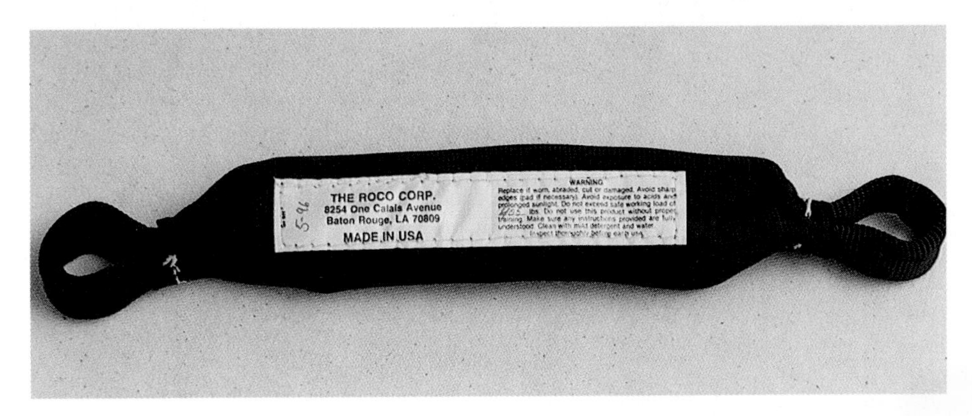

Figure 3.10 Shock absorber

it! When you do something with the equipment the manufacturer hasn't recommended, you assume the liability for it. Log everything you do on the history card. This certainly applies to general use as well. Use the equipment in a manner for which it is designed. Do not use it in any other way without written approval from the manufacturer.

- Hardware is not designed to be used without rope or some other flexible member in the system. Hardware does not give and therefore does not absorb shock. Avoid nonflexible attachments of hardware in a rescue system (hard-linking). If torsion occurs in the system and the hardware cannot flex, damage or failure of the hardware might result. As long as there is rope or other flexible equipment in the system, everything should be all right. As with all equipment, before using hardware rescuers should seek proper training from a competent person.
- Hardware items usually do not absorb shock well. Therefore, they do not withstand long falls onto hard surfaces well either. If you drop a hardware item to a hard surface from any distance, inspect it (if that is possible with the naked eye) according to manufacturer's recommendations for impaired operation or visible signs of damage. It may be that the only means of inspection appropriate is X ray or dye penetration to rule out hairline cracks. These tests can be expensive. Unless the manufacturer recommends otherwise, it is best to destroy and replace questionable item. If in doubt, throw it out!

Carabiners

Carabiners are metal load-bearing connectors with a self-closing gate used to join other components of a rope system. These metal snap links are also commonly referred to as biners or crabs. The NFPA has specific requirements for carabiners.

Design

Most carabiners are shaped like an oval, a D, or an offset D (see Figure 3.11). For industrial rescue, the D-shaped carabiners are recommended. The majority of a carabiner's strength is in the spine (major axis). When other equipment is clipped into a D-shaped carabiner, it has a tendency to slip into a position near the spine when loaded. This puts the majority of the load where the strength of the carabiner lies—in the spine. A carabiner is weakest when side loaded across the gate (along the minor axis). Oval carabiners do not distribute the load through the spine nearly as well. This makes them a weaker link and more likely to be damaged or fail under severe conditions.

Some carabiner shapes and sizes are better suited for certain industrial rescue applications. It is best to use a carabiner large enough to easily accommodate the introduction of $\frac{1}{2}$-inch rope, webbing, and other rescue equipment commonly used for two-person loads.

Some applications, such as those requiring the movement of a hitch tied around a carabiner with rope, may work better with a larger carabiner. Some carabiners are designed with a larger body and an "offset" (also called "modified") D shape, which more easily accommodates the movement of a hitch within the carabiner.

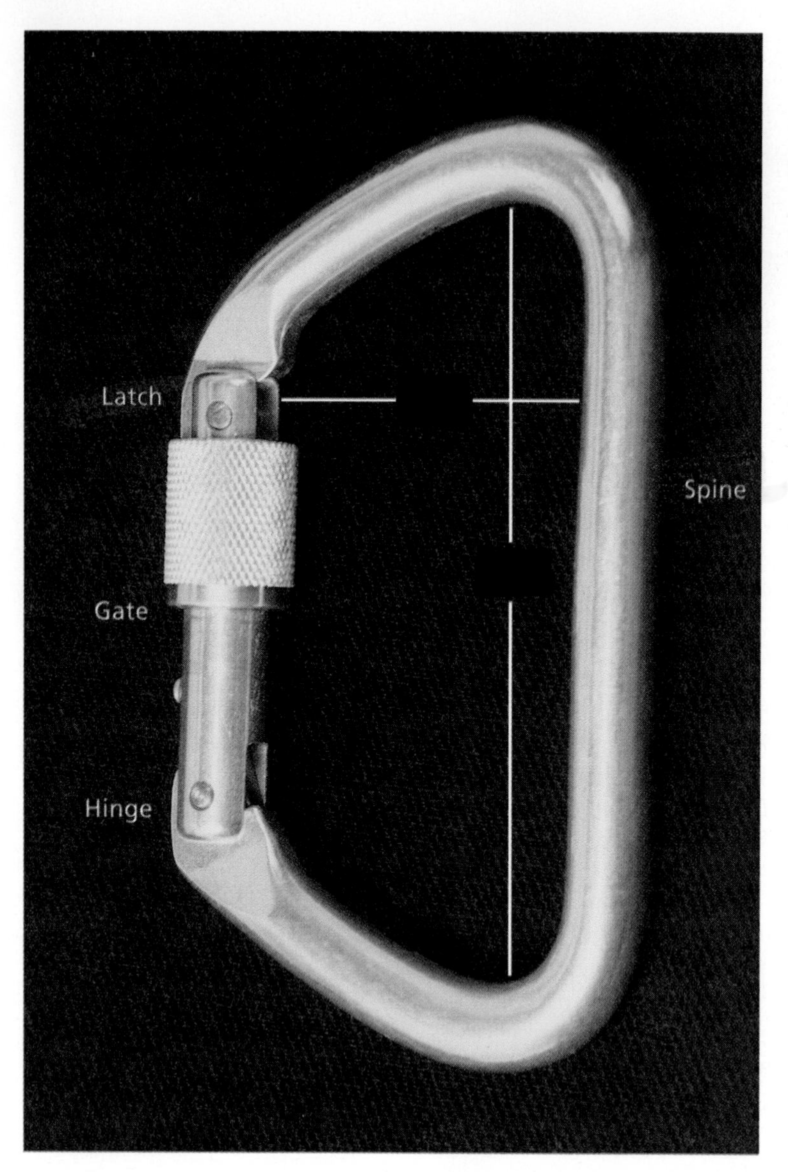

Figure 3.11 Parts of a carabiner

Materials

With the variety of metals used to manufacture carabiners, the most commonly recommended materials used in construction are either stainless steel or aircraft alloys. However, special considerations must be allowed for both potentially flammable environments where nonsparking hardware must be used and also chemical environments where the chemicals present could cause metal degradation.

Components

The parts of the carabiner are the (see Figure 3.11):

- **Spine.** This is the long axis of D-shaped carabiners and is always opposite the gate. The majority of the carabiner's strength is in the spine, therefore, rescue system components should always be loaded along the spine.
- **Gate.** The gate allows the carabiner to open for attachment to various components of the rescue system. The NFPA 1983 requires that the gate be self-closing and of a locking design so it cannot be opened accidentally. There are several types of gate locks although the most common are the screw type. The lock should be screwed completely closed and then backed off $\frac{1}{8}$ to $\frac{1}{4}$ of a turn. Once loaded, avoid additional tightening of the lock (unless it has come open) even though it may appear a little loose. Too much tightening compounds the difficulty of unlocking the gate once the system is unloaded. If you cannot get the gate open, either reload the gate or use a pair of pliers.
- **Hinge.** This is the attachment of the gate to the body of the carabiner. The hinge is usually spring loaded or otherwise designed to close the gate automatically when it is released.
- **Latch.** The latch is the way the terminal end of the gate connects to the body of the carabiner. There are basically two types of latches: the pin latch and the claw latch (see Figure 3.12). The pin latch has a pin on the end of the gate that seats into a slot in the body of the carabiner. This kind of latch usually can be opened under load. While this is not a desired feature for rescue, it is desired by some rock climbers. The claw latch looks like the gate was cut away from the body of the carabiner with a little saw. The claw at the end of the gate looks like a piece of a puzzle that fits into a matched slot on the body of the carabiner. The integrity of the carabiner actually relies on the positive connection of the latch. These types of latches should not be loaded while open. Both latches are used in various brands of general-use (two-person load) carabiners. Regardless of the latch type, the carabiner gate should always be locked before life loading the rescue system. If the gate remains locked, it cannot come open.

Strength Requirements

The NFPA 1983 (1995 edition) has specific requirements for minimum breaking strengths of carabiners along the major axis as well as the minor axis (see Figure 3.11). The tests are performed with the gate open and the gate closed. These requirements differ for personal use (one-person loads) and general use (two-person loads). The tensile tests for personal-use carabiners indicate:

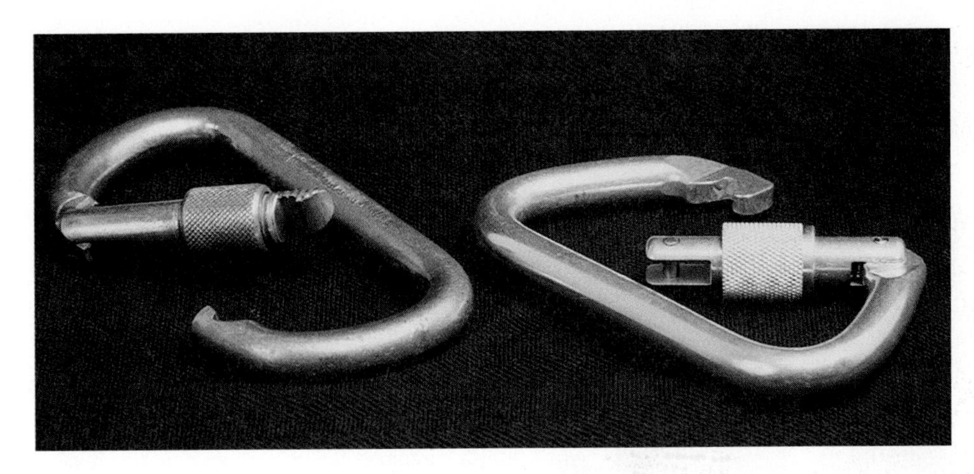

Figure 3.12 Pin latch vs. claw latch on carabiners

- Minor axis—minimum breaking strength of at least 1,500 force pounds
- Major axis, gate open—minimum breaking strength of at least 1,650 force pounds
- Major axes, gate closed—minimum breaking strength of at least 6,000 force pounds

The tensile tests for general-use carabiners indicate:

- Minor axis—minimum breaking strength of at least 2,400 force pounds
- Major axis, gate open—minimum breaking strength of at least 2,400 force pounds
- Major axes, gate closed—minimum breaking strength of at least 9,000 force pounds

Many rope rescue authorities recommend general-use carabiners for all rescues to avoid accidental use of a personal carabiner with two-person loads.

Operation

Carabiners are designed to be loaded along the long axis (spine), which is the strength of the carabiner. It should be noted that carabiners meeting the requirements of NFPA 1983 (1995 edition) for general use are so strong that under normal circumstances failure is highly unlikely. If carabiners are properly positioned and overloaded to failure, the long axis will begin to elongate into a bananalike shape. To create this type of force in a system would require monumental effort. The greatest chance of failure occurs when a carabiner is side loaded (short axis) rather than along the spine (long axis). In break tests with side-loaded carabiners, failure usually takes place at the gate. Do not load the short axis (gate) side. If a carabiner somewhere in the system has turned and is now side loaded, there is no cause for panic. A rescuer should correct the situation if reasonably possible. If not, he or she must get off the rope system as soon as possible so the problem can be corrected. This will happen often. Unless otherwise specified by the manufacturer, simple side loading of a carabiner does not require retirement.

As simple as it may seem, linking objects such as knots and rigging points with carabiners can sometimes be difficult. The latch opening may not end up in a position that makes hookup to the other object easy. One method that makes carabiner connections easier is the Fish Hook Method:

1. Simply hold the carabiner in the grip of your strong hand with the latch opening up and away from your palm.
2. Open the gate by squeezing it near the latch with your fingers. In this position, the opened gate gives the carabiner the appearance of a hook.
3. Bring the hook down to connect with the object desired.
4. Once the connection is made, release the gate allowing it to close.
5. Rotate the carabiner 180 degrees causing the gate to be up with the latch opening nearest you. This makes it easy to attach a knot or other object into the carabiner's latch opening, which is readily available in this position.

As previously mentioned, always lock the gate on the carabiner before life loading

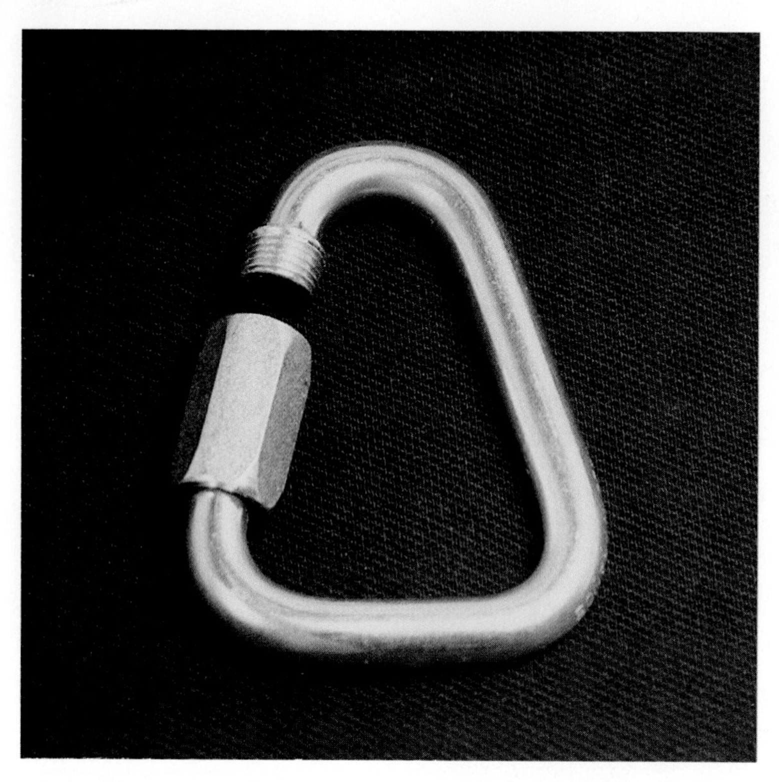

Figure 3.13 Triangular screw link

it.

Do not overtighten screw-type locks. Overtightening these locking gates can cause them to bind once they have been loaded. Tighten the screw lock with your fingers as far as possible and then back off $\frac{1}{8}$ to $\frac{1}{4}$ of a turn. This will keep the gate locked but will prevent overtightening.

Some trainers recommend that a screw-lock gate carabiner be positioned with its latch opening down to prevent gravity from unscrewing the gate. The theory is that if gravity causes the gate to turn, it will turn to lock the gate further if the latch is down. This is a fine theory and has some legitimacy. The problem is that a carabiner can change its direction relative to the earth's gravitational pull any time during the rescue. As a rescuer or system components move, so might the carabiners. What starts out with the latch positioned downwardly may end with the latch positioned upwardly. The rescuer should be more concerned about the potential for movement over projections and edges placing pressure on the screw lock, rolling it open and possibly opening the gate.

For example, this directional change might occur while a rescuer rolls over the parapet of a building while attached to a descent control device via a carabiner to the harness. If the gate is in a position to make heavy contact with the building edge as the rescuer crawls over, it may cause the lock mechanism to roll unlocked and the gate to open.

Consult the manufacturer's recommendations on additional information concerning use, inspection, maintenance, and retirement of carabiners.

Screw Links

Screw links are metal load-bearing connectors without a gate (see Figure 3.13). Instead of a gate, these links rely on a screw-type sleeve for closure. Triangular or D-shaped screw links (tri-links) can be used instead of carabiners when multidirectional pulls are encountered in a rescue system.

Three-directional pulls are common in rescue. For example, a utility belt has been wrapped around a large beam to form an anchor system for a rope. The D-rings at the ends of the belt, which barely touch each other due to the size of the beam, are fastened together with a carabiner. A knot in the end of the rope is now attached to the carabiner as well. Because of the tight angles formed by the belt, which is barely long enough to make it around the anchor point, a three-directional pull is created. The two D-rings of the utility belt are pulling in different directions on the carabiner (more along the short axis than the spine). The rope is pulling in an entirely different direction on the same carabiner. All forces should be applied along the spine. A three-directional pull places improper force on a carabiner; carabiners are designed to take pulls in only two directions.

There are a few ways to eliminate this problem. The rescuers could get a longer anchor sling (if they had one) so that the angle created by the webbing when wrapped around the beam is narrow enough to allow the two ends of the loop to load along the spine when attached to the carabiner. They could use the rope itself to attach to the anchor point if they have enough rope to do so. They might decide instead to use a tri-link to attach the ends of the utility belt to the rope. Tri-links are designed to take pulls in any direction.

Design

Triangular screw links are the most popular screw links for rescue although screw links also come in oval and semicircular shapes. The semicircular and triangular screw links are the only ones designed to take multidirectional pulls.

Materials
Tri-links are usually manufactured of galvanized steel or aluminum alloy. The steel screw link is the only version that should be used for industrial rescue; the aluminum screw link will not meet the NFPA strength standards for auxiliary equipment. Additional considerations must be taken for potentially flammable environments that require non-sparking tools or chemical environments that might degrade certain metals.

Components
The screw link has few components. There is the body of the screw link and the screw-locking sleeve. The sleeve should be finger tightened completely to maintain the integrity of the link. Overtightening, such as with a wrench, might crack the locking sleeve.

Strength Requirements
Screw links have no specific requirements but fall under the category of auxiliary equipment. The minimum breaking strength requirement for personal use (one-person loads) is 5,000 force pounds. The requirement for general use (two-person loads) is 8,000 force pounds.

As previously mentioned, the screw-locking sleeve must be tightened completely. If it is left open and loaded, the structural integrity of the unit is severely compromised. Even with a high breaking strength of over 9,000 force pounds, if left open and loaded, a screw link might bend and create permanent damage. It may be necessary to have a wrench or accessory cord available to open a screw-locking sleeve once it has been loaded.

Operation
Using a screw link is simple: completely tighten the screw-locking sleeve. If the sleeve is not closing properly or the tri-link has been bent, get rid of it. Always follow the manufacturer's recommendations on use, inspection, maintenance, and retirement of screw links. Always store the screw link closed to protect the threads and prevent misalignment.

Descent Control Devices
Many types of descent control devices are used today in rescue. In this section we will look at two of the most popular: the brake bar rack and the figure-8 plate. The NFPA 1983 (1995 edition) has specific requirements for descent control devices.

The Brake Bar Rack
The brake bar rack (also known as "rappel rack" or simply "rack") is a descent control device consisting of a series of short metal bars fixed to, and sliding along, a U-shaped metal rack with an eye at one end for attachment (see Figure 3.14). This device is attached to a rope by weaving it through the metal bars, thus producing friction and allowing control of the load as the rope moves through them. The greater the number of bars engaged, the greater the friction/control produced. The eye of the rack is attached to an anchor point or life safety harness, depending on the application. The device is extremely versatile and well suited for rescue. Some advantages and disadvantages of the rack are:

- It disperses heat well, making it ideal for both short or long distances (100 feet or more) in rappeling or lowering.
- The friction can be varied by adding or removing bars even while loaded, which makes it easy to adjust quickly to either one- or two-person loads when on line.
- Unlike many other descent control devices, racks do not twist the rope during operation.
- If they become worn, the brake bars attached to the rack frame are replaceable.
- The brake bar rack is bulkier and heavier than most other descent control devices and may take slightly longer to attach to the rope.

The brake bar rack, like any descent control device, is used for both rappelling and lowering. If required, most racks can accommodate two ropes at the same time.

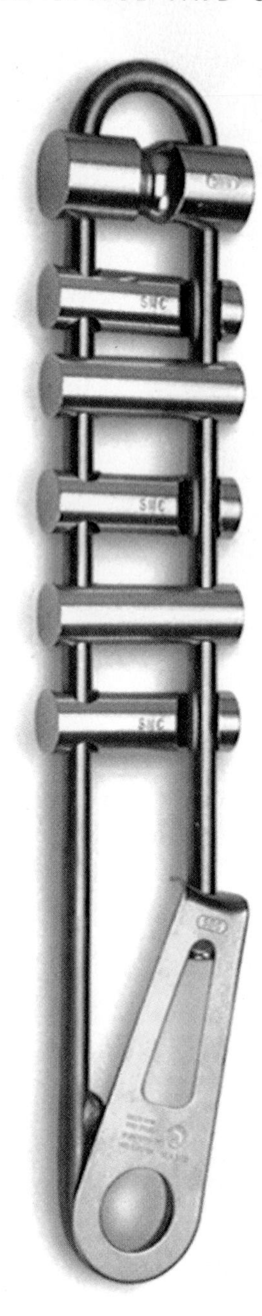

Figure 3.14 SMC version of NFPA brake bar rack

Design

Rack frames are made in a variety of sizes but generally maintain the same inverted U-shape. The most popular rescue rack frame is the six-bar size. There are other sizes, although they are not common in industrial rescue. All racks have some method of attachment to an anchor system or harness. Most have rounded eyes formed at the base of the inverted U-shaped frame. One type of rack actually uses the base of its U-shaped frame as the attachment point. It is important to note the construction of rounded eyes on the inverted U-shaped frames. The eye should be welded into the frame for maximum strength in rescue. When welded eye racks are placed on breaking machines and pulled apart, they generally fail at the base of the eye, not at the weld. The weld is actually stronger than the metal to either side of it. Racks with wound eyes (sometimes called pigtails) may allow the eye to unwind under stress. This has been known to occur with as little as 800 pounds of force. This type of rack is not recommended for industrial rescue.

The rounded bars that attach to the rack frame are available in different types and sizes. Most bars have a hole through one end and a slot cut in the other end (see Figure 3.15). The hole side of the bars slip onto one side of the rack frame for attachment and are secured by a lock nut to keep them from falling off. The slot side of the bars are slipped on or clipped in to the other side of the U-shaped rack frame as the rope is wrapped around them.

There are different kinds of brake bars (see Figure 3.15). Top bars are usually slightly larger than other bars and have a groove (training groove) in the middle of one side that is intended to train the rope down the center of the bars as it runs through the rack. The training groove also indicates to rescuers which side of the rack they should start on when rigging the rope through it. Straight slot bars also aid the rescuer in rigging the rack properly. The slot side of these bars is not clipped in or held in place when slipped onto the rod of the U-shaped frame. Instead, these bars are designed to unclip from the frame if a rescuer attempts to rig the rope improperly. For this reason, a straight slot bar is desirable as the second bar on a six-bar rack. The angle slot bars clip into the rod of the rack frame and are held in place by the angled slot cut into the bar. The top bar also has an angled slot to hold it in place. The straight and angle slot bars have no training groove. Top bars, straight slot bars, and angle slot bars are all available in both stainless steel and aluminum. Most stainless-steel bars are hollow or shaped like half moons to provide lighter weight and better heat dispersement than solid bars. Aluminum bars are solid.

Materials The rack is an assembly of components. The rack frame is constructed of stainless steel. The brake bars are made from either stainless steel or aluminum. The rack is very strong regardless of the material used for the brake bars. The two materials have certain advantages and disadvantages.

Aluminum Bars

- Provide more friction (equates to better descent control) than steel bars.
- Are lighter weight than steel bars.

- Are less expensive than steel bars.
- Heat up more rapidly but disburse heat better than steel.
- Wear faster than steel and have to be replaced sooner.

Stainless Steel Bars

- Last much longer than aluminum bars (virtually a lifetime).
- Are heavier than aluminum.
- Are more expensive than aluminum.
- Retain heat longer than aluminum.
- Provide considerably less friction and, therefore, less control.

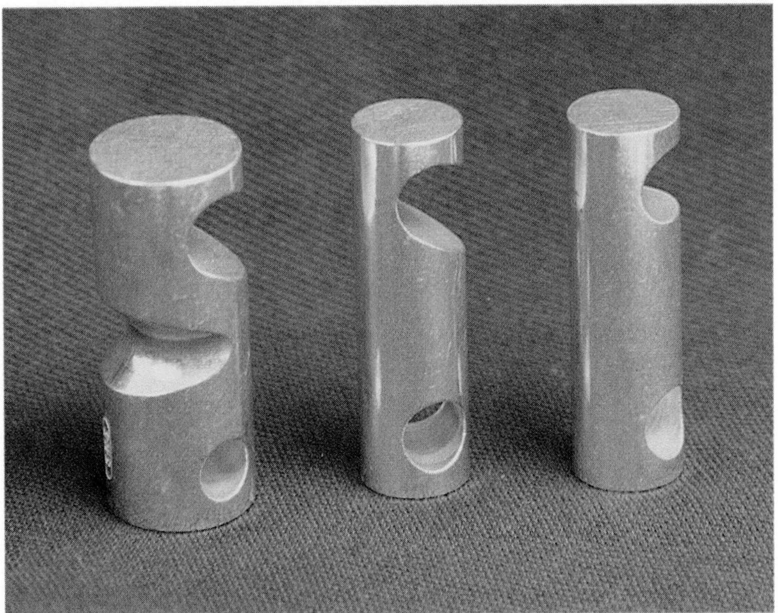

Figure 3.15 Bars used on a brake bar rack

Components

- **Stainless-steel rack frame**—Most are very strong and shaped like a U or an inverted U.
- **Top bar**—Some rack manufacturers use a grooved top bar to train the rope through the center of the rack during rappelling or lowering operations. The grooved side of this bar is where the rope should be placed to begin rigging.
- **Straight slot bar (second bar)**—These are used with racks whose bars are positively attached on one side to the rack frame, allowing the slot in the other end of the bar to slip onto the opposite side of the frame. The straight slot allows one end of the bar to fall off the frame if the rope is rigged improperly.
- **Angle slot bars (third through sixth bars)**—These are used with racks whose bars are positively attached on one side to the rack frame, allowing the slot in the other end of the bar to clip onto the opposite side of the frame. The angle slot clips into the rack frame, preventing it from falling off when unattended.

Strength Requirements The NFPA 1983 (1995 edition) has specific strength requirements for descent control devices intended for personal use (one-person load) or general use (two-person load). Personal use descent devices are required to sustain a minimum test load of 1,200 force pounds without permanent damage to the device or rope and a minimum test load of 5,000 force pounds without failure. General use descent devices are required to sustain a minimum test load of 1,200 force pounds without permanent damage to the device or rope and a minimum test load of 6,000 force pounds without failure.

Operation The safety and preparatory procedures concerning operation of the rack will be covered in later chapters. For the basic rigging of a common rack (see Figure 3.16), follow the manufacturer's recommendations. The following example is for rappel rack in widespread use by industrial rescue teams.

1. To rig the rack for lowering or rappelling, simply place the proper point of the rope (See chapter 7 for more information on attachment to rope.) across the training groove of the rack's top bar.
2. Push the second, straight slot bar up and wrap the rope across it. If loaded incorrectly, this type of bar will fall off. This provides an additional safety check for rack operation.
3. Continue to wrap the bars with the rope until all six bars are racked in. The number of bars used depends on many factors but, in general, no fewer than six bars should be used when first placing a load on the rack, and no fewer than five bars should be used at any time during rappelling or lowering with a single rack. There are very few exceptions to this rule. If necessary, the brake bar rack can be locked off to leave it unattended while loaded.

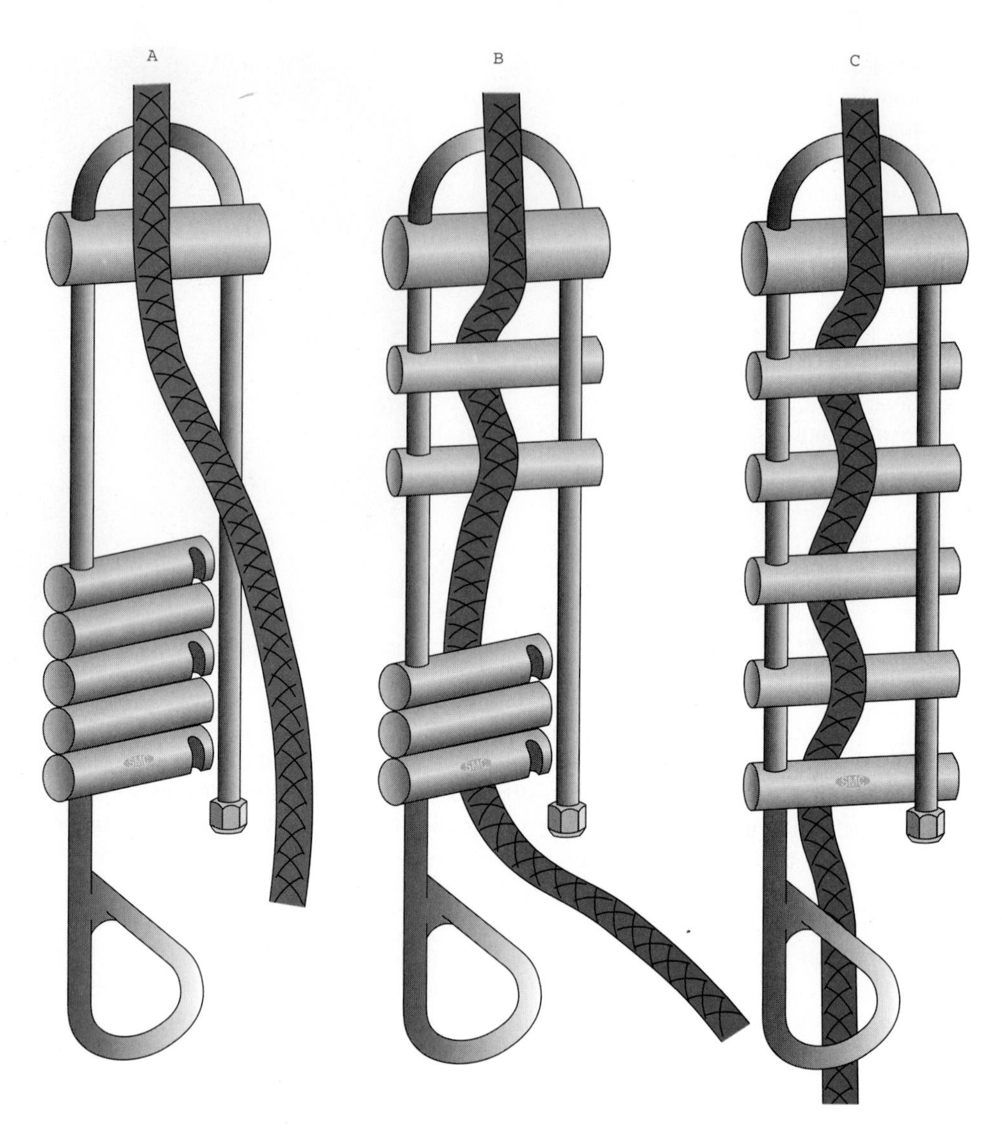

Figure 3.16 A, B, C Basic Rigging of Rappel Rack

As with the steel carabiners recommended for rescue systems, a rack that meets the descent control device requirements and is properly used and maintained simply should not fail under normal rescue circumstances. Consult the manufacturer's recommendations on additional information concerning use, inspection, maintenance, and retirement of brake bar racks and their components.

Figure-8 Descender with Ears

A figure-8 descender (also known as a "figure-8 plate" or just "8-plate") is a descent control device used for rappelling and lowering (see Figure 3.17). The rope is wrapped around the body of the eight-shaped unit, which creates friction as the rope moves through it. Although most are strong enough to meet NFPA 1983 (1995 edition) standards for general-use descent control devices, most authorities recommend limiting them to one-person loads. This is due to the control limitation associated with these devices. Some advantages and disadvantages of figure-8 descenders include:

- The figure-8 descender is lightweight and easy to attach to the rope.
- It builds up heat rapidly and disburses it poorly. It is not recommended for long rappels or lowers because it can build up enough heat to actually melt into the rope's sheath (glazing) and cause permanent damage.
- Friction cannot be varied while the device is loaded. This makes it difficult to adjust from one- to two-person loads when on line. It also provides much less control than a brake bar rack. For this reason, some authorities recommend it be used only for one-person loads.

- Figure-8 descenders can cause significant twisting and kinking of the rope during operation. This is due to the acute bending of the rope around the body of the device during operation.

The figure-8 descender is a versatile device and can be used for rappelling and lowering. It is sometimes used as a belay device although this is not recommended for rescue applications. The NFPA 1983 standards for descent control devices apply to the figure-8 descender. As with all rescue equipment, the figure-8 descender should be used only in a manner approved by the manufacturer.

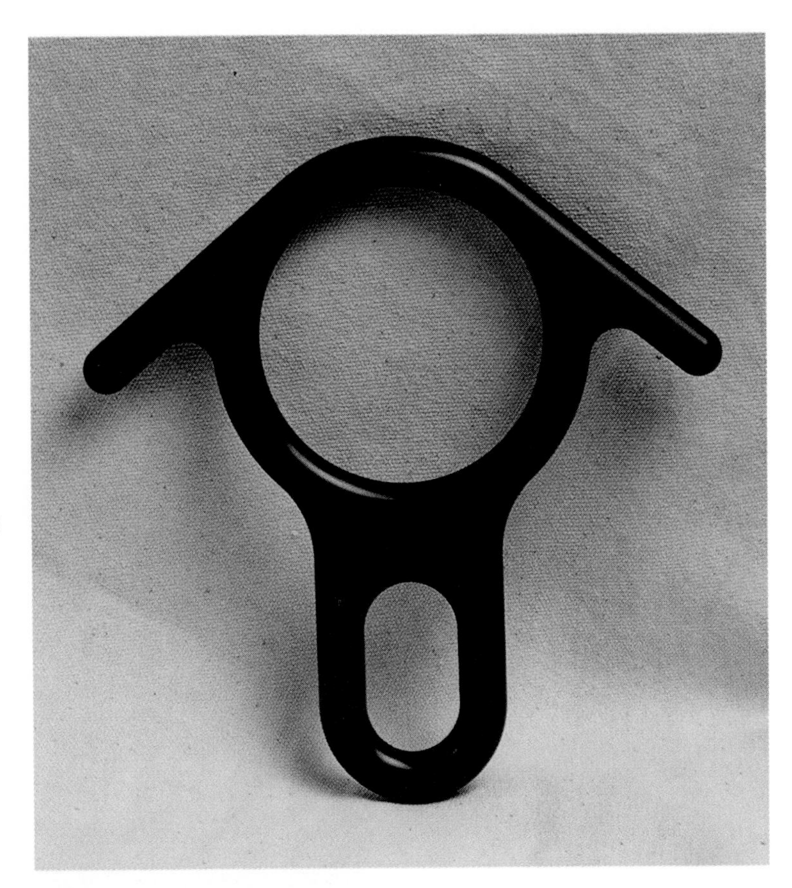

Figure 3.17 Figure-8 descender (with ears)

Design The figure-8 descender is shaped like an 8 with a large ring to create friction on the rope and a smaller ring for attaching to a seat harness or anchor point. There are many variations of the standard 8 shape. Rounded figure-8 descenders are the common variety. There are also figure-8s with squared edges (referred to as straight 8s), ovals, and even wire-body figure-8s designed to dissipate heat rapidly.

Regardless of the shape of the figure-8 descender, it should be equipped with "ears." Ears are short projections extending from either side of the large ring of the figure-8 body. These ears prevent a problem that was prominent with standard round figure-8 descenders. These 8-plates were notorious for allowing the bend of the rope, which creates friction around the body of the device, to slip up toward the top of the big ring, creating a girth hitch (see Figure 3.18). This hitch would bind the figure-8 to the rope and prevent further movement. The ears keep the bend of the rope from riding up over the big ring, effectively stopping the problem of girth hitch.

Materials Figure-8 descenders are most commonly made of anodized aluminum alloy or stainless steel. There are some very strong figure-8 descenders in both materials, though the stainless steel is the strongest version available and is more resistant to wear. With heavy use, the anodized coating on most aluminum alloy descenders eventually wear through to the base metal. Some anodized coatings (hard anodized) actually wear slower than the base metal. Hard anodized figure-8 descenders, once worn through, can create sharp edges as the base metal wears quickly in comparison. Some manufacturers will allow these sharp edges be filed down for continued use of the device. DO NOT use a descent control device if there are sharp edges. Repair or replace the device in accordance with manufacturer's recommendations.

Most figure-8 descenders today are "soft anodized." This means that the coating wears faster than the base metal, which prevents sharp edges. However, this may require more frequent replacement of the device.

Components The figure-8 descender is of unibody construction. The body has a large ring, a small ring, and may have ears or other openings.

Strength Requirements The requirements of figure-8 descenders are the same as those for brake bar racks and other descent control devices. Many manufacturers make both steel and aluminum figure-8's with minimum breaking strengths well over 6,000 force pounds.

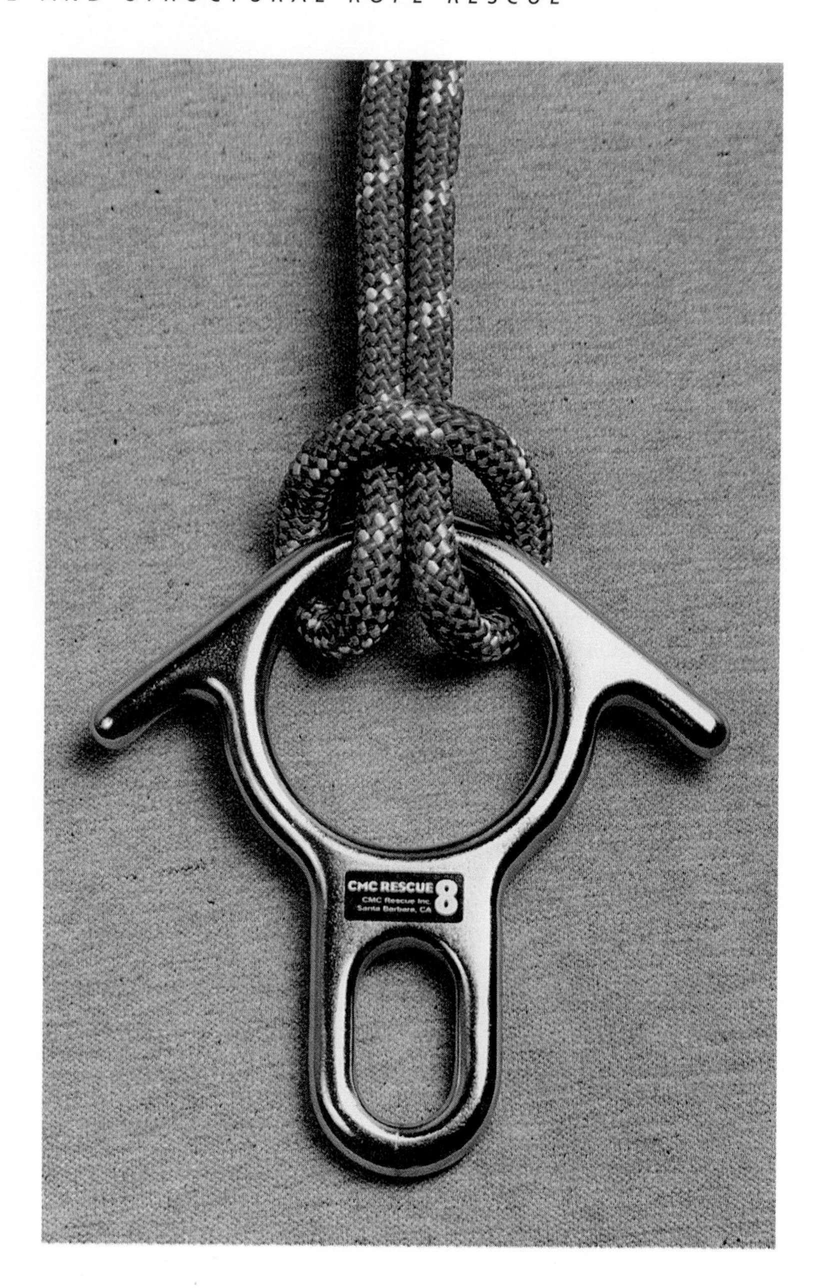

Figure 3.18 Girth hitch

Operation The rigging for a figure-8 descender can be varied for specific applications. The standard procedure is performed by creating a loop (bite) in the rope and feeding it up through the large ring from the bottom (see Figure 3.19). The loop is then placed over the top of the small ring, coming to rest on the narrow section of the body. The loaded end of the rope should always project from the top of the large ring. The loose end of the rope is used for controlling the friction of the device and issues from near the bottom of the large ring during operation. Friction is varied by changing the position of the control rope in relation to the body of the device. Moving this rope forward (toward the top of the large ring) reduces the friction, allowing the rope to move through the device more quickly. Moving the rope back (toward the small end of the device) creates additional friction and slows the rope's movement through the figure-8. The rigging of the rope through the figure-8 descender can be doubled to add friction for heavier loads. However, the friction cannot be varied easily while the figure-8 is loaded.

If necessary, this device, like the brake bar rack, can be locked off to leave it unattended. The proper operation and other preparatory procedures for the use of the figure-8 descender will be covered later in the text.

Figure-8 descenders are sometimes used as rigging points for litter bridles and anchor systems, which may be contrary to their intended use. Rescuers should use fig-

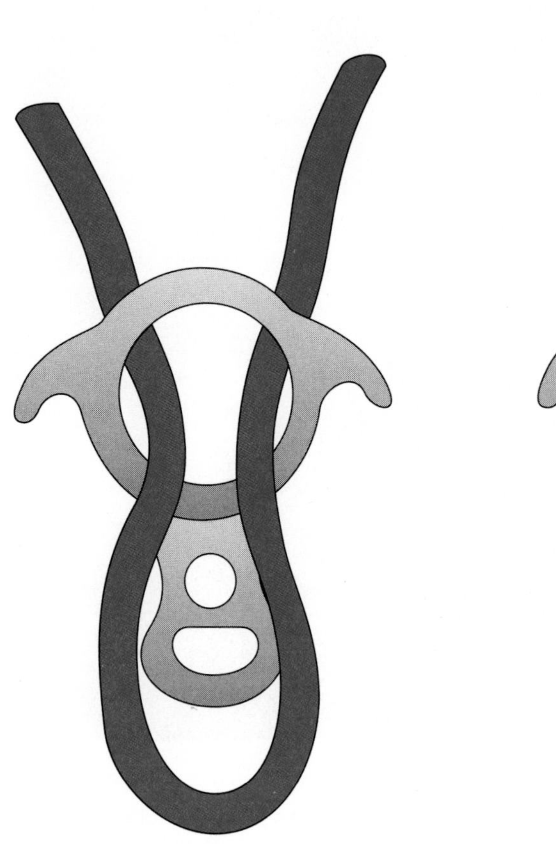

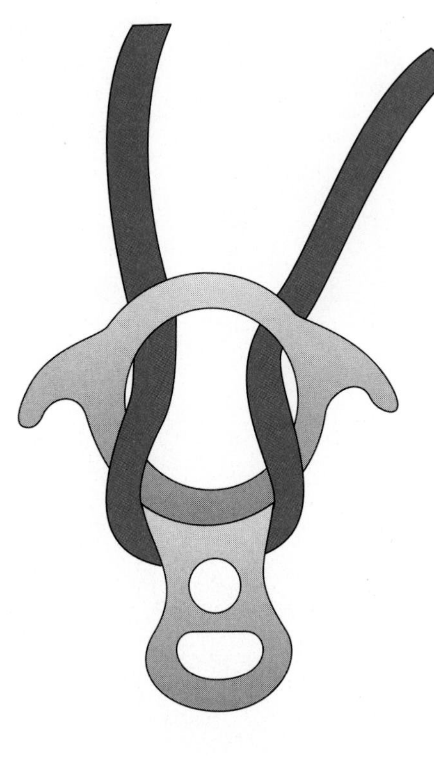

Figure 3.19 Basic rigging of figure-8 descender

ure-8 descenders only in the manner for which they were designed. Consult the manufacturer's recommendations for additional information concerning use, inspection, maintenance, and retirement of figure-8 descenders.

Ascent and Rope Grab Devices

Ascent devices are used to travel up (ascend) a fixed rope. Their mechanisms allow them to slide freely (at least in one direction) when unloaded but locks them in place or grabs when force is applied. In industrial rescue applications, there is little need for a rescuer to ascend a rope. There is, however, quite a need for a device that will grab a rope when attached to a load for hauling. Most manufactured ascent devices can be used as rope grab devices and vice versa. For this reason, we will address both ascent and rope grab devices interchangeably in this section.

There are two basic types of ascent devices: mechanical ascenders and soft ascenders. Mechanical ascenders are manufactured hardware items for ascending or grabbing a rope. They can be classified further as personal and general use ascenders (see Figure 3.20). Although they may not operate in exactly the same way, the action is the same.

Soft ascenders are Prusik loops made of accessory cord that can be used in the same way as mechanical ascenders to climb up or grab a rope. There is some controversy as to which is better for rescue applications. Both mechanical and soft ascenders have advantages and disadvantages.

Mechanical Rope Grabs

Not all mechanical ascenders are suitable for use as a rope grab during a rescue. These devices should meet the requirements of NFPA 1983 (1995 edition) for ascending and rope grab devices designated for general use (two-person loads). A major disadvantage of most mechanical ascenders is their tendancy to damage or fail a rope if severely shock loaded. For this reason, they should not be used in belay systems designed to catch a falling load. They should be used for steady pulls only. If a mechani-

WARNING

Avoid using mechanical ascenders where shock loading may occur.

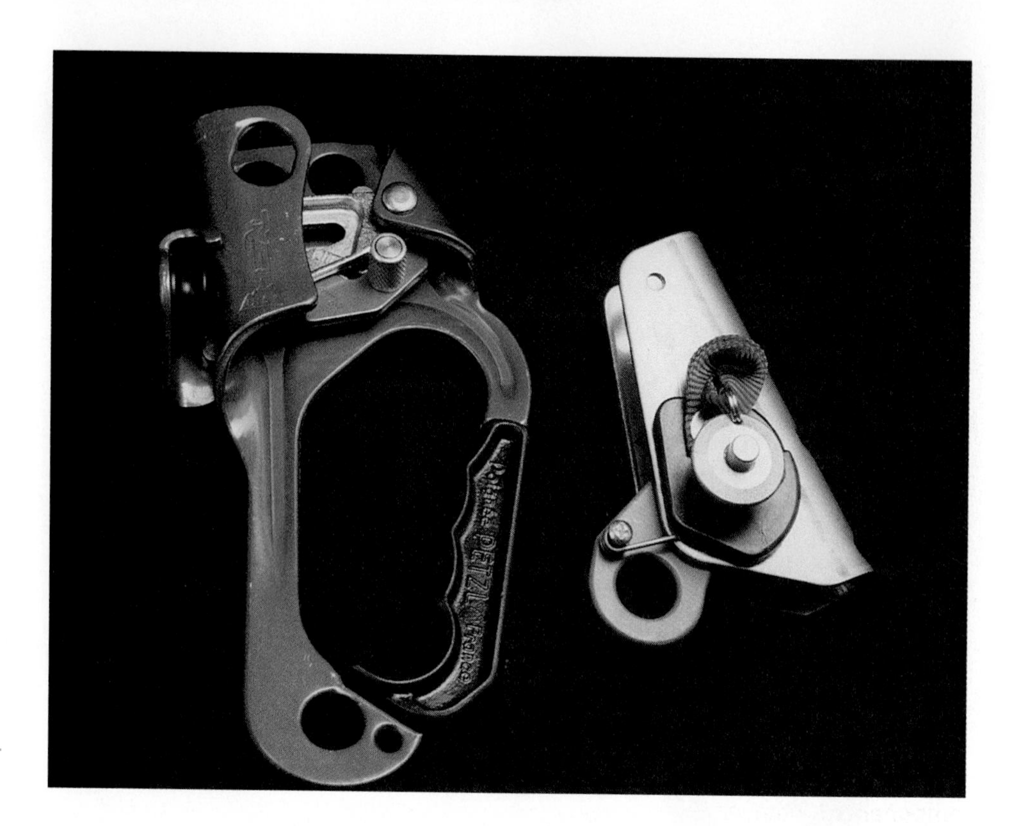

Figure 3.20 Examples of ascent device and rope grab device.

cal ascender is placed in a system that might be subject to a significant impact load, it should be backed up by a safety line belay system. This back up is recommended in training and actual rescue operations.

Some advantages and disadvantages of mechanical ascenders include:

- Proper application can be taught easily. This is an advantage for industrial rescuers who may have limited time for training.
- When properly applied, they activate and grab the rope the same way every time. They do not rely on the formation and dressing of a knot to hold the load.
- They are heavier and more expensive than soft ascenders.
- Some brands require more time to apply than soft ascenders.
- Most cam-type mechanical ascenders have the potential to damage or fail a rope when subjected to severe shock loading.
- Some types do not meet NFPA strength standards.

General use ascenders and rope grab devices function by squeezing the rope between a metal housing (shell) and a round-toothed cam or metal press. These devices are the only type of mechanical ascenders recommended for rescue and should meet the appropriate NFPA requirements. The more surface contact with the rope, the better the device since the load can be distributed over a larger area. The cam or press devices of most brands range from $\frac{1}{4}$ inch to 2 inches of rope surface contact area. The more surface area, the more likely the rope will be able to survive an unexpected impact load without damage. Some of these devices are designed to slip on the rope to prevent failure in the event of a shock.

Design Mechanical ascenders vary significantly in size but most have the shape of a rectangle with one tapered side, giving it the appearance of an arrow (see Figure 3.21). Some brands have versions that accommodate up to a $\frac{3}{4}$-inch rope. With the ability to accommodate a larger rope comes increased bulk, weight, and expense of the device.

Material Mechanical cam-type ascenders are made in a variety of metals including aluminum alloy and stainless steel. The stainless-steel versions are usually the strongest, although some aluminum alloys used in aircraft are stronger.

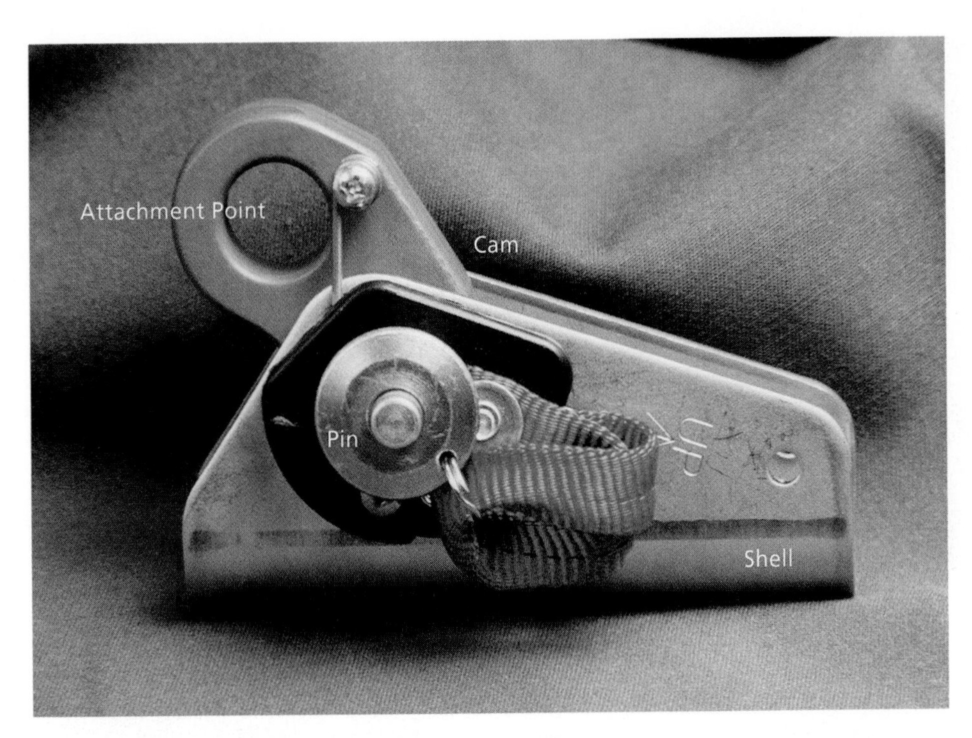

Figure 3.21 Different parts of the rope grab device.

Components Although these devices have slightly different designs, most general use mechanical ascenders have a form of the following components (see Figure 3.21):

- **Shell**—This is the casing of the device through which the rope travels while attached. Most shells are imprinted with an arrow that designates the direction of free travel.
- **Cam or press**—This part of the device grabs the rope by pressing it, usually by a cantilever action, against the shell. The size of the cam or press in relation to the shape of the shell largely determines the amount of surface contact with the rope. This component usually has a set of smooth or rounded teeth to help grab the rope while limiting the destructive potential. The cam can be spring loaded or free running. Spring-loaded cams are under slight tension at all times, making them grasp the rope even when no force is applied to the attachment point. This is desirable when a rescuer is ascending the rope but has little importance when used as a rope grab device. Some brands are designed to be interchangeable.
- **Pin**—This component is used to attach the cam or press to the shell. Pins are usually provided with a locking mechanism to prevent it from accidentally falling off.
- **Attachment Point**—This is the ring or hole used to attach the device to a hauling system or harness. When force is applied, the cam or press activates, causing the device to grab the rope. The attachment point may be part of the cam.

Strength Requirements The NFPA 1983 (1995 edition) implies that devices used for rope grabs should meet the general-use requirements. Personal-use requirements are intended for ascending applications with one-person loads.

Ascending and rope grab devices are required to meet a strength test in the manner of function. The test requires a minimum test load of a specific force without permanent damage to the device or rope. The NFPA does not designate a minimum breaking strength for ascending and rope grab devices.

- Personal use (ascending)—A minimum test load of at least 1,200 force pounds is required.
- General use (rope grab)—A minimum test load of at least 2,400 force pounds is required.

Most brands of mechanical general use ascenders designed for $\frac{1}{2}$-inch or larger rope meet the general-use requirements.

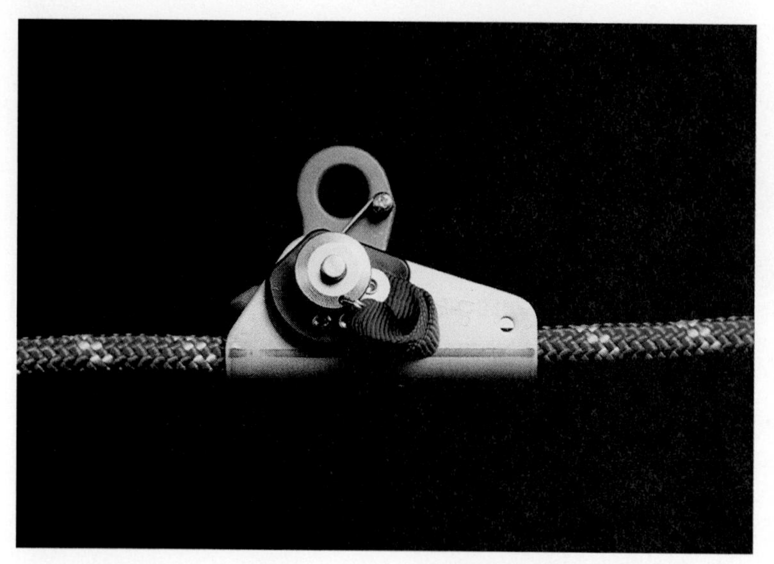

Figure 3.22 Rope grab attached to rope.

Operation Safety and other preparatory requirements for ascenders will be covered later in this text. The rope grab application and operation are very similar for most general use mechanical ascenders. The following example is for operation of a popular brand of ascender (see Figure 3.22).

The shell should be attached to the rope with the arrow pointing in the direction of free travel. In most cases, this means the arrow is pointing toward the load. The stainless-steel screw (or screw hole in the absence of a screw) in the cam should face the same direction as the UP arrow inscribed on the outside of the ascender shell. The mnemonic "Screw UP so you won't screw up" may help you remember this cam position. Before life loading cam-type ascenders, always test them for function by pulling on the attachment point to ensure they will lock.

The following procedures for use of this example of ascenders have been approved by the manufacturer:

- Use for slow, steady pulls only. Do not use these ascenders as a safety belay system to catch a falling load, only to hold a static load in place.
- Any time this ascender is used in a system where serious impact loads are possible, an additional independent safety line belay system should be used. This will catch the falling load in the event of rope failure due to an accidental shock load to the primary system. This applies in both training and actual rescues.
- The number of haulers with mechanical advantage systems constructed using these ascenders should be limited to prevent overstressing the system should the load become entangled. It is recommended that no more than four persons be allowed on a haul line in a system with a mechanical advantage of 4:1 or less. For systems with greater than a 4:1 mechanical advantage, the allowed number of haulers is reduced to two.
- An independent rescuer should be assigned to "load watch" in all hauling systems, regardless of the mechanical advantage. The scope of this team member's responsibility is to immediately stop the haul effort by physically alerting the haul team of a problem involving entanglement of the load. Haul team and other team members must be taught to react immediately to the load watch's alert.
- No more than two people should ever be loaded on a single system. The maximum two-person load is considered to be 600 pounds, which includes equipment and personal protective clothing.

If all of the above safety procedures are enacted, they will help prevent damage to the patient or rope that might result from overloading or shock of an ascender used as a rope grab in a system. It also provides a positive backup in the event of system failure.

Consult the manufacturer's recommendations for additional information concerning use, inspection, maintenance, and retirement of mechanical general use ascenders.

Ascent Devices

Personal ascenders are designed for light duty, that is, ascending with only one person's weight (see Figure 3.20). Two or three of them are generally used together to create climbing systems. They are structurally weak and have been known to fail with as little as 1200 pounds of impact force. Personal ascenders are not recommended for industrial rescue.

Soft Rope Grabs

Prusik loops are tied loops of accessory cord that can be looped around a larger-diameter rescue rope with a Prusik hitch. (Chapter 4 addresses knots.) Depending on the application, a Prusik hitch can be double or triple wrapped, causing it to tighten up and bind when loaded. It works basically the same way as the mechanical ascender device except that it will bind when pulled in either direction and, once it is bound, must be loosened manually to allow it to slide freely on the rope. Soft ascenders can be used effectively to ascend rope, perform self-rescue from a rope, and be a rope grab in hauling systems. Soft ascenders are also used commonly as belay devices in safety line belay systems. Some of the advantages and disadvantages of soft ascenders are:

- They absorb shock better than mechanical ascenders. They slip and fuse into the rope rather than destroying it when overloaded.
- They are lighter and less expensive than mechanical devices.
- Prusik loops must be tied and applied properly to the rope to operate well in hauling systems. If incorrectly applied, the Prusik knot may slip when loaded.
- Even when properly applied in hauling systems, Prusik loops can be difficult to operate, requiring constant attention to prevent binding.

Design For ascending and hauling system rope grabs, it is recommended that Prusik loops be made of 6-millimeter or 7-millimeter accessory cord tied in a loop with either a figure-8 follow-through knot or a double fisherman's knot. These recommendations are based on use of the Prusik loop with ½-inch rescue rope. Prusik loops used in ascending or self-rescue should be tied from 6- to 7-foot lengths of accessory cord. Prusik loops used as rope grabs in hauling systems are commonly operated in tandem, requiring one loop to be shorter than the other by 2 to 3 inches. The common lengths for accessory cord used to create tandem Prusik loops are 4½ feet and 5½ feet. In Prusik belay systems, the accessory cord should be 8-millimeter or 9-millimeter in diameter and always used in tandem. The lengths of the loops are the same as listed for tandem rope grabs in hauling systems. This is based on triple-wrap Prusik knots on ½-inch rope.

Design Accessory cord of 100% nylon is recommended for strength and durability.

Strength Requirements It is recommended that Prusik loops used as ascenders and rope grabs meet the same requirements as cam-type mechanical ascenders.

There are no NFPA recommendations for belay devices since the standard was written for applications involving fall factors no greater than .25. When used for belay systems, Prusik loops should be constructed of larger-diameter accessory cord than that for general-use rope grabs for increased strength. Using 8-millimeter or 9-millimeter in tandem will provide approximately the same strength as ½-inch nylon static kernmantle rescue rope.

Operation The operation of Prusik loops for self-rescue, rope grabs in hauling systems, and tandem Prusik belay systems will be covered later in this text.

Pulleys

A pulley is an auxiliary device with a free-running, grooved metal wheel (sheave) used to reduce rope friction (see Figure 3.23). It has side plates to which a carabiner can be attached. The "swing" side plates allow attachment of the pulley anywhere along the rope's length. Pulleys are used to develop mechanical advantage in rope hauling systems and to redirect the path of a rope for convenience or to prevent abrasion. Although used to reduce friction, all pulleys add some friction (as much as 10%) to the system. For a more efficient system, the number of pulleys should be limited. Rescue pulleys should meet NFPA 1983 (1995 edition) requirements for personal-use (one-person loads) or general-use (two-person loads) auxiliary equipment.

Design

Pulleys come in a variety of designs including specialty pulleys such as knot-passing pulleys, edge rollers, and pulleys with built-in cams (see Figure 3.24). There are many

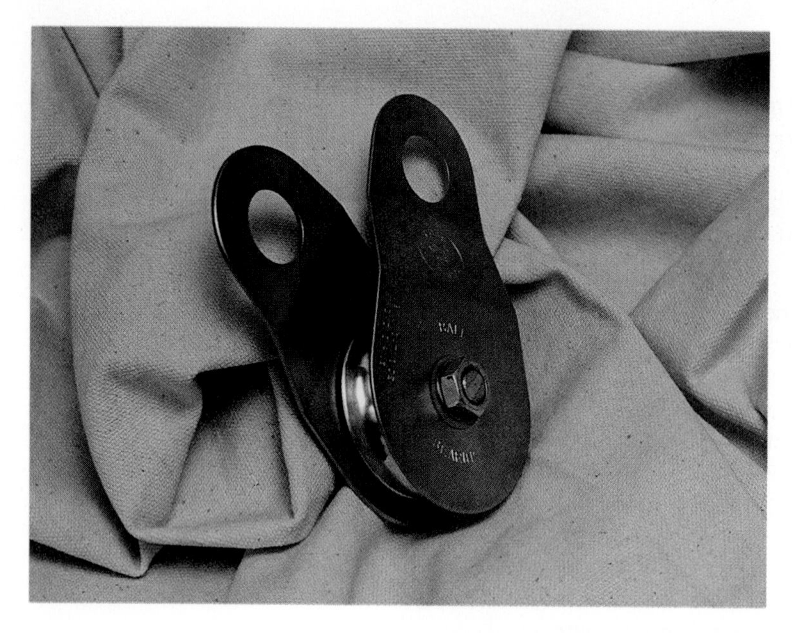

Figure 3.23 Basic pulley

standard rescue pulleys designed to fit $\frac{1}{2}$-inch rope. Most pulleys are shaped like a teardrop. Pulleys are generally classified by the number of sheaves and their sizes. There are single-sheave (one wheel), double-sheave (two wheel), and even triple-sheave (three wheel) pulleys. Double- and triple-sheave pulleys can be used as single-sheave pulleys as long as all of the side plates are fastened together. Pulleys are available in many sizes although 2-inch, 3-inch, and 4-inch pulleys are the most popular for rescue. The diameter of a pulley's sheave is usually smaller than the pulley. For example, a 2-inch pulley can have a sheave diameter of only $1\frac{1}{2}$-inches.

The sheave's size is very important to a pulley's efficiency. This is because of the effect of acute bends on rope. When a rope is bent around an object smaller than four times its diameter, a loss of efficiency occurs (see Figure 3.25). This is the "four-to-one rule." There will be no loss of rope strength if rescuers follow this rule. Since $\frac{1}{2}$-inch rope is common in rescue, it means the pulley sheave should be at least four times that, or 2 inches in diameter, for maximum efficiency. This does not preclude the use of smaller-diameter sheaves, but they are not as efficient with the rope. In general, the larger the pulley sheave in relation to the rope, the more efficient the pulley.

Some pulleys have an additional attachment point at the base of the pulley called a becket (see Figure 3.26). The use of this and other special features of pulleys will be covered later in this text.

Material

Rescue pulleys are made from stainless steel or anodized aluminum alloy. Pulleys with great strength are available in both materials.

Components

Most basic rescue pulleys are comprised of the following component parts (see Figure 3.26):

Figure 3.24 Various types of pulleys

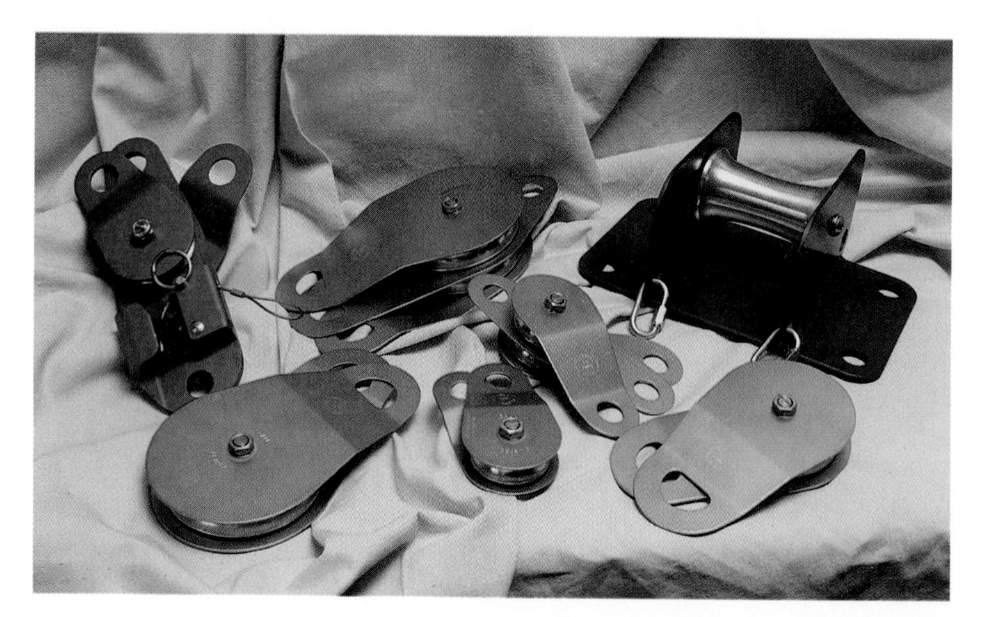

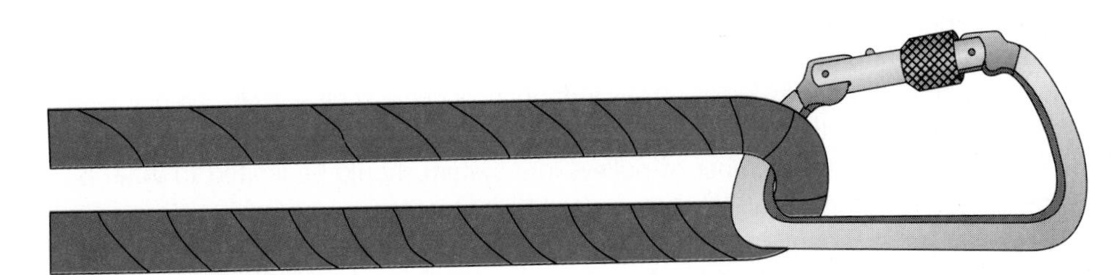

Figure 3.25 An acute bend in the rope

- **Sheave (wheel)**—Pulleys with a sheave diameter larger than 2 inches are recommended for maximum efficiency.
- **Bearings**—The bearing provides the surface on which the sheave spins. There are two main types of bearings common to rescue pulleys: (1) Bronze bushings are strong, removable, and can be taken apart and cleaned when dirty. They also hold up well to abuse. Since this bushing is not sealed, dirt and grit can affect the sheave' ability to spin freely. (2) Sealed ball bearings are not exposed to dirt and grit. They spin more freely than bronze bushings, although they are slightly heavier and more expensive. The problem is that sealed bearings do not handle abuse quite as well as bronze bushings and are subject to damage. Sealed bearings are highly recommended in industrial rescue applications.
- **Axles (pins)**—The axle secures the bearing to the side plates. Most pulleys have an aircraft steel axle for maximum strength. In some earlier aluminum pulleys, the pin was stronger than the side plates. If these pulleys were overstressed, striations and other visible signs of damage usually appeared in the side plates around the axle. Many modern pulleys have side plates as strong as the axle.
- **Side plates**—Side plates are made of steel or anodized aluminum alloy. Rescue pulleys are of "swing-side" design, which means that the side plates can swing open for easy attachment anywhere along the rope's length. The side plates attach to the axles and have openings at the top of the plates for attachment to other rescue system components. Most side plates are as strong as the rest of the pulley's component parts. When pulled to failure, these pulleys usually do so by pulling the carabiners through the attachment openings at the top of the side plates.
- **Becket plate and becket (double- and triple-sheave pulleys only)**—These are usually formed from an additional side plate or side plates in or near the center of double- and triple-sheave pulleys. The plate extends below the base of the pulley and has an opening designed for attachment of other rescue system components. This attachment point is referred to as the becket. Its use will be discussed more thoroughly in later chapters.

Other specialty pulleys are available and may have slightly different or additional component parts.

Figure 3.26 Parts of a pulley

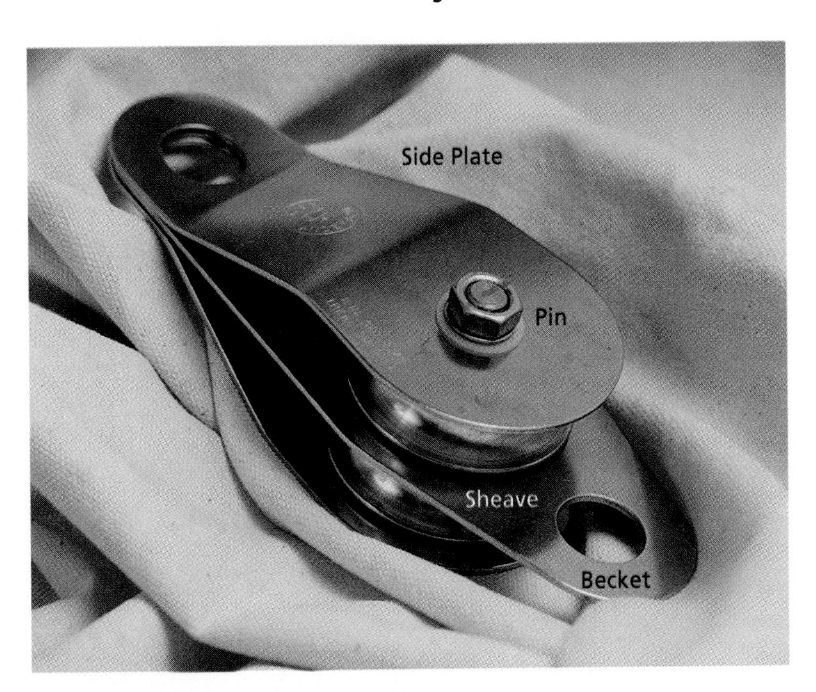

Strength Requirements

Rescue pulleys have no specific requirements but fall under the category of auxiliary equipment. The minimum breaking strength requirement for personal use (one-person loads) is 5,000 force pounds. The requirement for general use (two-person loads) is 8,000 force pounds. There are pulleys of various types and sizes that meet these requirements.

Operation

To operate most pulleys, simply open the side plates and attach them to the rope. Close the side plates and clip them together at the attachment openings with a carabiner or tri-link. Then the pulley can be attached to an anchor system or other rescue system component.

Do not allow the ropes issuing from a double- or triple-sheave pulley to pull in an outward direction on the side plates. Pulleys are not designed to withstand this type of force. Remember, the number of pulleys in a system should be limited to what is needed. Keeping it simple will make a more efficient system.

There are several generic things to look for when inspecting pulleys. Be sure the attachment holes line up properly when the side plates are closed. Check the sheave to ensure proper spin. Look at the side plate openings for signs of bending or striations that might indicate damage from improper use or excessive stress. More information will be provided later in this text on proper use of pulleys in various rescue systems. Consult the manufacturer's recommendations for additional information concerning use, inspection, maintenance, and retirement of pulleys.

Summary

Getting the right equipment for the job at hand is only half of the battle. The other half is learning how to use it. The following chapters will address this issue. Remember that all rescuers should seek proper hands-on training from a competent trainer before attempting any of the techniques shown in this book.

CHAPTER 4

Rescue Knots

The information in this chapter is provided as a basis for continued training. Each rescuer should consult with his or her own team leader for the correct SOGs for the team. Topics covered in this chapter include:

- Knot Efficiency
- Tying Knots
- Terms
- Applications

Introduction

A knot is a fastening made by tying together pieces of rope or by intertwining a rope. For rescuers, it means attaching a rope to anchors or other components of a rescue system. Some things described as knots in this chapter may not be "knots" by popular definition; however, they serve to attach the rope to other components of the system.

If we had to describe the most important ideas in knot tying, they would be

1. PRACTICE.
2. PRACTICE.
3. PRACTICE!

You have probably heard the phrase, "If you don't use it, you lose it." This saying is particularly true when it comes to tying knots. If you think you can tie these knots in a hurry, under the pressure of an emergency, and maybe even in the dark without practice, you are probably mistaken. Every chance you get, tie knots. Get a small piece of rope. Carry it around with you. Practice at work. Practice at home. Just practice!

Knot Efficiency

What is the really important thing common to all knots? It is the fact that *the rope is bent.* How acutely the rope is bent determines how efficient the knot is.

A sharp bend in a rope causes a loss of efficiency, not a loss of **strength** but of **efficiency.** When a static kernmantle rope is bent around a tight corner, as over a carabiner (see Figure 4.1), the core strands are pulled very tightly on the outside of the bend. The strands inside the bend are bunched up, almost loose. This means that only some of the core strands are supporting the load. This results in a loss of rope efficiency so that only part of the rope's strength is being used.

Now if that rope is straightened, and has not been damaged, it will be just as strong as it was before it had the bend in it. This is why the loss in strength due to knots is a loss of efficiency.

Four-to-One Rule

How do rescuers get maximum efficiency from knots? The previous chapter on equipment mentioned the four-to-one rule in relation to pulley size. According to this rule, if a rope is bent around an object at least four times its diameter, there will be no loss of efficiency. So if a knot has bends no smaller than four times the diameter of the rope (2-inches for $\frac{1}{2}$-inch rope), the rope maintains 100% of its strength.

This is a good idea. However it is usually impossible to tie most knots and still maintain the four-to-one rule. The goal is to use knots that are the most efficient, that

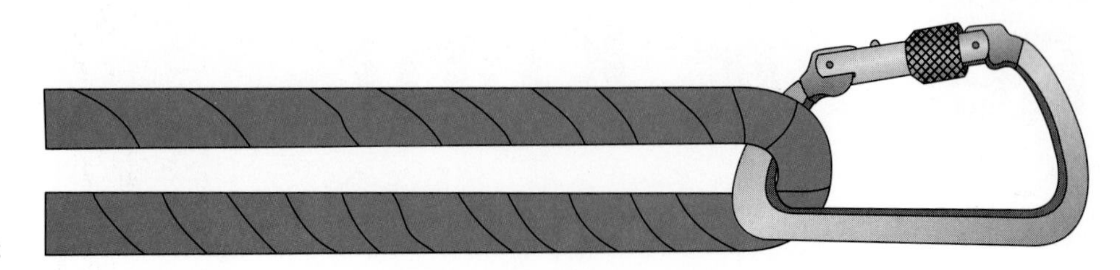

Figure 4.1 Rope bent around object

is, knots with large lazy bends rather than tight bends. The lazier the bends, the more efficient the knot.

One reason the NFPA established a safety factor of 15:1 for rope was to compensate for the loss of efficiency expected with knot tying. All of the knots discussed in this chapter are good knots, but some are more efficient than others. Still, a rescuer should never be so concerned with knot efficiency that he or she refuses to tie a knot he or she knows well because it might be slightly less efficient than another knot.

Consider the following scenario: A rescuer has been lowered to a patient who is wearing a harness. Other rescuers have lowered a rope to the rescuer to attach to the patient's harness. All the rescuer has to do is tie a knot in the rope and attach it to the patient's harness with a carabiner. The rescuer remembers that one of the most efficient knots is the double-loop figure-8, which has about 18% efficiency. But under pressure he suddenly cannot remember how to tie a double-loop figure-8. Fortunately, the competent rescuer knew the figure-8 on a bight very well. He quickly chose to tie it although, at about 20% loss, it is slightly less efficient than the double-loop figure-8. He did the right thing. If the rescuer had wasted time with attempt after attempt to tie the knot he could not remember, it might have been at the patient's expense.

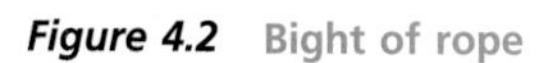

Figure 4.2 Bight of rope

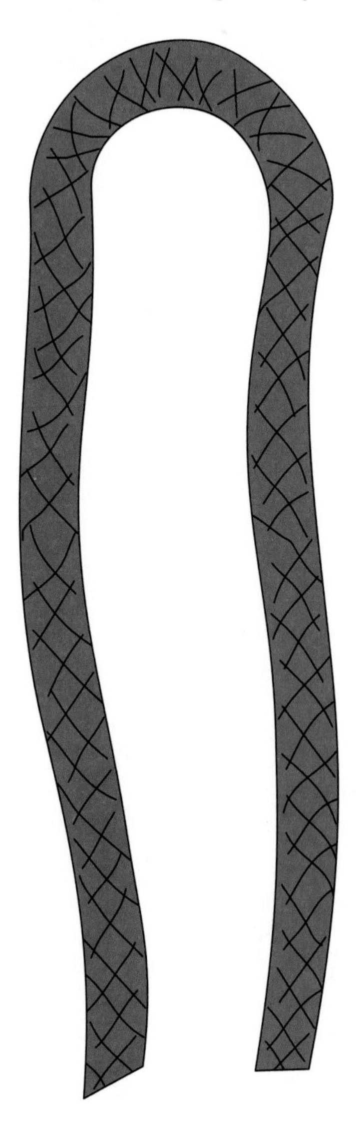

The point is, do not focus only on knot efficiency. Rather, base your choice of knots on all important factors. Knot efficiency is only one of them. Remember that most rope failures are not a result of overstress, but from cutting by exposed sharp or abrasive edges. Life safety ropes usually do not break; they get cut.

Knot Tests

Break test data is not available for every knot mentioned in this chapter. This is particularly true for knots using $\frac{1}{2}$-inch static kernmantle rope of 100% nylon. Most of the older knot efficiency charts were based on tests performed with ropes of braid-on-braid and laid construction. Some testing was conducted in 1987 by CMC (California Mountain Company). The tests were performed using Wellington Puritan's $\frac{1}{2}$-inch low-stretch nylon Rhino Rescue Rope. The tests showed that most knots listed in this chapter have efficiency losses somewhere around 20% to 40%, depending on the knot and its use.

As we cover the various knots in this chapter, we will include information (when available) derived from this and other testing conducted by PMI (Pigeon Mountain Industries). Keep in mind that these figures should be considered rough guidelines. The testing was not always performed scientifically. We cannot always verify the control of the tests or their repeatability. We simply cite them as a general guideline. Information concerning tests of knots is available from companies or persons who sell the ropes.

It is important to mention that loss of rope efficiency due to knots is not a cumulative process. In other words, in a rope with several knots, the total efficiency loss in the rope is approximately equal to the amount of loss from the least efficient knot. It is like a chain, only as strong as the weakest link.

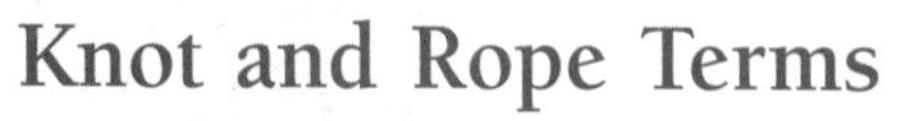

Knot and Rope Terms

The three elements of a knot are the bight, the loop, and the round turn. All knots consist of one or more of these three elements.

- **Bight**—A U-shaped bend in the rope (see Figure 4.2)

- **Loop**—A turn in a rope that crosses itself to create a closed loop (see Figure 4.3)
- **Round turn**—A full wrap of a rope around an object so that both ends emerge from the same side (see Figure 4.4)

There are several other important terms to understand before embarking on knot tying. Many traditional knot and rope terms used in the fire service provide a basis for this terminology. Some of these terms may be altered slightly for simplicity.

There are usually two ends, or legs, of rope issuing from any knot. If the knot is not tied in the middle of the rope, there is one short and one long leg (see Figure 4.5). For the sake of simplicity, we will refer to the longest rope (the one leading to the running end) as the long leg. We will refer to the other leg (actually part of the working end used to tie the knot) as the short leg or the tail. This terminology should make things a bit easier to understand when reading the knot tying procedures later in this section.

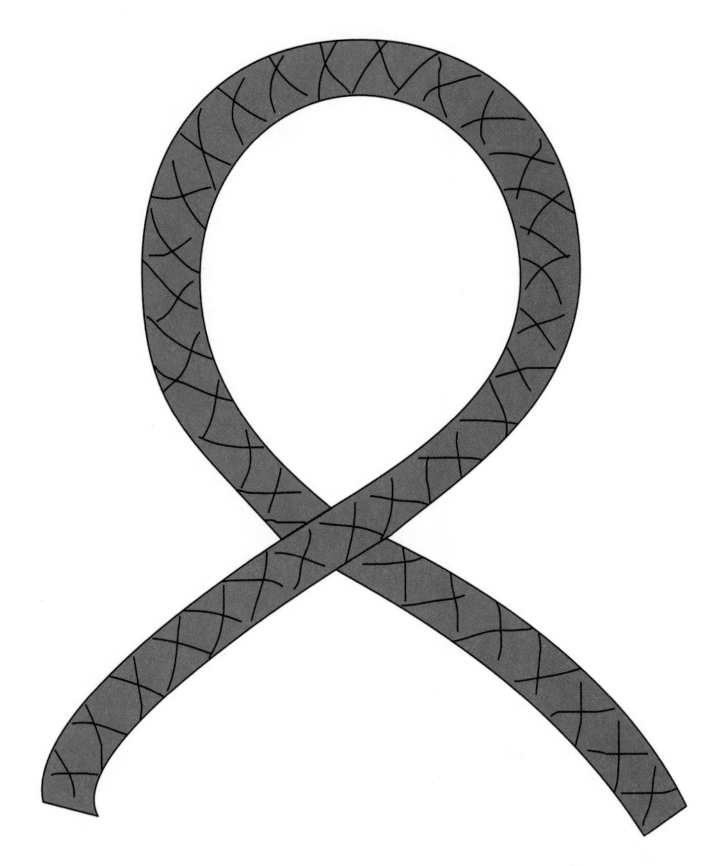

4.3 Loop of rope

Tying Knots

There are three important steps to tying most of the rescue knots in this chapter. The steps are (see Figure 4.6):

1. **Dress the knot.** Physically arrange the ropes in the knot to remove improper crossovers or kinks. Proper dressing of a knot makes the knot more efficient. It also makes the knot easy to recognize. Recognizability is important because it helps you know if you've correctly tied the knot. If the knot is poorly dressed, it is difficult to see if you have properly tied the knot.
2. **Load (or set) the knot.** Tightly pull all the rope ends emerging from the knot so you remove any slack from within the knot. This makes the knot more compact, prevents slippage, and helps to dress it. You should pull the knot in the same way it will be loaded in the system.
3. **"Safety" the knot.** Secure tail ends of rope emerging from the knot. If the knot has a tail, or tails, tie them around the long leg to prevent them from slipping through the knot and untying when loaded. Acceptable safety knots are listed later in this chapter. Midline and certain other knots do not require safeties.

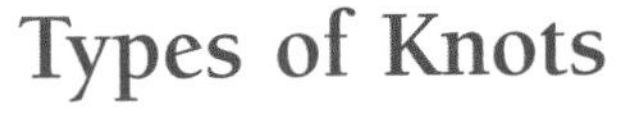

Types of Knots

There are different types and applications of knots. This text uses the common, recognizable names and groups knots according to use. Types of knots include:

- **Loops**—Any knot that creates a loop for attachment

  NOTE: *In confined spaces use, the loops created in some knots should be just large enough to make the necessary connection easily. Large loops can take up rope and space, possibly shortening the distance a patient can be moved before the rope system butts against the knot. Keep knots compact!*

4.4 Round turn of rope

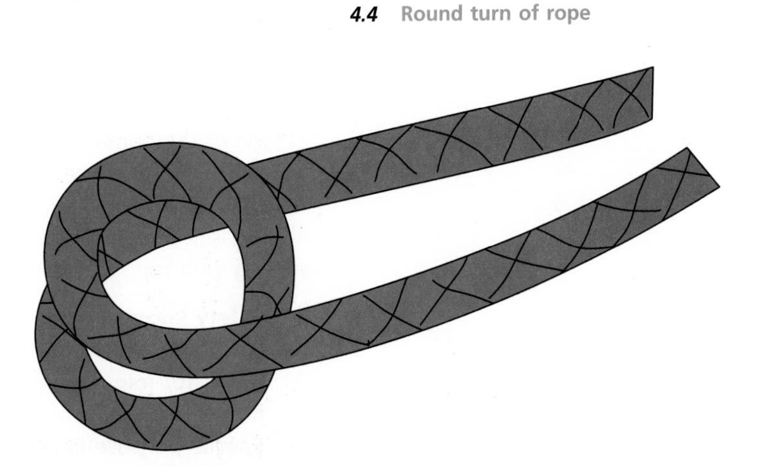

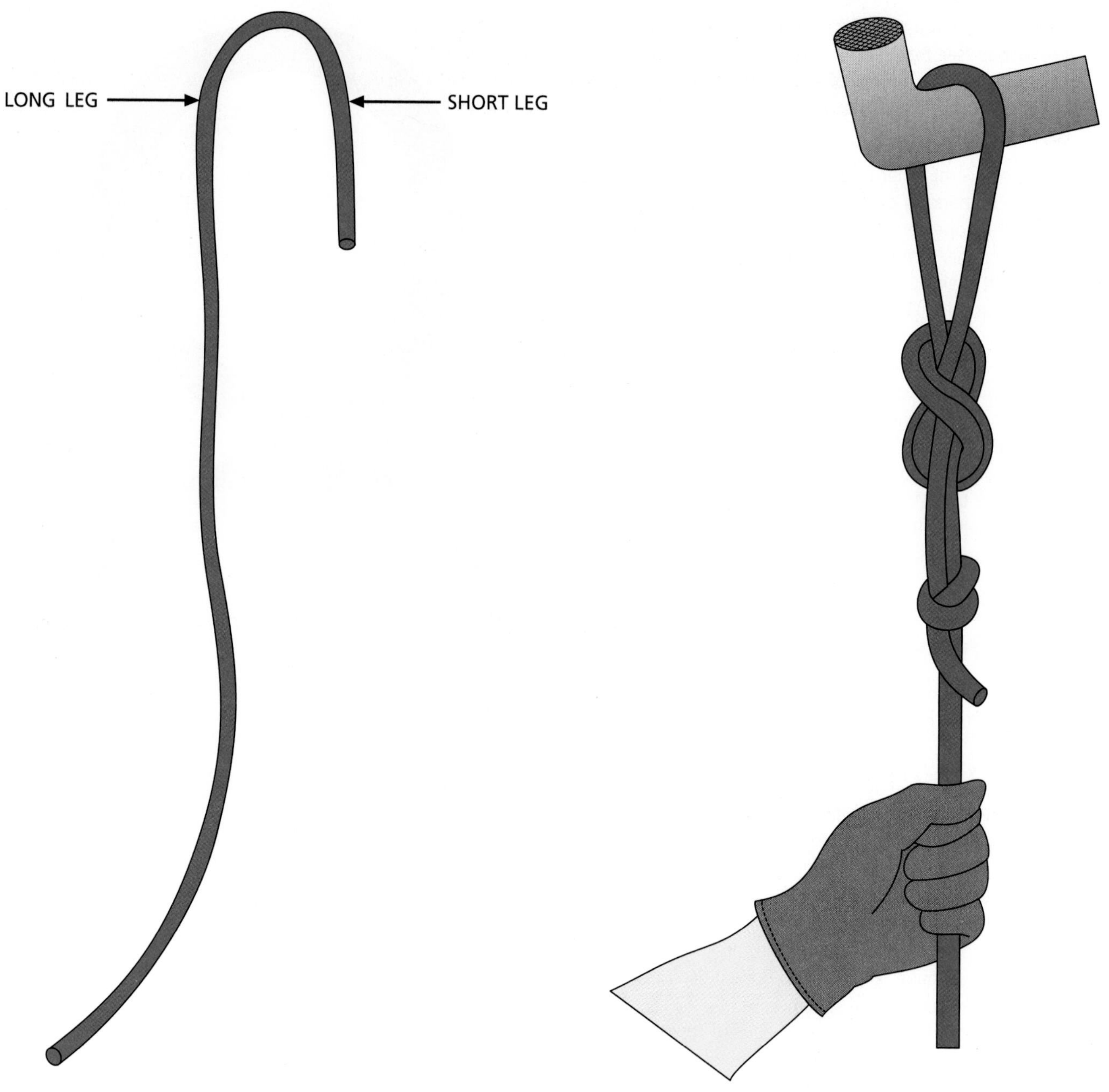

Figure 4.5 Long and short leg of a rope

Figure 4.6 Dress, load, and safety ALL knots

- **Hitches**—Any knot used to attach a rope to an object or anchor
- **Bends**—Used to join ropes (see Figure 4.7)

One of the primary families of knots is the figure-8 family. The figure-8s are very efficient (usually between 18% and 25% efficiency loss) and recognizable. They are also very similar, so someone who knows one figure-8 knot can probably learn the others easily. There are many other knots, however. The knots shown here focus on working with rope rescue systems. They fall into one of the following groups:

- **Safety knots** are used to create some type of safety or backup in a rope or knot.
- **Anchor knots** are used to attach a rope to an anchor point or system.
- **Knots for joining ropes** join ropes of equal or unequal diameter. These knots are further classified as load-bearing or non–load-bearing.
- **Special purpose knots** are used for specific applications in rope rescue systems.

Illustrations show, step by step, a method of tying each knot. There are many recognized methods of tying almost every knot known to human beings. Based on the experience of leading rope rescue trainers, the methods shown here seem to work well for most beginners. If you have a method that works best for you and achieves the same result, use it!

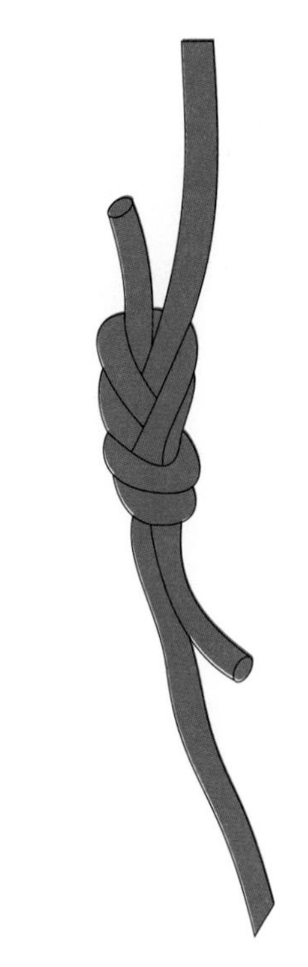

Figure 4.7 Example of a bend knot

Safety Knots

As previously mentioned, safety knots are used to tie a short, loose end emerging from a knot around the long leg of rope to prevent slippage. Traditionally, half hitches have been used in the fire service to create safeties. They have proved unreliable, however, because they easily untie when the rope travels over edges. Modern practice recommends overhand or barrel knots for safeties. Neither of these knots requires additional safety backup. They should be tied so that they rest very near the primary knot. If the tail begins to pull through, it will stop quickly if the safety has been tied close. Safety knots are not required with the double fisherman's knot or midline knots because there are no short, loose ends. A different type of safety knot used to put a stopper in the end of a rope (should it be too short to make it to the ground) is the figure-8 stopper.

Overhand Knot

The overhand is a safety knot used to secure loose ends. It is very much the same knot used to begin to tie shoe laces. Tie this knot with the tail end of the rope emerging from the primary knot around the long leg of the rope. The overhand creates an efficiency loss of approximately 15%.

How to Tie the Overhand Knot

1. Tie the overhand knot with the tail end of the rope. Tie it around the long leg.
2. Form a small loop around the long leg with the tail end near the primary knot.
3. To create the overhand, cross the tail end over the loop and back through the center.
4. Load the knot as close to the primary knot as possible.

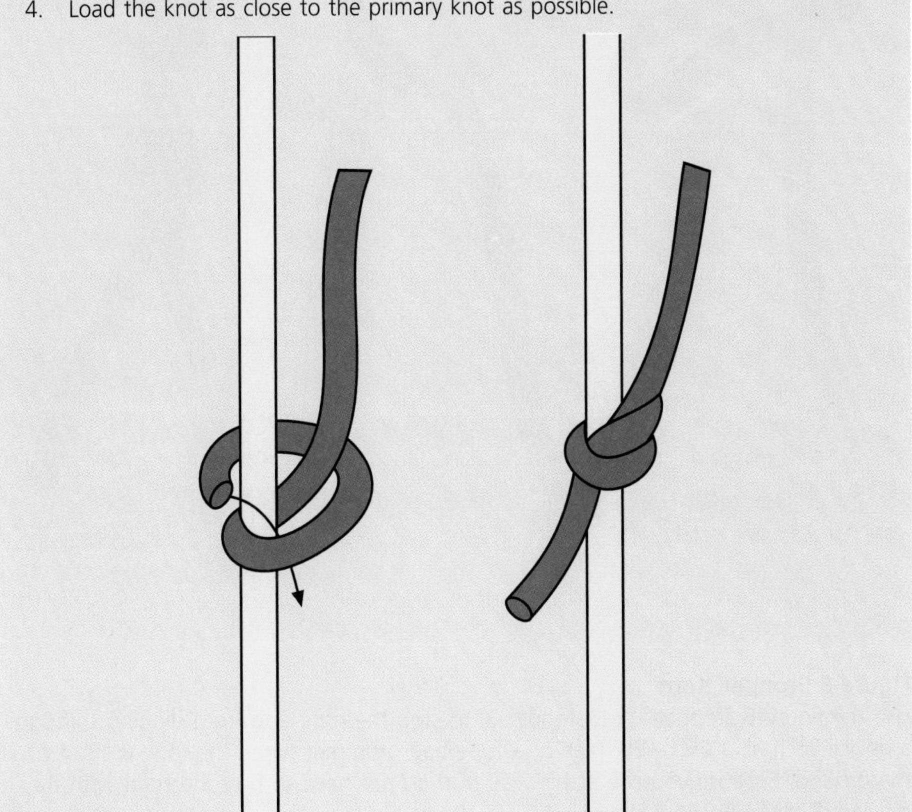

Barrel Hitch

The barrel hitch (fisherman's knot, double overhand) is a safety knot used to secure loose rope ends. Tie this knot like the overhand, with the tail end of the rope emerging from the primary knot around the long leg of the rope. The exact efficiency loss is not known.

How to Tie a Barrel Hitch

1. Tie the barrel hitch with the tail end of the rope. Tie it around the long leg.
2. Form a round turn around the long leg with the tail of rope. Allow the round turn to cross over itself, forming an X.
3. Continue to wrap the tail end around on the same side of the X until it has crossed itself a second time.
4. Pass the tail end through the center of its own loops. Pass it parallel to and directly beside the long leg, and pointing away from the primary knot.
5. Load the knot as closely to the primary knot as possible.

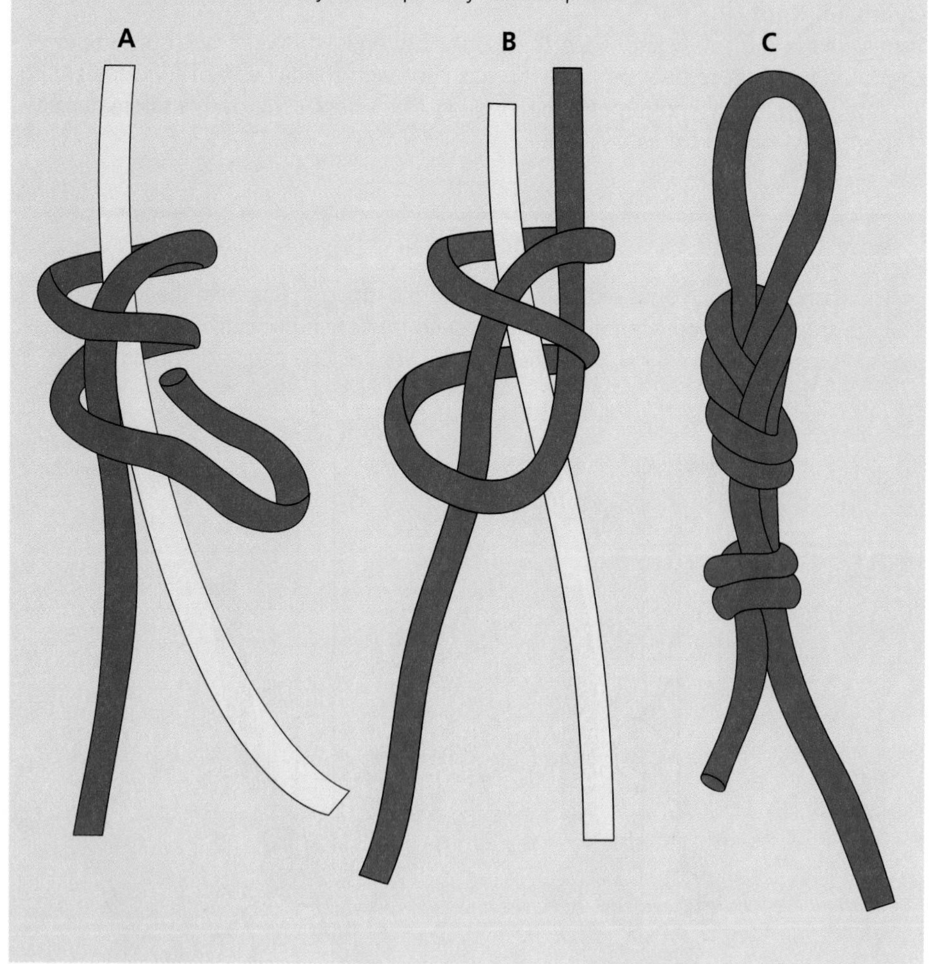

Figure-8 Stopper Knot

Use the figure-8 stopper knot (stopper-8) to stop the rope end from slipping through a device such as a brake bar rack or a rope bag grommet when the rope is short of the ground. Because you use it this way, you do not have to be concerned with the efficiency of the figure-8 stopper.

How to Tie the Stopper Knot

1. Tie the stopper knot in the running end (end of the long leg) of the rope.
2. Form a bight with this end of the rope and hold it in front of you. It should look like a hanging inverted U.
3. While holding the bight with one hand, wrap the short leg around the long leg one full turn to create a loop at the bottom of the forming knot.
4. Pass the end of the short leg through the original bight.
5. Load the knot by pulling the long leg and the short leg in opposite directions. When you do this, the knot should automatically dress itself.

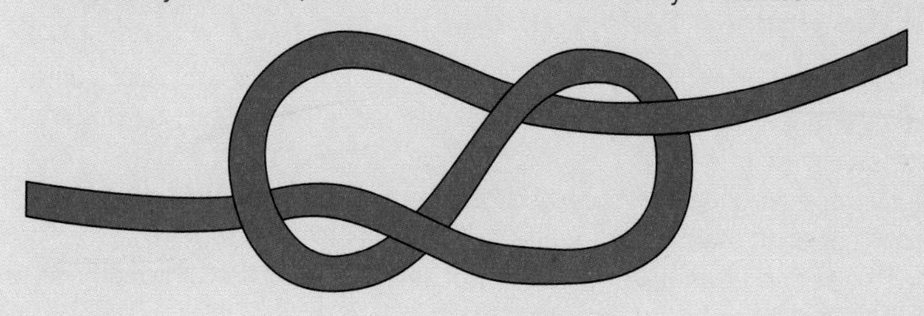

Anchor Knots

Most anchor knots are tied directly around an object. Some, however, are designed to be attached to rope system components via a carabiner or screw link. These knots are grouped as anchor knots. However, rescuers can use them to attach a rope to almost any point in a rope system.

Figure-8 on a Bight

A rescuer can attach this anchor knot (figure-8 loop with a bight, single-loop figure-8) to various components of the rope rescue system with a carabiner or screw link, or can slip it over an object with an open end such as a post. It creates a loop in the rope that will not slip. Rescuers should not forget to include a safety knot if there is a loose end. The figure-8 on a bight creates an efficiency loss of approximately 20%.

How to Tie the Figure-8 on a Bight

1. Tie the figure-8 on a bight in the same way as the stopper knot. The difference is that you tie this knot on a bight. This means you use a doubled rope to do it.
2. Double the rope back on itself a couple of feet. This should form a bight.
3. Squeeze the bight tightly to make it appear more like a rope end. Consider this bight the loose end (working end) of the rope.
4. Form a bight with this doubled rope and hold it in front of you just as you did with a single rope when tying the stopper knot. It should look like a hanging inverted U.

   NOTE: *There is some speculation about whether this bight should be formed by bending the rope toward the short leg or long leg of the doubled rope. Do not worry about this detail. If you dress it properly, the ropes will be in proper position for maximum efficiency.*
5. Hold the double-rope bight with one hand. Wrap the short leg (the tight single-rope bight you formed initially when you doubled the rope) around the long leg (also doubled rope) one full turn to create a loop at the bottom of the forming knot.
6. Pass the end of the short leg (the original single-rope bight) through the double-rope bight to form a loop for connection to another rope system component.
7. Dress this knot carefully to ensure that the ropes in the knot run parallel and do not cross. This can make a significant difference in efficiency.
8. Load the knot by pulling the loop and both legs in opposite directions. You can set the knot even tighter by pulling on the individual ropes in opposite directions until all slack is removed.

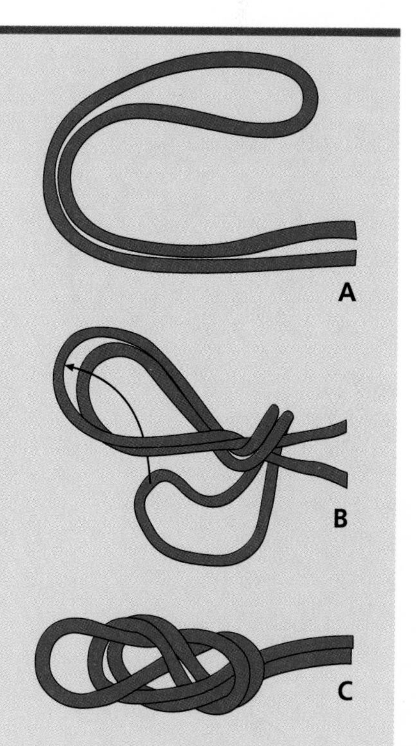

Figure-8 Follow Through

The figure-8 follow through (Figure-8 loop follow through, tracer-8) is virtually the same knot as the figure-8 on a bight. The difference is that the "follow through" allows you to tie the knot around an anchor point with no open end. A structural column between floors would be an anchor point with no open end. Be sure to include a safety knot if there is a loose rope end. Since this is the same physical knot as the figure-8 on a bight, it has the same efficiency loss of approximately 20%.

How to Tie the Figure-8 Follow Through

1. Start a figure-8 follow through by tying a loose figure-8 stopper knot. Use about two feet plus enough tail rope to wrap completely around the object to which you will be attaching it.
2. Wrap the tail rope around your point of attachment. Begin feeding it back into the stopper knot at the same point where the tail exits it.
3. Now allow the tail end to follow every bend of this rope as it goes through the stopper knot. That is the follow through. Wherever the stopper goes, so goes the tail end.
4. When it has been completely followed through the short leg (or tail end), the long leg should be issuing from the same side of the knot, so the legs are parallel. It should look exactly like the figure-8 on a bight. It results in the same finished product. You should have enough tail rope to tie a safety.
5. Dress and load this knot in the manner previously described for the figure-8 on a bight.

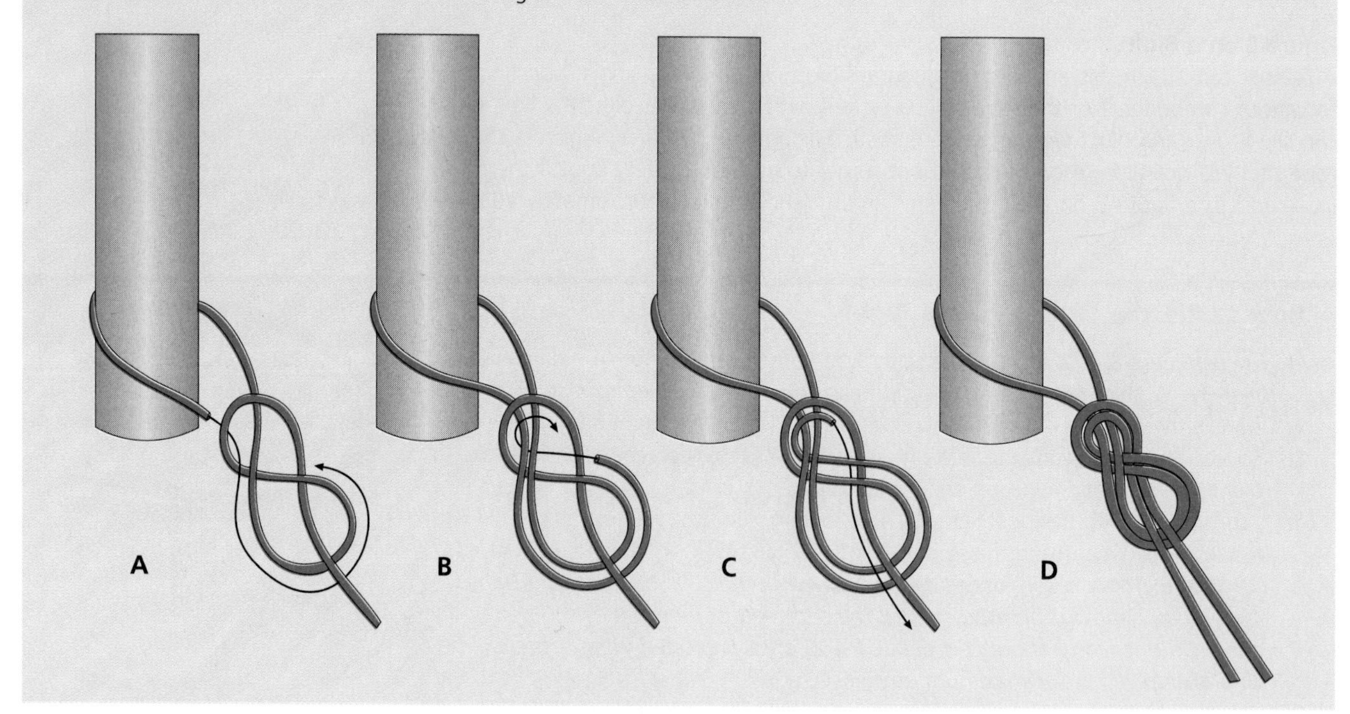

Double-Loop Figure-8

This knot (also called double figure-8 loop) is another anchor knot in the figure-8 family. It is like the figure-8 on a bight, but has two loops instead of one. Rescuers commonly clip these knots into small-diameter carabiners (much too small to meet the four-to-one rule). Using two loops provides more load-bearing surface and slightly better efficiency. The double-loop figure-8 creates an efficiency loss of approximately 18%. Be sure to include a safety knot if there is a loose end.

How to Tie the Double-Loop Figure-8 Knot

1. Start this knot exactly the same way you start the figure-8 on a bight. Use doubled rope and continue until you reach the point where you pass the single-rope bight through the double-rope bight.
2. Grasp the doubled rope about 10 inches or so short of the single bight.
3. Push this part of the doubled rope through the double-rope bight a few inches to create a set of handles. Hold these handles with one hand while holding the single-rope bight with the other.
4. Reach the fingers of one hand through the single-rope bight from the bottom.
5. Continue to bring these fingers over the top of the double-rope bight and grab the two handles created in earlier steps. Release the handles from the other hand.
6. The single-loop bight should now be positioned over the top of the double-rope bight and around the two handles.
7. Continue to hold the handles with one hand. Pull the single-rope bight downward to a point below the base of the knot.
8. Release this single-rope bight and grasp the two legs of the rope with the same hand.
9. Load the knot slightly by pulling the handles (which form the loops for attachment to other components) and the two legs in opposite directions.
10. Dress the knot carefully before completely loading it. This may be one of the most difficult knots to dress. One good way to help dress this knot is to keep the doubled ropes free of twists as you tie it.

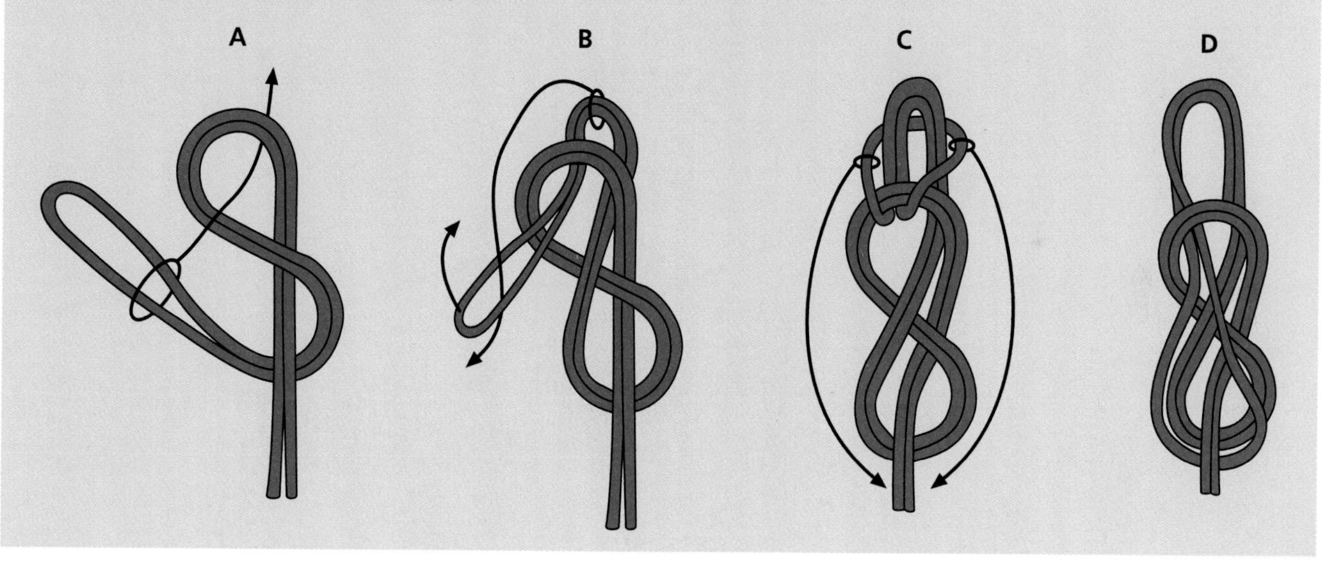

Tensionless Anchor

The tensionless anchor (four-to-one wrap) provides the least loss of strength when anchoring a rope to a rounded, secure anchor point at least four times the diameter of the rope. Since the rope is wrapped around the anchor point, there is no knot in the loaded rope. This means no strength loss due to bends. It should make a minimum of three full wraps. Once loaded, the rope should bind on the first couple of wraps. This leaves the tail rope without tension (thus the term "tensionless"). Thus, a rescuer can tie a secondary or safety knot without losing efficiency in the loaded part of the rope. More wraps may be required on a smooth surface such as a round pipe. Rescuers should be sure to include a safety knot or secure the loose end to a separate anchor system as a backup. They can also use the tensionless anchor on other

WARNING

Be cautious when tying the tensionless anchor around large objects. This can require a significant amount of rope to wrap around the object several times. If the anchor point fails in these situations, the load will drop the length of the rope wrapped around the object. The fall distance may be significant and possibly create a force more than a fall factor of .25.

than round objects. It is recommended that squared edges be rounded out with padding or other material to prevent significant loss of efficiency due to acute bends in the rope.

How to Tie a Tensionless Anchor

1. To tie a tensionless anchor simply wrap the rope around the object until the long leg binds when you pull it. There should be a minimum of three wraps.
2. Leave enough tail rope to create a backup. You can form backups in more than one way. Two common methods are:
   A. You can take the tail end back to a second anchor point and secure it with another anchor knot.
   B. You can tie the tail end with a loop-type knot and clip it back into the long leg of the rope using a carabiner or screw link.
3. Avoid tying the tail end around the long leg because this wrap is subject to movement with constant loading and unloading. Although not likely, this loose moving connection could allow heat damage to the rope from nylon rubbing across nylon.

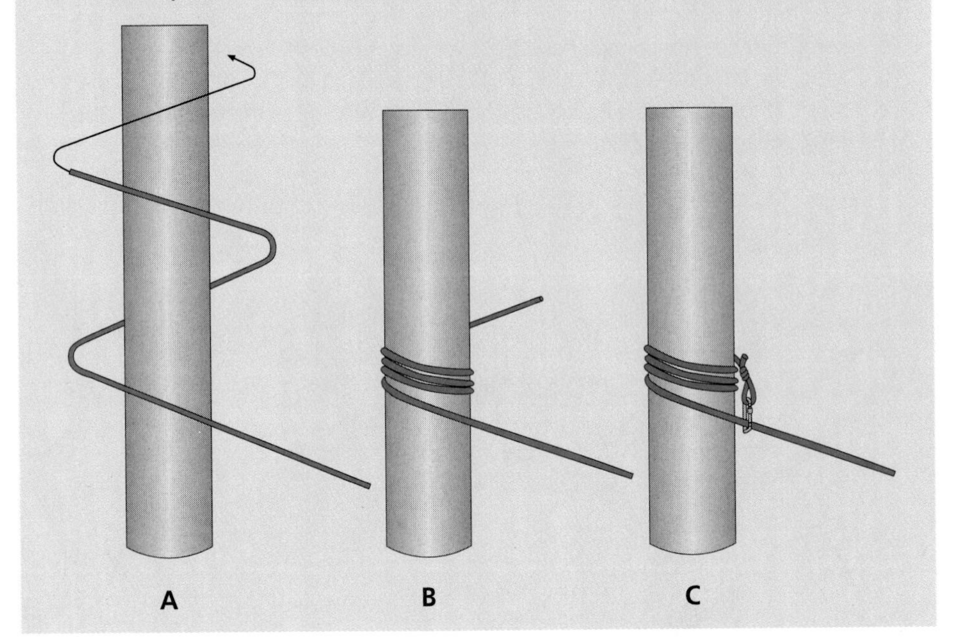

Bowline Knot

This is a traditional fire-service knot that creates a loop that will not slip. Rescuers use it for the same general purpose as the figure-8 anchor knots. It is a good knot for some applications.

There is a great deal of controversy about the bowline knot. When efficiency tests were conducted with laid and braid-on-braid ropes, it was thought that a bowline reduced the efficiency of the rope by 40% to 60%. Modern testing with kernmantle rope indicates the bowline has between 27% and 33% loss. This is only slightly more than knots of the figure-8 family. A bowline knot requires very little rope to tie and works very well in most anchoring applications.

The bowline does have a serious disadvantage. Rescuers should never use it as a running knot (one moving over an edge). It is possible for a bowline to hang on an edge and become untied. Rescuers should only use the bowline in static (nonmoving) applications, and always tie off its tail end with a safety.

How to Tie the Bowline Knot

Whatever method you use, tie the bowline knot around a closed-end object. It is not always possible to tie the knot and slip the loop over an open end. The following method works around a closed-end object. Remember the phrase "equal opportunity knot" as you use the following method.

1. Start by wrapping the tail end of the rope around the object to which you will attach.
2. Allow the short leg to cross OVER the long leg, forming a loop.
3. Bring the tail end under and around the long leg to form a big overhand knot around the object.
4. Hold the short leg in one hand while supporting the long leg in the other. DO NOT pull or hold tension on the long leg of the rope.
5. Pull quickly and steadily on the short leg of the rope until it rolls. This should create a loop in the long leg of the rope with the short leg running through it.
6. At the beginning of this knot the short leg was passed over the long leg. Since this is an equal opportunity knot, now pass the short leg UNDER the long leg.
7. Continue to wrap the short leg of the rope around the long leg and pass the tail end through the loop in the long leg from the top.
8. The short leg should end on the inside of the large loop formed around the object to which you are attaching the rope.
9. Carefully load the knot by grasping the tail rope and the part of the loop beside it with one hand while pulling on the long leg with the other hand. Pull in opposite directions until loaded tightly. This knot usually dresses itself well as long as all the slack is removed from all ropes within the knot.

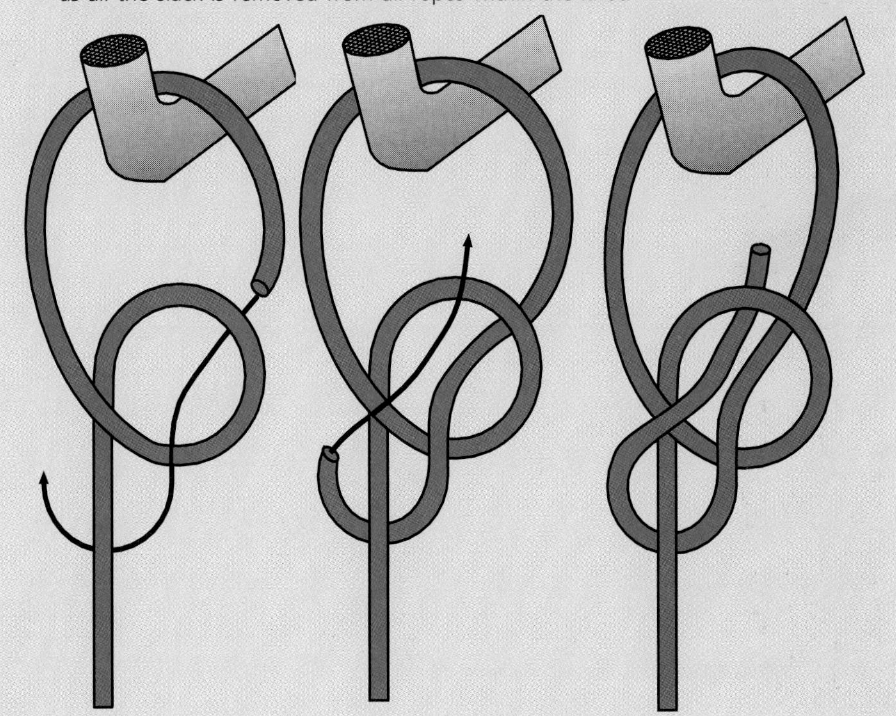

Clove Hitch

Another traditional fire-service knot, the clove hitch is an anchor hitch often tied to rounded, horizontally or vertically configured anchor points. This hitch is sometimes tied with webbing as well as rope. Rescuers should always back up this hitch with a knot by wrapping the tail end around the anchor again and securing it back to the long leg of the rope with a safety. Or they can secure the loose end to a secondary anchor system. The same word of caution about tensionless anchor applies to the clove hitch. If anchored around very large objects it may take a great deal of rope. This could create significant falls if the primary anchor point fails and allows the rope to unravel. Rescuers should consider this factor when choosing anchor points.

How to Tie the Clove Hitch Knot

We will present two methods for tying this knot. In the midline method, you tie the knot in the middle of the rope and slip it over the anchor point. In the other technique, you tie the knot in the end of the rope around a closed-end anchor point. You should learn both methods.

Midline Method

1. To follow the midline method, start by holding the rope in front of you with both hands to form a horizontal plane.
2. Form two counterclockwise loops, one with each hand. You should end up holding the top of a loop with each hand.
3. If you formed the loops with counterclockwise twisting, you should pass the right-hand loop in front of the left-hand loop. This forms the clove hitch.
4. Carefully holding the loops together, slip them over the object to which you wish to attach. Pull both legs of the rope to tighten.
5. If a tail end is present, tie a safety as described in the following method.

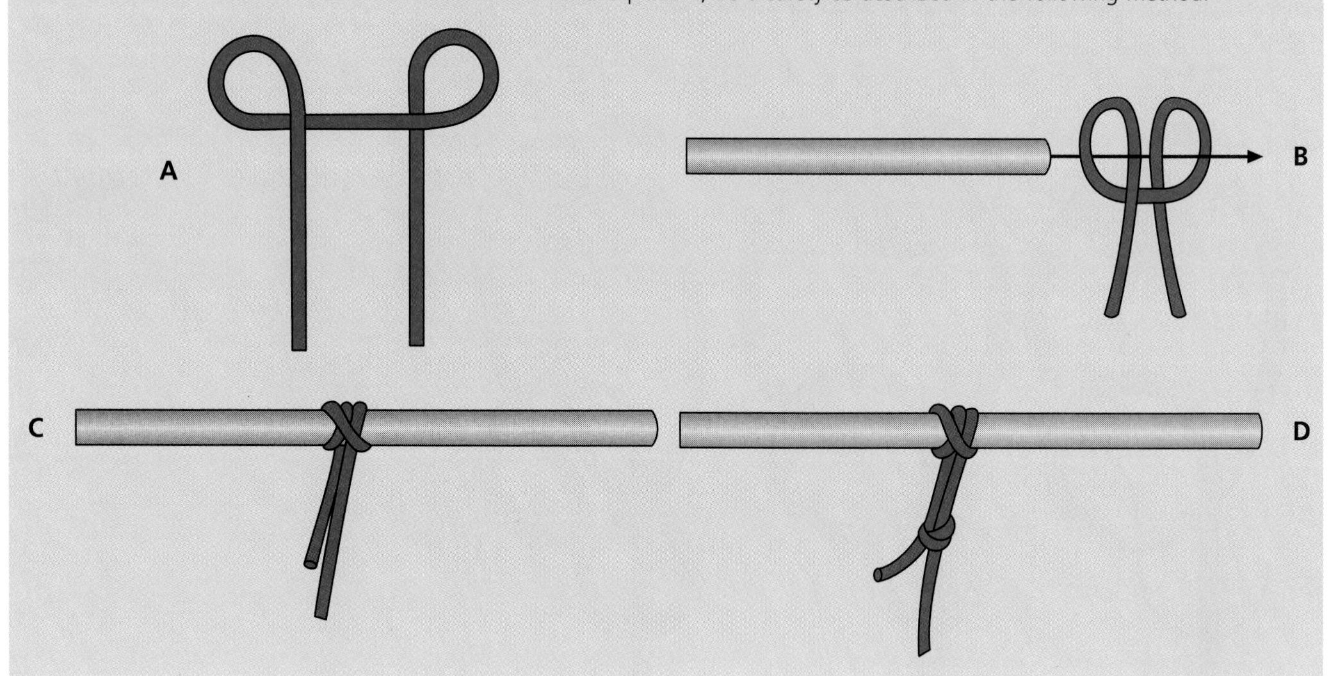

Working End Method

The working end method is most easily tied around a horizontal object such as a beam or pipe.

1. Starting from the top, wrap the end of the rope around the object used as an anchor point.
2. Continue to pass it around the object to create a round turn. The rope should cross over itself in a half hitch, forming an X.
3. Hold the X with the fingers of one hand while continuing to wrap the rope around the object again.
4. Pass the tail end through the underside of the second loop to form another half hitch on the other side of the X.
5. To tighten, pull the long leg and short leg in opposite directions.
6. Safety the tail end. Bring it back to a second object and secure with another anchor knot. Or wrap it around the object again and tie a safety knot around the long leg.
7. Before you tie a safety knot around the long leg, first wrap the tail rope around the object again. If you do not take this extra wrap, the knot will open slightly when loaded, possibly creating slippage.

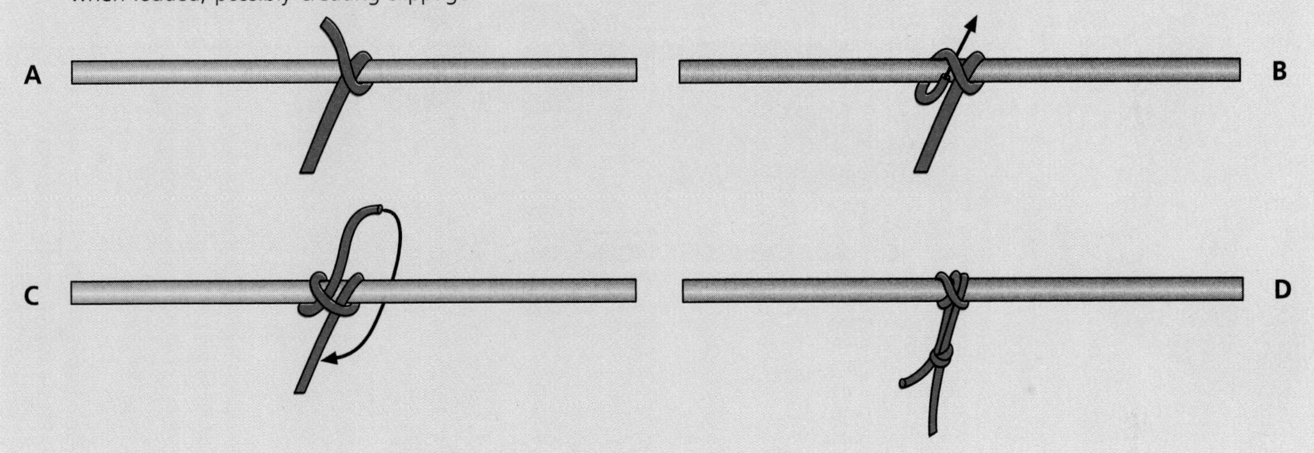

Joining Ropes

Knots used for joining ropes meet the classification of a "bend," although they may not include the term in their names. Bends are commonly used to form a loop of rope such as the Prusik loop. Rescuers can also use a bend to tie two ropes together when a single length of rope is not long enough. The bends in the following section include those intended for load-bearing applications, except the square knot, which is absolutely discouraged for life loading. It has specific applications that will be addressed later in this text.

Figure-8 Bend

Rescuers use the figure-8 bend (Flemish bend) to join two load-bearing ropes of equal or slightly unequal diameter. This knot is a more secure knot than the traditional fire service knot known as the "becket" or "sheet bend." It is formed in much the same way as the figure-8 follow through. The difference is that the rope feeds through in the opposite direction to create two tail ends instead of one. Rescuers should secure both of these tails with safety knots. The figure-8 bend creates an efficiency loss of approximately 19%.

How to Tie the Figure-8 Bend Knot

Tie the figure-8 bend knot in almost the same way as the figure-8 follow through.

1. Tie a loose figure-8 stopper in one rope. Leave about a foot of tail to later form a safety knot.
2. Pass the end of the other rope into the stopper knot at the point where its tail end exits.
3. Follow every bend of the stopper knot with the tail end of the other rope.
4. When complete, the tail ends of the two ropes should exit opposite sides of the knot.
5. Dress the knot carefully and tie safety knots in both tail ends.

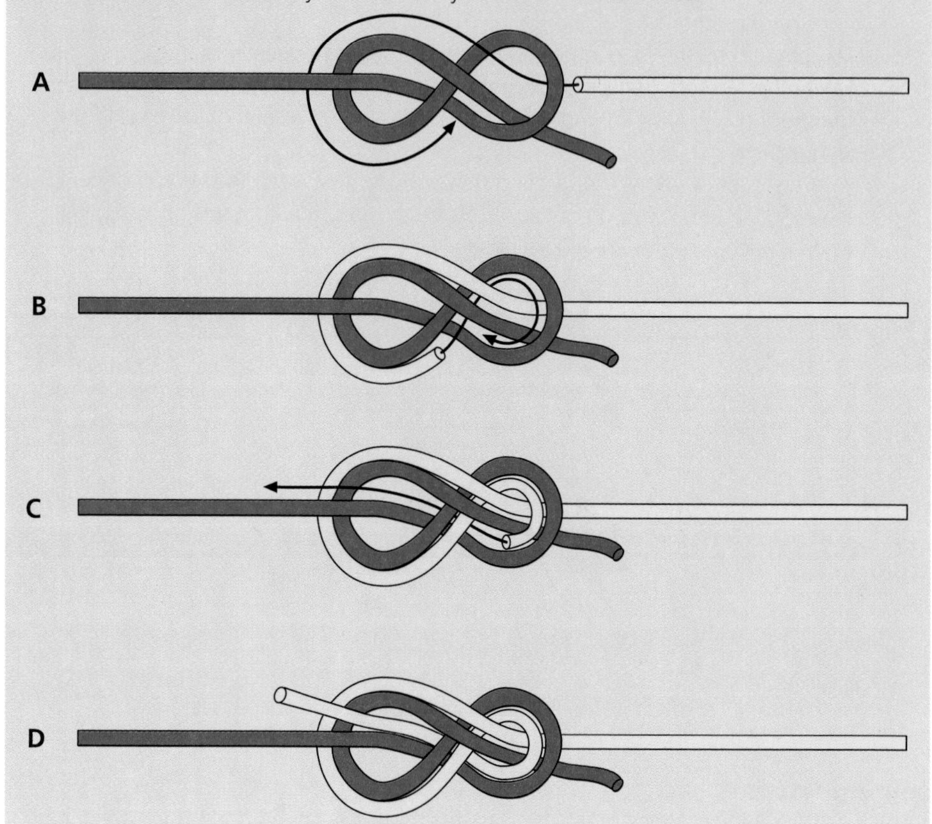

Double Fisherman's Knot

This is another knot (also called grapevine knot) used to tie two load-bearing ropes together. This knot is more suited to ropes of equal diameter. Because of its compact nature, it is commonly used in Prusik loops or when knots must be passed around objects. The double fisherman's knot has the advantage of requiring no safeties. This makes it extremely compact in comparison to the figure-8 bend. The double fisherman's knot creates an efficiency loss of approximately 21%.

How to Tie the Double Fisherman's Knot

To tie the double fisherman's knot:

1. Hold the two ropes horizontally and parallel to each other with the tail ends pointing in opposite directions.
2. Using one tail rope, tie a barrel hitch around the second tail rope. This knot slides on the rope.
3. Repeat this process on the other side by tying another barrel hitch with the second tail rope.
4. Be sure you tie the second barrel hitch in the opposite direction from the first barrel hitch.
5. Dress and tighten both barrel hitches well.
6. Create the double fisherman's knot by pulling the long legs of each rope in opposite directions. This should allow the barrel hitches to slide together, forming the knot.
7. Safety knots are not required on barrel hitches.

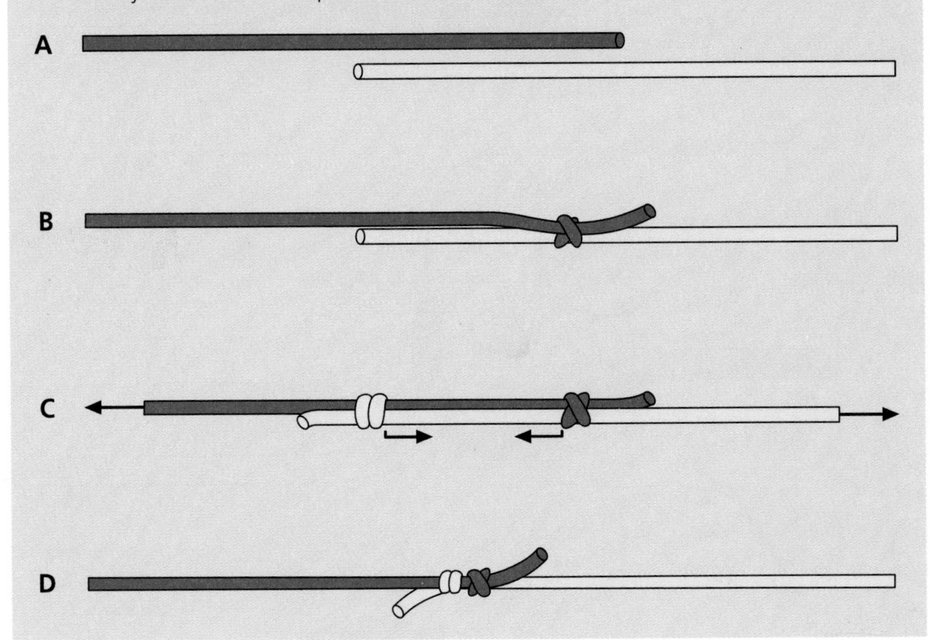

Square Knot

Use this knot to bind together two rope ends of the same diameter.

Like the figure-8 bend, the square knot has two tail ends that must be secured with safeties. Rescuers can use the square knot for tying loose ends of rope together when they must remove all slack. Examples include certain rope bridles for litters rigged in a vertical position. You must configure these bridles so the square knot will not take the load of the litter. Since the square knot should not be load bearing, inefficiency is not a concern.

WARNING

The square knot is responsible for more injuries than any other knot. Do not use it for bearing human loads.

How to Tie the Square Knot

Use a traditional fire service method to tie the square knot.

1. Start by holding the ends of both ropes, one in each hand.
2. Pass the left over and around the right to form an overhand.
3. Change hands.
4. Pass the right over and around the left forming a second overhand on top of the first.
5. Pull the two tail ends tight to form the square knot.
6. Always tie each tail around its respective long legs with safety knots.

This is the safest method of tying the square knot. It can also be tied starting with the right over the left and following with the left over the right.

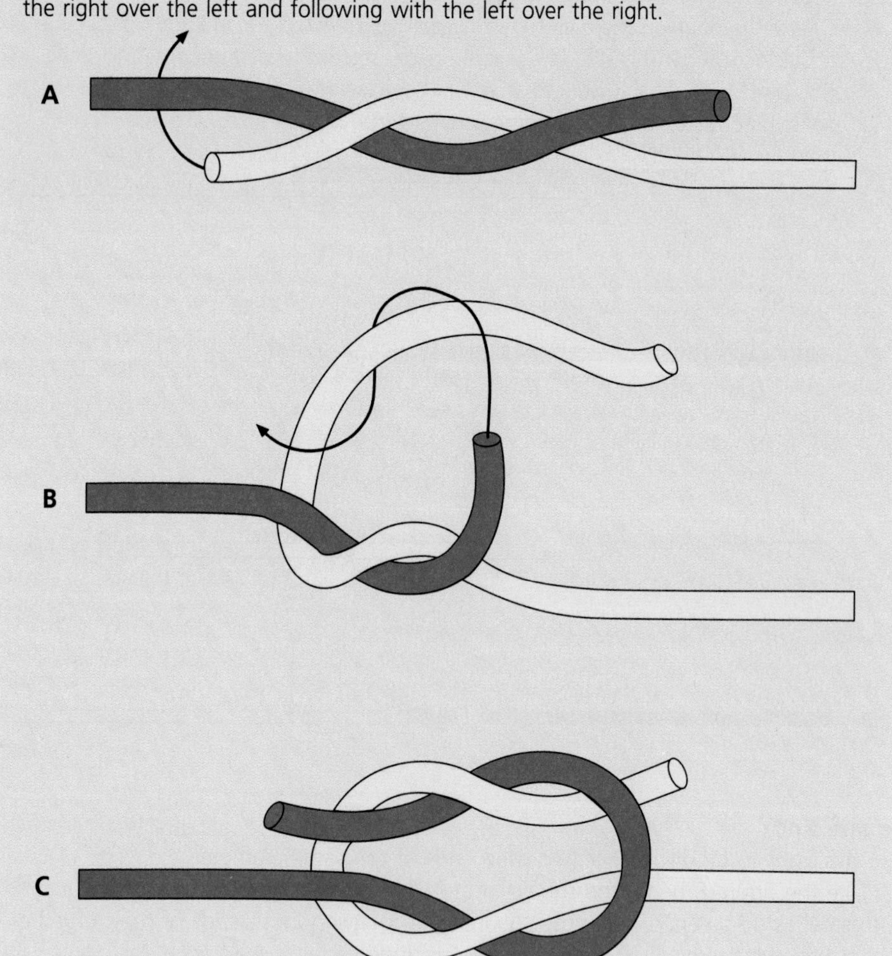

WARNING

Whatever method you use to tie a square knot, you must finish with both tail ends emerging from either the top or the bottom of the knot. If the tail ends issue from opposite sides (one from the top and the other from the bottom), it is not a square knot and will slip easily when force is applied to the long legs in opposite directions.

Special-Purpose Knots

Butterfly Knot

The butterfly knot is designed to take a pull in three directions. It is to knots what the triangular screw link is to hardware. To rig anchoring systems, rescuers can sometimes use a butterfly to create a bridle to change the rope path. They can tie off a rope to two anchor points, leaving slack rope between. They can then tie a butterfly in this slack line at the desired location to form an anchor point for a rope or rope system. The legs of the knot that create this bridle should be maintained at an angle less than 120 degrees to prevent overstressing the rope and its anchors. This application is discussed further in chapter 5, Rigging.

You can use the butterfly anytime a pull in more than two directions is required. It is considered to be a midline knot, so no safeties are required. The butterfly knot creates an efficiency loss of approximately 25%.

How to Tie a Butterfly Knot

To tie a butterfly knot:

1. Start by placing any part of the rope in the palm of one hand. It does not matter which end goes in what direction. Position your hand horizontally with the thumb side up and the palm facing you.
2. Wrap the rope so it loosely emerges from the top of your palm around the width of your hand. Allow the rope to cross itself in the palm. The rope should cross toward the wrist rather than toward the fingers.
3. Wrap the rope around loosely again making sure this loop is nearest the wrist. Make sure the loop at the bottom is on the same side of the long leg as the first loop where they emerge from the bottom of the palm.
4. There should now be three wraps of rope in your palm, each one progressively closer to your wrist.
5. Pull the middle wrap away from your palm, toward your wrist and over the one loop. This creates somewhat of a bight with the middle wrap of rope.
6. Now push the bight underneath the remaining wraps in the palm. The bight should travel between the wraps and the surface of your palm and in the direction of the fingers, away from the wrist.
7. Tighten the knot slightly by pulling the bight (which creates the attachment loop for the knot) with one hand while pulling the two legs of rope in the opposite direction with the other hand.
8. To form the butterfly, grasp the two legs, one in each hand, and pull them in opposite directions. This forces the knot to "roll," creating the butterfly. If you have trouble making the knot roll, popping the legs apart several times should do the trick.
9. Load the knot by pulling the loop and rope legs in all directions until all slack is removed. This knot usually dresses itself.

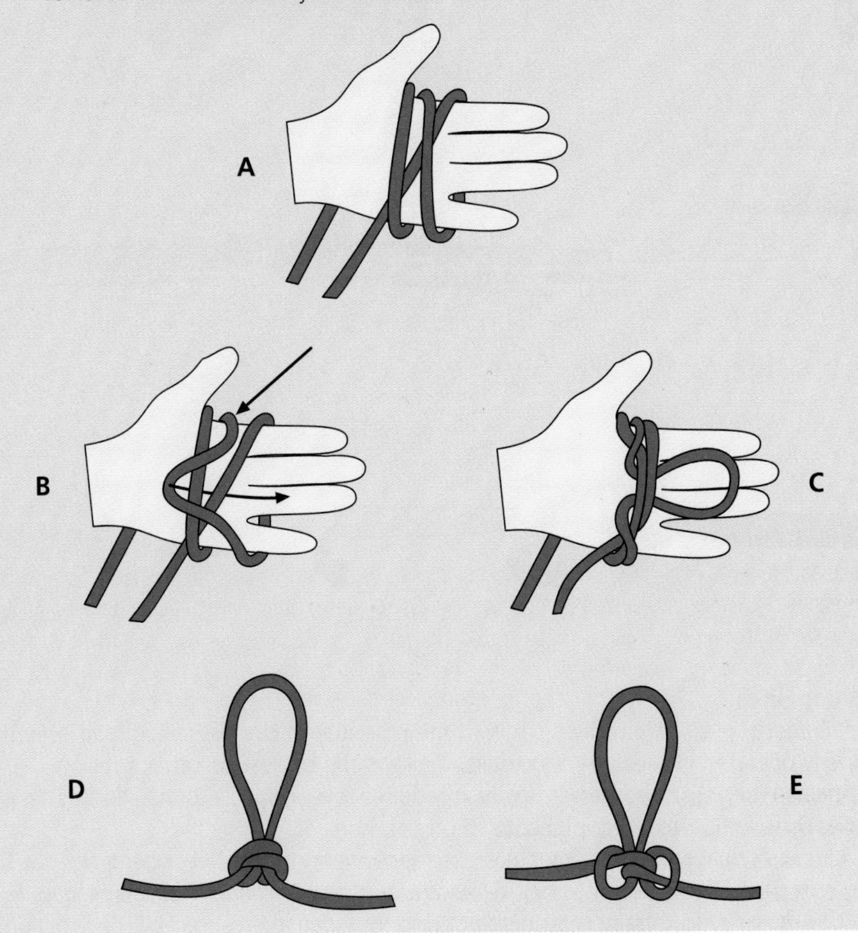

Water Knot

Rescuers use this knot (also called ring bend, tape knot, ribbon knot) specifically to tie two pieces of webbing together for bearing human loads. It is the most appropriate knot for this purpose. It is, in effect, an overhand bend. It is very important to properly dress the water knot and tie both tail ends with safety knots. If the webbing twists in the knot, the webbing can slip. The water knot can create an efficiency loss up to approximately 36%.

How to Tie the Water Knot

To tie the water knot:

1. Using one of the webbing ends, tie a loose overhand knot. Flatten the knot to avoid twists. Leave 8 to 10 inches of tail for a safety knot.
2. Feed the end of the other piece of webbing into the overhand knot at the point where the tail end exits.
3. Follow each bend of the webbing in the overhand knot with the tail end of the other piece of webbing.
4. When completed, a tail of webbing should emerge from each side of the knot.
5. Dress the knot carefully to ensure that there are no twists in the webbing.
6. Load the knot by pulling the long leg and short leg on each side of the knot in opposite directions.
7. Secure with tail. Do this by tying each tail around the long leg on the respective side with an overhand knot.

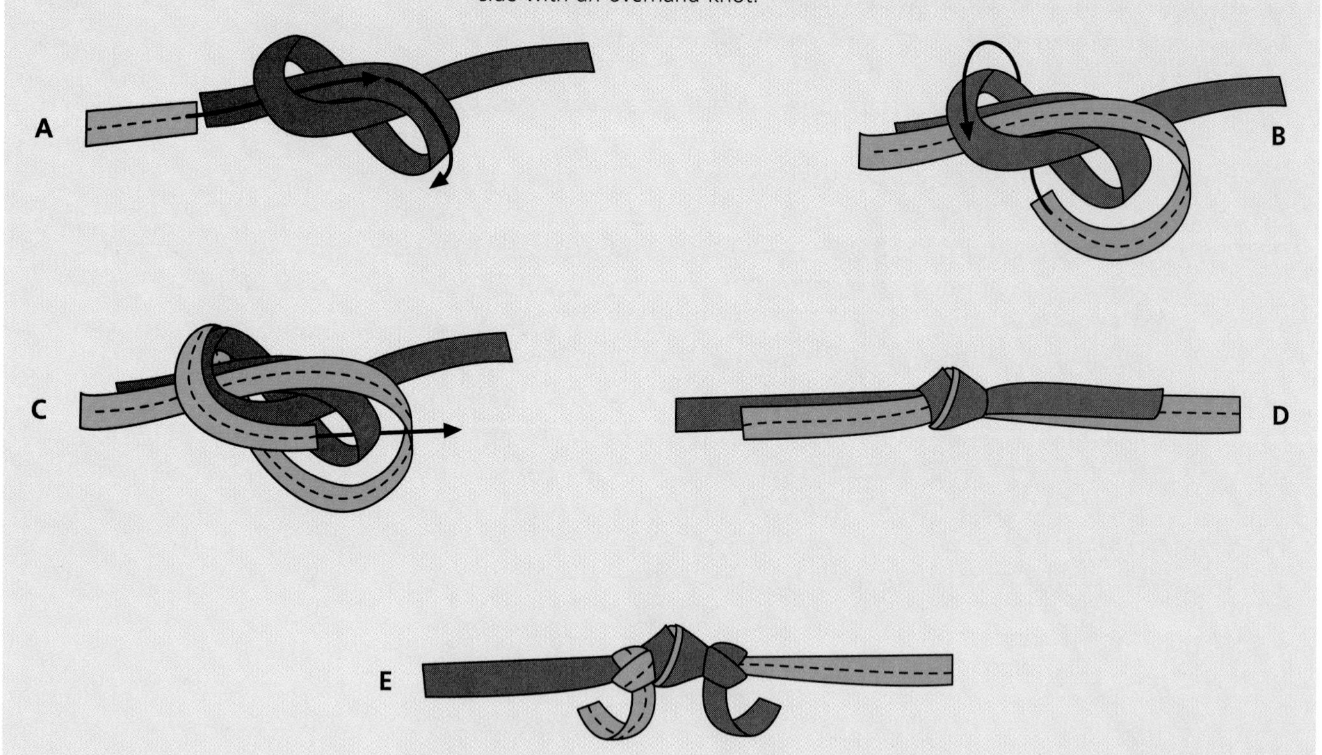

Munter Hitch

The Munter is used as a belay hitch with the potential to catch a falling load. When properly operated in relatively short falls, it allows the belayer to catch a falling one-person load. For two-person loads, it requires several special precautions. These applications will be covered in chapter 6 on belaying.

Although the Munter is sometimes used for lowering a load, it is generally not recommended for this use. It might damage the rope when operated under load. In addition, some rescue trainers suspect possible rope damage caused by rope friction within the hitch when operated under load. At this time, this concern is not supported by testing. Further testing is required to reach a more objective conclusion.

The efficiency of the Munter hitch is not known. However, it survived significant repeated impacts with two-person loads during belay competency testing conducted in early 1994. Since the hitch is used in a belay system that should only be loaded if the primary system fails, this reaction to impact loading is very significant.

How to Tie the Munter Hitch

To tie the Munter hitch:

1. Start the Munter in the same way you would tie a midline clove hitch.
2. Instead of passing one loop in front of the other, fold the two loops together in either direction. It does not matter which direction.
3. Clip the doubled rope at the top of the hitch into a carabiner for belaying. An extra-large carabiner is preferred. The Munter's operation will be covered in the chapter on belaying. Safety knots are not needed.

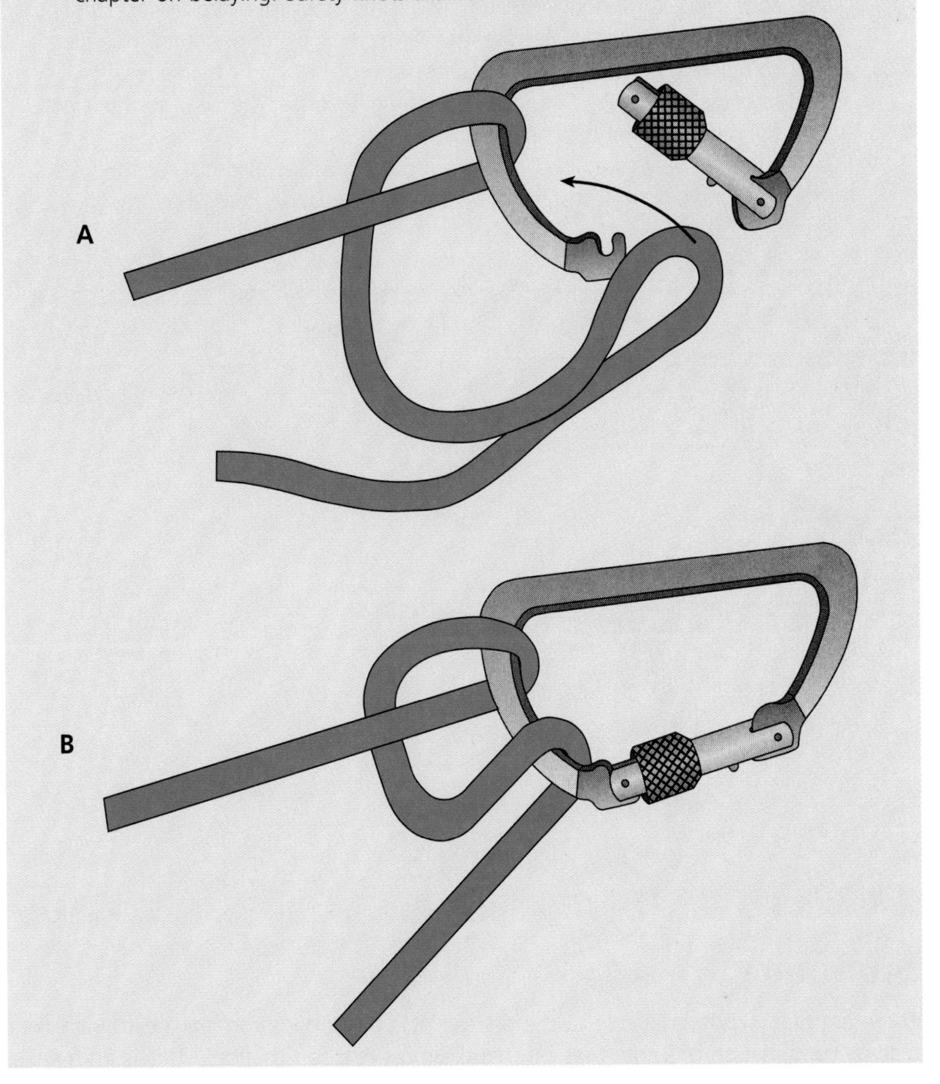

Prusik Hitch

The Prusik hitch is formed with a loop of small-diameter accessory cord wrapped around a large-diameter rescue rope. Lengths, diameters, and number of wraps can vary depending on the specific application. A girth hitch (lark's foot) is basically a single-wrap Prusik. Rescuers can use it in a variety of applications for hitching rope and webbing to a point in the rope system. The double-wrap and triple-wrap Prusik hitches are used to form rope grabs in various rope systems. Some of these applications include certain types of self-rescue, ascending a rope, and rope grabs in hauling systems. Tandem triple-wrap Prusiks can also be effective as a belay device for one- and two-person loads. These applications will be covered later in this text.

The knot used to tie the accessory cord in a Prusik loop (usually a double fisherman's knot) should be offset to prevent it from being dead center of the loop for attachment. The exact efficiency of Prusik hitches are not known but both the double- and triple-wrap Prusiks usually slip before breaking.

How to Tie a Prusik Hitch

To tie a Prusik knot:

1. Place the bend used for creating the accessory cord loop at the desired point on the rope.
2. Wrap this bend around the rope the appropriate number of times. (Once for a lark's foot, twice for a double-wrap Prusik, three times for a triple-wrap Prusik). Be sure that the bend stays between the wraps as they form around the rope.
3. After completing the wraps, pull the accessory cord toward either side of the bend to complete the Prusik knot. This will slightly offset the bend so it will not be in the middle of the attachment point.
4. Dress this knot very carefully. If it is not properly dressed, it can slip on the rope instead of grabbing it. Constantly reassess the Prusik knot to ensure proper form.

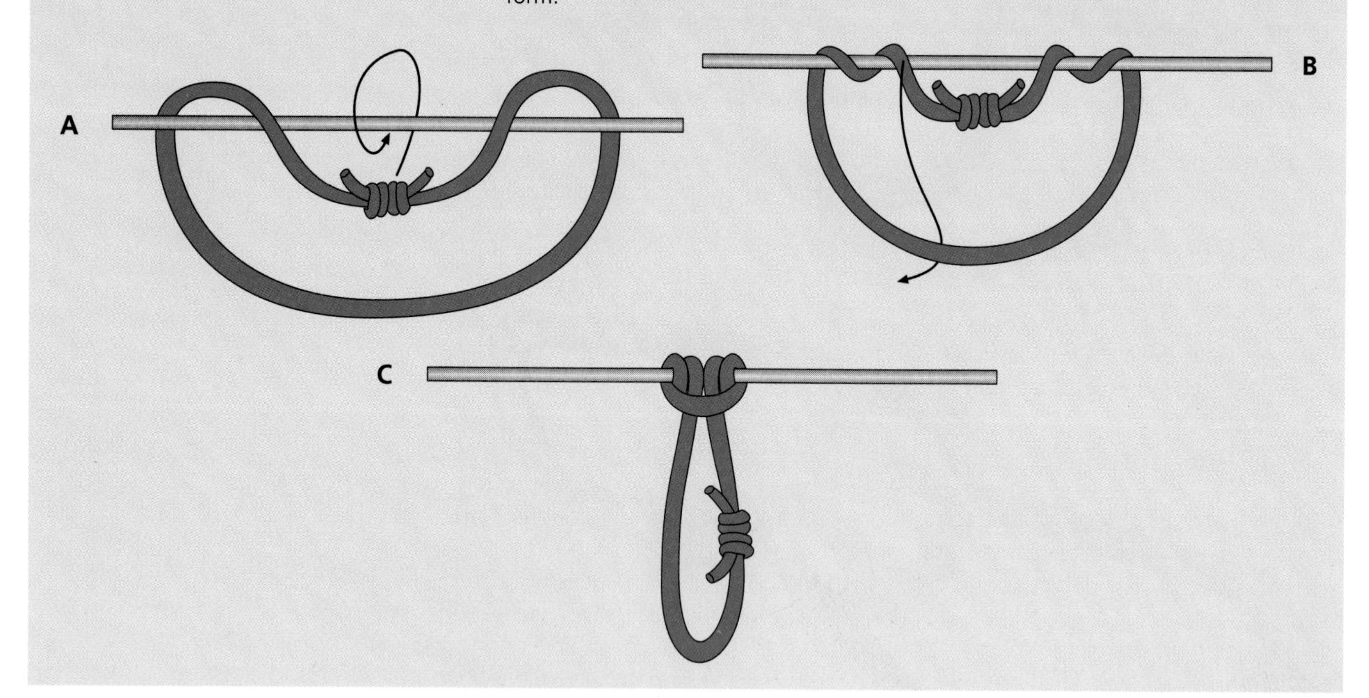

Summary

There are many knots available to the rescuer. It is a good idea to learn extremely well a small combination of knots that can handle most rescue situations. This is preferable to learning many knots that have the same purpose and learning none of them well. Remember . . .

1. PRACTICE.
2. PRACTICE.
3. PRACTICE!

CHAPTER 5

Anchoring & Rigging

The information in this chapter is provided as a basis for continued training. Each rescuer should consult with his or her own team leader for the correct SOGs for the team.

Topics covered in this chapter include

- Principles of Anchoring
- Anchoring Configurations
- General Rigging Precautions

Introduction

Rigging, a term constantly used in rescue work, is the assembly of rope and hardware used to form anchoring and associated rope rescue systems. Or, more simply put, rigging is a group of components used together to create a rope system.

Rigging is not an exact science. Deciding the best way to rig for a particular situation requires experience, ingenuity, and good judgment. Because there are so many ways to accomplish the same task, it is important for rescuers to become very familiar with rigging techniques. In deciding which method to use, the rescuer must base their decision on all the factors surrounding the incident.

Most importantly, rescuers should not make things complicated. Remember KIS—keep it simple. Don't start by building the most complicated and equipment-intensive system possible. Start with the simplest, most efficient method.

With the many choices available, rescuers must have a solid grasp of the safety principles involved in rigging so that they can use their ingenuity and experience to put these principles into practice. Practice and preplanning will enable both rescuer and the trainer to sharpen skills and create the most efficient, safe, appropriate rigging system for the incident at hand.

Principles of Anchoring

With the strength of modern rigging components, one could overlook the real foundation of the entire rope rescue system: the anchor system. It does no good to have components with breaking strengths more than 10,000 pounds if the strength of the system to which they are anchored is only 1,000 pounds. This section will look at materials and construction of anchor points, along with some common anchoring systems and configurations tailored to the industrial environment. There are other types of anchoring systems, some more suited to wilderness applications, however this text will focus on systems that streamline the rescue operation in the industrial environment.

Anchor Points

Anchor systems are the foundation of the total rope rescue system. The term here is anchor system rather than anchor points because rescuers usually rig more than one point in some combination to form the completed anchorage to which they will attach the rest of the rope system.

Most industrial facilities have plenty of strong anchor points. Consequently, industrial rescuers should not use anchor points considered too weak to hold the entire load. This does not mean that rescuers should never worry about the possibility of failure. On the contrary, they consider most anchor points as questionable at best and back them up. Considering all anchor points as having the potential to fail makes it harder for a rescuer to make errors in judgment when trying to decide whether to back them up. A point to remember about anchors: things are not always what they appear to be.

Steel

Structural steel is usually the strongest material for anchors. There is usually plenty of this around industrial sites in the form of steel beams and beam projections. Beams are the most desired anchor points. Other structural steel items may include:

- **Stairwell support beams**
- **Supports for large machinery**
- **Davits**—These are boom arms designed for use as anchor points when lifting large pieces of machinery and certain other heavy items. A plant engineer can verify that a particular davit is in good shape and designed to hold the expected system loads. They may look great, but wear and abuse can make davits poor choices for anchor points.
- **Welded steel handrails**—There are many very strong handrails in existence. Examine the construction and securement first. Check the following:
    - Is it heavy-gauge steel? Avoid lightweight, weak metals such as aluminum.
    - Is it welded or bolted securely to structural members? Check the welds or bolts to see if they are broken or otherwise insecure. When you kick the handrail, is it shaky or does it shake you? These methods are not conclusive but will help you evaluate the handrail's strength.
    - How many points of attachment to structural members does the handrail have? The more of the railing secured to structural members, the better.
- **Large-diameter steel pipe**—It should be well supported. Make sure it is welded or bolted at the joints. Look for the same things in pipe you would look for in handrails. Try to anchor near the more stable attachment points. If you use standpipe risers, avoid attachment near joints. Try attaching near the floor, if possible.

Some metal items *to avoid* using as anchors include:

- **Insulated pipe**—The insulation is there because the pipe is either hot or cold. It might be too hot for your rope. Besides, the metal housing often used to cover the insulation can crimp under a load, possibly creating a sharp edge that will cut your rope or webbing. Also, insulation can disguise the pipe's actual diameter and other factors that determine strength.
- **Lightweight or unsupported handrails**
- **Instrument stands**—These are often designed only to hold a gauge or another instrument in place and may not be structural. Check to see whether they are properly attached to a structural member such as a beam or whether they are only welded to the deck plate.
- **Fire hydrants or monitors**—The flanged connections of these pipes are often secured with Break-away bolts to prevent vehicles from damaging them severely when run over. These flanges may be below grade and not visible for inspection. It is also possible that they may need to be used for fire suppression while you are using them for an anchor point.
- **Corroded metals**—This applies to any potential anchor point, despite its construction. Chemicals may degrade structural steel over a time, making it unreliable or abrasive to rope or webbing. If you decide to use it anyway, pad sharp edges that the rigging may cross.
- **Cast-iron or small-diameter threaded pipes**—Cast iron is a brittle metal and should always be avoided for anchorage. You should avoid small-diameter threaded pipes because corrosion can eat through the thin threaded interior wall without visible warning and cause failure.

- **Rooftop air-conditioning units**—These are present on many standard building roofs. Before considering them as an anchor, be certain they are large and structurally attached to the roof. These units have been known to slide across a roof under the weight of a two-person load.
- **Vent pipes**—These are on roofs of many standard buildings. These ventilation pipes are not structural and absolutely must be avoided.

Masonry

Masonry is generally the second best material for anchor points. But not just any old masonry will do. Rescuers should only use structural masonry with large bulk. Here are some good examples:

- **Reinforced structural concrete columns or beams.** Be certain the beam you think is solid is not hollow. Many hollow beams with masonry materials appear to be huge structural members. Tap them with a hammer or other solid object. Often you can tell by the sound that is made. If you are not sure, ask the building engineer.
- **Brick or other masonry work with large bulk.** An example is the whole corner wall of a building or something similar to it. When rigging around a brick or block wall section, the section should be larger than life. Watch out for a brick or block parapet. Wrapping through a drain opening and around the brick or block may not provide enough bulk. Make sure the parapet is very large and well supported. You must also judge its condition according to age and exposure to weather and chemicals.

Avoid the following types of masonry:

- **Brick or block work without bulk.** A few rows of brick or block will not do; it is not stable or strong enough to be an anchor point.
- **Masonry that shows signs of degradation.** Look for signs of structural instability such as crumbling, cracks, spalling, and other degrading.

Vehicles

When there are no other anchor points, rescuers may be able to use vehicles for anchoring. The advantage of vehicles is that they can be placed where needed. When possible, use large vehicles such as fire apparatus. There have been reports of smaller vehicles sliding on the smooth surface of a parking garage during rope rescue incidents. This is not usually a problem in the industrial environment, although some warehouses have very smooth floor surfaces. Just be aware of this possibility and be cautious. There are some strict safety guidelines that you must follow when anchoring to any vehicle.

- **Secure the vehicle**—Use the following methods.
  - If possible, position the vehicle at a right angle to the direction of pull. This should provide maximum protection from vehicle movement.
  - Set the parking brake.
  - Place the transmission in "Park" if it is an automatic, in "Reverse" (if the pull is from the front of the vehicle) if a manual transmission.
  - Chock the wheels on both the front and back.
  - Remove the keys from the ignition. There are true stories about training exercises in which rescuers died when an emergency call was received and the fire chief drove off with the anchor point. Do not let it happen to you! Many emergency vehicles do not need keys for starting. In these cases, always station a guard with the vehicle. If you are short of personnel, you can turn off the master switch with all lights and sirens in the "on" position. This can alert the driver when the battery switch is turned on.
- **Anchor to structural parts** such as axles and cross members in the frame. Avoid tow eyes unless they are of closed construction and structurally welded to the frame. Do not tie off to bumpers.

- **Avoid sharp edges, battery acid, axle grease, oil,** and so on when rigging with rope or webbing. You will encounter all these nasty little problems when anchoring to a vehicle. If your software gets saturated with oil or grease, get rid of it. If it contacts battery acid (the silent killer), get rid of it. It is better to replace it than risk using damaged equipment. The manufacturer of the software can provide information on cleaning or decontamination procedures, if they are even possible.
- **Watch out for hot exhaust pipes, mufflers, and other heat sources**—These can cause serious heat damage to nylon software.

Natural Anchors

Large rocks are not usually found in the industrial environment. But there may be a few trees around. If there is a choice between a tree and the steel beam beside it, use the stronger anchor point—the beam. You can get more information on natural anchors from a wilderness rescue book. But, in general, trees should have the following characteristics before you consider them for rescue anchor points:

- **They should be LARGE and rooted deeply.** Some apparently big trees have very shallow root systems and may not hold up to the demands of the rope rescue system.
- **They must be alive.** Dead trees, even big ones, can crack and break. There have been cases in which the anchor point collapsed under its own weight during moderately windy conditions. Inspect the tree for greenery and other signs that suggest life.

Window Washer Eye Bolts

Some industrial facilities have multistory office buildings with engineered rooftop anchor points for window-washing equipment. These window washer eye bolts are engineered to be very strong if they are constructed according to building codes governing their installation. Consider the following precautions first:

- **You can often use window washer eye bolts,** but back them up. These bolts are most often designed to be used with a cantilever device that creates a straight up pull. These bolts work well when pulled from the top but not as well when pulled from the side. Unfortunately, that is how rescuers usually attach to them—from the side. Window washer eye bolts have been known to bend when pulled from the side. To be safe, back them up to another anchor point just in case.
- **Do not confuse window washer eye bolts with guy wire hooks.** Window washer eye bolts are usually $\frac{3}{4}$-inch closed-eye steel bolts with a bevel design planted in around 9 inches of structural concrete, double washered and double nutted. Guy wire hooks are used to secure guy wires to stabilize such items as antennae. Guy wire hooks are usually $\frac{1}{2}$-inch (or smaller) open-eye bolts. They are not designed to be attached to anything of significant bulk or weight.

Wooden Building Structures

Wooden structures can be good anchor points but many considerations are necessary. Follow the same rules for brick and block: GO FOR BULK! Grab a whole corner wall or something really big. Also consider the age and condition of the building.

Certainly there are other anchor points not mentioned here. Good anchor points are usually abundant in industry. As many as there may be, all anchor points generally fall into one of two categories: questionable or bombproof.

Anchor Point Safety—Questionable or Bombproof

As already discussed, always be suspicious about any anchor point. Use only good strong anchor points, but always assume the potential for failure. Some anchor points are so structurally significant that, if they were to fail, it would cause the collapse of the structure. These are generally called "bombproof anchors." In industrial and structural environments they would be large steel I-beams or structural concrete columns. Remember, if there is a question in the mind of any person on a rescue team, consider the anchor point questionable. In this case, the term "questionable" is not meant to imply that an anchor point is weak or likely to fail. This "questionable" anchor point is expected to be individually strong enough to support the entire load. We have referred to the two types of anchor points as "questionable" and "bombproof." But in the rescue environment it may be more appropriate to call them "strong" and "indestructible." Make sure all the anchor points in your system qualify as either strong or indestructible.

Backing Up Anchor Points

As strong as anchor points might be, most authorities still recommend some form of backup to compensate for extraordinary circumstances. Any questionable anchor point should be backed up with an additional anchor point. With the bombproof anchor points, no backup is required since the anchor point is not in question. Classifying an anchor point as questionable or bombproof is a subjective process. It is a good idea to err on the side of safety by backing up any anchor point that might have the slightest possibility of failure. If you have any doubt as to whether the anchor point you have chosen is bombproof, treat it as questionable and back it up.

A backup system for an anchor point involves the use of at least one other anchor point. Usually, a primary anchor point is backed up by a secondary anchor point. It is a very simple and practical system for the industrial/structural environment as long as certain conditions are met:

- **Do not use multiple poor anchors in an attempt to create one strong anchor.** Choose anchor points individually that are strong enough to support the potential forces produced by the entire rope system.
- **Secondary anchor points should be at least as strong as the primary anchor point.** If the secondary is weaker than the primary, the chances of it holding if the primary point fails are not good.
- **The secondary anchor point should be, as much as possible, directly behind and in line with the primary anchor.**
  - If you do not position the secondary anchor behind the primary, there could be a serious shock load in case of failure.
  - Try to make the secondary anchor point in line with the direction of the system's pull. If the secondary is far enough out of line and the primary fails, there will be at least some degree of pendulum and a serious potential for shock loading.
  - Pendulum of the rope can be very dangerous. Consider, for example, if you have placed rope over an edge covered with metal flashing. This may work if you protect the edge sufficiently at that point to prevent rope damage. If however, the primary anchor point fails and the secondary is not in line, the rope will swing into alignment with the second anchor point from the force of the load. If you have not protected the entire edge that the rope travels across, it will slide across the sharp metal flashing, severing the rope. If you cannot get directly in line, anticipate the expected travel of the rope and protect sharp edges along the entire path before you load the system. It is not always possible to get the secondary in exact alignment with the primary, but get the best alignment you can.

Backing up Bombproof Anchor Points

Anchor points considered bombproof are not in question and, consequently, require no backup. Before deciding to rig to any single anchor point, consider carefully your choice. If anybody doubts the integrity of the anchor point, consider it questionable and back it up as described above. In training students, it may be desirable to treat all anchor points as questionable since proper assessment of anchor point integrity is largely a matter of experience and judgment.

Extending Anchors

Anchor points are not often located in the desired position. Any of the previously mentioned anchor points can be effectively extended or redirected using rope and other rigging components. In multistory structures, rescuers can easily use an anchor system several floors below or above the working floor (see Figure 5.1B). Do this by attaching a rope to the anchor and directing the rope from the system floor through a window or other opening. Now run the anchor line up or down to the working floor and attach it to the primary rope system.

Directionals

One common solution to locating an anchor point is to direct rescue ropes through anchored pulleys rigged high above an edge or opening. These directionals can serve two purposes. They can prevent abrasion by running a rope over an edge. They can make it easier to negotiate edges or openings when lowering and hauling rescuers or patients.

The term "directional" refers to any rigging that redirects the path of a rope. Although here directionals primarily relate to anchor systems, they can be used anywhere along the length of a rope. One example of the use of directionals in anchor rigging is where two anchor points are positioned several feet apart on the roof of a building (see Figure 5.1). The rescue team needs to position a lowering line directly over a window three floors below to rescue a trapped occupant. The problem is that the window is located at a point between the two anchors. The rescue team must use both of the anchor points in a way that redirects the path of the rope directly over the window. One way they can do this effectively is with a load-sharing bridle.

Load-Sharing Bridles

Load-sharing bridles are configurations of rigging that can distribute a load over two or more anchor points. They are not recommended in rescue as a means of creating a

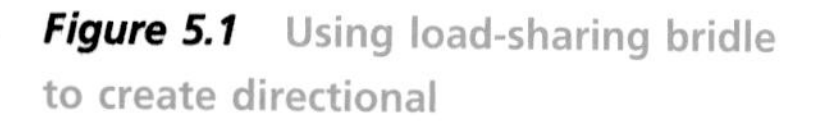
Figure 5.1 Using load-sharing bridle to create directional

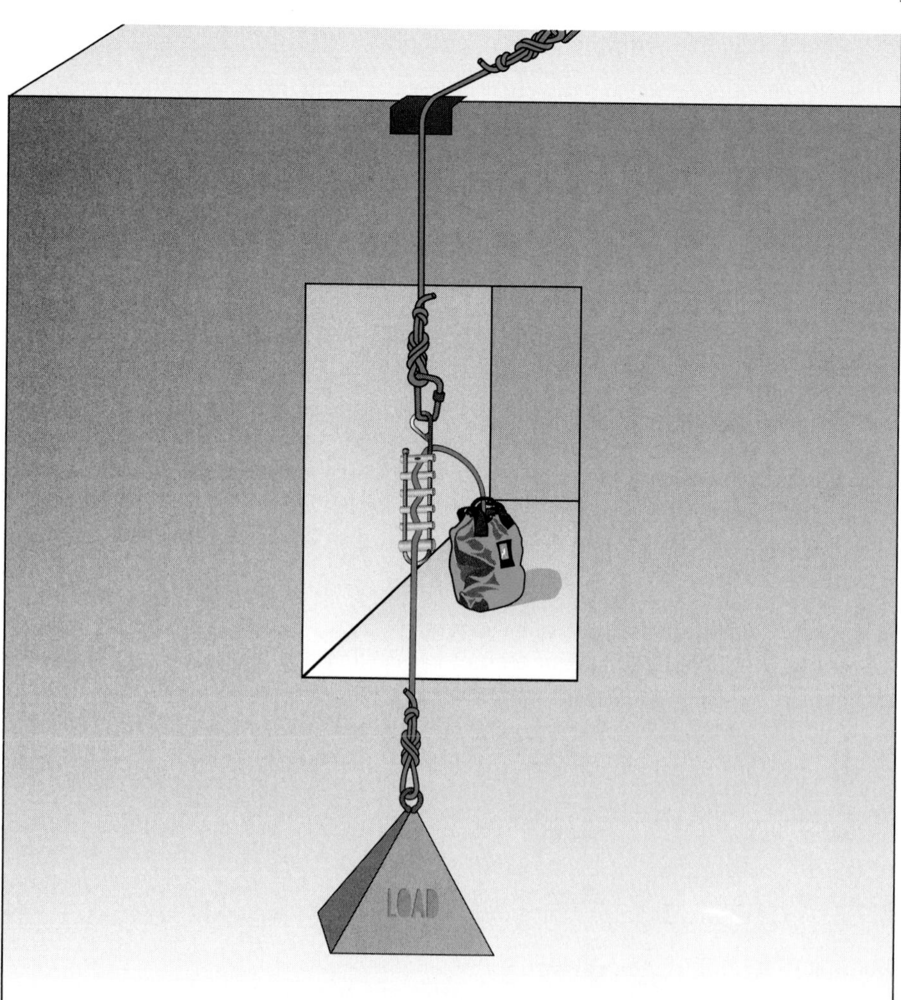

strong anchor by linking multiple weak anchor points together. In rescue, bridles are most commonly used to redirect the path of a rope at the anchor system. However, simple bridle configurations can be placed anywhere in the system to do the same thing.

"Load-distributing" or "self-equalizing" anchor systems are not discussed here. Equal distribution of the load depends on many factors, two of which are the direction of pull and the angles created within the bridle structure. Studies suggest that these systems cannot be counted on to truly equalize the load between multiple anchor points.

Rescuers can configure these bridles in several ways. All of the methods shown in this book involve the use of only two anchor points or systems.
Other methods exist. The rescuer's choice depends on the rescue system, and ingenuity to build a system that best fits a situation.

When used for anchor systems, this bridle configuration has one advantage over the other type we will discuss later in this chapter. This system has a built-in backup for the anchor points. In short, one anchor point backs up the other. Rescuers must

Configuration 1

To create the first configuration:

Option A:

1. Attach webbing slings (configured properly for two-person loads) to each anchor point.
2. Then, depending on the angle between them, connect them with a carabiner or screw link for attachment to the rope or rope system.

Option B:

1. Attach the ends of a rope to each anchor point. Leave enough slack to tie a butterfly knot in the rope between the two anchor points in the position needed.
2. Attach the butterfly knot to the rope or rope system with a carabiner or screw link.

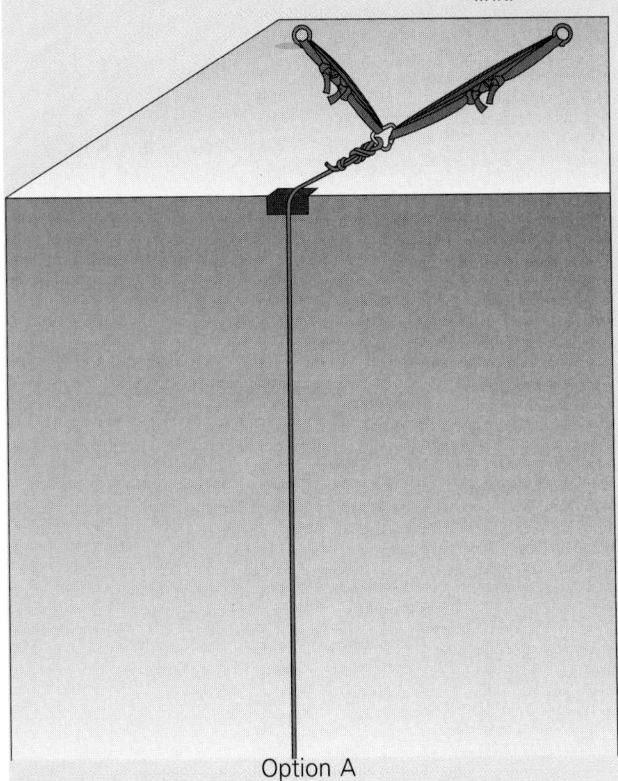

Option A

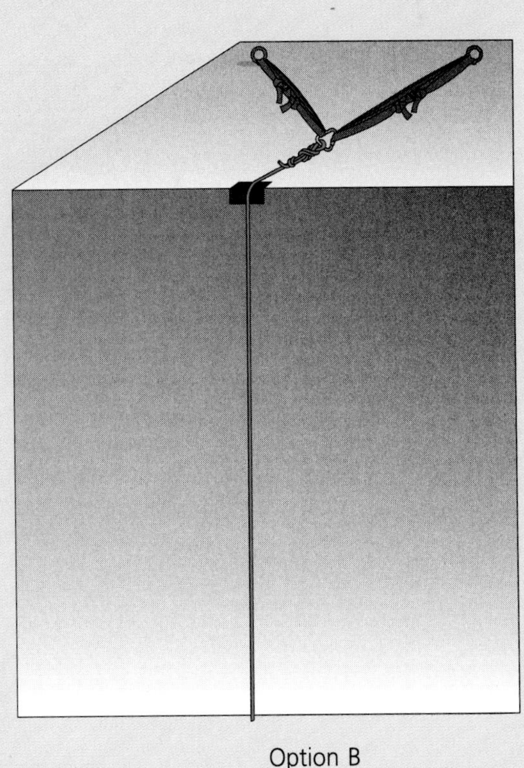

Option B

rig them so that if one anchor fails, the other will take the load. If these anchor points are separated by much of a distance, pendulum and shock load may be as prominent as with a secondary anchor point not in line with the primary. Rescuers must consider the advantages and disadvantages carefully before deciding to use this directional system for anchoring.

The directional rigging pulls the rope system into a little different alignment.

Although not usual, it is a good idea to use the same backup anchoring for the directional rigging as for the main rope system. The force exerted on the directional anchor system depends primarily on how far the rope system deviates from 180 degrees or straight line. In general, if the main rope system is directed 60 degrees or more out of line, the directional rigging anchor is receiving at least the weight of the load and should be backed up.

Configuration 2

In contrast to configuration 1, the second type of bridle configuration does not create a backup system for a questionable primary anchor point. However, depending on the angles created, it does allow the load to be more evenly distributed (not equalized) between the anchor points.

1. Using the previous scenario, start by creating the appropriate backup for the anchor system (questionable or bombproof).
2. Anchor the rope or rope system.
3. Take an appropriate length of rope or a webbing sling and attach it to the other anchor point.
4. Use this directional rigging to redirect the main rope by attaching to it a pulley or simply clipping onto it with a carabiner. (You may wish to use two carabiners to create less of a bend in the main rope).

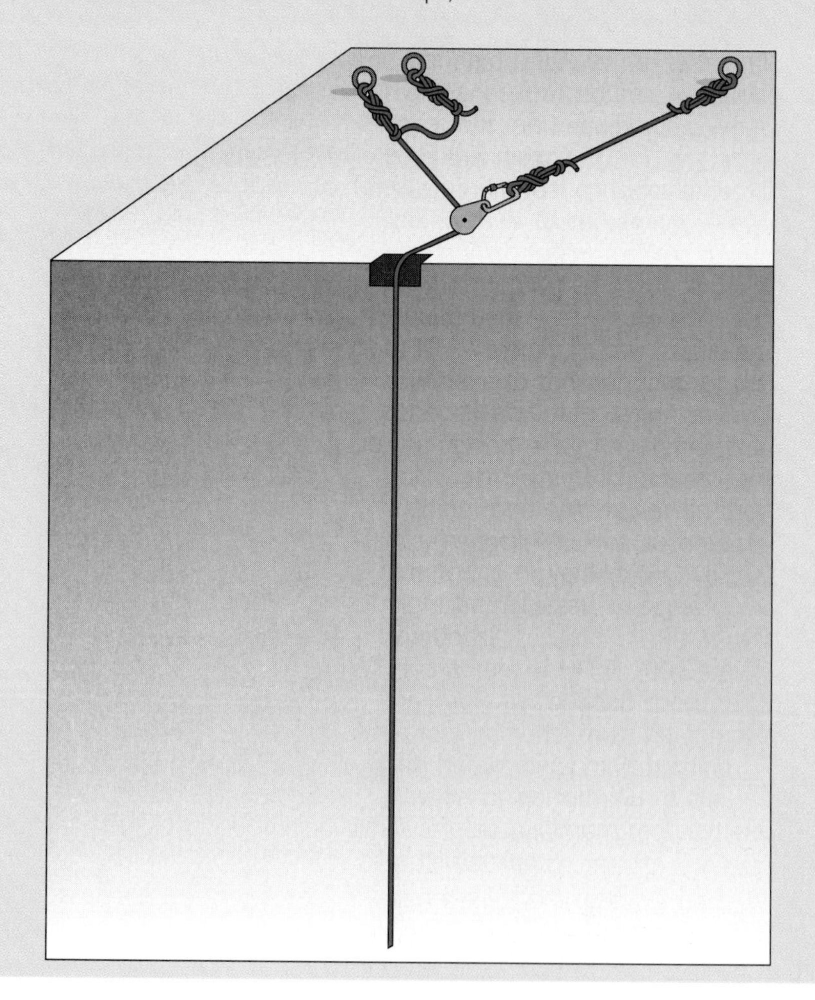

Angles

One important consideration when creating directionals of any type in a rope rescue system is the angle formed by the directional. The more the rope is pulled away from its normal path, the more force is exerted on the anchor points because of the increasing angle in the directional rigging.

A bridle is formed by the two legs of rope or other rigging extending from the anchors and forming a junction to redirect the path of the rope or rope system. We will assume for this scenario that the bridle rigging is formed in a way that distributes the load equally on both anchors.

It might seem reasonable that a 100-pound load attached to the main system would distribute 50 pounds of force to each of the two anchor points and their associated rigging. This is rarely true.

The actual force on the anchor point depends on the angle between the bridle's legs. In principle, the wider the angle between bridle legs, the greater the force exerted on the anchor points and the associated rigging.

Consider the example of a 100-pound load attached to a bridle with a 45-degree angle between the legs (see Figure 5.4). The theoretical force exerted on each of the anchor points is not much more than half of the total weight of the load.

Now if the angle widens to around 90 degrees, the forces increase significantly to around 71 pounds on each anchor point. At 120 degrees the entire weight of the load (100 pounds) is exerted on each anchor point and its associated rigging. If the angle widens any further, it will create system stresses greater than the load.

If this just does not seem possible, a simple little experiment can verify it. Take a short section of rescue rope and have a couple of big strong rescuers pull on the ends like a tug-o-war. Challenge them to pull tight enough that you cannot move the rope. When their muscles are bulging and their faces are beet red, grasp the rope in the center (between the two strongmen) with two fingers and make a quick pull perpendicular to the rope's alignment. It should cause the two rescuers to stumble slightly and fall forward.

Now have the rescuers stand side by side with the same ends of rope in their hand. Try pulling on the center of the rope with both hands and all your might. You will quickly see that you are easily overpowered.

What changed in this experiment? The angle formed by the bridle legs. Again, the wider the angle, the greater the force exerted on the anchor points and the associated rigging. So, what does this mean to rescuers?

Avoid angles greater than 120 degrees when rigging any bridle. At 120 degrees, the force of the entire load is on each point. Rescuers never want to exceed this amount of force. It is even more desirable to keep the angle at 90 degrees or smaller. This does not mean they carry protractors in rescue gear to measure angles. A practical way of viewing angles is to create an angle that looks like a nice narrow V (see Figure 5.5).

Rescuers can also use a pulley to redirect the rope anywhere in a system. In a hauling or lowering system, pulleys are commonly anchored at a high point above an edge (see Figure 5.6). This prevents the main line from dragging over the edge and makes it easier to get the load over it. Depending on the configuration of the directionals and the angle created by them, a single high-

Figure 5.4 Diagram of forces related to the anchor point position

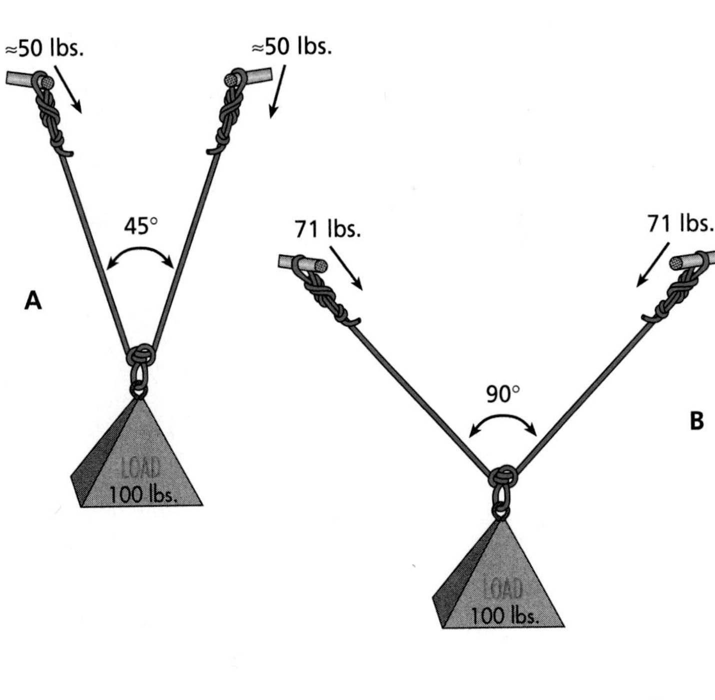

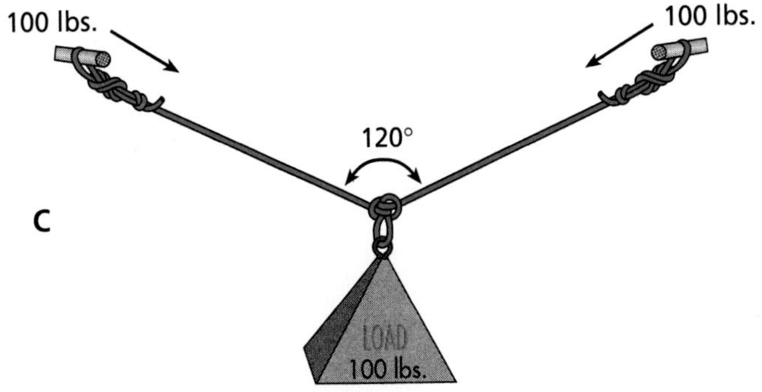

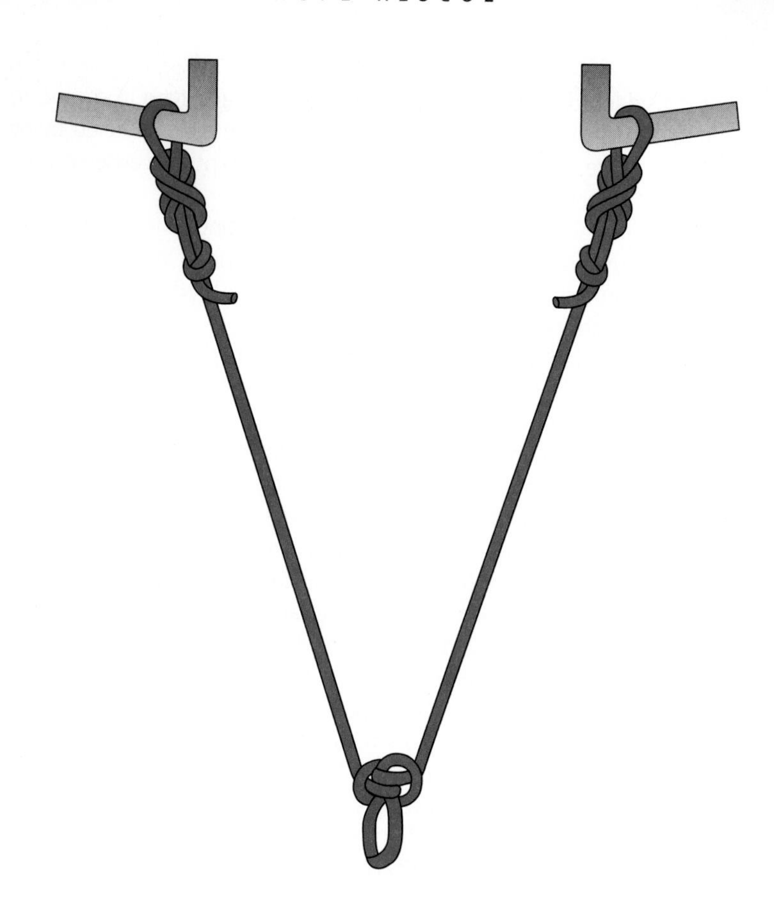

Figure 5.5 Ideal angle for anchor bridle

als and the angle created by them, a single high-point pulley supporting the entire load can have the force of the load pulling from one side of the pulley and an equal force from the rescue system pulling from the other. This will produce forces on the pulley and its associated rigging as much as twice the load. Pulleys and other rescue equipment used in this capacity should meet NFPA 1983 (1995 edition) strength standards for general use (where they apply) whether being used for a one- or two-person load. Any rescue hardware or software serving this purpose and not configured to meet the general-use standard (see Chapter 3 on Related Rope Rescue Equipment) should be reconfigured or backed up with components that do.

Anchoring Configurations

There are endless rigging configurations for rope rescue anchor systems. However, when rescuers are rigging any system for rescue they should keep in mind the two legs on which every rescue stands: safety and efficiency. As previously discussed, simplicity generally brings about both results. This section will review several rope configurations that employ some of these principles very efficiently.

Based on analysis of actual industrial rescue cases, it appears that the majority of vertical rope rescues are performed within 30 to 40 feet of the ground or safe area, and strong anchor points are usually plentiful.

These observations can help rescuers develop systems that will streamline rigging, at least most of the time. The following rigging systems work well in most cases for vertical applications where two single lines are required in the rescue system. Other configurations are possible. But these systems are generally used for a combination of one rappel line and one safety line belay, one lowering line and one safety line belay, or two lowering lines. Depending on the distance to the anchor points and the distance to the ground or safe area, one 200-foot rope may be sufficient to rig both lines and their anchor systems. This makes the rigging more efficient. Remember, keep it simple!

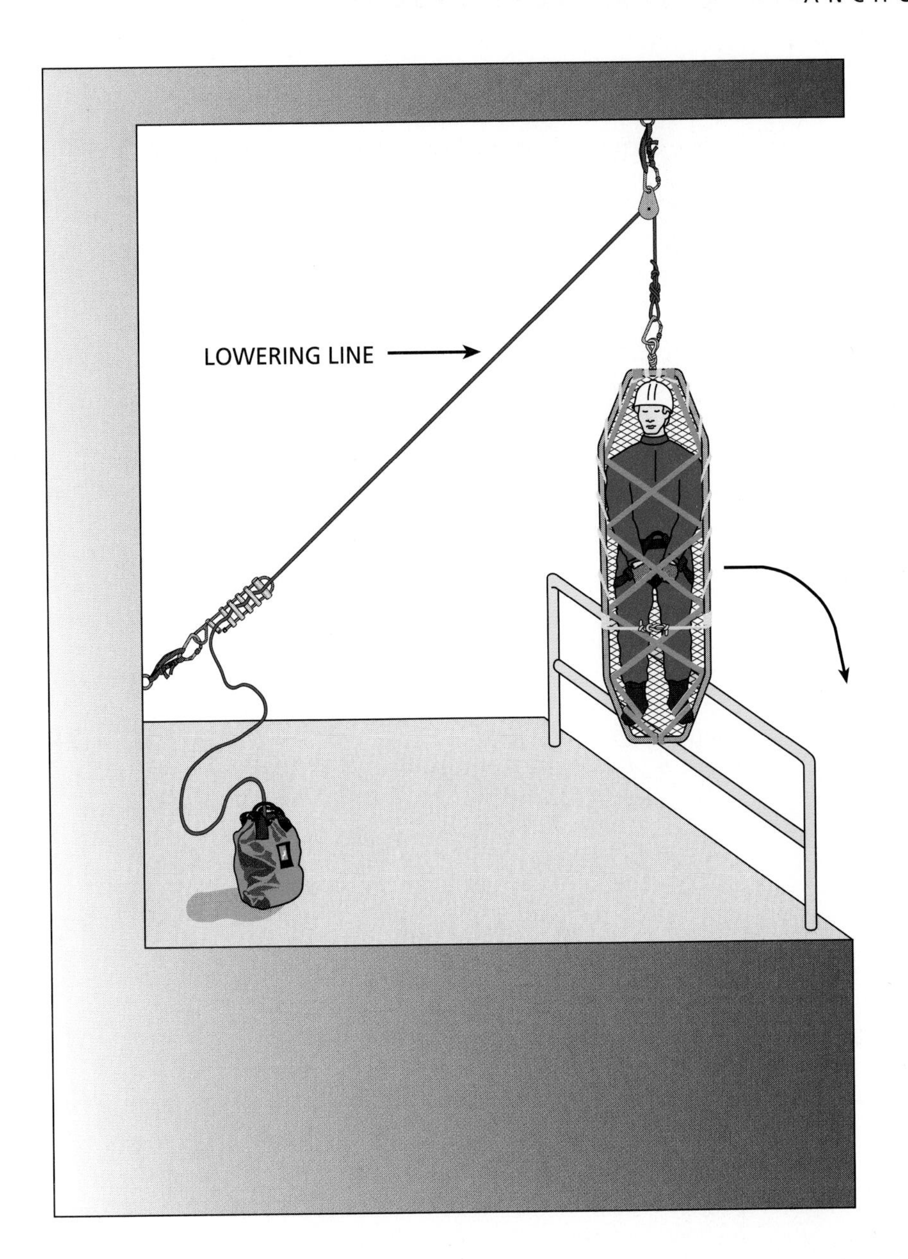

Figure 5.6 Using a pulley to direct rope from a high point anchor. (Brakeman, secondary anchor point and safety line not shown)

Anchoring Two Lines with One Rope

Depending on rope length, distance to anchors, height of the drop, and the rescue system, a rescuer may rig two lines from one rope length. By finding the center of the rope, the rescuer can effectively divide the rope in two halves, then use these two halves to create an anchoring system for two lines. However, it may be possible to form both the lines and their anchor riggings with the same rope. Again, this depends on many factors. There are several methods of rigging these two rope halves, depending on the configuration of the anchor points. The methods shown here assume that the primary anchor point should be backed up with a second anchor point. Rescuers can often use one or more of the following examples.

Rescuers can successfully use these configurations and their variations in most industrial anchor rigging. They do not always expect to find anchors positioned just right. Rescuers should use standard primary and secondary systems to back up anchor points following the principles presented in this chapter.

Remember these principles of anchor rigging. It is acceptable to use one anchor point for one system's primary and another system's secondary. It is acceptable to use one anchor point as a common secondary for two different primary systems. It is NOT acceptable to use one anchor point as a primary for more than one rope system. Theoretically, this does not apply to bombproof anchor points. However, it is a good idea to apply this principle to all anchor points just in case of a mistake in judgment.

Two Anchor Points, Sharing Primary and Secondary

When there are two anchor points side by side and near each other (2 to 3 feet apart), one anchor point can provide the backup for the other anchor point. In other words, the primary for one line is the secondary for the other line and vice versa. For purposes of this text, it is considered acceptable practice to use one anchor point as the primary for one system and the secondary for another.
To rig this configuration:

1. Tie anchor knots in the middle of the rope just far enough apart to allow a little slack between the two anchor points.
2. Attach one knot to each anchor point using any proper combination of hardware and software. Utility belts or webbing loops can make the job easier.
3. You can tie additional knots in the two lines to anchor descent control or belay devices.
4. If enough rope is left (after tying knots) to reach the final destination of the rescue system, you can use the remaining line from each half of the rope for lowering or belay lines.
5. Remember, DO NOT allow more than a few inches of slack between the two knots once they have been attached to the anchor rigging. However, there should be no tension in the rope connecting the two anchor points together.
6. If the anchor points are too far apart or one anchor point is several feet in front of the other, shock loading and/or pendulum can occur if one anchor fails. A pendulum may cause damage to the rope by allowing it to slide across unprotected sharp or abrasive edges. If these circumstances exist, do not use this method.

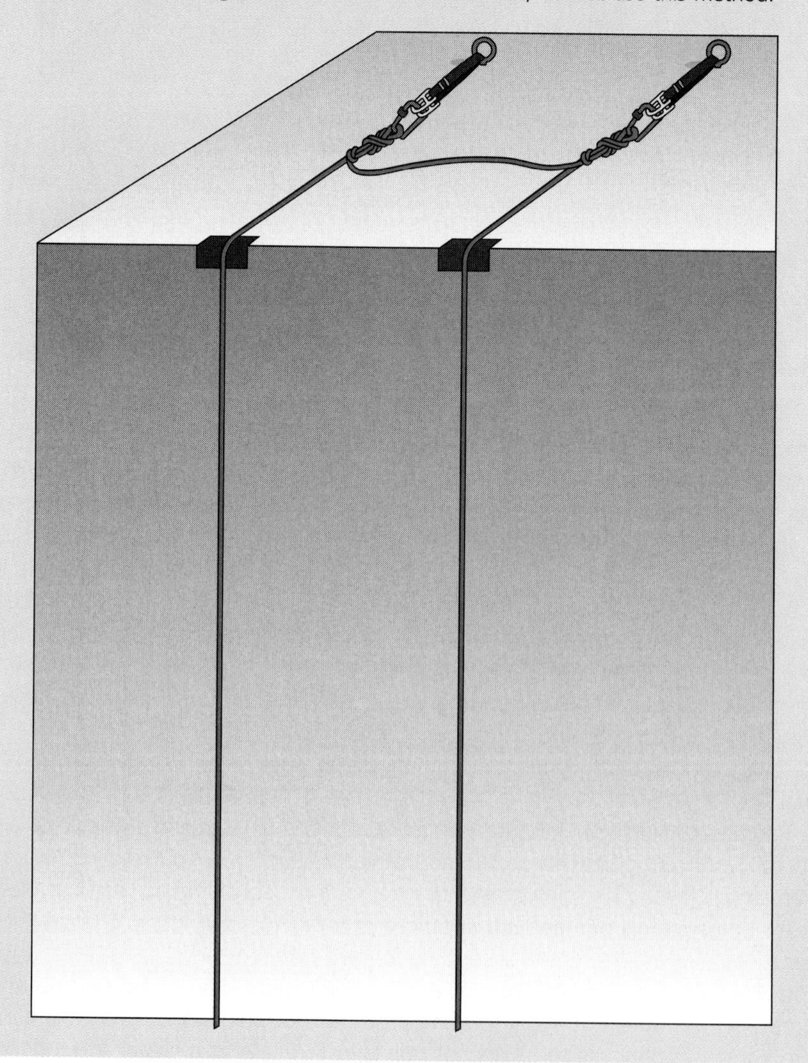

Three Anchor Points, Common Secondary

If the two anchor points are too far apart or uneven, rescuers can use a similar method for splitting one rope into two lines. This configuration requires a third anchor point located some distance behind and relatively in line with the other two. This third anchor point will serve as a common secondary for the two primary anchor points. It allows minimum shock and pendulum should one anchor point fail. For purposes of this text, it is considered acceptable practice to use one anchor point as the secondary (backup) for two different systems. To rig this configuration:

1. Find the middle of the rope. Select an anchor behind the two anchor points you have already chosen. This anchor point should be nearly in line with the two front anchor points to avoid pendulum and shock in case the primary anchor fails.
2. Tie a knot in the middle of the rope and attach it to this secondary anchor point with proper combination of hardware and software.
3. Extend the ropes from the secondary anchor point toward the two primary anchor points, one rope toward each primary anchor.
4. Tie a knot in each line at its primary anchor point and attach it to the anchor with proper combination of hardware and software. Leave as little slack possible between the primary anchor points and the secondary. However, there should be no constant tension on the secondary point.
5. You can tie additional knots in the two lines to anchor descent control or belay devices. If enough rope is left (after tying knots) to reach the final destination of the rescue system, you can use the remaining line of each half of the rope for lowering or belay lines.
6. In this system, both ropes use the same secondary anchor point. If the primary anchor point fails, the rope loads on the secondary anchor point behind it rather than swinging across to the other primary as in the first system.

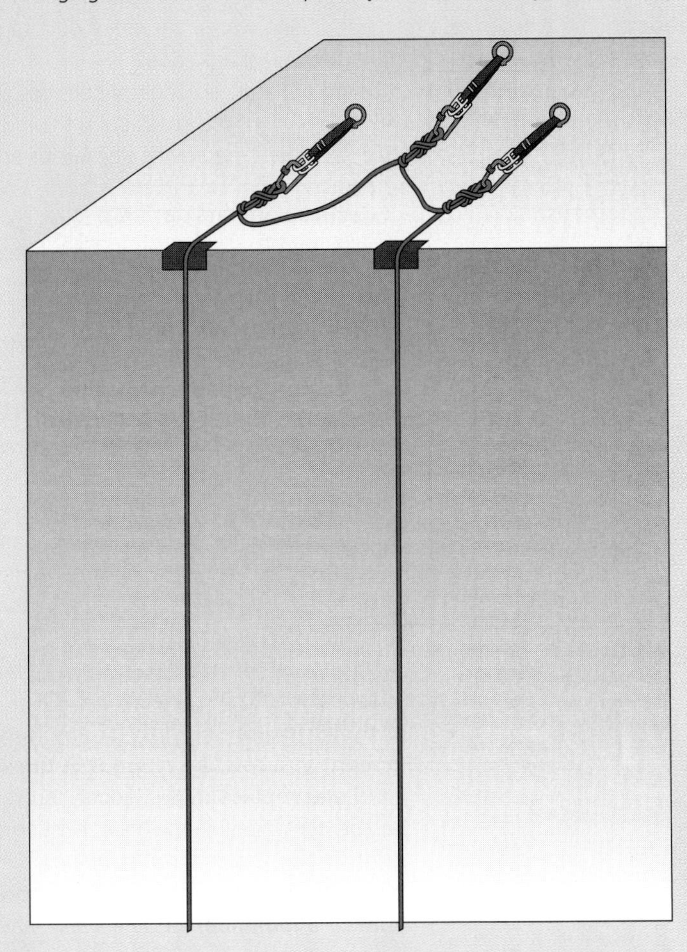

Streamlining

Rigging efficiency considers not only the efficiency of equipment, but the conservation of time and physical effort associated with the rigging. In other words, it may be possible to rig two rappel lines and a hauling system from one 300-foot rope without using a single piece of hardware or additional software. But if it takes two hours to rig it, it is not an efficient system. The term "streamlining" describes a sound rescue principle. Based on the known surroundings and activities in the industrial environment, rescuers use methods that enhance efficiency in a balanced way, thus streamlining their operations.

General Rigging Precautions

There are several important considerations when rigging rope rescue systems. Always follow these basic safety principles:

- **Backup all questionable anchor points with a second anchor point of equal or greater strength.** Bombproof anchor points are not in question and require no backup. If any member of a team doubts the integrity of a bombproof anchor point, treat it as questionable and back it up. It is better to err on the side of safety.
- **Protect all abrasion points or sharp edges with padding or other means and inspect these points frequently** (see Figure 5.9). There are many types of edge protection.
  - Padding comes in many forms. Some of them include prefabricated rope pads or guards, carpet samples with jute backing (Do not use the synthetic front of the carpet with moving rope. It will melt.) You can use pieces of canvas, fire hose, heavy felt, blankets, or similar materials. Even cardboard can be used as padding in a pinch. These materials, along with a big roll of duct tape, protect rescue software against most abrasive and sharp edges.
  - Use thick layers of padding to round out squared edges when rope is being bent over them (see Figure 5.9). These edges are common in the industrial envronment, frequently I-beams or angle-iron. Padding them creates a less acute bend, allowing more of the rope's core fibers to hold the load. Webbing distributes its load-bearing fibers somewhat evenly over squared edges and does not require the same consideration.

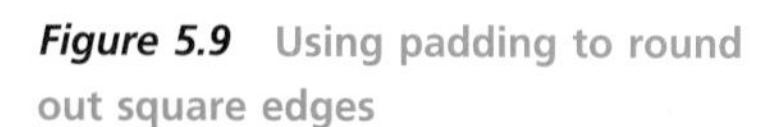

Figure 5.9 Using padding to round out square edges

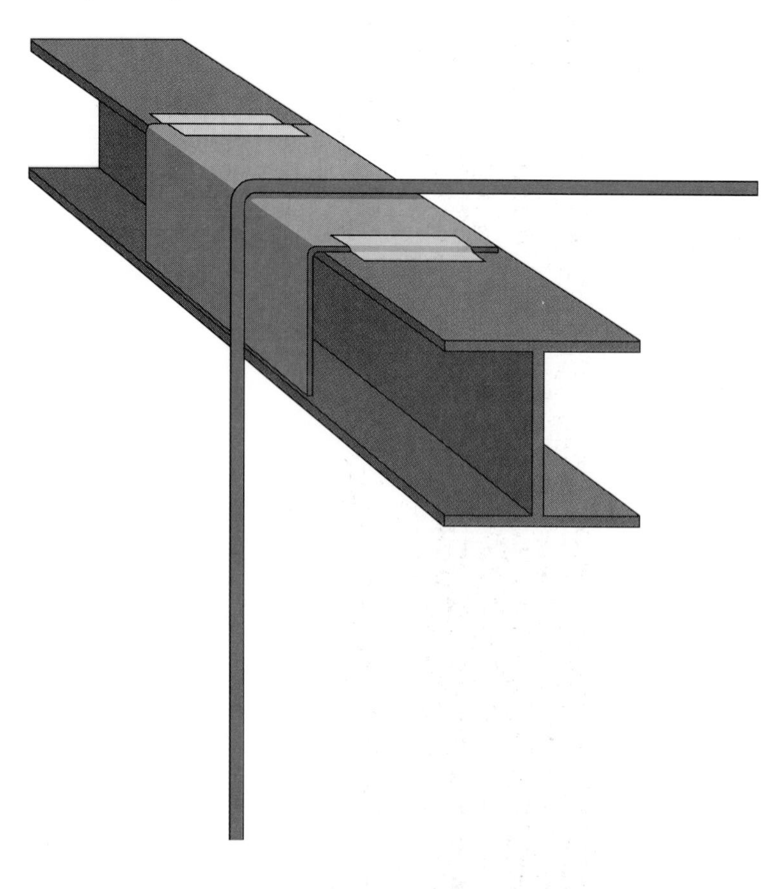

  - Many other prefabricated hardware items are designed to provide edge protection for rope and webbing. Do not use common hose rollers for edge protection with rescue software. Hose rollers are designed to reduce friction when hauling or lowering fire hose over an edge. They are not designed to use with live loads and can develop sharp edges or collapse under load.
  - As rope systems are loaded and unloaded, things change; padding can shift. Frequently recheck all protected points in a system to make sure they stay protected.
- **If the structural integrity of any rigging component in a rescue system is in question, discard and replace it.** If in doubt, throw it out! All rescue equipment should meet existing applicable construction and strength standards.
- **Keep the components of the anchoring system to a minimum.** This generally makes it a safer and more efficient system. Keep it simple!

- **Avoid nonflexible links (hard links) with hardware items.** These may be created by linking rigid components without allowing for normal twisting and movement (see Figure 5.10). Linking three or more carabiners together can create a hard link. Hardware is not designed to be used without rope or other flexible software. It also relies on this component for shock absorption.
- **Do not use webbing where it might receive even small dynamic loads (impact or shock loads) without including rope or shock absorbers in the system as well.** Remember, a fall factor greater than .25 is unacceptable for low-stretch rescue rope. Webbing stretches even less than rope.
- **Check all the rigging in your system after each use.** We already mentioned protected edges. Also check anchor and system rigging to make sure it is still okay. Remember, things can change.

  NOTE: *This does not apply in cases where both parts of nylon are moving, such as in a Munter hitch (see Figure 5.11).*
- **Do not use knives or scissors around loaded ropes.** Under load, it takes very little contact with a sharp object to cut a rope in two. There are ways to do things that will virtually eliminate the need for knives and scissors in rope rescue. Scissors and shears have certain emergency medical applications. Do not use them when suspended on line.

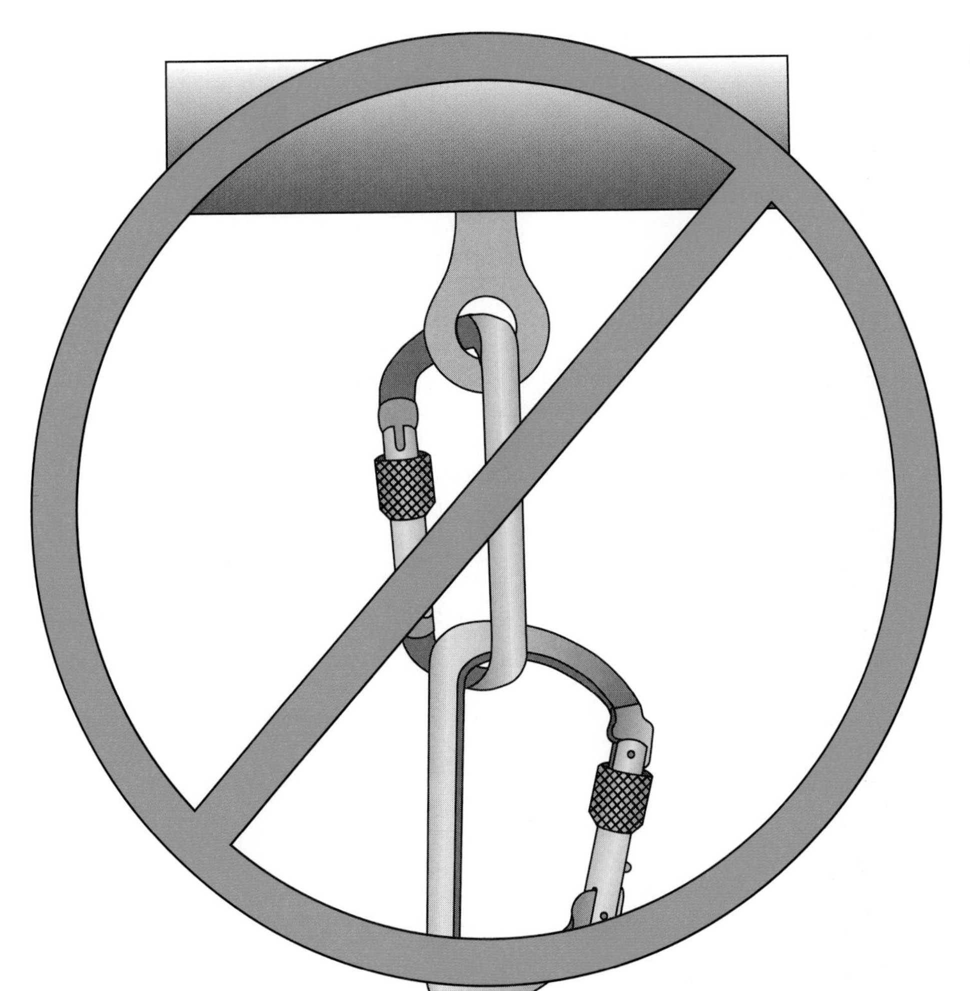

Figure 5.10 Example of hard link

WARNING

Avoid nylon-on-nylon in rigging. This can happen when nylon ropes cross or nylon rope crosses nylon padding. This applies to moving (running) nylon on one spot of non-moving (static) nylon. When certain synthetic materials run over other static synthetic materials the friction creates a great deal of heat. Under load, a piece of nylon rope or webbing can be severed quickly when exposed to this heat. If you see this in a rope system, STOP the operation immediately. This is a true emergency.

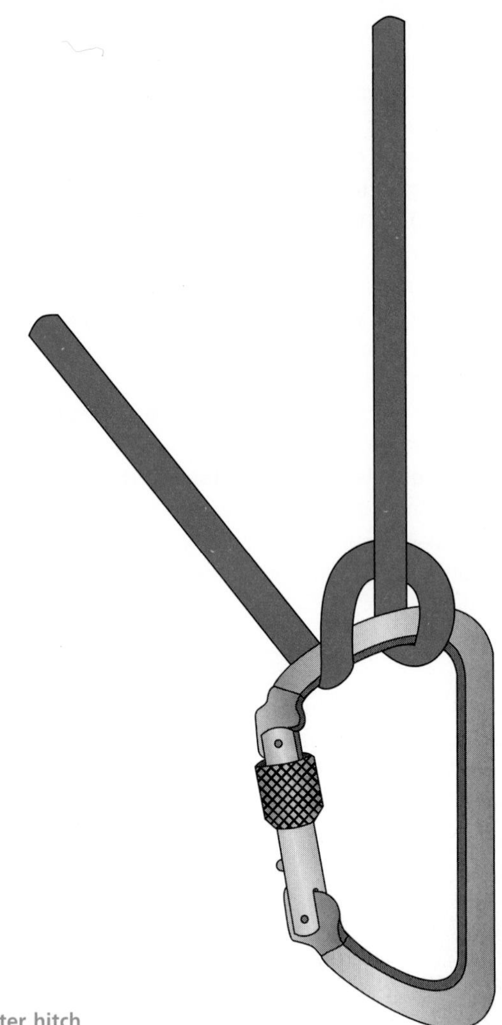

Figure 5.11 Munter hitch

Summary

There are many ways to create safe and effective rigging. This book does not attempt to present all possible rigging considerations or configurations. The goal of this text is to provide you with a basis from which to work. Use the safety principles presented here to develop your own rigging practices. You must base your rigging on the particular situations and circumstances you face as a rescuer.

CHAPTER 6

Belaying

The information in this chapter is provided as a basis for continued training. Each rescuer should consult with his or her own team leader for the correct SOGs for the team.

Topics covered in this chapter include

- Belay Cautions
- OSHA Mandates
- Types of Belay Systems

Introduction

The word "belay" comes from the days of sailing vessels. On those ships, belaying pins were set in the rails of the vessel. When sailors raised heavy objects such as sails they would attach a rope to the load. They would then take a turn of the rope around the belaying pin to prevent the line from slipping away from them.

The principle is the same in the high angle environment. However, instead of a sail, a person is belayed. This person is attached to a rope and the rope is managed in such a way, or belayed, that it prevents him or her from falling far enough to be harmed should something go wrong.

Belaying ability is a necessary skill for anyone operating in the high angle environment. If you accept the assignment as a belayer, you have made a very serious commitment. It means that the well-being, perhaps even the life, of the person at the end of the rope is in your hands. To say that you can belay when you cannot or to allow your attention to lapse from the job of belaying could mean severe injury or death for the person at the end of the rope.

Belay Cautions

There are several types of belay systems available to the rescuer. Whatever the methods used, all belay systems have one thing in common. They are all intended as a type of backup to the properly operating rope rescue system. If something out of the ordinary happens, such as a primary system failure, the belay must function to save the person or persons who might otherwise fall. In this text, we will discuss two principle types of belay:

- **Bottom Belay**—Bottom belays are used usually with a rappel sequence (see Figure 6.1). The technique involves tensioning a rappel line (usually around the belayer's body) to control the descent of rescue personnel. It acts as a backup to the rappeller should he or she lose control of the descent device. A rescuer can also use the bottom belay to lower or assist the rappeller.
- **Safety line belay system**—As the name implies, this system incorporates a safety line to the belay (see Figure 6.2). This safety line is a separately anchored rope system attached to a control device. It is designed to catch any person suspended on the primary rope system should a failure occur. Although many methods are taught for controlling the safety line belay system, we will present two in this text.

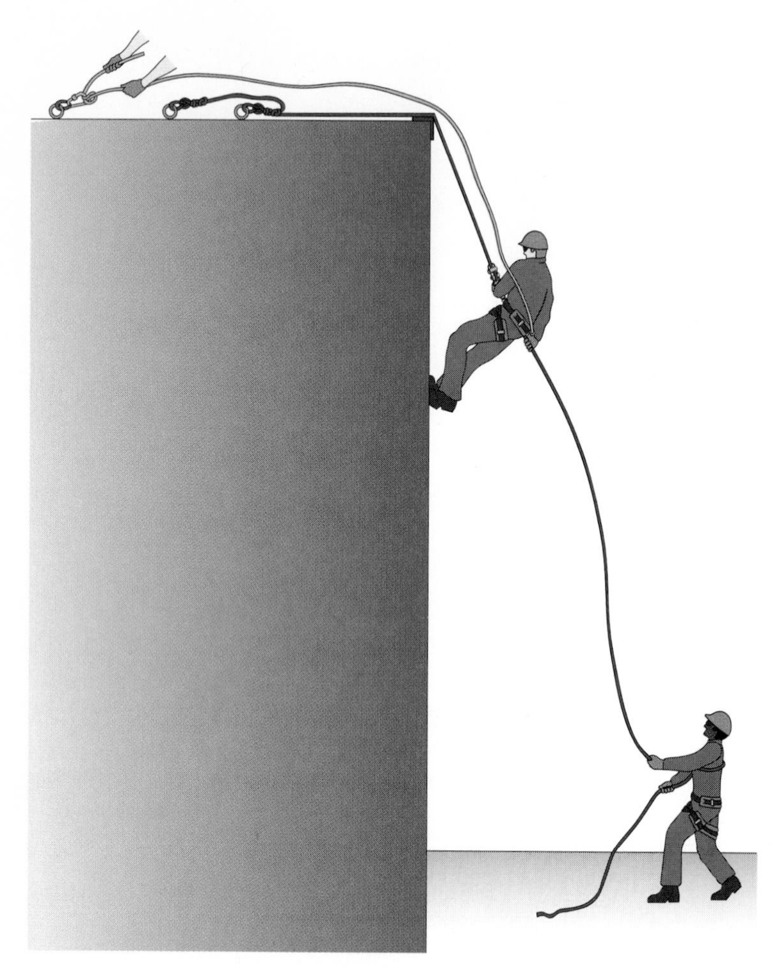

Figure 6.1 Bottom Belay (Backup anchor on safety line not shown.)

Belay System Slack

During normal operation, there should be slack in all belay ropes (see Figure 6.1). Belay ropes should be tensioned only to catch a falling load or, in special cases, when the rescuer calls for "tension." A good recommendation is to allow no more than 18 inches of slack in the belay ropes at any time.

The reason for the 18-inch limit is simple. Too much slack will allow the person being belayed to fall a significant distance before he or she can be stopped. This rapid fall and sudden stop can generate high-impact forces. Much of this force can be transferred to the person on line, causing serious injury or even death. Additional injury can occur if the person strikes the ground or some other object while falling.

In contrast, too little slack can create a "jerky" ride for the person on the line. If there is any question, it is much better to err on the side of safety. A jerky ride is better than a smooth but uncontrolled fall! In other words, the goal is to keep as much of the slack out of the system as possible without impeding the normal operation of the system.

Over the Edge

One more important note on belaying. It seems that when things go wrong, they often do so while the person is going over an edge. This can be attributed to many things such as the apprehension the person feels while climbing out into thin air, or maybe even the physical difficulty in climbing over an edge. Whatever the cause, the belayer must always be ready to catch a falling person should something go wrong (see Figure 6.3). This is especially important while the person is moving over an edge to load the rope system. Be ready! Don't lose sight of the importance of your mission for even one second. The person you're belaying cannot afford it.

The edge can present problems for the person negotiating it. It can also be a serious danger for the belayer if he or she is near it unprotected. Always take the time to protect yourself (whatever your rescue function) if you are working near an edge. If you are close enough to fall over an edge, you should be secured properly to an appropriate anchor system. Always wear the proper personal protective equipment including helmet, gloves, and safety glasses. Remember, your safety is number one.

OSHA Mandates

The Occupational Safety and Health Administration (OSHA) has mandated requirements for the protection of employees who work at heights greater than 6 feet off the ground. This Fall Protection Standard contains much information pertaining to harnesses and fall protection equipment for industrial workers. It does not specifically address that needed for rescue or by rescuers. Belay systems are simply a form of fall protection. Any competent industrial rescuer should research all applicable standards to make the job safer. Although it may have no direct reference, this standard may at least have some relevance to the belay systems used in rescue. The Fall Protection Standard and some others that might relate to rescuers are covered in chapter 18, "Regulatory Compliance."

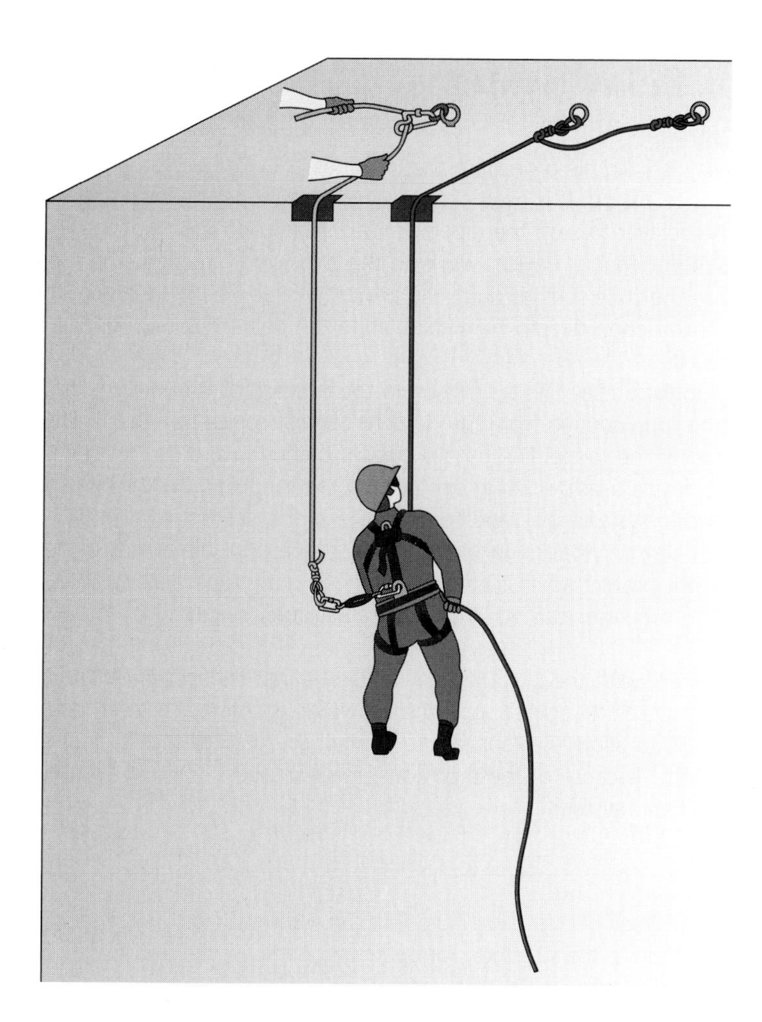

Figure 6.2 Use a safety line belay system on a separate anchor (Pictured systems may not portray ideal anchorage.)

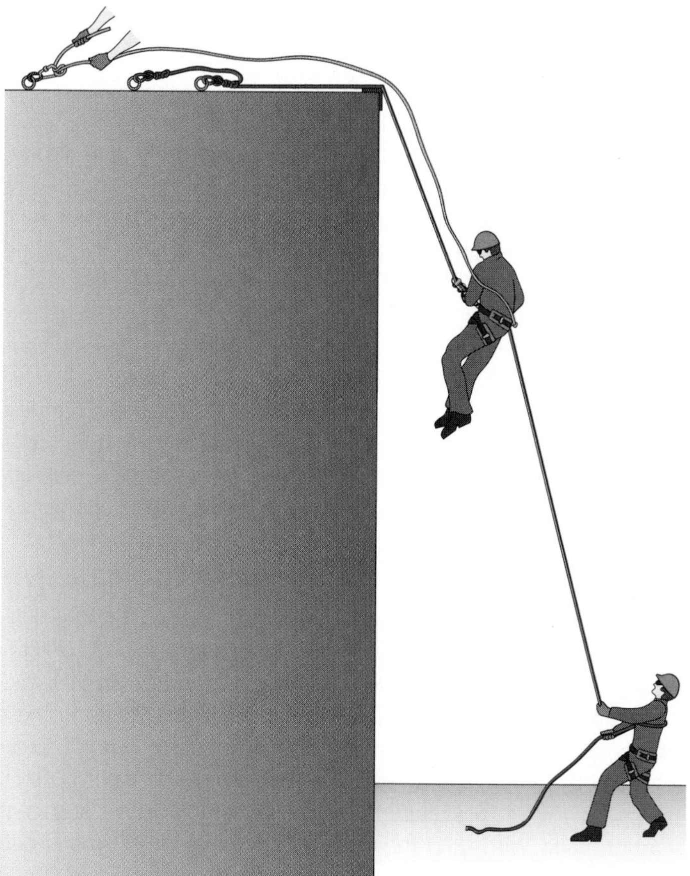

Figure 6.3 Stopping a falling rappeller (Pictured systems may not portray ideal anchorage.)

Types of Belay Systems

Bottom Belay

The bottom belay is a simple procedure that requires only one person and no additional equipment to set up. It is used exclusively during rappelling exercises. A bottom belay allows the belayer to stop the rappeller who loses control of the descent control device. Most descent control devices work on the principle of friction. The more friction produced as the rope runs through the device, the slower the descent. The rappeller controls this friction directly by manipulating the descent control device or the rope attached to it.

Similarly, a bottom belay creates friction in the descent control device. You do this by pulling on the rope coming from the descent control device. In other words, pulling on the loose end of the rappel line usually creates friction in the control device (depending on the device used), slowing or stopping the rappeller. Variations of this technique with lowering systems give additional safety to the descent control.

The bottom belay only backs up the rappeller as the principle means of descent control. It does not protect against a failure of the primary rope system. There is only one thing a bottom belayer can do in case of catastrophic failure . . . GET OUT OF THE WAY!

Another problem with the bottom belay system is that it depends on the belayer's reaction time for successful operation. If the belayer is distracted for even one second, it could be enough to allow the rappeller to contact the ground should an incident occur at that moment. Because of these obvious disadvantages, it is wise to use an additional safety line belay system.

Procedure

1. The bottom body belayer (see Figure 6.1) can assume almost any position necessary in relation to the structure. For optimum operation, the belayer should stand at the rappeller's general landing zone.
2. Face the structure at 45 degrees (or less) from its base. This may not always be possible. Nearby process units or other obstructions can seriously limit the standing room in the industrial environment.
3. Do the best you can but avoid standing directly under the rappeller. If a rope failure were to occur, it might be difficult to get out of the way.
4. It is also possible to provide a bottom belay while standing at levels at or above the rappeller. Although this can be done, slight modifications may be necessary to operate this system safely. One such method involves bending and attaching the rope that is below the rappeller to an anchor or an anchored friction device instead of to your body. This prevents the belayer from being pulled over the edge by the falling rappeller.
5. Stand facing the rappeller with your feet slightly offset. The foot on your dominant side (strong side) should be a little farther back than the other. Keep the feet about shoulder width apart. This belay stance will provide a stable platform from which to work. One common mistake among body belayers is to stand with the body turned sideways rather than facing the rappeller. This is a very unstable position and can allow you to be pulled over when attempting to stop a falling rappeller.
6. Wrap the running end (loose end) of the rappel rope around your torso at the level of the armpits. It will give you the best chance of making the stop should something go wrong.

Remember, the rappeller will be falling. Falling fast! When you finally react by pulling on the rope, you are going to get somewhat of a shock load. If you are holding the rope loosely in your hand(s), you will likely lose it. By wrapping the rope around your body, you provide additional surface friction, which might prevent it from getting away. If you have the rope around your waist or under your buttocks, the initial shock may knock you off your feet. By wrapping it high above your center of gravity, you can probably withstand the force of the initial impact much better while remaining in position. Of course, there will be a second shock to your body as you finally arrest the person's fall. If you are standing and stable (rope around upper torso), you should maintain the control required. Proper rope positioning is critical in stopping the falling rappeller.

Emergency Stopping

To stop a falling rappeller, bottom body belayers simply bring their hands together to grasp both lines as they roll to one side (see Figure 6.3). This should rapidly take up all slack in the rope and apply tension to the descent control device, slowing or stopping the fall. Although the technique works rolling to either side, it seems more stable when the belayer rolls to his or her stronger side. Having the loose end of the rope on the belayer's weaker side also seems to help a bit. In this configuration, the loose end of the rope actually wraps around the rescuer's body during an emergency stop. If you have allowed too much slack in the rappel line prior to the emergency, you may not be able to tension the rope in time to stop the falling rappeller. As a rule, you should allow enough slack in the rope so that it drapes loosely below the rappeller without pulling at an angle from his or her body. If the rope is pulled at an angle or otherwise tensioned, you will apply some belay and you might impede the rappel. If you are below the rappeller, standing closer to his or her landing zone can help prevent this problem. Make sure you don't allow so much slack that you cannot quickly tension the rope in case of an emergency.

Lowering the Rappeller

As you tension the rope, you create friction in the rappeller's descent control device. Once the belayer has arrested the rappeller's fall, he or she may lower the rappeller to the ground by allowing a small amount of rope slack. This will reduce the friction in the control device enough to allow movement. This is a very basic form of lowering system. Be careful with the slack. A little goes a long way. As the rappeller descends, the belayer can walk forward (while maintaining control) to meet the rappeller on the ground for initial medical assessment and treatment as required.

Assisting the Rappeller

Certain situations could require the rappel rescue of a victim who has no other means of escape. In this case, rappelling might take place with both rescuer and victim's weight on one descent control device. Depending on the control device, this can make the descent very difficult for the rappeller to manage alone.

A bottom body belayer can provide some assistance to the rappeller in these situations. By applying tension to the rope, additional friction is created in the control device, making the descent much easier for the rappeller. The rappeller can call for this assistance by giving a verbal command such as "TENSION" or some other appropriate signal. Whatever the command, good communication is extremely important.

You can use a modification of this technique where you need a backup in safety line belay, lowering, and hauling systems. Instead of wrapping the rope around the torso under the arms, the rope is wrapped further down near the buttocks. This is no problem since an impact load is not expected. This "line tender" simply helps the primary operator of the control device if he or she loses control (see Figure 6.4).

Communications

Communication is extremely important. If a body belayer is not ready, it will not help the rappeller who is crawling over the edge. If there is no communication between belayer and rappeller to ensure this readiness, accidents are sure to happen. We will cover the important aspect of communications during the rappel sequence in the next chapter.

Bottom Belay Summary

This type of belay system is a very efficient use of both personnel and equipment because it requires only one rescue team member and no additional equipment. The tech-

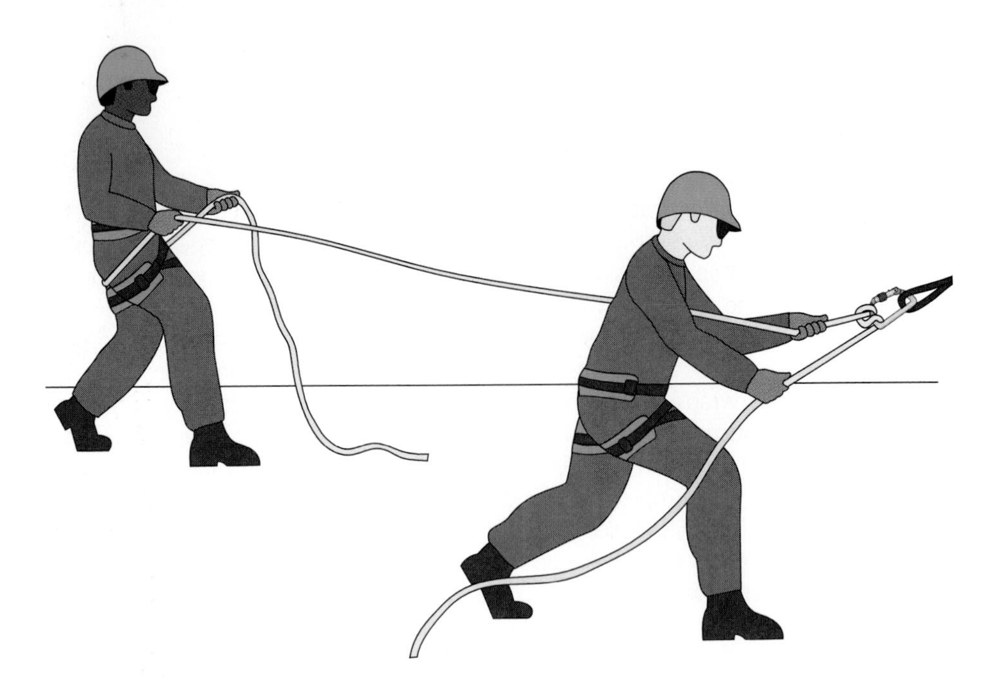

Figure 6.4 Line Tender

nique is also very simple to learn and operate. However, its effectiveness depends on the reaction time of the belayer. Therefore, it is not 100% reliable. For this reason, it is good in training to use the bottom body belay with a separate safety line belay system.

Safety Line Belay

There are many effective ways to create a safety line belay system. Most systems incorporate a separate safety line attached to anchorage with rigging separate and apart from the primary rescue system (see Figure 6.2). This type of belay system must have an anchor system that can withstand a shock load should the primary rope system fail. The belay rope should have no more than 18 inches of slack and be attached to a device capable of slowing or stopping a falling one- or two-person load.

As mentioned previously, there are many control devices in use these days. Some of these devices are not well suited for catching falling loads. Rescuers should avoid mechanical ascenders or any other device that may be destructive to the belay rope when shock loaded. Some devices are difficult to control and rely heavily on belayer reaction time. Devices like the figure-8 or rappel rack descenders and stitch plate personal belay devices fall into this category and should also be avoided. Two of the most popular control devices for safety line belay systems are the Munter Hitch (Figure 6.5) and the tandem Prusik belay (Figure 6.6).

Figure 6.5 Munter hitch

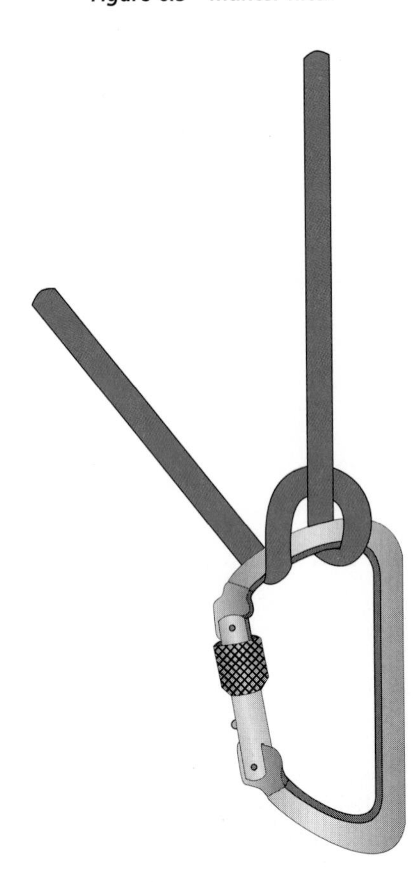

Both methods will operate during raising or lowering operations. Both will work with a high degree of accuracy. However, both depend heavily on proper setup and operation. Controversies exist about which of these methods is best. Both control devices have certain advantages and disadvantages and their use should be based largely on the circumstances surrounding the incident. Both require strict adherence to certain guidelines for safe operation.

Setup

All safety line belay systems are identical in setup and operation except for peculiarities associated with a particular control device. To provide the safest backup, the belay line system should have an anchor system completely separate from that of the primary rope system (see Figure 6.2). The control device is attached to this anchor and to a point on the belay rope (commonly called the "safety line"). The safety line is then attached to the person(s) to be belayed. Remember, maintain the suggested maximum length of 18 inches of slack in these safety lines. Attempt to use the least amount of slack that will not impede the normal operation of the system.

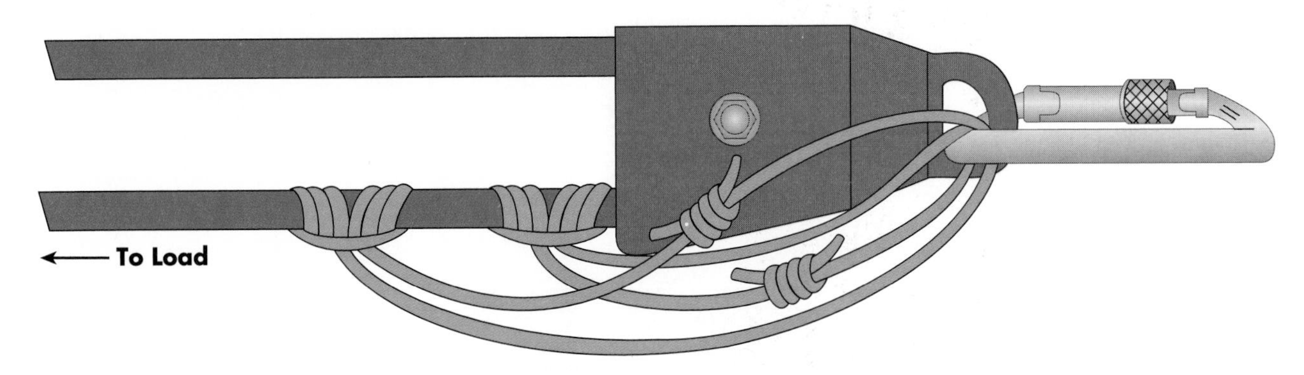

Figure 6.6 Tandem Prusik Belay

Shock Absorbers

Since these systems are intended to catch falling loads, it is reasonable to assume that significant impact forces will be produced. This constitutes dynamic loading. Some rescue teams use dynamic ropes exclusively for their safety belay lines. These ropes are designed to stretch when shock loaded, absorbing much of the dangerous force produced by rapid deceleration. This reduces the chances of injury by preventing transfer of these forces to the person being belayed.

Some rescue teams prefer to use ropes that will maintain the strength of the system and handle the potential weight of a two-person load. Most dynamic ropes have a breaking strength of about 6,000 force pounds, so they might not be considered adequate. The problem is, static (low-stretch) ropes do not absorb high-impact forces well enough to prevent injury to the person being belayed.

Many industrial rescue teams use shock absorbers (also called "load limiters'' or "force limiters") to provide a dynamic effect in their static rope. These shock absorbers are placed directly inline between the belay rope and the load (see Figure 6.7). The purpose is the same as the dynamic rope—to absorb shock in case of a fall.

When two persons are being belayed with the same rope, each should have an in-line shock absorber. If this is not possible due to the circumstances of the incident, a single shock absorber should be placed in-line at the first point of contact with the load. Since this is the first place to receive the impact force in a fall, it would be the best placement of a single shock absorber. If shock absorbers are not available, be extra cautious to keep nearly all of the slack out of the belay system. Should a fall occur, this is extremely important.

Figure 6.7 Shock absorber placed directly between belay rope and load

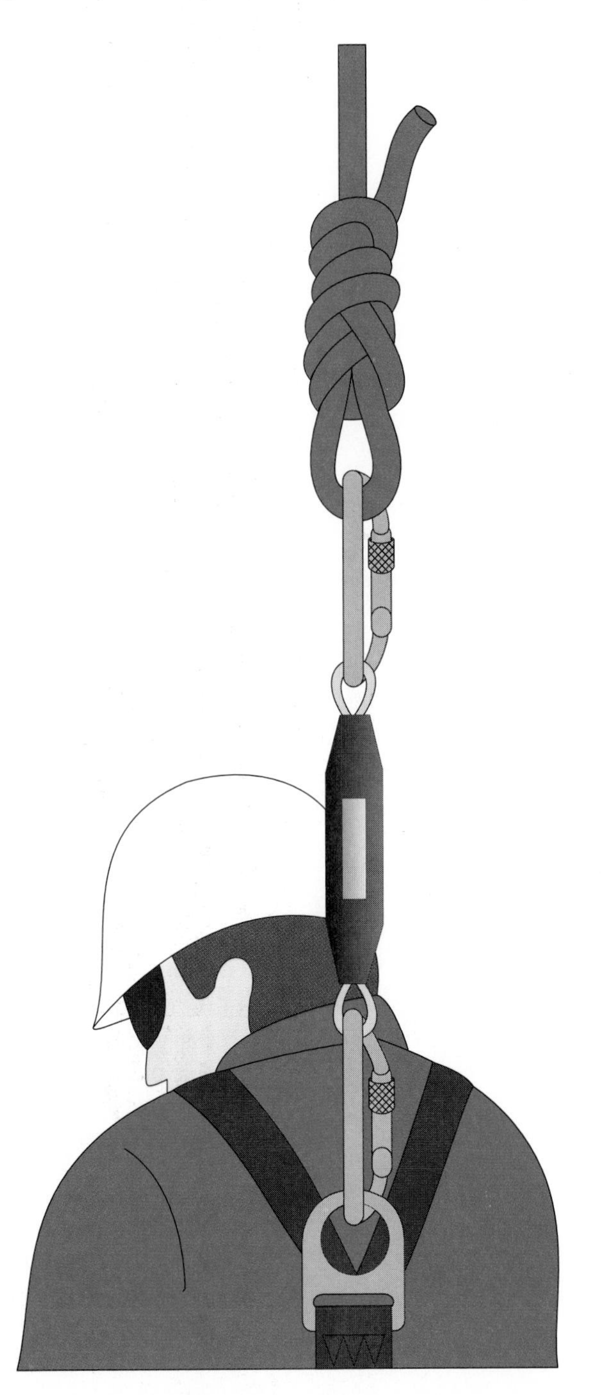

Communications

As with bottom belays, proper and clear communication is essential to the operation of a safety line belay system. The system should be attached to the person to be belayed first, before any other prepa-

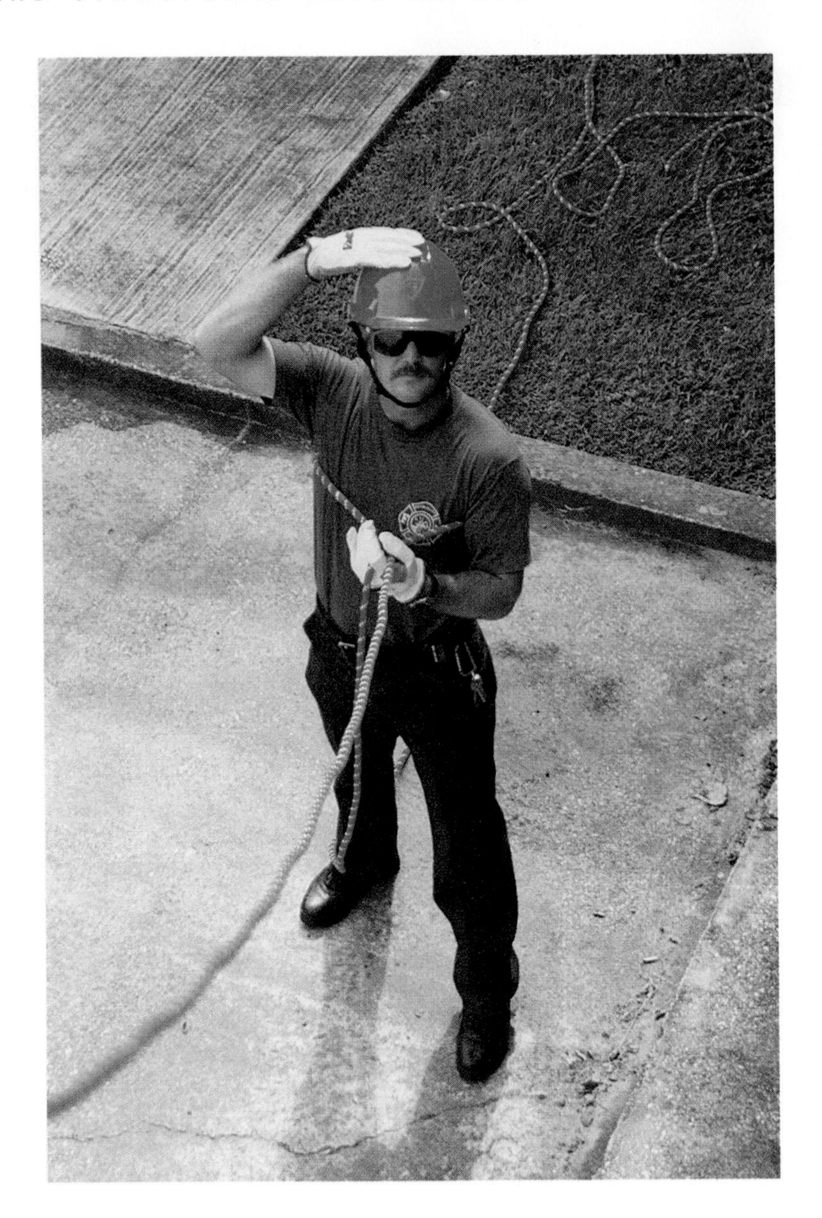

Figure 6.8 Visual belay signal—patting the top of the head with an open palm

ration is made. This "safety first" approach will prevent injury should a fall occur before the primary rope system is completely attached. The attachment and readiness of the belayer should be indicated by a signal either verbal or visual. Common verbal signals are "ready on safety" and simply "on safety." It is issued as soon as the belayer (also known as "safety man") has the system attached and is ready to operate it. In a very noisy environment, rescuers use hand signals to communicate. One such signal involves patting the top of the head with an open palm (see Figure 6.8).

In either case, proper communication lets the person being belayed know that it is safe to begin the procedure of attaching to the primary rope system. The signal is usually repeated once the primary rope system is ready and the person to be belayed is prepared to load the system. This procedure may vary slightly depending on the specific rescue and belay system. Whatever the signals, proper communication is extremely important to the successful application of safety line belay systems.

Configuration

Rescuers usually rig these systems with the belay device at the same level as or above the person to be belayed (see Figure 6.2). The systems can be run from any level. When necessary, rescuers can use directional pulleys to redirect the path of the rope. With these directionals, they can even operate the belay device on the

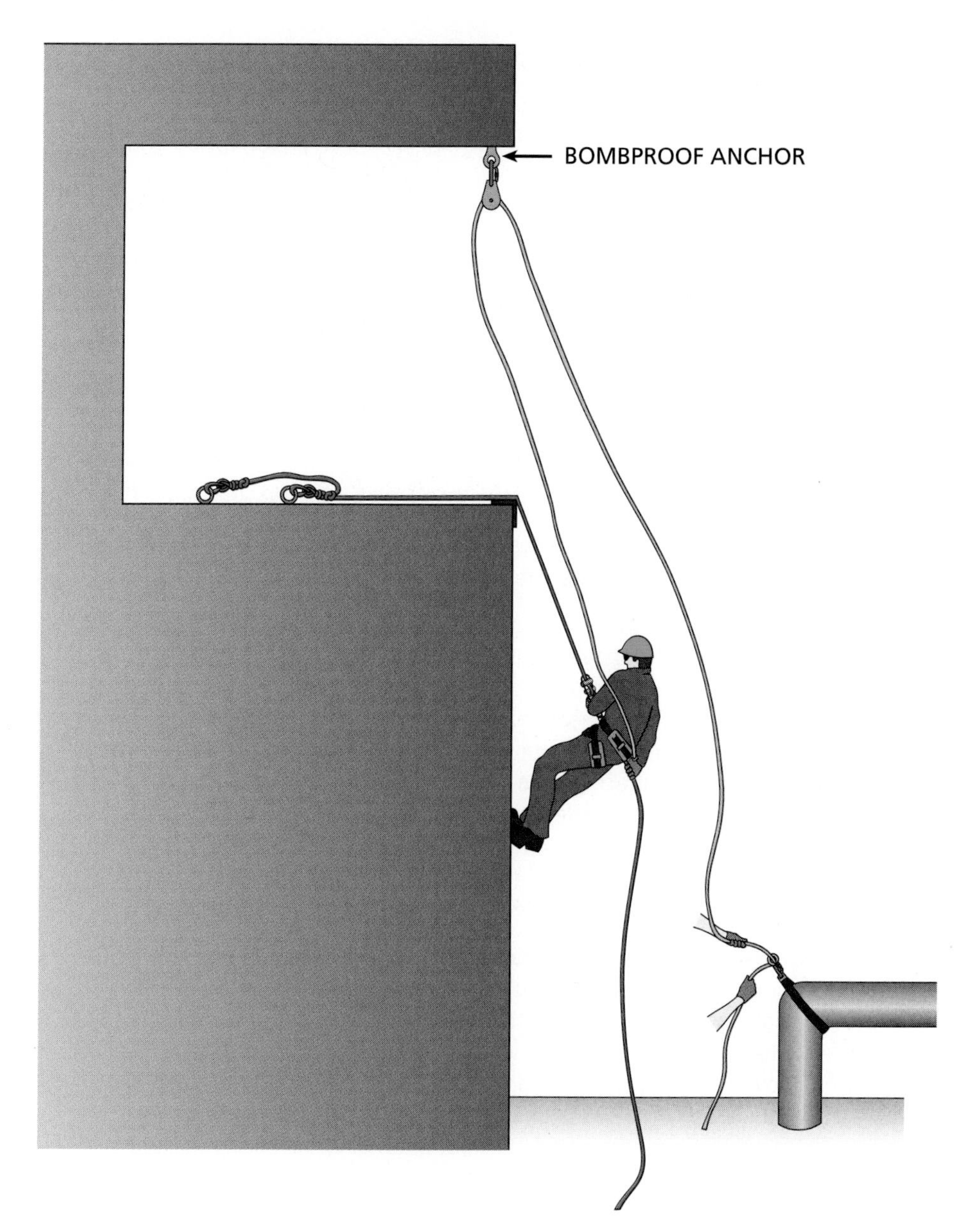

Figure 6.9 Running a belay line using a directional pulley

ground while running the rope through a free hanging pulley anchored above the level of the load (see Figure 6.9). This configuration usually allows the belayer to see the person being belayed. This advantage eliminates the need for an additional person to spot the load for the belayer, making the system more efficient in use of personnel.

Redirecting the rope's path from below requires about twice as much rope as belaying from the top. This loss of equipment efficiency somewhat counters the gain in personnel efficiency, but this technique is still highly recommended, especially for training. The decision to vary the system configuration must be based on the situation at hand and the type of belay device being used. The ability to move the system around is quite advantageous, particularly in the industrial setting where positioning of personnel in one location might be difficult.

Munter Hitch Belay

One effective safety line belay device is the Munter hitch (see Figure 6.5). The Munter is a hitch that, when loaded, binds on itself to stop the falling load. A Munter hitch is very effective for one-person loads and is simple to learn and operate. When operated properly, it catches the falling load with a high degree of reliability. It can be used to give or take up slack quickly and easily.

Operation The Munter hitch as a belay device is simple and quick to rig and operate.

1. Anchor a carabiner using proper rigging technique. Larger carabiners are usualy better for running the Munter hitch.
2. Tie and attach the Munter hitch to the carabiner and grasp both legs of rope issuing from the hitch, one in each hand.
3. The belayer should face the hitch positioned approximately 2 feet away. For maximum effectiveness, the angle between the two legs of rope issuing from the hitch should be no greater than 45 degrees. The wider the angle on this hitch, the less effective it will be. Keep the two legs as close together as possible during operation.
4. The belayer should feed the rope into the hitch with one hand while pulling slack with the other, keeping the hitch loose. Do not just pull the rope through with one hand. This would create unnecessary friction and subsequent buildup of heat in the rope's sheath.
5. You can change the direction of the rope (from taking up to giving slack or vice versa). Simply roll the hitch on the carabiner by pulling on the appropriate rope while feeding with the other hand to reverse the direction of the movement.

Belaying Two-Persons If possible, run one Munter hitch safety line belay system for each one-person load. However, due to constraints of equipment or personnel, it is often necessary to support two-person loads with a single Munter hitch safety line belay system. With a static kernmantle rope that meets NFPA standards for two-person loads, both persons can be attached to a single safety. If this situation arises, a rescuer must take several precautions in order for the Munter hitch belay to work effectively. This information is based on a series of nonscientific tests conducted in early 1994, which suggested that the Munter hitch, by itself, was not capable of catching a two-person load dropped approximately 3 feet. Additional measures are required:

- **To increase friction, run the Munter safety line over an edge** (see Figure 6.2). The tests quickly showed a free-hanging Munter hitch to be incapable of providing enough friction to hold two people easily and steadily, much less stop them when they fall. However, it was discovered that when the belay rope was passed over a properly padded edge (such as angle iron or a toe plate), the edge absorbed enough of the initial shock to allow the belayer time to brace for and catch the falling load. This measure is instrumental in the effectiveness of a Munter hitch to catch a falling two-person load should a system failure occur.
- **Place a shock absorber at the first point of attachment to the load.** This will activate a delay during the fall and allow the belayer to prepare to catch the falling load. The shock absorbing device (load limiter) should be placed as near to the load as possible. If it were placed at the anchorage of the Munter hitch (on the belay device side of the edge), the edge would most likely isolate the effect of the shock absorber to the belay device side of the system. This would allow the load (people) to take a significant impact, possibly causing injury. Shock absorbers are a good idea in any safety line belay system that stops the load suddenly. Reports by OSHA indicate that impact forces as little as 1,800 force pounds could cause the death of persons wearing full-body harnesses. The impact forces during this series of tests were distributed between two-person loads. However, they appeared sufficient to cause injury to the persons being belayed had shock absorbers not been used. If possible, use one shock absorber for each person attached to the belay line. If this is not possible, use one shock absorber at the first point of attachment to the patient, rescuer, litter, and so forth.
- BE READY! Keep alert to the possibility of system failure at all times. One thing evident in all of the tests was the importance of the Munter operator's readiness. The belayer who is not ready is not able to stop the falling load very quickly (within 6 or 7 feet). Be alert; be ready; be truly on belay.

If a separate safety line is not used for each person being belayed, then a line tender should be a backup for the belayer operating the Munter hitch (see Figure 6.4). As

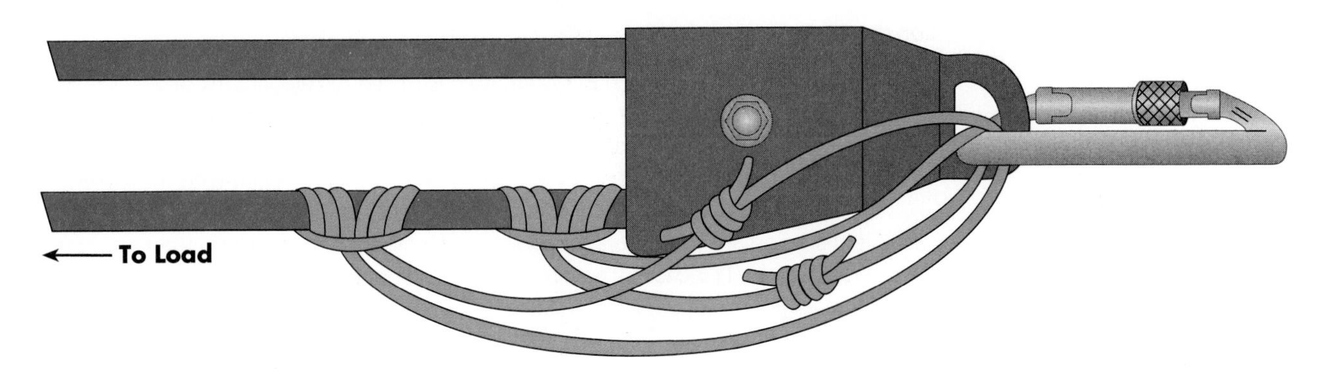

Figure 6.11 Tandem Prusik Belay

previously described, this person performs a kind of body belay with the rope wrapped around the body at the level of the buttocks. This prevents the rope from burning through clothing and into skin. This back-up person helps slow the falling two-person load if the belayer is having trouble. Although belaying a two-person load with a Munter hitch is not recommended, it is possible for rescuers operating within these configurations to stop a falling two-person load.

Lowering It appears feasible that the Munter could be used to lower or rappel with one-person loads. However, there is currently some opposition to that idea. This contention is based on some limited testing that indicated permanent degradation of the rope could occur if it were allowed to slide through the Munter hitch while under load. Until more testing is completed, it is not a good idea to use the Munter hitch to lower or rappel in a rescue. Thinking about the many possible rescue scenarios, a rescuer might ask, "What if the primary system fails and the load is hanging on the Munter safety belay line? Can we lower the load to the ground on the Munter?" The answer (as with the answer to most rescue questions) is that it depends on the circumstances surrounding the incident. If the victim is hanging on for dear life and there is no time to send another rescuer down, it may be less risky to simply lower the victim on the Munter hitch. If, however, the victim is calm, alert, and oriented and there are no compromises in the system due to the fall, rescuers might choose to send another rescuer on a separate rescue system to complete the rescue. It is impossible to give an unconditional approval to run loaded rope through a Munter hitch. Each situation is different and rescuers must consider all variables to make an informed decision. It is widely suspected that a Munter hitch could be used with loaded rope without serious degradation.

The nonscientific testing mentioned in the previous paragraph was performed by dropping a load and allowing the rope to slip through the Munter hitch as it caught. A reduction of strength was reported in the area of rope that slipped through during the fall arrest. This is precisely the type of thing NFPA 1983 addressed by requiring a 15:1 safety factor—that conditions might be such to create significant loss of rope strength. Knots, abrasive edges, and other conditions could reduce significantly the effective rope strength. While rescuers may choose to lower on this system following a fall, they must destroy the rope afterwards because of the impact forces it was subjected to.

Tandem Prusik Belay

Another effective belay device for one- and two-person loads involves the use of small-diameter accessory cord. These cords are tied into loops (Prusik loops), attached to the safety line with a special Prusik hitch (see Figure 6.11), and anchored securely. If utilizing $\frac{1}{2}$-inch rescue rope, the Prusiks should be used in tandem, triple wrapped, and equalized using 8-millimeter accessory cord for the best effect. They work by binding in case of failure, acting as a rope grab and stopping the fall. While this method is very effective, it requires practice and effort to learn and operate properly. The tandem Prusik belay system is not a lowering system.

Construction

1. The tandem Prusik belay (TPB) system is constructed of two lengths of very supple 8-millimeter ($\frac{5}{16}$″) kernmantle accessory cord. Follow manufacturer's recommendations in selecting accessory cord for Prusiks. The cord should be supple enough to make a very small radius bend (no space inside the bight) when pinched with the fingers. The minimum breaking strength of this cord should be about 4,000 force pounds.
2. Tie the accessory cord into a loop using a double fisherman's knot. The tails should be as close to $1\frac{1}{2}$ inches as possible on each side once the knot is tied, dressed, and tightened.
3. Make one Prusik loop from a $5\frac{1}{2}$-foot length of 8-millimeter cord and the other from a $4\frac{1}{2}$-foot length of 8-millimeter cord.
4. When you attach the Prusik loops, wrap them three times around the $\frac{1}{2}$-inch static (low-stretch) kernmantle safety line to make a triple-wrap Prusik knot (see Figure 6.13).
5. Wrap the longer of the two Prusiks around the safety line between the anchor and the load.
6. Wrap the shorter of the two Prusiks around the safety line between the first Prusik and the anchor.
7. Wrap both Prusiks in the same direction around the rope. Position the double fisherman's knots between the Prusik knot and the carabiner (not in the Prusik knot or touching the carabiner).
8. After they are tied and properly dressed, attach both Prusik loops to the anchor system.
9. The anchorage for a TPB should consist of the anchor system itself, a general-use steel locking carabiner, a load releasing hitch (discussed later), and another general-use steel locking carabiner to which the Prusiks are attached. Link these in the order described.
10. After the Prusiks are attached and properly dressed, there should be 2 to 4 inches between the Prusiks. If the Prusiks are too close to each other, they may not operate properly to arrest a load.
11. It is equally important to keep the Prusik hitches tight on the safety line during the entire operation. Should they become loose at any time, stop the operation and tighten the Prusik hitches before resuming.

Prusik Minding Pulleys During raising operations, rescuers can use a Prusik minding pulley (PMP) to make the operation of the Prusiks easier (see Figure 6.11).

1. Attach a Prusik minding pulley to the same carabiner as the Prusiks.
2. The Prusiks should be attached closest to the carabiner's spine with the pulley next to them. This assures the load is transmitted through the strongest part of the carabiner.

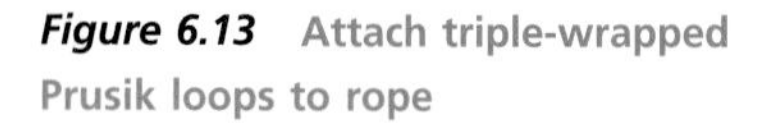
Figure 6.13 **Attach triple-wrapped Prusik loops to rope**

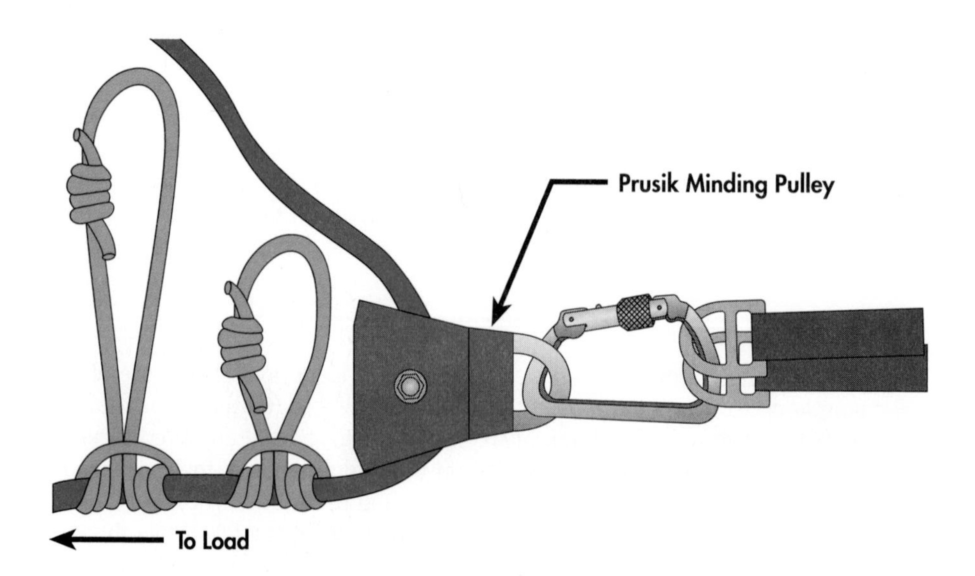

3. Complete the setup by running one end of the rope through the pulley and then attaching the Prusiks.
4. Attach the load to the Prusik side of the belay rope.
5. For a stronger system, attach the carabiners with the gates down to keep the load along the spine.
6. If you use a screw-type locking carabiner in any configuration other than horizontal, the locking sleeve should be in a position to allow closure should vibration loosen it.

The Load Releasing Hitch The load releasing hitch (LRH) (see Figure 6.14), which is constructed from 33 feet of 9-millimeter low-stretch kernmantle accessory cord, is used between the anchor and the Prusiks for two principle reasons:

1. Due to its configuration, it provides some shock absorbancy if there is a failure in the main system.
2. It allows the load to be transferred back to the main line if the tandem Prusiks become accidentally loaded.

A LRH can also be useful in nonbelay applications. When used at the anchor of certain rope rescue systems, it expedites changing from a raising system to a lowering system and vice versa. As with all rope systems, the load releasing hitch should be replaced if it is shock loaded.

Lowering

1. Operate the TPB in lowering operations by placing one hand on the Prusik farthest from the anchor.
2. While this hand holds the Prusik in place, the other hand grabs the safety line where it issues from the Prusiks and pulls enough slack to make a "Z twist" (usually 8 to 12 inches).
3. During lowering, the weight of the load will straighten out the Z twist.
4. Just before the Z twist is straightened, the hand holding it will release the rope and pull more slack to make another Z twist.
5. Repeat this process throughout the lowering procedure.
6. If the lowering operation stops for any reason, the Prusiks should be pulled tight and all slack taken up in the system.
7. Before resuming the operation, start with a new Z twist. It is very important that the Prusiks remain tight on the safety line at all times to ensure proper activation of the belay system. Keeping the Prusiks tight also helps to keep excess slack out of the system.

Remember to wear gloves to protect your hands should the belay be activated by a failure of the primary rope system. During operation, allow no slack between the Prusiks and the anchor system. Slack can make the shock load much greater if the primary system fails.

Hauling As previously discussed, a Prusik minding pulley will be incorporated into the system during hauling operations. The side plates of this specialized pulley are designed to keep the Prusik knots sliding on the rope without binding in the sheave.

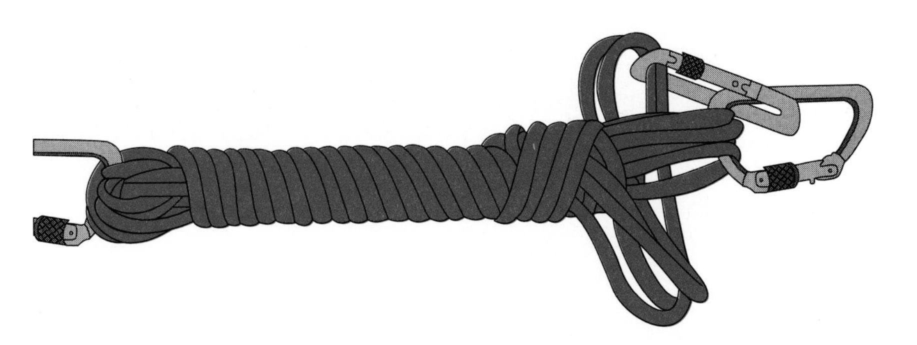

Figure 6.14 Load releasing hitch

1. As the load is raised by the hauling system, you must pull the safety rope through the PMP. This involves keeping one hand on the load-bearing side rope (the rope feeding into the pulley) while pulling the rope through from the opposite side with the other hand.
2. As the hand on the load-bearing side of the pulley grasps the rope, it will travel toward the Prusik knots.
3. As your hand nears the Prusik knots, grab them, sliding them toward the load to prevent excess slack between the anchor system and Prusiks.
4. As with a lowering system, take the opportunity to retighten the Prusik knots and remove the slack each time the operation is interrupted for any reason.
5. It is also important to keep the angle between the ropes feeding in and out of the pulley as close to 0 degrees as possible in order for the PMP to properly mind the Prusiks.
6. It is recommended that the belayer be located no further than 3 feet from the PMP to tend the Prusiks properly.

Safety Line Belay Summary

There are new products coming to the rescue market (some still on the drawing board) that might someday eliminate the controversy over control devices for belay systems. Rescuers hope these devices will allow belay of two-person loads with minimal effort and maximal operational finesse. The competent rescuer constantly looks for safer, more efficient ways of accomplishing rescues. Effective solutions can often be found in new technology.

Summary

The techniques presented here require much training and practice to properly deploy and operate. It is important to seek training from a competent source in order to perform safe rescues.

The concept of a belay system is just one step that can be taken by a rescue team to ensure a high degree of safety in training and rescue operations. Again, it is highly recommended that all industrial rescue teams utilize applicable belay systems in their training operations. Although optional, many carry this policy into their actual rescue operations as well. The determination of when and where to apply these systems is ultimately the responsibility of the rescue team. Whatever the decision, it must be based on the two most important aspects of any rescue issue–safety and efficiency.

Authors' Note: Information on the Tandem Prusik Belay System was provided by Mark D. Baker, Fire/Rescue Captain, Wichita, KS Fire Department.

CHAPTER 7

Rappelling and Self-Rescue

The information in this chapter is provided as a basis for continued training. Each rescuer should consult with his or her own team leader for the correct SOGs for the team. Topics covered in this chapter include:

- Personnel Assignments
- Commands
- Starting the Procedure
- Attaching to the Rappel Rope
- Safety Check
- Rappelling Position and Ledge Negotiation
- Descent Control
- Self-Rescue

Introduction

Rescue capabilities are similar to a tool box. Each technique represents a different tool. You use the right tool for the job at hand. Rappelling is just another tool. It might be useful in certain situations. Understanding when and when not to use this technique helps put rappelling in the proper perspective for industrial rescue.

Rappelling is a way to instill confidence in rescue personnel and teach them the proper use of a particular descent control device. But rappelling should be considered less effective than a lowering system for most rescues. In general, when given a choice between a lower or a rappel, *choose to lower.*

Rescuers sometimes use rappelling to retrieve victims from exposed or dangerous high places such as buildings and windows. Rappelling is a self-lowering technique based on the rescuer's controlled sliding on a rope, with friction created by rope passing through a descent control device.

Control is a vital goal in any rappelling operation. So, the technique of belaying is closely related to rescue rappelling. The previous chapter discussed in detail safety line belay systems to back up the primary rope system in case of failure. It also previewed the body belay technique to stop a falling rappeller. This chapter discusses the application of these techniques within the rappelling operation.

Body belays only back up the rappeller; they do not back up the rope system. For this reason, many trainers strongly recommend the use of an additional safety line belay system. This discussion assumes that the rescue team has chosen to use both body belays and safety line belays with their rappel system.

Rappelling is an important industrial rescue technique. Most people really enjoy the experience and actually consider it fun. But because it is fun, rescue teams can spend too much training time on this barely practical technique. "Barely practical" because, although rappelling seems very dramatic and exciting, it actually has limited practical use in industrial rescue.

Almost any rescue that can be performed with a rappel can be much more safely and efficiently done with a lowering system. For example, a rescuer being lowered to a patient who may panic (possibly beating you about the head and body) could have full use of both hands and legs for self-defense, or could rappel to the same patient, having to use one or both hands to control the descent.

One of the biggest advantages of the technique is that it can provide for a very efficient rescue in terms of equipment and personnel. For example, a worker that has taken a fall on a fall-arrest system and is hanging suspended (and possibly unconscious) requires immediate rescue because of the physiological dangers of hanging in a harness that is severely restricting blood flow to the victim's limbs. Rappel rescue, in this case a line-transfer technique, requires only one rescuer with one rope (a safety line is preferred but not mandatory to effect the rescue) and a few pieces of equipment found in most rescuers' personal rescue tote bags. "Pick-off" techniques like this will be further discussed in the next chapter.

Rappelling can also provide a multitude of benefits to the developing rescue team. Some of these advantages are that it

- teaches new team members to deal with their natural fear of heights.
- reinforces the team's confidence in the equipment and in teammates.
- establishes the importance of teamwork and intrateam communications.
- allows the development of proper techniques for the controlled use of descent devices.

Sometimes, it may be necessary to rappel. The following are some situations where rappelling might be preferred:

- Someone must escape from a height.
- The rescuer must stop precisely at a specific location that cannot be seen by the lowering system operator and communications are poor.
- A situation requires instant adjustments of descent control in reaction to the patient's actions.

These scenarios are generally considered "worst case" and do not represent the norm. However, rescuers must be prepared for the worst case and should therefore practice all potentially useful techniques including rappelling.

Personnel Assignments

To staff the positions previously discussed requires four team members (if using a safety line belay). In summary, the necessary positions are:

- **Rappeller** is obviously the person doing the actual rappelling. The rappeller is also responsible for issuing the "on rappel" commands to the belayer.
- **Body belayer** is the person at the bottom of the drop designated to help slow or stop the rappeller if out of control. The body belayer will respond to the verbal command "on rappel" with the signal "on belay." The body belayer's ability to stop a falling rappeller depends on reaction time. The body belayer must *always* be ready when the rappeller is on line.
- **Safety line belayer** operates the safety line belay system that backs up the primary rope system in case of failure. The safety line belayer is sometimes called a "safety man" for short. This position should be a requirement in training and is a highly recommended option in actual rescues as well.
- **Rappel master** is responsible for the general safety of the rappeller, though all team members should share in this task. A rappel master has two basic functions: (1) to check the rappeller and have the entire system rechecked before life loading the system, and (2) to act as the eyes and ears of the safety line belayer, if applicable. If the belayer cannot see the rappeller directly, the rappel master must advise the safety man of his or her position and the amount of slack or tension needed in the belay rope.

Commands

As noted, intrateam communication is important. Rescuers must develop commands that make the operation run smoothly. These commands should be clear, simple, and to the point. This text does not dictate the commands rescuers should use but suggests some common terms. The commands rescuers use probably are not so important as making sure all members of a team use the same ones. Uniform communications are essential for efficient and safe rescue. The suggested verbal and nonverbal commands throughout this text are common. Industrial rescue teams can use them effectively. However, each team should meet to discuss the most appropriate use of verbal and nonverbal commands based on its circumstances.

Obviously proper commands (signals) are an integral part of this and other rescue processes. To recap the verbal commands suggested so far and introduce a few:

- **"On safety"**—The rescue master asks this question of the safety line belayer. Or it can be a response from the safety line belayer to the rescue master and rappeller. This should be issued before starting the rappel sequence and before going over the edge or anytime before preparing to rappel.
- **"On rappel"**—The rappeller gives this command twice in the rappel sequence. It first comes before attachment to the descent control device. It comes next after receiving a final safety check but just before climbing over the edge or anytime before preparing to rappel. This signal should always receive a response from the bottom belayer. It should also incite a response from the safety line belayer when used just before starting to rappel. "On line" is a common alternative.
- **"On belay"**—The body belayer gives this command in response to "on rappel." The first time the belayer gives it, it means the belayer is protecting the rappeller's rope from bystanders. The second time it is given it means absolute readiness for the rappeller to begin loading the line. A command "belay on" is commonly used in place of "on belay" for this second signal.
- **"Locked-off"**—This signal should be given by the rappeller once he or she has locked off the descent control device for hands-free operation. It is a courtesy to the body belayer. It means the belayer can relax rather than look up for an extended period while the rappeller is locked off. The body belayer is ineffective as a belayer while the rappeller is locked off. Before unlocking, the rappeller should give the "on rappel" signal. Then rappeller waits for the body and safety line belayers to respond with "on belay" and "on safety" before unlocking the device.
- **"Off rappel"**—The rappeller gives this signal after reaching the ground and after detaching completely from the rappel line. The commands "off line" or "off rope" are used synonymously.

If noise is excessive or the height is great and radios are not available, rescuers have to use hand signals in place of voice communications. One simple signal that all personnel can use is tapping the top of the head with one hand (see Figure 7.1). Rescuers can use this in the same sequence as the verbal communications. It is generally a good idea to use a combination of verbal and visual signals to ensure good communications.

Figure 7.1 **Tapping head to communicate**

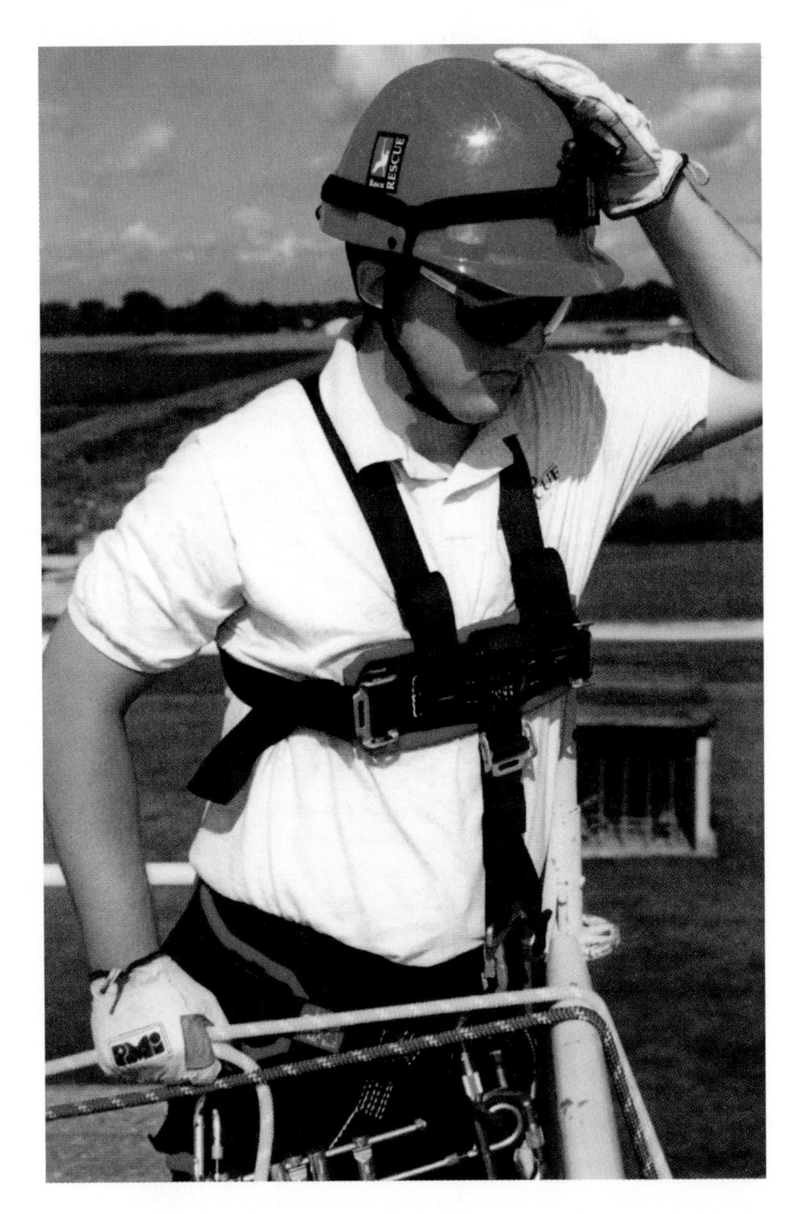

Whenever possible, use radios or some other positive means of communication between crews that are out of sight from each other.

Starting the Procedure

If you are using a safety line belay system, attach it with a carabiner to the rappeller's harness. The safety line belay system should be completely prepared before the belayer gives the ready signal. For this discussion, the verbal signal "on safety" indicates readiness. This "safety first" practice helps prevent rappellers from injuring themselves by going over the edge before attaching to their descent control devices.

The rappeller then looks at the bottom belayer, grasps the rope and gives a command such as "on rappel." It is important that the rappeller wait for a response from the body belayer before doing anything else. After grasping the loose end of the line on the ground, the body belayer looks up and says something like "on belay." This ensures that a bystander does not pull on the rope while the rescuer is attaching to the descent control device, which could drag the rappeller over the edge. In effect, the rappeller has just told the body belayer "I'm getting ready to start attaching myself to the rappel line." The body belayer has, in turn, told the rappeler "Okay, I'll keep people away from your line down here so they won't pull you over the edge." It is not necessary for the body belayer to keep his or her eyes on the rappeller during this phase. He or she only has to control the rope by keeping a hand on it and staying alert. Once this is done and everybody is ready, it is time to attach the descent control device to the rappel rope.

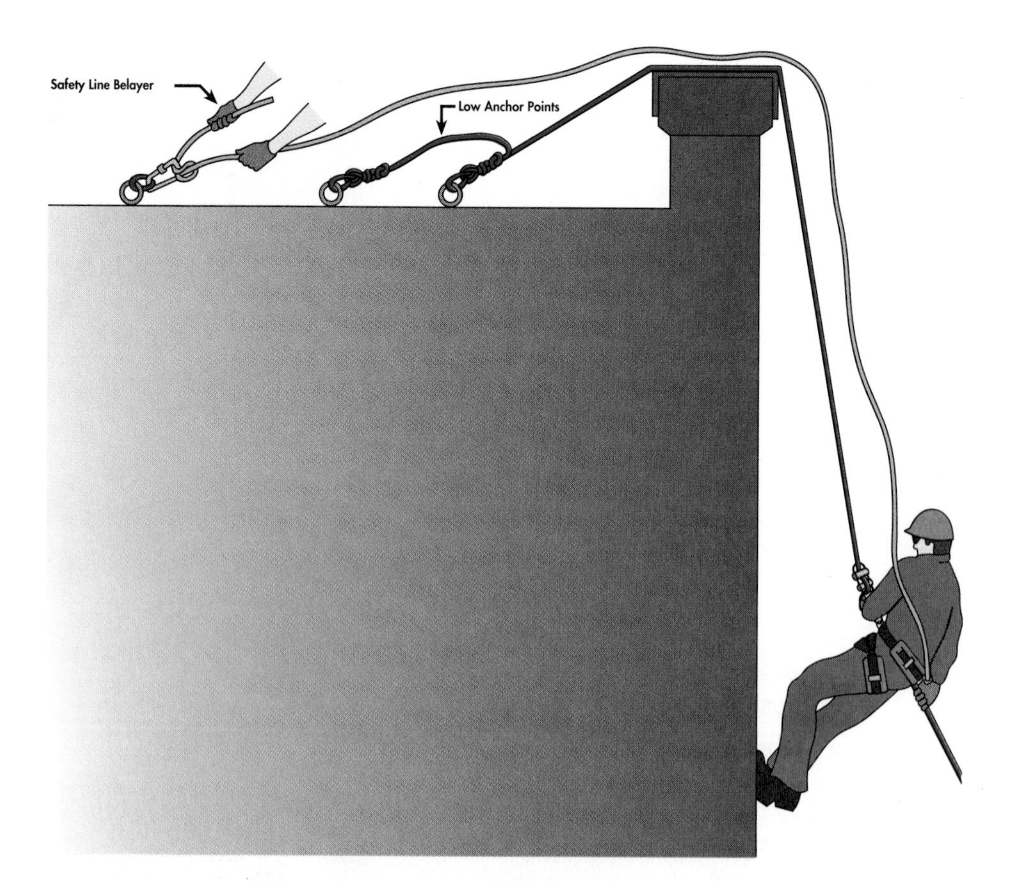

Figure 7.2 Low-point anchor

Attaching to the Rappel Rope

Decide how and where the rappeller attaches to the rope. This depends primarily on the location of the rappeller in relation to the anchor system. If the rope is anchored at or below the level of the rappeller, it is considered a low-point anchor (see Figure 7.2). The rappeller should pull the rope tightly away from the anchor and over the edge, grasping it at the plumb point. The plumb point is an imaginary point on the rope located approximately 1 inch over the edge. With a low-point anchor, attaching at the plumb point will ensure that the descent control device will clear the edge when a rescuer crawls over to load the line. This method also prevents the rappeller from shock loading the rope as it limits the distance the rappeller has to travel over the edge before the line is loaded.

An anchor located above the rappeller is considered a high-point anchor (see Figure 7.3). When using a high-point anchor, you should attach to the highest possible point on the rope. Stand on your tiptoes if you must to make this attachment. Usually, the higher the attachment point, the easier it is to get over the edge. If given a choice of a high- or low-point anchor for rappelling, go for the high-point anchor every time. This is because there is less chance for shock loading the rope and it is usually easier to climb over the edge.

After receiving the reply from the bottom belayer, the rappeller completes the attachment of the descent control device to the rappel rope and to his or her harness. Chapter 3, "Related Rope Rescue Equipment," covered the basic operation of two of the most popular descent control devices, the rappel rack and the figure-8 plate. We will quickly review the process of attachment for both devices.

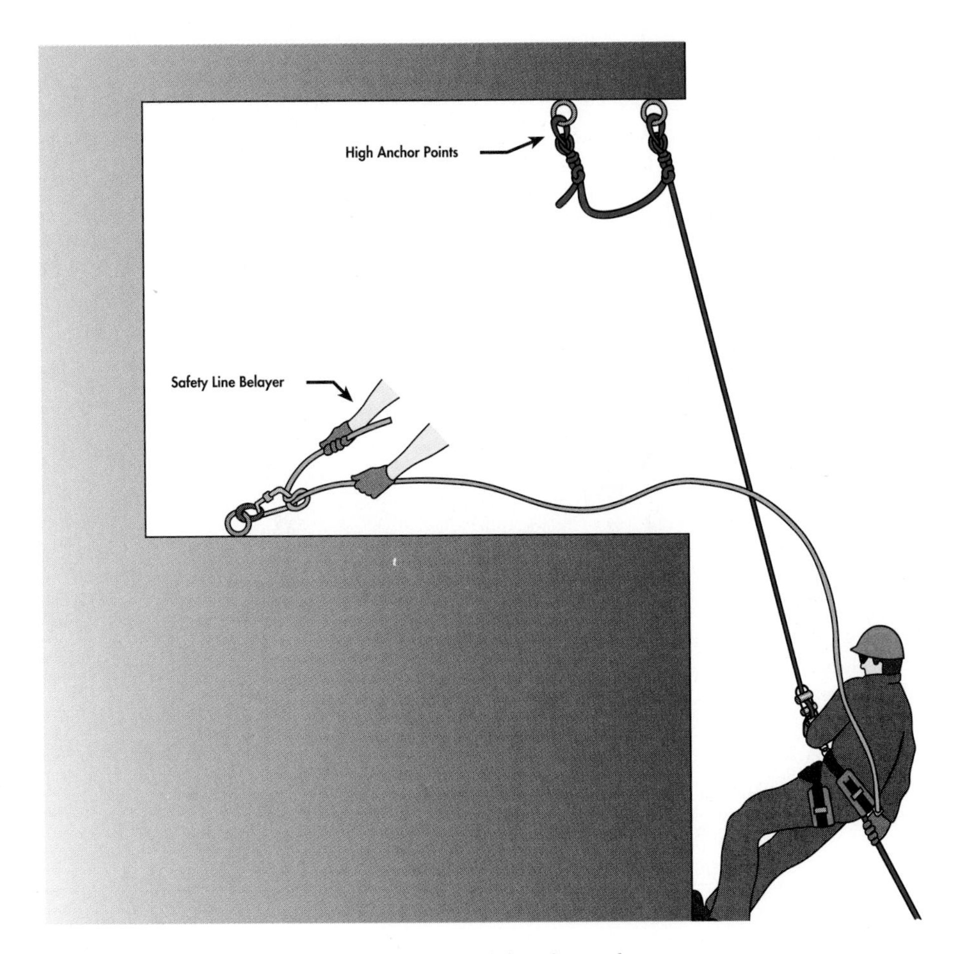

Figure 7.3 High-point anchor

The Rappel Rack

The rack should be preattached to the harness of the rappeller with a carabiner.

1. The rappeller begins to "rack in" by placing the plumb point across the top bar of the rack. If the top bar has a "training groove," the rope should go across the groove.
2. With a high-point anchor, pull out all the slack through the rappel rack, attaching to a point as high as possible on the rope.
3. Push the second, straight slot bar up and wrap the rope around it. If loaded incorrectly, this type of bar will fall out of place. This provides an additional safety check for rack operation.
4. Continue to wrap the bars with the rope until all six bars are racked in.

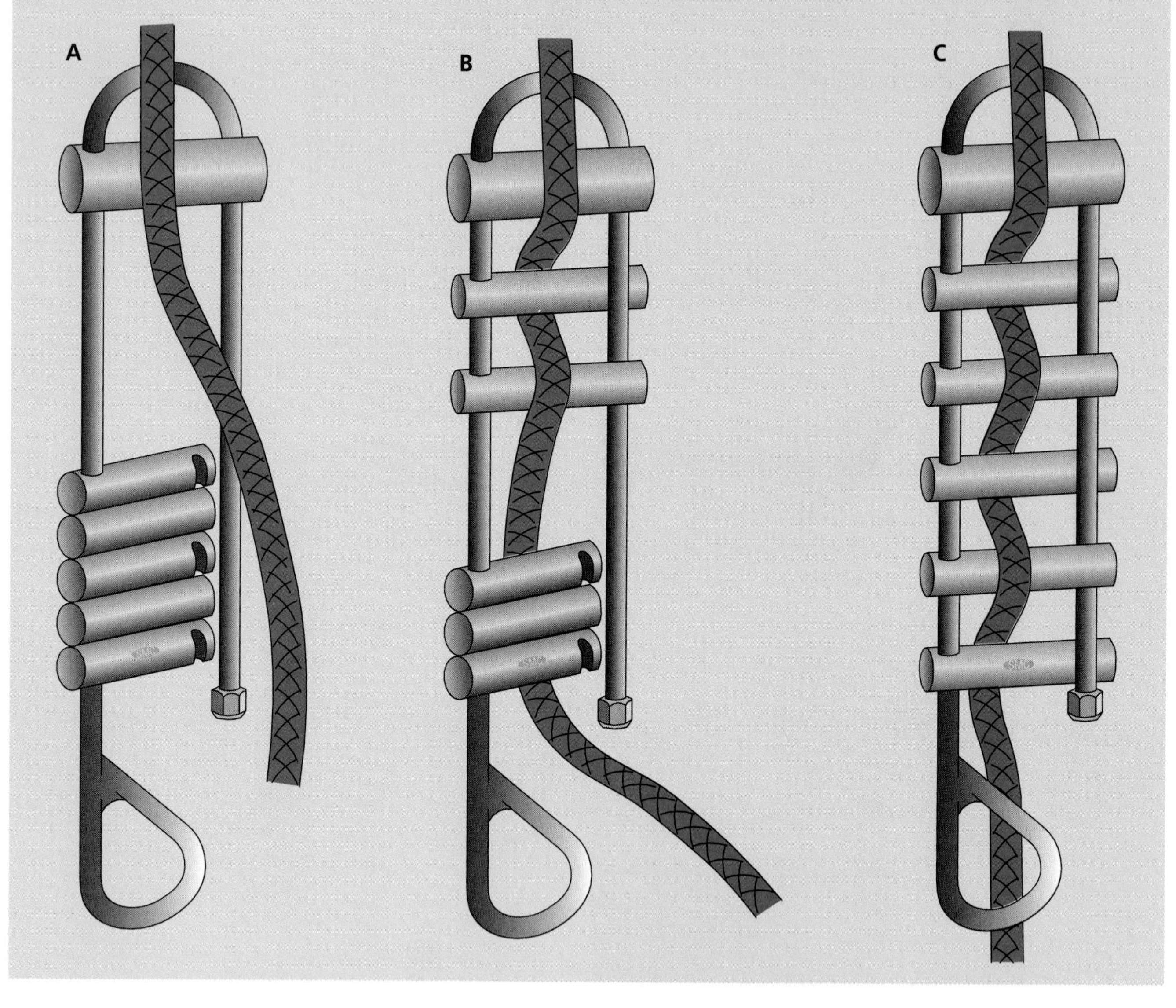

The Figure-8 Plate

Most figure-8s require removal from the rappeller's harness before attachment to the rope.

1. If you use a low-point anchor, form a bight in the rope below the level of the plumb point. If using a high-point anchor, form a bight in the rope somewhere at the rappeller's waist level.
2. Place the bight through the large ring of the figure-8 (from the bottom side) and over the small end of the body of the device.
3. Attach it to the rappeller's harness with a carabiner. When using a low-point, do not allow the figure-8 to move on the rope. This can cause you to end up in an undesirable position when trying to negotiate the edge. If using a high-point anchor, try to pull out all the slack between the anchor and the figure-8 to get in the highest position possible.

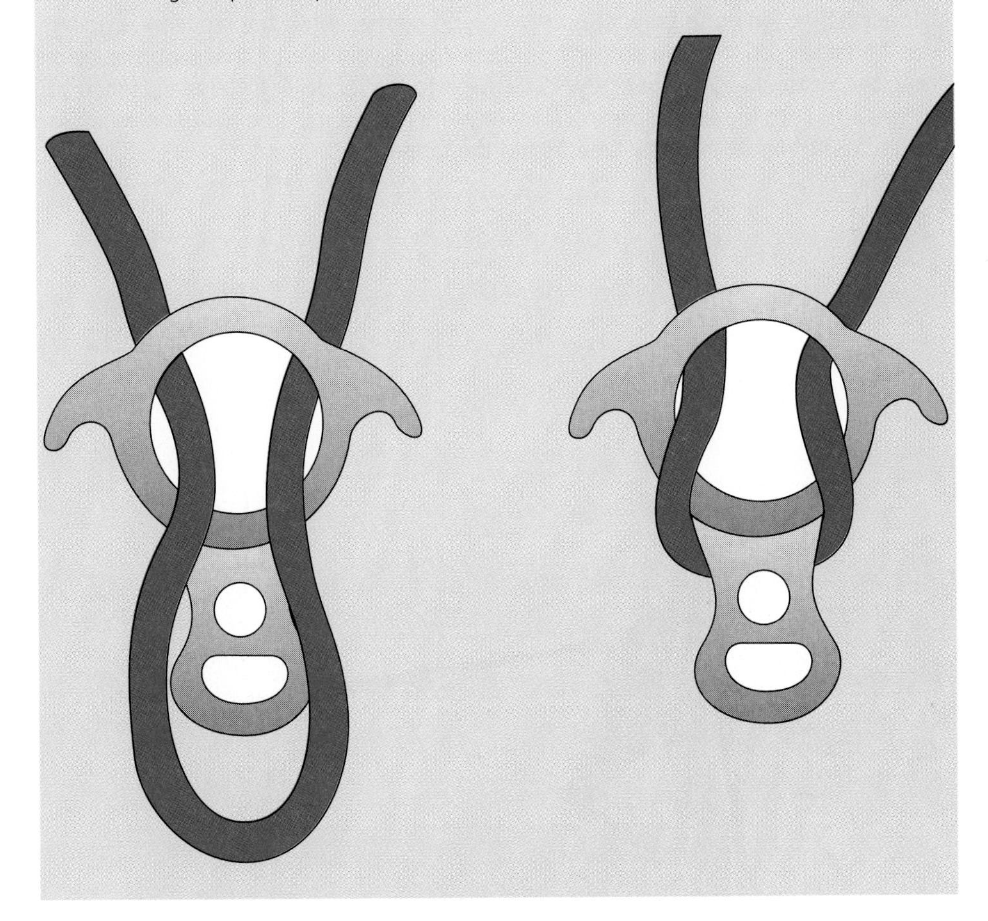

Safety Check

A team member designated the rappel master should perform a final safety check. The safety check should ensure at least the following:

- The rappeller is wearing the proper personal protective equipment.
- The rack and safety lines are properly attached to the rappeller's harness.
- All carabiners are locked.
- The harness is adjusted properly and all webbing ends secured.

The rappel master is also responsible for communicating to the safety line belayer the need for more or less slack in the safety line. This is because the belayer cannot see the rappeller directly. If working near an unprotected edge, the rappel master may also need a safety line. Any person working near enough to an opening or edge to fall should tie off properly to an anchored system (see Figure 7.6). The tie off must support the person(s) in such a way to prevent them from falling. Appropriate positioning can also eliminate the chance of falling over an edge. For example, a person lying prone on a flat roof looking over the edge is less likely to fall than when standing.

Before going over the edge, the rappeller gives the command "on rappel" again and waits for the belayer's response. Once the safety line and bottom belayer are positioned properly, the belayer issues the "on belay" signal for the second time, showing his or her readiness. This signal is very important. The rappeller must hear it before negotiating the edge.

If you are the body belayer, take your job seriously. When the rappeller yells "on rappel," you should get ready to catch him or her should something go wrong. Before you yell back that you are ready, MAKE SURE YOU ARE!

If anything is going to go wrong, it is likely to happen while the rappeller is going over the edge. You must be properly positioned with your eye on that rappeller before giving the signal that you are ready. You owe it to the rappeller to be ready when you say you are. Both the body belayer and safety line belayer must be alert and ready to catch a falling rappeller at any time during the rappel.

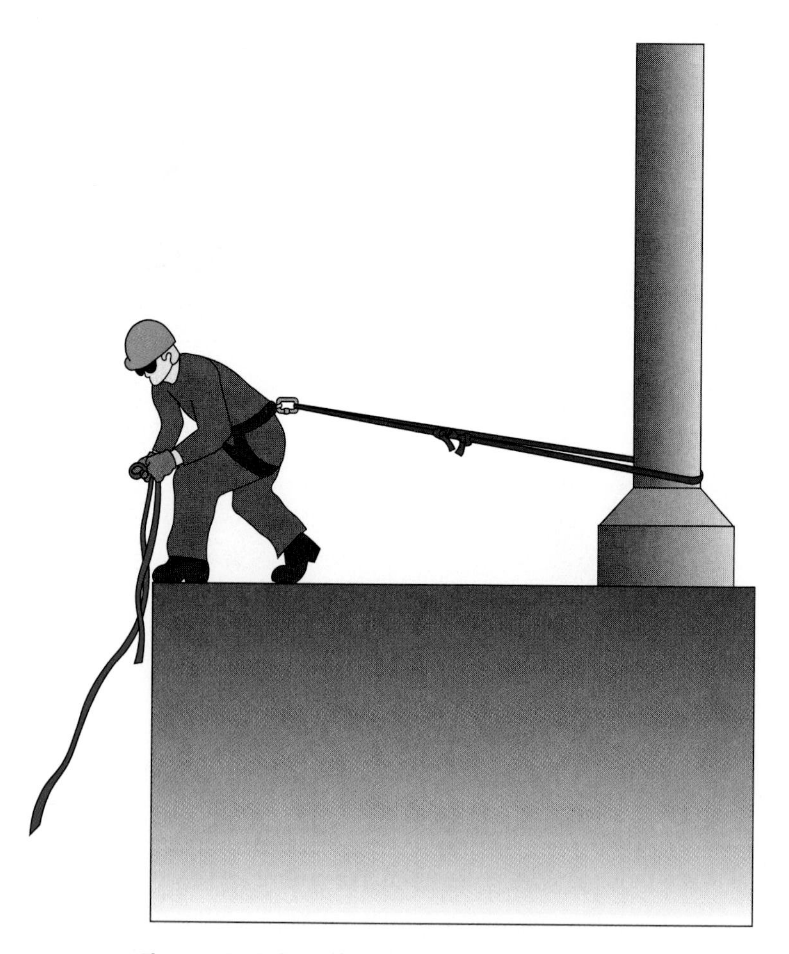

Figure 7.6 Tying off while working near an edge

Negotiating the Edge

After completing the safety check, the rappeller is ready to negotiate the edge. If the anchor is high enough above the edge to be negotiated, the rappeller simply attaches to the rope as high as possible before stepping over the edge (see Figure 7.7). If the anchor is at or below the level of the edge, the rescuer must rack in at the "plumb point." He or she must then crawl over the edge (see Figure 7.8). While doing this the rappeller must keep control of the rappel device, making certain not to crush hands beneath the rope or device. Note the instruction to "crawl over" not "walk over" or "jump over" the edge. Rappelling in rescue differs significantly from tactical or "sport" rappelling. Fundamental to rescue rappelling is *control.* Walking over the edge on a

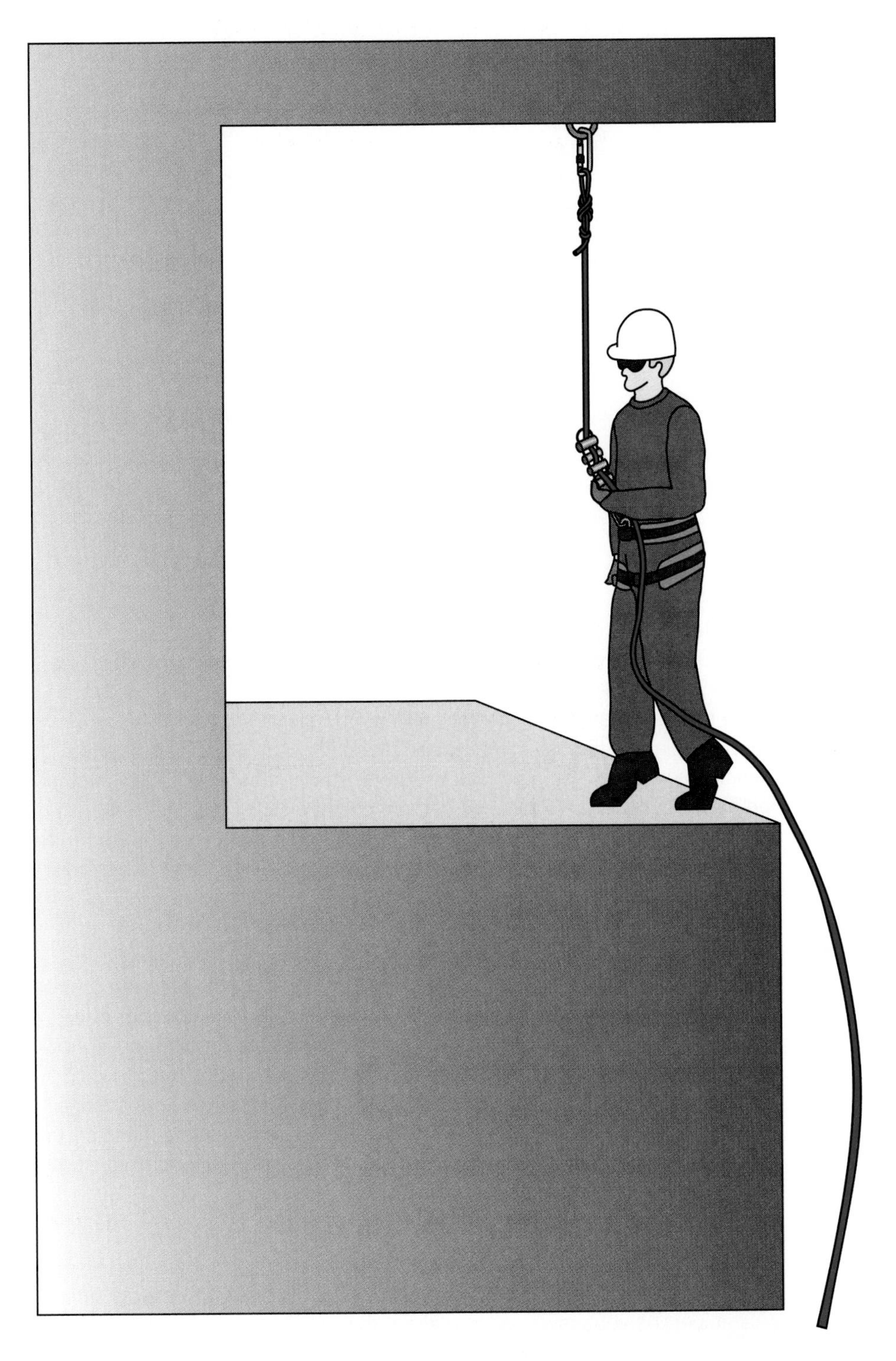

Figure 7.7 **Attaching as high as possible (Safety line belay not shown. Pictured systems may not portray ideal anchorage. Team members not shown.)**

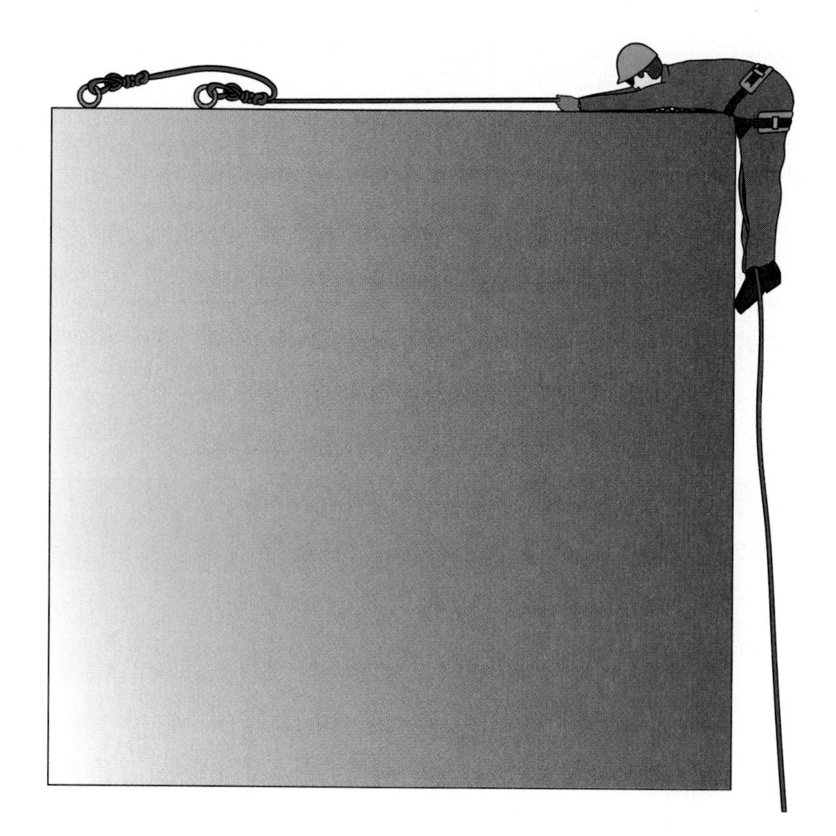

Figure 7.8 Crawling over the edge (Safety line belay not shown. Team members not shown)

low-point anchor can be tricky and probably should be avoided. Jumping over an edge anytime is an uncontrolled and dangerous act, especially on static kernmantle rope. Do not jump to negotiate an edge during a structural rescue operation.

There are a few fundamental differences in the use of descent control devices while loading the line for rappelling. Here are some for the rack and figure-8 devices:

The Brake Bar Rack

1. Make certain you are racked in on all six bars before going over the edge (see Figure 7.9). It is seldom necessary to lock off the device since, with six bars, there is usually plenty of friction to prevent movement.
2. Most people find they can let go of the rack and not move if all six bars are jammed tightly with the rope. This is extremely helpful because it frees the rappeller to use both hands and legs to climb over the edge.
3. Once you are over the edge, place your right hand on the rope trailing from the device (the control rope). Have your left hand cupped around the bottom two bars of the rack for additional control.

The Figure-8 Plate

1. When rappelling with the figure 8, make certain that you hold onto the control rope with your dominant hand at all times. The figure-8 plate does not offer nearly the control of the brake bar rack. If you release the control rope, the figure 8 allows you to fall at a rapid rate.
2. To crawl over on a low-point anchor, hold the control rope with your stronger hand and pull the rope downward, over the wall. Plant the weaker hand on the edge or window sill by crossing it over the rope. This will keep you from crushing your hand beneath the rope while crawling over the side.
3. Drop one leg at a time over the edge. Allow each leg to fall over the side while holding tension on the control rope.

When negotiating the edge with either the rack or "8," be careful to avoid side loading the carabiner. As you crawl over the edge, the carabiner will become un-

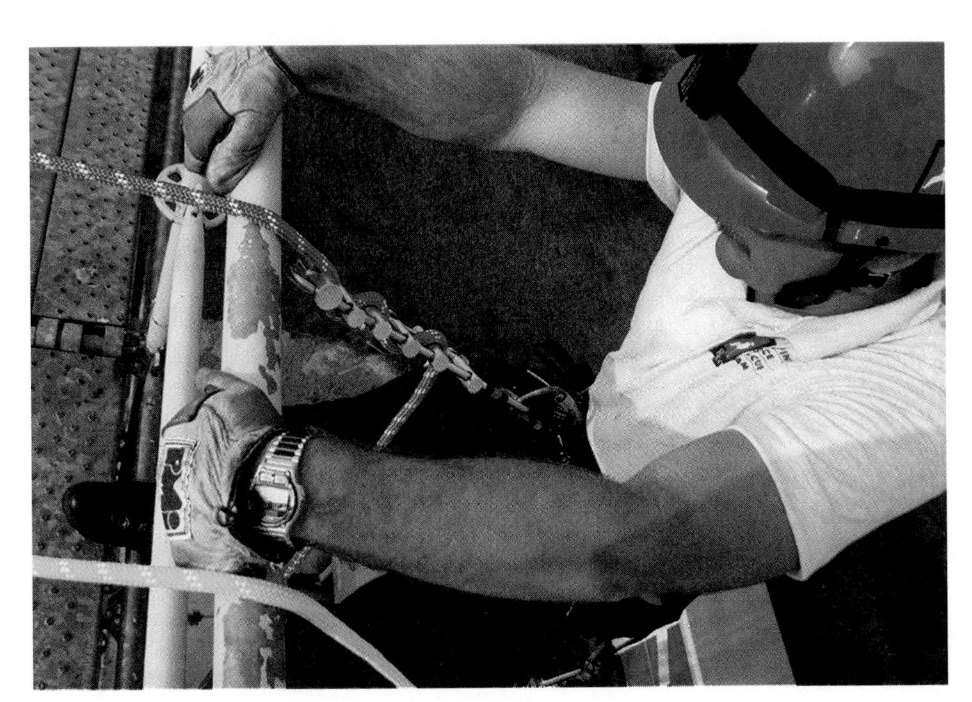

Figure 7.9 On all 6 bars while going over the edge

loaded and can turn sideways (see Figure 7.10). This may cause it to be loaded along the short axis (on the gate) once your weight is placed on the system. If this happens, do what you can to correct it. If you cannot correct it while on line, rappel to the nearest area that will allow you to take weight off and correct it. Do not panic, just fix it when and if you can.

Another important precaution concerns harnesses. Harness D-rings that are vertically configured allow the carabiner gate to be either up (on top) or down (on bottom) once it is attached. When crawling over the edge with a harness of this type, always position a screw-lock carabiner with the gate on the side next to your body (see Figure 7.11). If the gate is on the bottom, it will probably contact the edge as you

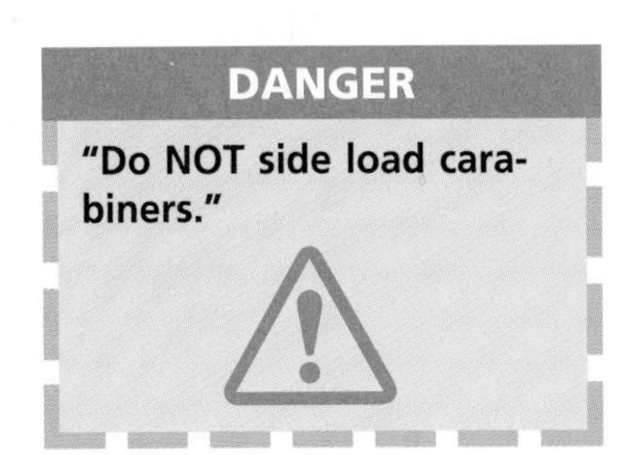

Figure 7.10 Side loaded carabiner

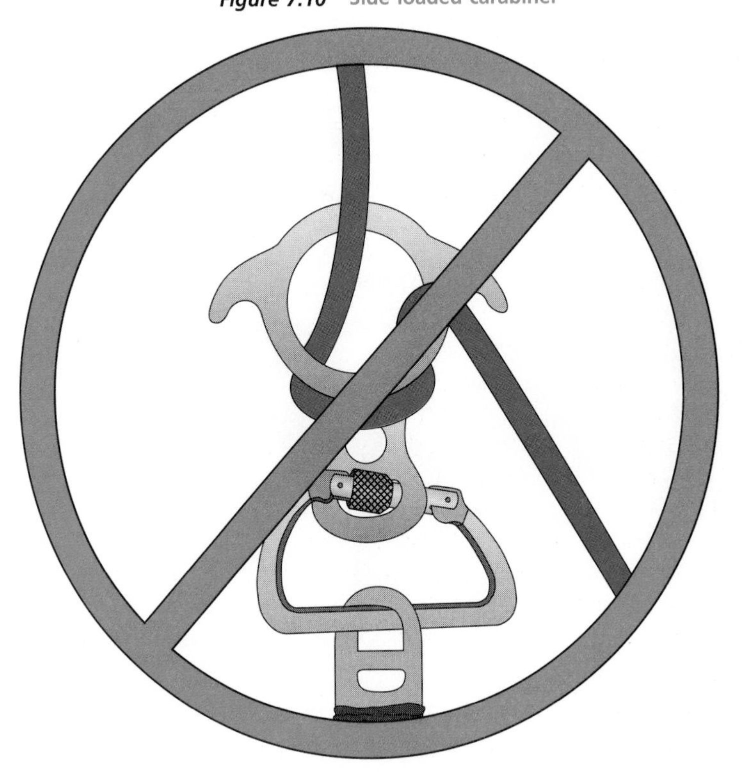

Figure 7.11 Carabiner gate on inside towards body

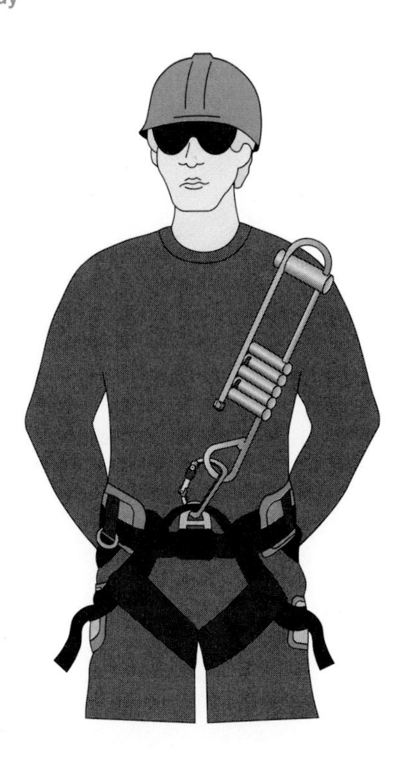

move across it. This contact can cause the screw mechanism to turn, possibly unlocking the gate. Always be conscious of this situation.

Rappelling Position and Ledge Negotiation

Once over the edge, lean back into rappel position and begin the rappel by walking slowly down the surface in a controlled manner. WALK down the wall. DO NOT JUMP, LEAP, ZIP, or FLY. This is *rescue,* where control is the key.

"Jumping" refers to jumping out from the wall while rapidly sliding down the rope, only to stop abruptly when your feet touch the wall again. This is far from controlled and can create significant shock loading (as in a fall) on the rope.

DO NOT jump.

The proper positioning of the rappeller's body should form an L-shaped posture in relation to the wall or surface that he or she is rappelling (see Figure 7.12). The feet should be shoulder width apart for balance and the knees relaxed and slightly bent.

Ledges or other projections can cause real problems for a rappeller. If you rappel to a ledge and drop your feet below it, your upper body tends to swing into the projection. A hard crash such as this will cause no small amount of pain and discomfort (see Figure 7.13). To pass over these projections without bodily injury, keep the balls of your feet on the lower lip of the projection while continuing to lower the upper body (see Figure 7.14).

Once you reach a nearly inverted position, you may drop your feet. This helps ensure that your upper body and hands clear the projection before you drop your feet. The reason for the nearly inverted position is to prevent swinging of the rappel line and possible abrasive contact with the projection once you drop your feet. By inverting, you place the rope nearly in line, thus preventing swing when you release your feet. Be sure to use a harness designed for inversion when performing this procedure (NFPA 1983 specifies Class III harnesses for inverting).

7.12 Ideal rappelling position—"L" position

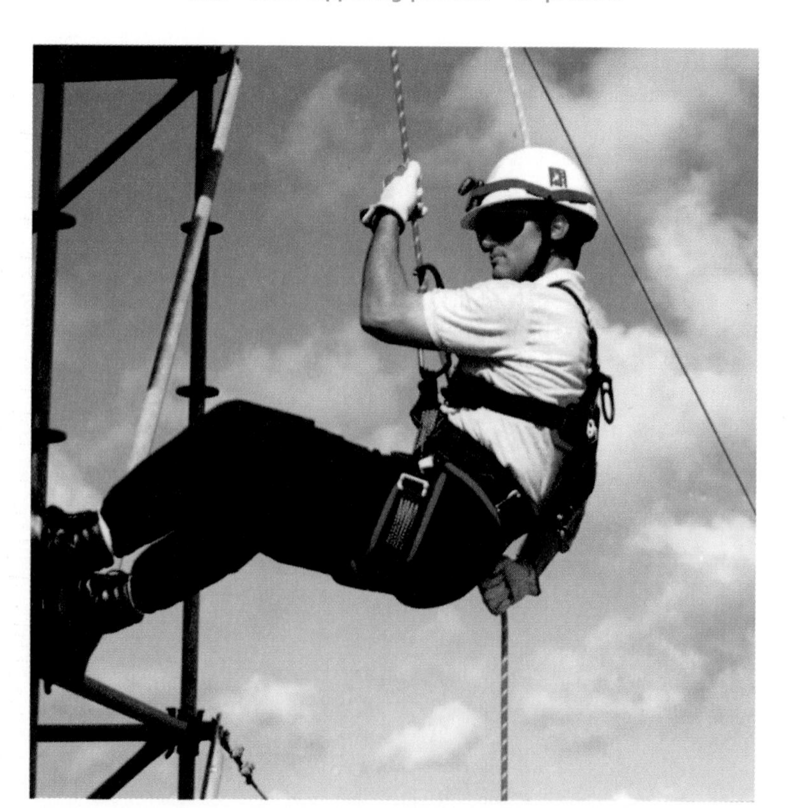

Once you go over the ledge and are no longer in contact with the structure, you will encounter what is known as a free rappel situation. Free rappels (those without a wall or surface to walk on) require no special positioning. It may be harder, however, to gauge rappel speed if there is no reference to the distance the rappeller is traveling. This is commonly the case when rappelling from helicopters. Free rappels require slow and steady movement. Again, control is the key.

7.13 A, B **Dropping feet below ledge can cause injury**

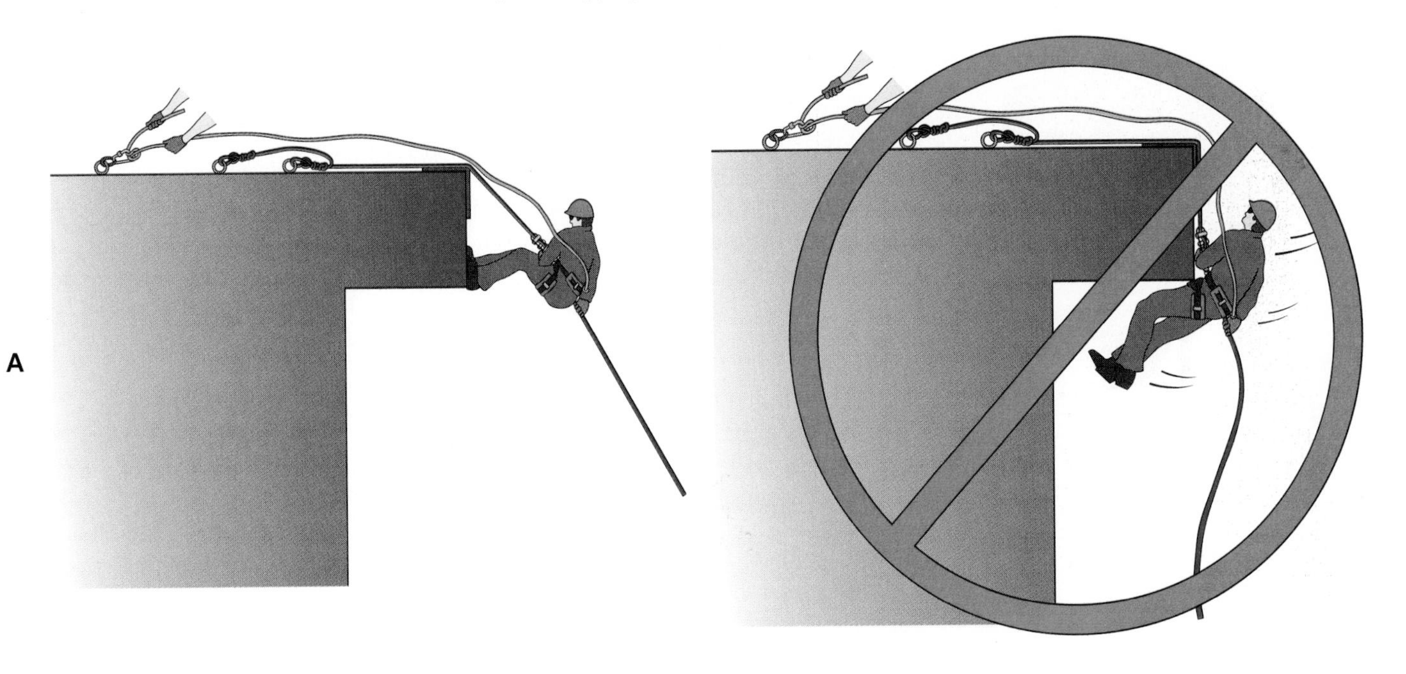

Figure 7.14 A, B **Clearing ledge before dropping feet**

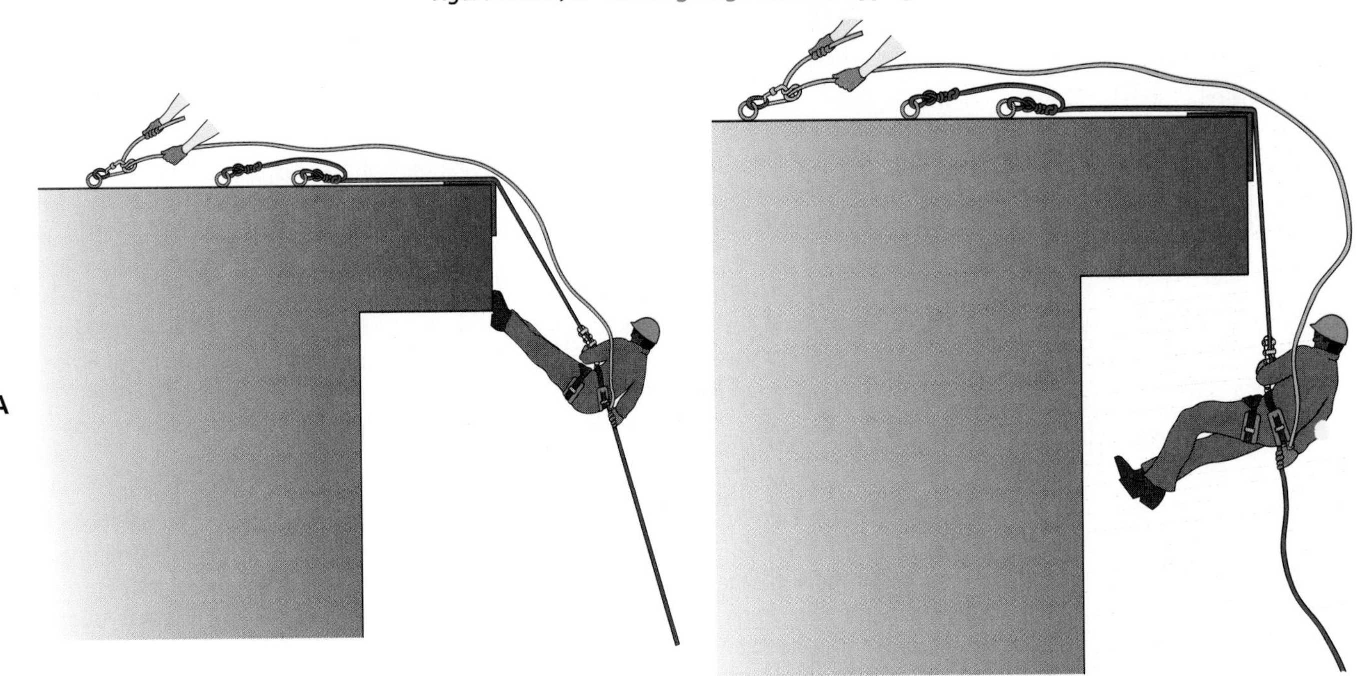

Descent Control

During the rappel, positioning and use of the hands is extremely important for proper operation of the descent control device. The methods used for control depend on the device.

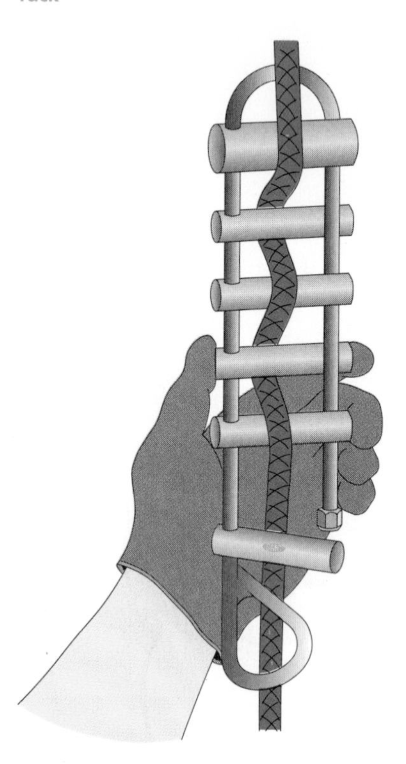

Figure 7.15 Controlling brake bar rack

Controlling the Brake Bar Rack

To control the rappel rack (see Figure 7.15), your right hand should grasp the rope below the rack near the level of the hip and act as the control hand. Allow the rope to flow through this control hand during normal rappelling. Another option is to hold the rope above the level of the bottom bar with the right hand. This requires feeding the rope downward into the rack to rappel. Although this method is more difficult for the operator, it allows quicker stops if needed. Either method is acceptable.

The left hand, or guide hand, should rest on the back side of the rack, cradling the bar ends between the thumb and fingertips. The hand and arm should be nonsupportive and relaxed to prevent muscle cramps. With the hands in these positions, there are two ways to slow or stop yourself as you are descending. You can jam the bars together with the left hand to create more acute bends in the rope, slowing or stopping the descent. An alternative method is simply to pull on the rope with the right hand. This creates friction in the device the same way a body belayer does when he or she tenses the rope. This also slows or stops the descent. The ability to use either hand for controlling descent allows the rappeller the use of one hand to negotiate obstacles if needed.

Rappelling with the rack is performed by spreading the bars with the left hand while relaxing the grip of the right hand to allow the rope to flow through. One advantage of the rappel rack is the ability to vary friction by adding or removing bars or changing the spacing of the bars.

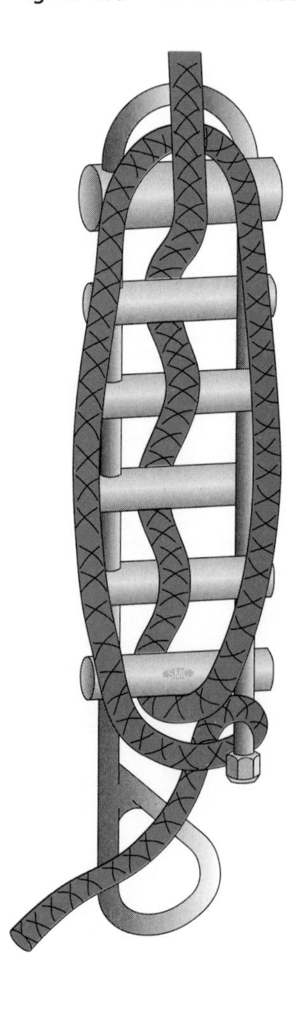

Figure 7.16 Locked-off rack

To add bars, lock in the bottom bar while wrapping the rope upward, around it. To remove bars, unwrap the bottom bar while unclipping one side of it from the rack. Once you have gone over the edge on six bars, you can remove the sixth bar to start your rappel. It is extremely difficult for most people to rappel on six bars. If you are moving too fast on five, just go to six. Remember, use SIX bars when going over the edge, a MINIMUM of FIVE bars when controlling the descent of a one-person load on a single rack.

If you have to work with both hands, you can lock off the rack to prevent movement (see Figure 7.16). Do this by clipping in all six bars. Loop the rope up and around the top training bar and then bringing it down across the front of the rack. There is an additional measure to prevent the lock-off from being loosened or knocked off the top bar. Secure the loose end of the rope coming from the top bar with a half hitch around the short leg of the rack. Pull upward on the rope to tighten the lock-off. After completion, the rappeller should issue the verbal signal "locked off" to the belayer. He or she should give the "on rappel" and await the "on belay" and "on safety" before unlocking. Unlock by reversing the process. Go back to five bars (if needed), and continue the descent.

Controlling the Figure-8 Plate

The positioning of the hands for rappelling with the figure-8 plate (see Figure 7.17) is essentially the same as with the rack. The difference depends on the preference of the rappeller. A right-handed rappeller grasps the rope below the device with the right hand. This acts as the control while the left hand is placed on the rope above the device for stability. A left-handed rappeller does the opposite.

Rig the figure-8 so the loose end of rope comes out of the device on the rappeller's control side (to the right for right-handed, left for left-handed). Control the figure-8 by pulling downward on the rope with the control hand. This creates friction just as the body belayer creates friction in an emergency stop. Keep your control arm locked and your guide arm bent and relaxed to allow rope to constantly slide through it. The control hand should grasp the rope with the thumb up and the palm facing inward, toward the body. Your control arm should move upward (bending as a unit at the shoulder) to go, downward to stop. The old military rappel method of putting your fist to your backside is generally not necessary with the figure-8. If it helps you feel more secure, though, you can use this method. Just remember, the figure-8 is not like a rack. NEVER let go with your control hand while on line unless you are locked off. You will fall . . . fast!

You cannot easily vary the friction of the figure-8 while loaded on the rope. But you can create additional friction in the initial rigging of the device. If, for example, you know that you will be supporting a two-person load on a figure-8 plate, you must double-wrap the device with the bight of the rope before going over the edge (see Figure 7.18). This creates a great deal of additional friction. However, it makes it really difficult while there is only a one-person load on the device. The rope tends to overlap in the device and jam. To prevent this, hold the control hand in a more forward position than normally used during rappelling. This keeps the wraps of rope in the device from overlapping. Remember, you cannot easily vary friction on the figure-8 while you are loaded on the rope. You should take the weight off the device, remove it from your harness, and rig it to suit your needs.

Just as with the brake bar rack, you can lock off the figure-8 plate for hands-free operation. The procedure is quite simple but requires precision. In other words, if not done right, the rope will slip (see Figure 7.19).

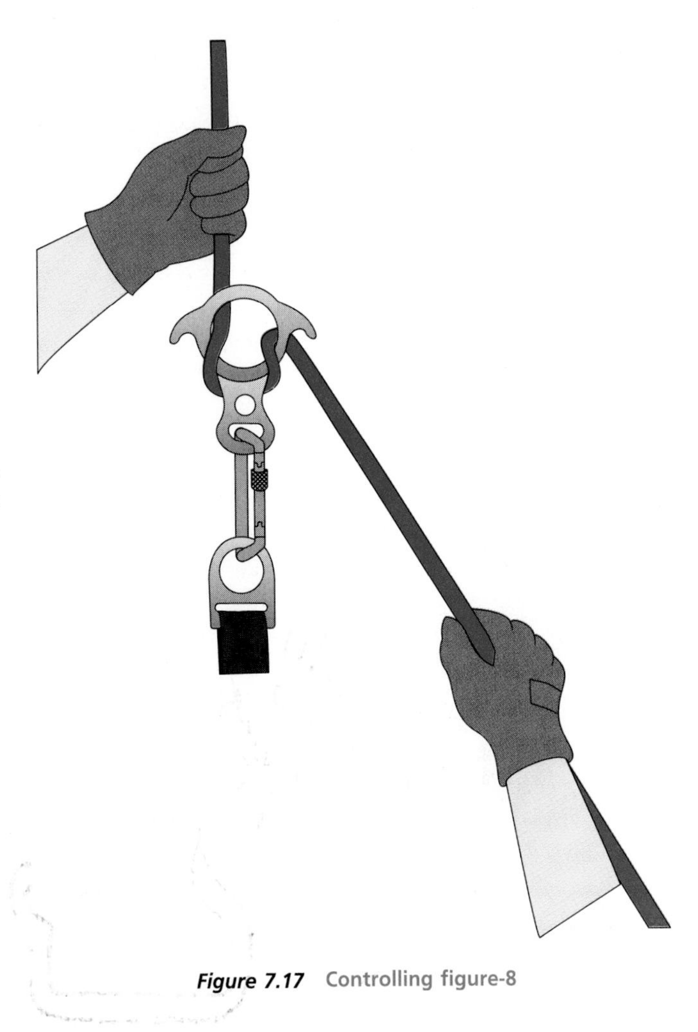

Figure 7.17 **Controlling figure-8**

Figure 7.18 **Double wrapped figure-8**

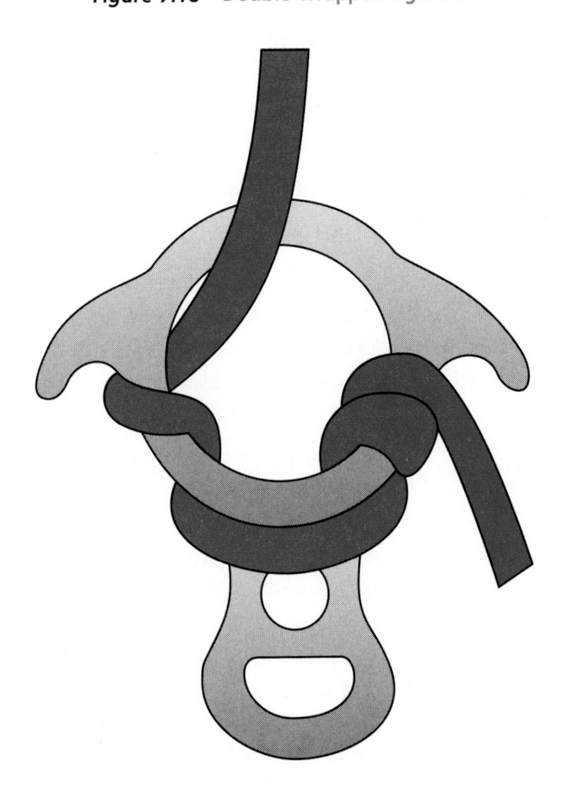

Locking Off

1. Allow your control hand to drift up to within about 8 inches of the device and then stop.
2. With the weaker (guide) hand, grab the carabiner that connects the device to your harness.
3. Hold the carabiner tightly to stabilize the figure-8 and keep it from turning during the lock-off.
4. Now, with the control hand (always keeping tension on the rope), quickly wrap the rope around the top of the large ring. Pull down hard to lock the control rope between the device and the loaded rope issuing from the top of the device. You should actually feel the control rope "pop" into place. If you get no "pop," you probably have no "lock."
5. Pull tightly on the control rope with both hands to make sure it is truly locked. Some trainers recommend a second or even a third wrap around the large ring of the device to ensure the lock-off is secure. For added security, you can form a bight with the control rope and tie the doubled line around the loaded rope with an overhand knot.

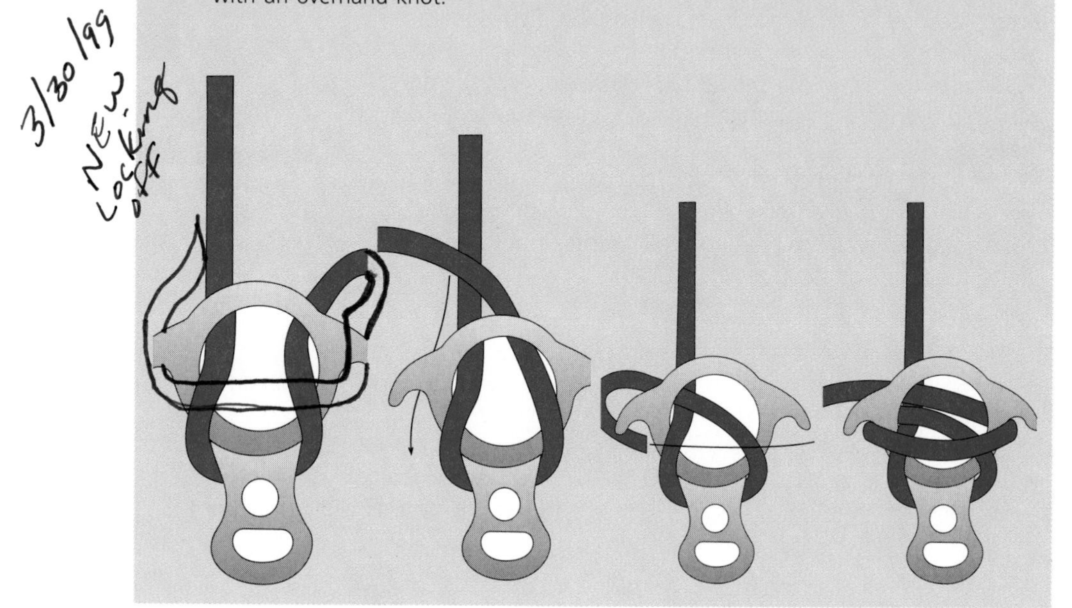

You can take all these extra steps, although most people find they are not necessary. Consult the manufacturer of the device for recommendations on locking off. The technique differs among manufacturers. As a courtesy to the body belayer, remember to call out that you are "locked off."

Unlocking the figure-8 plate requires more precision than does unlocking the rappel rack. Unlocking a figure-8 WILL create a slight shock in the rope due to a very short drop that will feel like at least 2 feet to the rappeller. The goal is to make this drop less than one inch. Here's how it works:

Unlocking

1. Call out "on rappel." Wait for the "on belay" and "on safety" signals before taking all those overhand knots and extra wraps off the figure-8 plate.
2. Take the last wrap of the control rope. Leave the small section of rope cinched between the loaded rope and the large ring of the device in place. Then unwrap it so that the control rope is again on the strong side of the rappeller.
3. Grasp this control rope with both hands close together (somewhat like holding a baseball bat), as close to the device as possible.

4. With one quick but smooth motion, pull on the control rope with both hands until it pops out of its lock. You must maintain tension of this device to prevent sliding once you have unlocked.
5. Return your hands to the normal rappel position and continue your descent.

Once the rappel has been completed, remove yourself from the device and the safety line belay system, and the device from the rappel rope. Give the signal "off rappel" once you are completely detached from the rappel rope. Take a deep breath and relax. You did it!

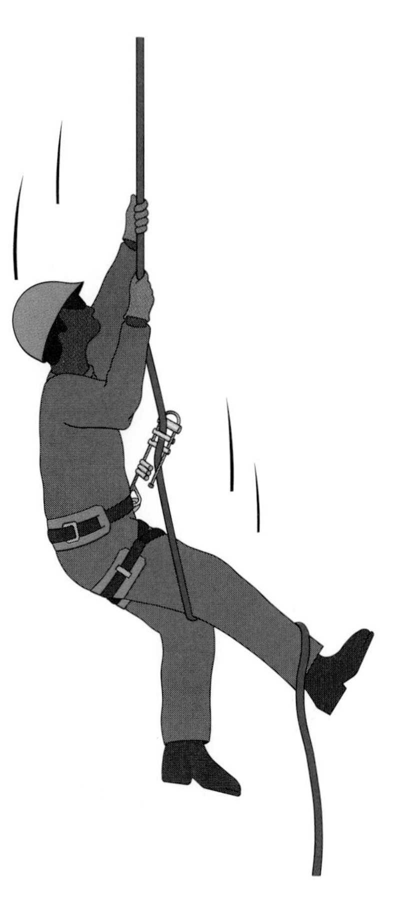

Figure 7.20 Emergency leg wrap

Self Rescue

Unforeseen things can happen in any rescue. The procedures rescuers use, as safe as they try to make them, are hazardous by nature. Although the wrong things may not happen to every rescuer, it is best to prepare for the worst.

Other than a system failure, there are two "worst" things that can happen during a rappel sequence: (1) being pulled off the building while in the early stages of attachment to a rappel rack and (2) getting something caught in a descent control device.

Leg Wrap

An accident may cause the rappeller to be pulled unexpectedly over the edge before the descent control device is completely rigged. If you are using a rack or similar device, you might be able to use an emergency technique called a "leg wrap" as a last-ditch effort to slow your fall and regain control of the rappel. This procedure, however, may produce severe rope burns on the leg. Practice it only while in a stationary position on rope.

Perform the technique by pointing the toe of the right foot and swinging the right leg clockwise around the rope trailing below you (see Figure 7.20). The hope is to catch the rope with your right foot. Once you have wrapped the line, flex the right foot and rapidly bend the right leg at the knee to produce additional friction. Enough friction will cause you to slow or stop. Your leg will act like a brake bar on a rappel rack. The rope will burn through your pants, your skin, and perhaps even the muscle tissue but you might still be alive. This is a better outcome than the sure alternative without a leg wrap. This technique must be practiced well enough to be automatic. If you have to think about it during an emergency, it is probably too late to practice it.

The leg wrap can be used by the rappeller to slow a rapid or uncontrolled descent with any device.

Figure 7.21 Prusik self-rescue

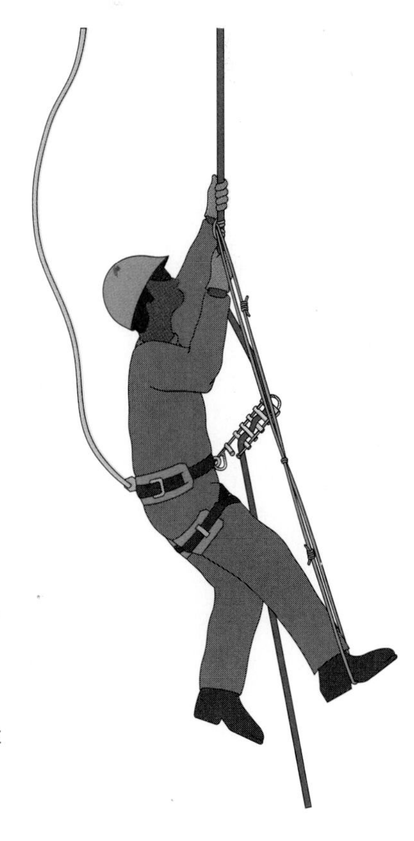

Prusik Self-Rescue

Another emergency self-rescue technique that a rappeller can use with any descent control device is the Prusik self-rescue. A rappeller might use this technique after somehow getting something stuck in the device. Objects such as loose clothing, gloves, or hair are most common. Don't even think about cutting yourself free. Others have tried it, only to find that even a dull knife quickly cuts through a loaded rope. Knives or other bladed objects (including scissors and seat belt cutters) should be considered dangerous around loaded ropes, since the slightest touch can cause rope failure. Do not use them; there are *usually* other ways. Here is one way (see Figure 7.21):

1. If possible, lock off your descent control device.
2. Take a 6- to 7-foot accessory cord tied in a loop. Attach it to the main line with a double-wrap Prusik knot positioned just a few inches above the descent control device.
3. Use two of these Prusik loops joined with a girth hitch to form a sling to step up into. This removes your weight from the device so the object can be freed from it by loosening the rigging.
4. DO NOT remove the rappel rope entirely from the descent control device. Just loosen it enough to free the entrapped object(s).

Summary

Rappelling may be necessary, though not frequently, for rescue. It is extremely helpful for teaching confidence in the equipment and the proper use of descent control devices. Practice the technique frequently enough to be proficient, but do not overdo it. Other techniques require your attention and practice that might be of more benefit to a patient. Helping the patient is one of the primary goals in rescue.

Again, do not try this or any other technique shown in this text without proper hands-on training from a qualified person or agency. The techniques can be dangerous and should not be learned exclusively from a book.

CHAPTER 8

Victim Pick-Off Techniques

The information in this chapter is provided as a basis for continued training. Each rescuer should consult with his or her own team leader for the correct SOGs for the team. Topics covered in this chapter include:

- Third-Man Pick-Off
- Line-Transfer Pick-Off

Introduction

This chapter reviews two methods of quick access to and rescue of a patient isolated from other persons. These rescue methods are called "pick-off techniques." To reach and rescue an individual who is conscious, communicative, and oriented and has no other way to escape, "third-man pick-off" is best. The "line-transfer pick-off" is designed to reach and rescue a patient suspended in space, no matter what his or her medical condition. Both of these methods are designed to be efficient and fast.

These rescue skills should be practiced with a four-member team (one rescuer) or a five-member team (two rescuers), although sometimes patients must be hauled up from their point of isolation. In a dire situation, either technique can be performed by a single, experienced rescuer. Either method can be completed in just a bit longer than it would take to set up and make a simple lower or rappel. Both techniques involve similar basic actions:

1. Getting close to the patient (usually from above)
2. Applying a harness to the patient, if needed
3. Removing the patient from the isolated location
4. Transferring the patient to a safe area, such as the ground

For quick packaging, these techniques use full-body harnesses on the patient. Ideally, pick-off techniques should be limited to patients without suspected spinal injury. A patient who might have a spinal injury should be packaged if possible, in a litter with appropriate spinal precautions. This type of packaging is very nearly impossible to do properly with only one rescuer and very difficult with two. However, we do not live in an ideal world and sometimes medical protocol must be "bent" to save a life. For example, a worker who has fallen several feet and is hanging unconscious in a full-body harness attached to a fall arrest system obviously may have suffered some spinal injury. One viable option for the rescuer is to rappel or be lowered down to the patient who is hanging immobile on line, transfer him or her to the rescuer's lowering system, and gently bring him or her to the ground level to be properly back-boarded for transportation. Every rescue must be evaluated as to what makes the most sense.

Comparison of Techniques

Both techniques have similar procedures. One technique involves the rescue of a person from a window, floor, deck, or other surface that can support the person's load. This technique is sometimes called a "third-man rescue" or "third man." One application would be a high-rise fire where fire blocks the victims' escape and they have to be reached and rescued from window openings. Although possible in industry, this type of rescue is more likely in a municipal environment.

The term "third-man rescue" was coined based on the use of a single-line technique with only one rescuer. With a lowering system, the rescue requires:

1. a rescuer,
2. a brakeman, and
3. a rescue subject (victim/patient).

In a rappel rescue it requires:

1. a rescuer,
2. a bottom belayer, and
3. a rescue subject.

In both cases, the third man (person) is the rescue subject. Hence, the term.

The main reason not to use a third-man pick-off technique with an unconscious or disoriented patient has to do with the difficulty of getting these patients over an edge. When there is only a single rescuer, a conscious and capable patient (e.g., a noninjured firefighter trapped above a fire floor) can provide assistance in getting over an edge. An unconscious or disoriented patient cannot provide this assistance.

The line-transfer pick-off, or line transfer, is more likely in the industrial environment than third-man rescue. It involves the rescue of a person who is suspended on a rope or lanyard. This could easily be the case when workers fall from scaffolding, pipe racks, or other heights and are caught by their fall protection devices. A rescuer has to get to the person, attach him or her to a rescue system, and remove or transfer the patient from the lanyard to the rescue system for safe evacuation.

Either of these techniques can be performed by only one rescuer who rappels or is lowered to the patient to perform the pick-off. While one-rescuer pick-offs are possible, it is less physically stressful to perform the techniques with two rescuers. With a one-rescuer operation, positioning is very critical. For example, to apply a harness to a panicky person in a window, the rescuer may find it necessary to enter the window opening and work inside the room at the patient's level. Once the patient is attached to the rescue system, the rescuer must help him or her out of the window. This is usually performed with both rescuer and patient attached to the same line. They must now try to get all of the slack out of the line and both crawl over the side without dropping a significant distance, shock loading the system, or hurting themselves. This is difficult, even for the most experienced rescuer.

Although two-rescuer operations do increase the personnel need, the same operation is actually made easier and safer. The first rescue responder makes access to the patient, comes into the room, and applies the patient's harness while rendering medical and emotional first aid. The second rescuer rappels or is lowered to a point just low enough to barely make the connection to the patient's harness. The first responder now helps the patient over the edge while the second rescuer remains stabilized on the wall with little or no slack in the connective rigging between rescuer and patient. The two-rescuer operation is safer and actually more efficient (in both speed and effort) than a one-person operation.

This chapter assumes the worst-case scenario—only enough personnel and equipment for one rescuer. Rescuers who can perform this rescue well with one rescuer, find it at least as easy to do when two are available. Rescue teams should practice this scenario both ways for maximum versatility.

Access to the Victim

Rescuers have at least two options to reach the victim. A pick-off technique assumes a rescuer can get above the patient to set up a rope system. The question then is, which lowering technique is best to reach the patient?

Rappelling (a self-lowering technique) exposes the rescuer to a possibly panicked patient who can (and often will) grab the rescuer's rope or body. It may take both of the rescuer's hands and feet just to defend himself or herself. The rappeller would also want to consider a "fanny pack" rappel to prevent the patient from grabbing the rappel line. Rappelling is a viable option, if (1) personnel is limited, and/or (2) there is not a good line of sight from the initial rappel to the victim, and/or (3) communication with the rest of the rescue team is limited.

The second option is for the team to lower the rescuer. This option for accessing the patient is usually more desirable. A team in a controlled area can slowly lower the rescuer to a point just above the patient. There the rescuer can talk to the patient without having to worry about control of the descent device. If the patient panics and jumps onto the rescuer, there is little worry about losing control of the descent. The team above has control. Additionally, the team has the option to raise/haul both patient and rescuer *up* to safety if necessary.

Lower or Rappel?

Although it is usually better to lower when performing a pick-off, there are situations in which a rappel may be necessary. One situation is where the patient is obscured from the view of the brakeman or rescue master. This might require the rescuer to operate the descent control device in order to stop at the appropriate position above the patient. This problem can be virtually eliminated with the use of radios or other communications systems.

If there is no communication between rescuers and the patient is hanging on a line below a ledge out of the rescue master's line of sight, a rappel is probably the preferred method. In this case, a few additional precautions should be noted.

- **Do not allow the rappel line to get anywhere near a patient who might panic.** Remember that a bottom belayer can stop a descent by pulling down on the rope . . . so can a panicky patient. As a result, the rescuer can become stuck in midair while the patient is screaming for help, desperately clinging to the rappel line. To keep the line out of the patient's reach, use a fanny pack or bag the loose end of the rope and attach the bag to your harness. A bottom belayer in this instance, cannot be used because the rappel rope does not reach the ground.
- **Prepare for a two-person load.** If adjustment of the descent control device is necessary, make that adjustment before the patient is placed on line. With the brake bar rack, make sure all six bars are used prior to loading the patient on line. DO NOT USE FEWER than six bars with a two-person load on one rack. When using the figure-8 plate, double wrap it before starting the rappel. Remember that friction cannot be adjusted easily after the figure-8 has been loaded. (One technique to add friction to the figure-8 is to clip in another carabiner to allow additional wraps in the trailing rope). While it may be difficult to rappel at first with only the weight of the rescuer on a double-wrapped figure-8, once the patient is added on line there should be no problem continuing the descent.
- **Stop well above the patient.** Positioning is everything with pick-offs, especially in a line transfer. If the rescuer gets too low, he or she may not be able to remove the patient's weight from the line. Stop at a point above the patient's head. Then gradually move down until connection to the patient is possible. This will ensure the best chance to transfer the patient. Stopping above the patient allows not only proper setup for the pick-off, but also time to prepare the patient for the rescuer's arrival.
- **If rappelling, once in position, be certain to lock off the descent control device to facilitate hands-free movement.** To extend the rescuer's reach without getting too low, it is often necessary to invert on line for patient attachment. If not locked off, the rescuer could accidentally slide down the rope while hanging upside down.
- **Always be ready for patients to suddenly panic.** They are usually frightened and just want to get down. While descending, the rescuer should observe and talk to the patient, noting any extreme apprehension.
- **If rappelling, be certain to give appropriate signals to the belayer(s) before unlocking the descent control device.** The bottom and safety line belayers

must be ready in case something goes wrong during the unlocking process. There will be two people's weight on the line so it is important to notify and wait for the belayer's acknowledgement BEFORE unlocking the device.

Evacuation

Once you make the pick-off, you must bring the patient to a safe area. In most cases, you can continue lowering or rappelling to a safe area. In some cases, it is necessary to access the patient, attach to the patient, and then haul him or her up. An example is a patient who is working over areas that are unsafe or are too far off the ground for your rope to reach. (Chapter 12 addresses how to attach a hauling system to a lowering system line to lift the load.) This will work if your method of evacuation requires a haul rather than a continued lower. The rescuer is lowered to make access, the patient is attached, and then, both the patient and rescuer are hauled up to safety by the rescue team. It works quickly and easily.

Third-Man Pick-off Technique

A third-man pick-off rescue is best performed as a two-person procedure with a lowering system rather than a rappel system.

The first rescuer is lowered to secure the patient and to attach a harness if needed. A prefabricated full-body harness is best, although a tied full-body harness made from webbing may be necessary in an emergency.

Figure 8.1 Rescuer rappelling to patient (third man)

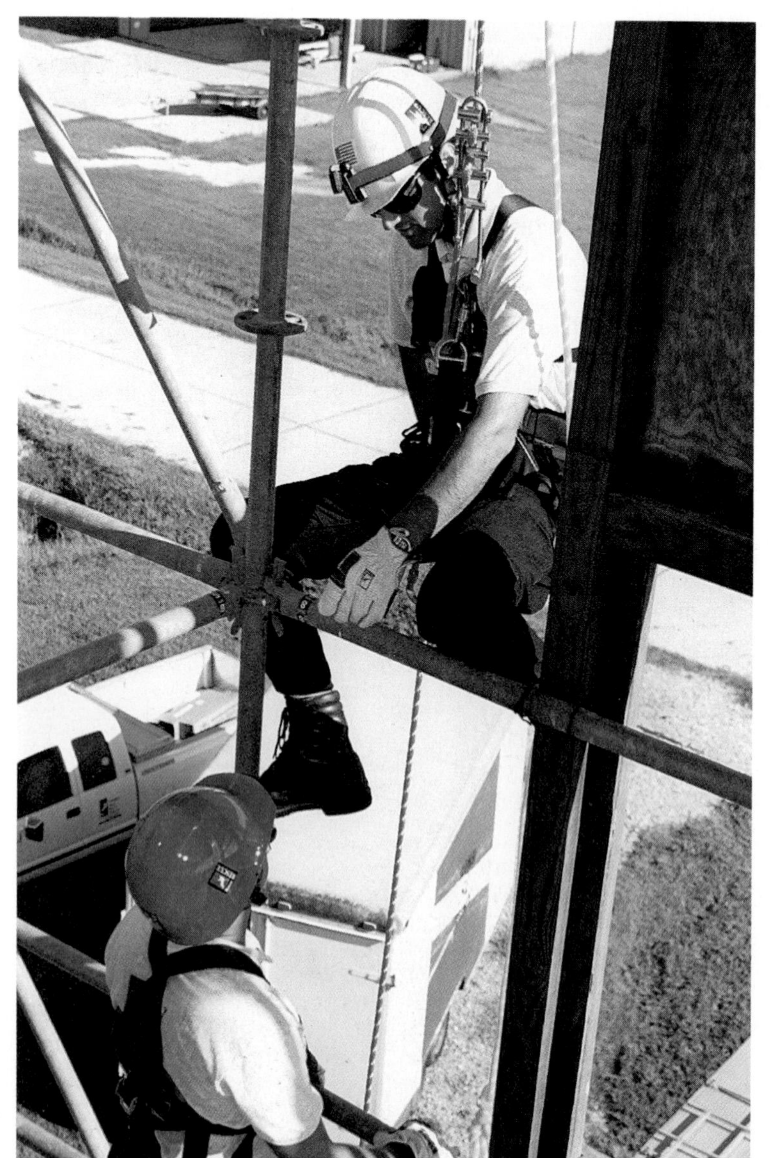

The second rescuer can then be lowered to attach to the patient and descend to the ground. Again, if communication between rescuer and the lowering system brakeman is impossible, use a rappel system. Webbing or other rescue auxiliary equipment can be used to make the attachment of the patient to the rescuer's rope system.

Although you can use many types of equipment, prefabricated adjustable webbing straps work well for this attachment. The length of these devices can be adjusted to separate the patient from the rescuer. This helps avoid injury should the patient panic while suspended below you. Always follow specific manufacturers' recommendations for use of their products. Regardless of what is used to connect the patient, it should be configured to place the load on the rope system and not on the rescuer. In a rappel, connect the patient's rigging to the attachment point of the rappel device. For a lower, attach it to the same knot from which the rescuer is suspended. This places the load of the patient on the rope system rather than on the rescuer's harness.

Attach the other end of the connective rigging to the patient's harness with a carabiner. This rigging allows you to be lowered or to rappel to a patient. There you attach the loose end of the belt to the patient's harness, and then rappel or be lowered to the ground with the patient suspended below you.

In training, always use a safety line belay system for persons suspended from rope. Instead of using a separate safety line for the patient and the rescuer, tie an in-line knot approximately 4 feet from the knot in the end of the rope. This provides attachments for the rescuer and patient. Since these ropes are rated for a two-person load, the one rope is acceptable.

Remember to attach a shock absorber between the safety line and the first point of attachment, in this case, the rescuer. If available, it is a good idea to include an in-line shock absorber for each person attached to the safety line belay.

To begin the rescue:

1. Rappel or be lowered to a point a few feet above the patient (see Figure 8.1). Allow the utility belt to dangle below the rescuer; it serves as a point of reference to measure distance to the patient.
2. Descend just enough to be able to make the connection to the patient's harness. This is critical if rappelling.
3. If the rescuer is being lowered and gets too low, a haul system can be applied to the lowering line up top. The rescue team can haul the rescuer up as needed.
4. If rappelling, lock off the descent control device.
5. If the patient is far below you, you may have to invert (turn upside down). This helps the rescuer remain high enough above the patient to prevent excess slack and to reach low enough to make all of the necessary attachments. Inverting on line actually extends your effective reach. There is one very important requirement for inverting. You can only invert if you attach the rope or device to your harness at a point on your waist. You must be able to pivot near your center of gravity. You may also want to consider the NFPA's recommendation to use only a Class III harness when inverting. (Although many manufacturers design their Class II harnesses to keep the rescuer from falling out when inverting.)

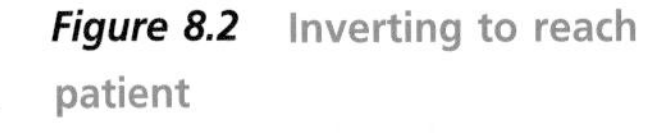

Figure 8.2 **Inverting to reach patient**

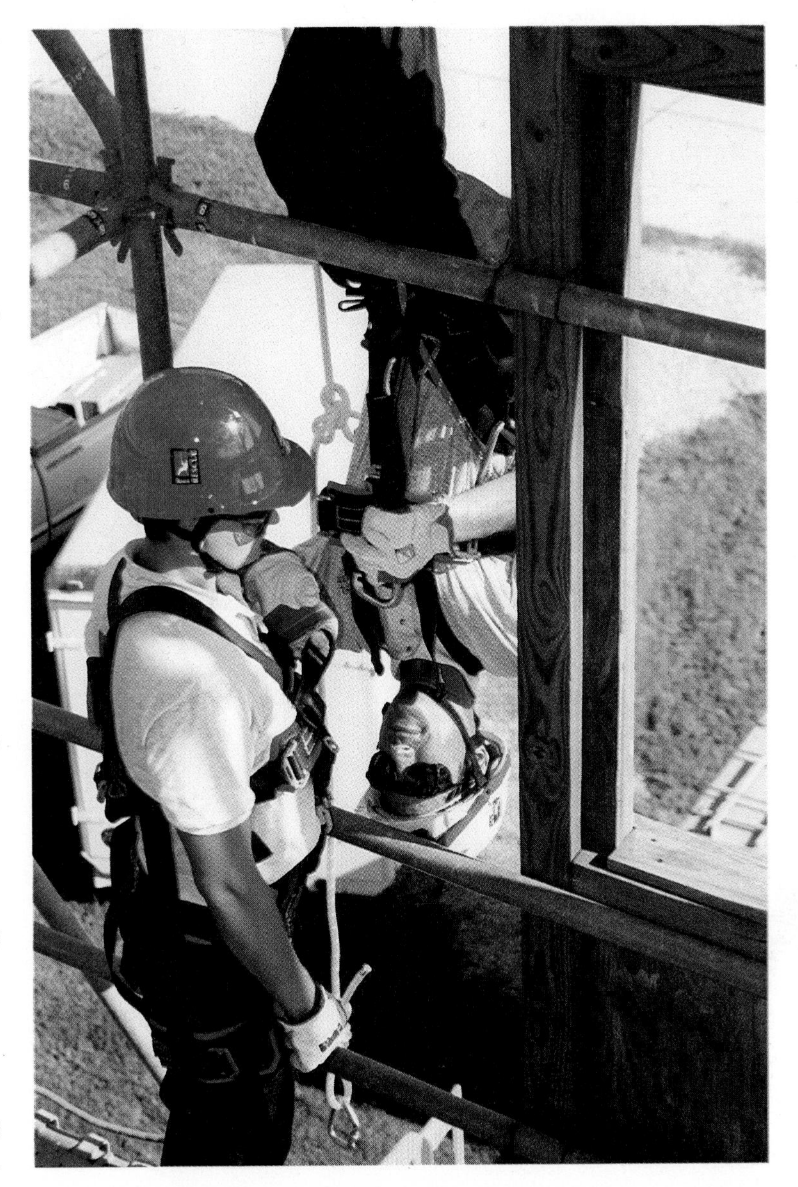

Inverted Pick-Off

Avoid lying backward in the harness to invert. Although many rescuers use this method successfully, it places a strain on the lower back and could lead to injury. Instead, try rolling to the side. Here is one method that works (see Figure 8.2):

1. Start by dropping the utility belt, or whatever you are using to attach to the patient, over the upper leg on the same side you are rolling to. If you leave this rigging dangling between your legs, it will end behind you when you invert.
2. Lower the knotted end of the safety line to the patient below you. In a real rescue with a panicky patient, tell him or her not to touch the line.
3. If you are rappelling, you may find it difficult to keep everything separated when you are hanging upside down with all those lines. One way to prevent tangling of the rappel line is to attach the trailing end to the side of your harness opposite the direction to which you will roll. Clip it into a carabiner on the side of your harness. This keeps the rappel line away from the safety line and other rigging hanging beneath you while you are inverted.
4. Pull your knees into your chest and roll slowly (in one fluid motion) to the appropriate side. You can wrap your legs and feet around the loaded line you are hanging from to stabilize yourself. Attach the main rigging and safety line to the patient before uprighting yourself. Check

all of your carabiners one last time by sight and touch. When you return to the upright position, be sure to turn in the opposite direction of the initial rotation (go back the way you came) to prevent tangling equipment.

Patient Harness

If the patient has no harness, or perhaps the harness has been damaged, you may have to apply a harness. The harness should be a full-body type with a high attachment point to prevent accidental inverting of the patient. A prefabricated harness is the ideal patient harness, although it may not be feasible due to difficulty in application. In a true emergency, when time is critical, you may tie a full-body harness out of webbing and quickly apply it to the patient for rescue. (For methods of creating these harnesses, see Chapter 9, Patient Packaging.)

Completing the Rescue

Once all the appropriate attachments have been made and the rescuer has reinverted, you are ready to load the patient on the system (see Figure 8.3). *NOTE:* If you are rappelling and using a figure-8 descent control device, unlock the device before loading the patient because the added patient's weight will make unlocking difficult. A rappel rack can be unlocked easily even after the patient has been loaded on the system.

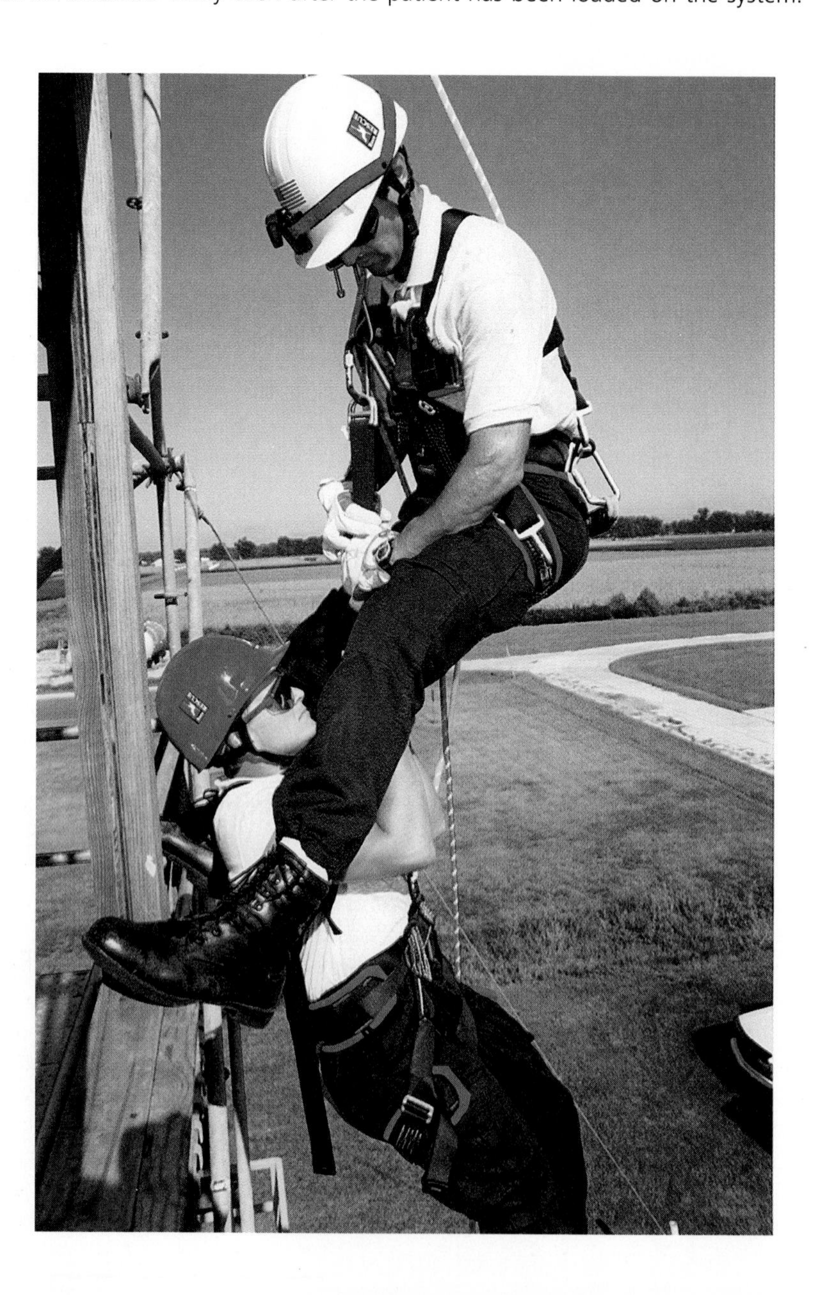

Figure 8.3 Loading patient onto system

Before you start to load the patient, it is extremely important to let the other rescuers know what you are doing. If anything is going to go wrong, it will probably happen as you load the patient's weight on the line. With another person's weight on the line, the descent can be harder to control. Make certain everyone is ready. If you are rappelling, call out "on rappel" and wait for the response from both the bottom and safety line belayers before loading the patient on the line. If you are being lowered, give a signal such as "ready to load" and wait for a response from the brake man and safety line belayer.

If you use a Munter hitch in the safety line belay system, remember the additional precautions that must be taken for two-person loads. Make sure you have them in place before you load the patient on the system.

When all rescuers are ready, load the patient onto the system. As he or she holds onto the main attachment rigging with both hands, have the patient slowly crawl over the edge. The patient can use this rigging as a slide pole to carefully load his or her weight onto the system.

The rescuer may wish to use both hands on the rigging as well to help keep slack out of the system (there should be very little) while the patient crawls over. BE CAREFUL! Lifting a load like this can strain the back. Only use this method to assist the patient, not to lift his or her entire weight.

When everyone is ready and the rescuer has loaded the patient onto the system and unlocked the descent control device (if applicable), move the patient to a safe area. It is not always necessary to evacuate the patient to the ground to reach a safe area. In most structural fires, a firefighter can reach a safe area within a few floors of the danger. This may also be true with industrial rescue. Get the patient to the nearest safe area. This may require a haul or it might require a lower. If it will not hurt the patient to ride it out, it may be more convenient to go all the way to the ground where the ambulance or other response unit is waiting.

During lowering or hauling, the rescuer keeps the patient away from obstructions to prevent snagging. If the rescuer is rappelling, he or she uses one hand to negotiate the obstacles while using the other for control of the device.

Rescuers should keep their legs at about a 45-degree angle from the torso rather than forming the usual L shape. This helps prevent pressure to the rescuer's groin area by contact with the utility belt or other rigging. If rappelling, the bottom body belayer may help control the speed of the descent, if requested by the rescuer.

Once on the ground, the rescuer and patient should be detached from the system and appropriate transfer of the patient should be made to more definitive care.

Line Transfer Pick-off Technique

The line-transfer technique is identical to the third-man rescue except that the patient must be removed from the line on which he or she is suspended. One method is to lower the rescuer on a rope to the patient, and attach both rescuer and patient to the lowering line as in a third-man rescue. Then have the team up top attach a haul system to the lowering line and haul just enough to unload or slack the patient's line. It is then a simple matter to untie or detach the patient from his or her lanyard. The transferred load can then be replaced on the descent control device and the patient lowered to a safe area, as in a third-man rescue.

Another method to use with a lower or a rappel system is also very similar to the third-man rescue. Instead of a utility belt or webbing, use a short simple mechanical advantage system (a 4:1 block-and-tackle system built with about 20 feet of $\frac{3}{8}$-inch rope) to haul the patient's weight off the line. The system should include a device to hold the load in place should the rescuer release the haul line. Some manufactured systems employ a specialized double-sheave pulley with a built-in rope grab to prevent the patient from falling back down when the haul line is released. These dedicated, prerigged systems are commonly referred to as "line transfer assemblies." These assemblies make the task of transferring the patient's weight much easier for the rescuer.

WARNING

Several years ago, a rope-cutting technique was being used by a firefighter to rescue a woman from a static line. The firefighter cut her line with a knife. When the drop and subsequent shock occurred, it caused the firefighter to thrust the knife forward, stabbing the woman in the cheek. In horror, he quickly withdrew the knife and, in his haste, stabbed himself in the buttocks. How he avoided cutting his own rope in the process remains a mystery to this day. DO NOT use bladed objects around loaded lines.

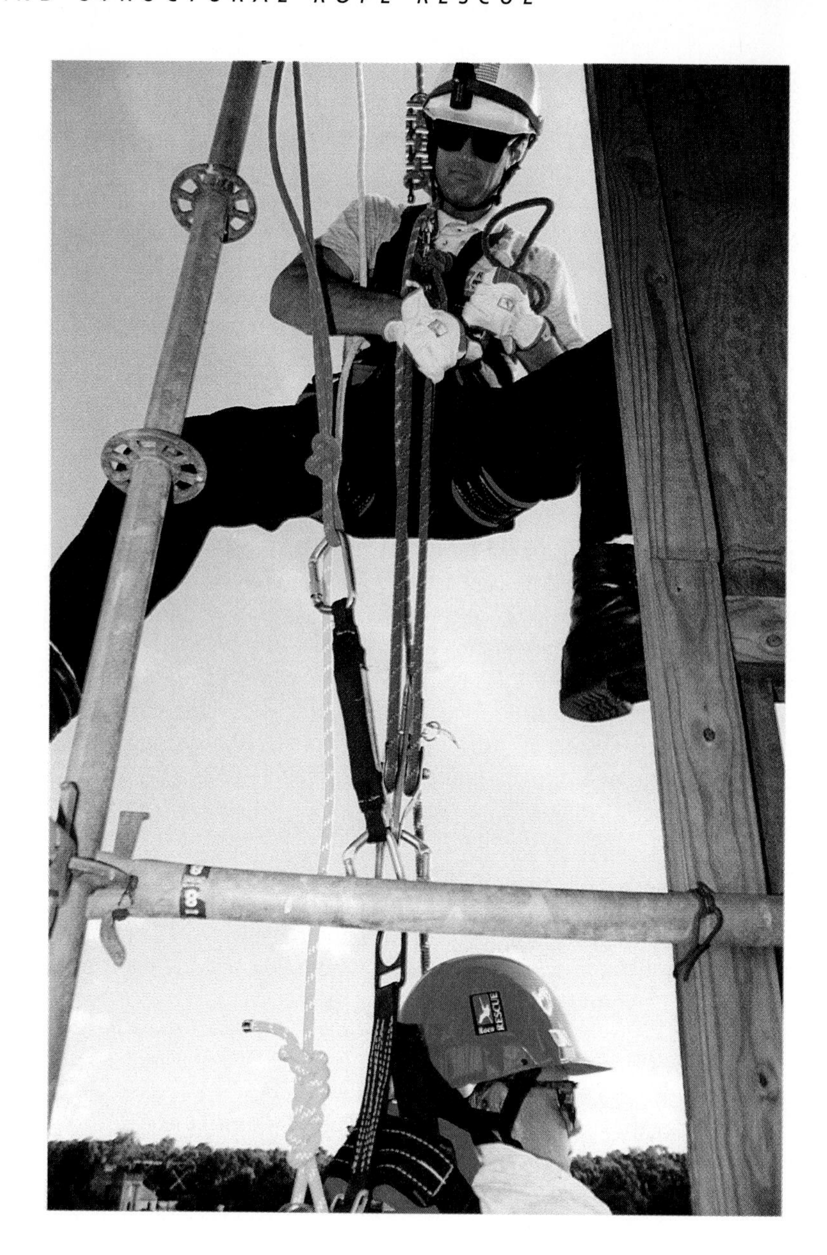

Figure 8.4 Rappelling down to a few feet above patient with line transfer attached

A third method involves attaching the rescuer to the patient with webbing or carabiners and then cutting the patient's line with a knife, scissors, or some closed-bladed object. The problem with this way of transferring the patient to the rescuer's system is that it can cause significant shock loading. When the line is cut, the patient's weight can be loaded suddenly onto the rescuer's line, causing a drop and a potentially serious impact load. If this were the only problem with the rope-cutting technique, it would be enough to avoid it. Unfortunately, there are other dangers associated with bladed objects around loaded ropes.

Line Transfer Assembly

1. To begin this rescue, the rescuer rappels or is lowered to a point a few feet above the patient (see Figure 8.4). Be sure that the line-transfer system is connected at the attachment point of the descent control device when rappelling or to the knot in the end of the lowering line when being lowered.
2. Attach the safety line and line-transfer assembly to the patient's harness with a carabiner, as is done in a third-man rescue.
3. The rescuer then hauls with the system to transfer the patient's weight to the rescuer's line and disconnects the patient's line (see Figure 8.5). Only haul the patient as high as needed to slack the line from which he or she is suspended.

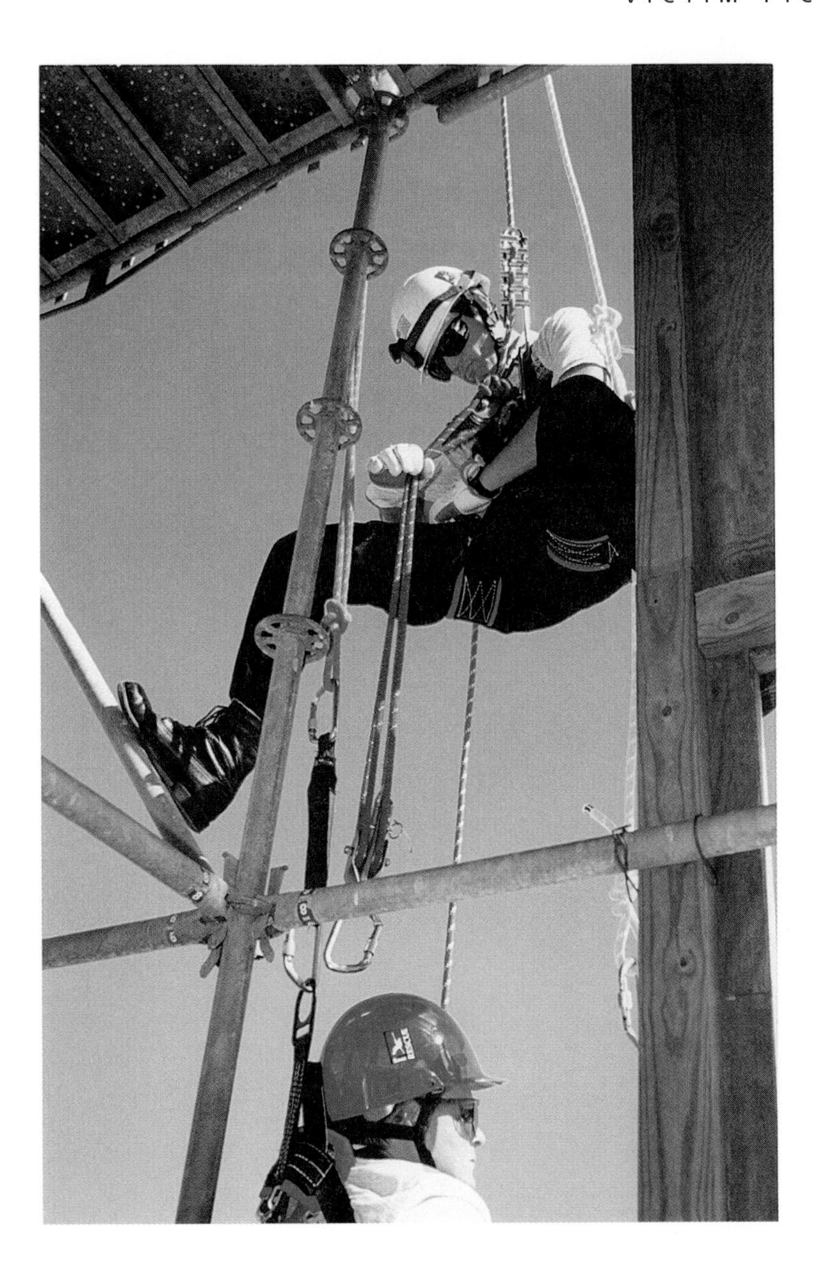

Figure 8.5 Using line transfer to get load onto system

4. Once you have hauled far enough, make sure the cam locks in place and tie off the end of the haul line to get it out of your way. All other procedures are identical to the third-man rescue technique.

Summary

Patient pick-off techniques are necessary tools in the industrial and structural rescuer's toolbox. Whenever possible, execute these techniques with a lowering system for better control. However, rappel rescue pick-offs are quick, efficient, and effective options. As always, PRACTICE, PRACTICE, PRACTICE!

CHAPTER 9

Patient Packaging

The information in this chapter is provided as a basis for continued training. Each rescuer should consult with his or her own team leader for the correct SOGs for the team. Topics covered in this chapter include:

- Choosing the Method of Packaging
- Spinal Injury Packaging
- Spinal Immobilization
- Angulated Extremities
- Monitoring the Patient
- Tied Full-Body Harness

Introduction

Before making a decision on the rescue system, rescuers must carefully consider the patient's condition and physical surroundings. A key concern in the decision-making process is *packaging* of the patient.

"*Packaging*" may mean different things to different people. In rescue, it means ***properly protecting the patient and injuries so he or she can be moved or transported without further harm.*** Packaging often involves common immobilization techniques such as splinting. It can also include specialized procedures and equipment for dealing with more technical forms of rescue. These procedures can involve the use of litters, short-spine immobilizers, and many other items of rescue equipment.

There is not much difference between the basic packaging considerations EMS (Emergency Medical Services) uses every day in the municipal environment and those rescuers use in the industrial/structural environment. Although basic treatment priorities and packaging considerations in rescue emergencies might be similar to those in other emergencies, they can be very different. What makes the difference is the relationship of a patient's condition to his or her surroundings. The physical surroundings are the structural and atmospheric environment through which an injured person must be transported.

Choosing the Method of Packaging

This chapter focuses on considerations of patient packaging that might not be normal to some environments, but are very common to technical rescues in the industrial environment. In industrial/structural emergencies, rescuers need different information and training to make decisions on the patient's transport vehicle. When they cannot use a litter, rescuers' options might include short-spine immobilizers, full-body harnesses, and even wristlets in some extreme cases.

Patient's Condition

The patient's condition should be the number one consideration in choosing the method of packaging. After all, it does no good to remove patients from the hazard if they die during the rescue. There are many horror stories detailing injuries, paralysis, and deaths resulting from improper attempts to rescue patients from hazardous areas without regard for their condition. Often, these injuries are completely preventable. Every rescuer dedicated to emergency patient care should determine to DO NO HARM!

Rescuers try to package patients with appropriate considerations for both their injuries and the environment. These ideals should always be the "Plan A" of patient packaging in the rescue environment. Unfortunately, many circumstances can seriously hamper the ability to use Plan A. These problems may cause rescuers to move to Plan B, Plan C, or maybe even Plan D.

Patient's Surroundings

The circumstances surrounding the patient during the rescue should have a major influence on the packaging plan. The wide variety of structural configurations and specialized hazards found in industry and structures can cause rescuers to modify packaging. A few of the concerns to consider in packaging for rescue include:

- extremely hot or cold exposures
- sharp projections
- chemical exposures
- operating machinery
- energized electrical equipment
- fire
- confined spaces
- narrow or obstructed passageways
- confined working areas

Figure 9.1 Worker injured at the bottom of a vessel

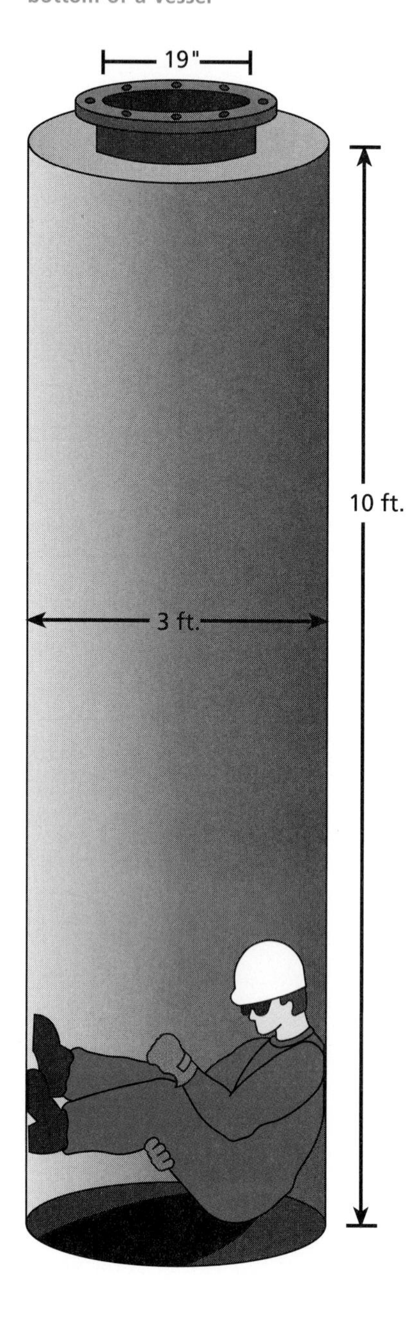

To protect a patient from hazards, rescuers might have to package him or her in a full litter to act as a shield. They might have to include an attendant to help maneuver the patient away from these problems. Rescuers sometimes have to use a particular type or configuration of litter to pass patients through a narrow passage or to keep them from further injury while dragging over and around rough or sharp projections. Packaging that uses special protective clothing and breathing apparatus may also be required to isolate the patient from hazards.

Determine the Rescue Technique

Once rescuers know the patient's condition and physical surroundings, they can make a decision on appropriate packaging. The following scenario is an example of a typical industrial rescue (see Figure 9.1).

> A male worker is lying in the bottom of a vessel and rescuers are not sure how he got there. From observations of the scene, they assume he may have fallen through the manway at the top of the vessel. This is a fall of about 10 feet. Knowing this about the patient's condition leads rescuers to suspect spinal injury. Because of possible spinal injury, full spinal immobilization and a horizontally configured litter would probably be suitable packaging for this patient. However, because the only egress is the round 19-inch manway in the top of the vessel, a vertical litter with full spinal immobilization might be better. Unfortunately, the vessel is only 3 feet in diameter, so it will not be possible to lay the patient on a full spine board. Also, the 19-inch manway is too narrow for the patient to pass through on an 18-inch wide spine board.
>
> The team plans to use a short-spine immobilizer with a full-body harness. This spinal immobilization would not be complete, as it would be with a full-spine board. But it would be possible to get the patient into the device and out of the vessel. They could then transfer the patient to a full-spine immobilizer and a horizontal litter and lower to the ambulance on the ground.
>
> Unfortunately, when the first rescuers reach the patient, they find him pulseless and breathless. They intend to just get him out as fast as possible to a clear atmosphere (out of the IDLH atmosphere) to provide more definitive care. The rescuers then throw a full-body harness on the patient (about 15 seconds to accomplish). Rescuers can then haul him out quickly so CPR can begin in a clear atmosphere.

During rescues, plans can change quickly. In this scenario, as the priorities changed, less desirable packaging plans became more acceptable. This theoretical, but realistic, scenario shows how the combination of the patient's condition and circumstances surrounding the incident can affect the priorities in patient packaging.

Prepared rescuers learn to meet the challenges of these decisions through training. Training helps them anticipate the unusual and keep priorities in place. In life, misplaced priorities can lead to much difficulty. In rescue, they can lead to death.

Personal Priorities

The following questions may at first appear unrelated to packaging, however, these questions are important to every rescuer. It does no good if rescuers ignore their own safety. A rescuer's personal priorities are

1. self,
2. my fellow rescuers, and
3. the patient.

An important rescue saying is, "Don't become a victim." Before attempting any rescue, answer the following questions:

- **Do you have the proper protective equipment, personnel, and training necessary to safely complete the rescue in this environment?** If the answer is "no," *DO NOT* consider the rescue. The idea of doing *anything*, as long as you are doing *something*, does not apply in modern technical rescue. It may be that your *best* action is *no* action until you can clear the environment and enter it safely or summon a specialized rescue team.
- **Is this a rescue or a body recovery?** Is it unlikely that the patient survived the hazard to which he or she has been exposed? Is it likely he or she could not have survived? It is not wise to place a team member at risk to perform a body recovery. This would be like allowing a firefighter to make a rescue attempt in a structure 90% involved in fire. It places the firefighter at unnecessary risk to recover a dead body. It is better to wait and make the environment safe for entry before attempting to recover the body. It may even be necessary to call in specialized rescue teams to remove the body if the hazard cannot be cleared. *DO NOT* risk human life for a body recovery!

Prioritize Injuries

Prioritize injuries appropriately. Consider the following scenario: EMS personnel stay on-scene with severely traumatized patients longer than they should. The EMS persons are trying to establish IV (intravenous) access at the scene; which should be done en route to the hospital. They should spend the valuable time while in rapid transport to a qualified trauma center. They should concentrate their initial effort on the immediately life-threatening issues such as airway and breathing, and spinal immobilization.

The same concerns apply to patient packaging. Rescuers must quickly assess injuries and circumstances and set priorities. For example, rescuers must not waste time splinting a simple fracture when the patient has a severe head injury. Prioritize and package appropriately.

Atmospheric Considerations

In a toxic, flammable, or oxygen-deficient atmosphere, rescuers may have to remove the patient immediately, before attempting resuscitation.

A patient sometimes faces imminent danger such as fire or flammable atmospheres, structural collapse, or other immediately life-threatening situations that cannot be stabilized. In these situations, rescuers should remove the patient in the quickest possible way, doing what they can to protect the spine and keep the airway open as they go. Again, rescuers should only make these attempts when they can adequately protect themselves with personal protective clothing and/or breathing apparatus.

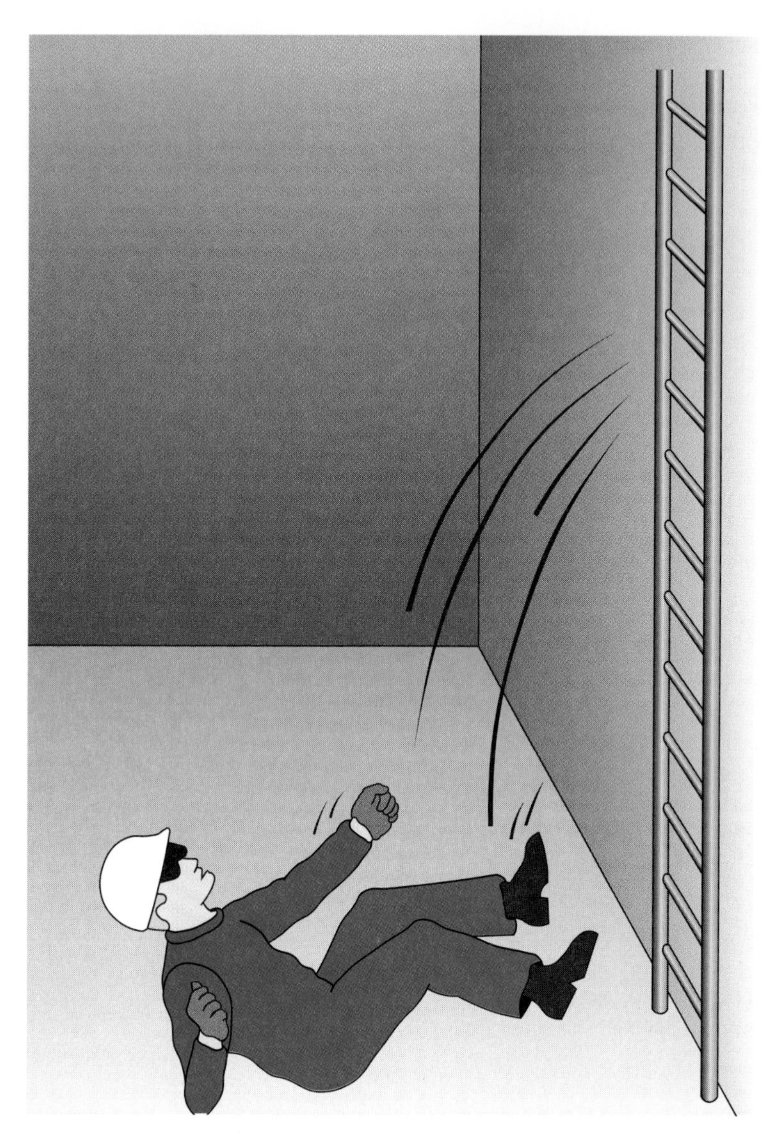

Figure 9.2 Worker falling—possible spinal injury

This is the same idea as having a patient with a spinal injury trapped in a burning car, in a burning building, or near the wall of a building ready to collapse. Rescuers cannot spend time doing anything but getting them out of that situation. If rescuers do not get them out, they *will* die; if they do get them out, they might live. Blanket drags, clothes drags, full-body harnesses, or even wrist or ankle hitches may work best in this situation, although they are far from desirable under normal circumstances. These are last-ditch efforts.

If the patient is in a bad atmosphere and is not breathing, it does them little good to put fresh-air breathing apparatus on his or her face. Unless the mask can provide positive pressure ventilation, the good air is not getting into the blood where it is needed. The time wasted applying the useless apparatus is time the patient does not have.

In these cases, remove the patient as quickly as possible, while considering the cervical spine to prevent unnecessary manipulation until the patient is in a clear area where rescuers can provide more definitive care. Remember, these atmospheres may be immediately life-threatening. Do not waste time on minor or otherwise stable injuries while the patient is exposed to the hazard. The extraction method of choice is any positive means of securement that you can apply quickly (less than 1 minute). A tied full-body harness or even wristlets, though undesirable, may be appropriate in extreme circumstances.

A patient breathing and in a hazardous atmosphere (not about to explode) can be isolated from the hazard by the application of fresh-air breathing apparatus. Put it on him or her and slow down a little. If the patient's vital signs are good and he or she is isolated from the immediately life-threatening problem (bad air), use the same means of packaging you would use for a patient in a more controlled environment. Consider the ideal packaging methods appropriate when time is not critical.

WARNING

Most short spine immobilizers are not designed to be hauled vertically by their prefabricated-fabric lifting handles. These handles are usually there to help maneuver the patient onto a long-spine board.

Spinal Injury Packaging

Consider any person who has fallen or might have fallen to have possible spinal injuries. This includes a person who is unconscious for unknown reasons. Even if the person has only fallen to the ground from a standing position, the force could produce a spinal injury. Do not assume that the conscious patient without neck or back pain is free of spinal injuries. If the mechanism of injury suggests a potential for spinal injury, assume it to be so (see Figure 9.2). With these patients, consider immobilization of the cervical spine simultaneously with opening of the airway.

The packaging plans for a patient with potential spinal injuries include:

Plan A

Fully and completely immobilize the patient with some sort of long (full) spine and cervical immobilizer (see Figure 9.3). Then secure the patient in a litter. A horizontally configured litter is usually better for a person with a spinal injury, although you could use a vertical litter if necessary.

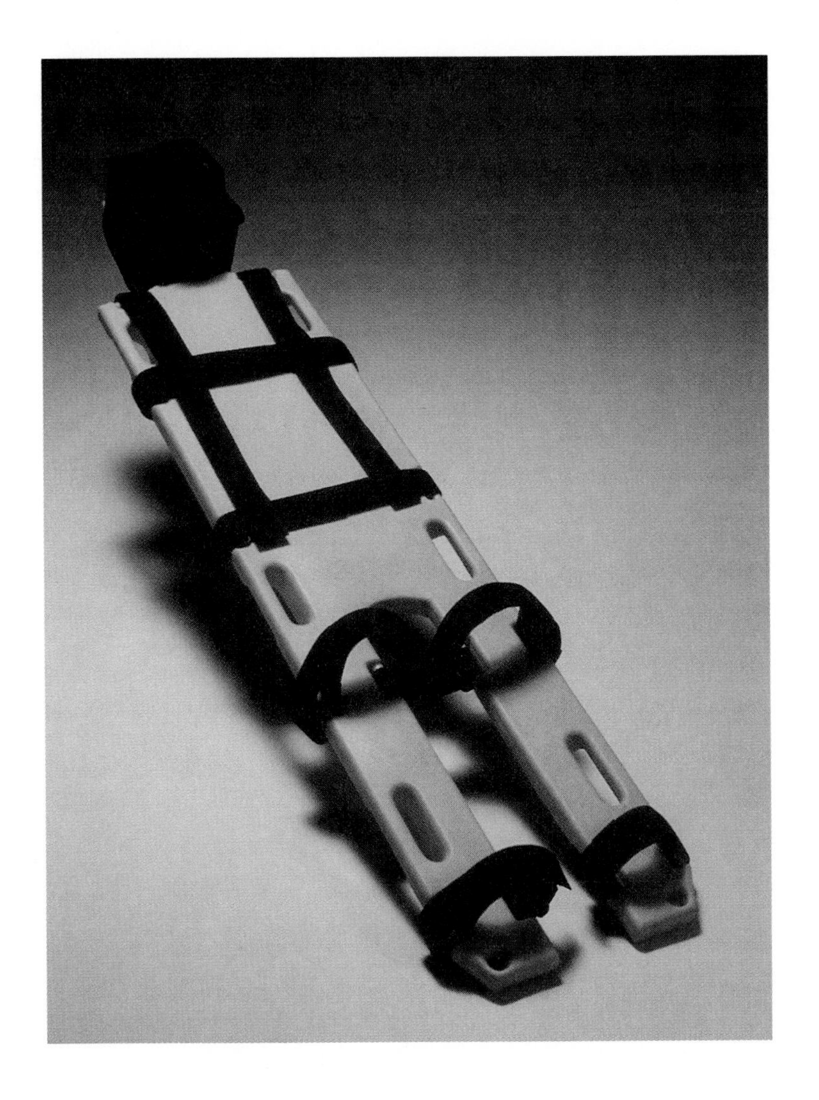

Figure 9.3 Long-spine immobilizer

Plan B

In some circumstances, your working area may be so restricted that a long-spine immobilizer is too wide or too long. Watch out when dealing with narrow openings! You may be able to get a spine board through the opening, but that doesn't mean you can get it back out with the patient on it. Most patients will not fit through an 18-inch round manway on a backboard (even if the board is only 14 inches wide). The board takes up too much of the opening. Consider a short-spine immobilization device for these situations (see Figure 9.4). They are easier to apply in confined areas and will conform to the patient's body to make it through tighter openings. If the manufacturer allows, you can secure a full-body harness around both the patient and the immobilization device for vertical lifting. Remember, short spine immobilizers are designed as a temporary measure in tight areas where long spine immobilizers will not fit. Whenever possible, the patient and short spine immobilizer should be placed on a long-spine immobilization device and secured in a litter for further technical rescue procedures.

Plan C

The final option could be just about anything the situation dictates. Use good judgment. Above all else, do no harm to the patient as you do what has to be done. Consult your medical control when at all possible for guidance.

Respiratory Considerations

In most cases involving respiratory hazards, the best treatment for the breathing patient is immediate administration of good air.

WARNING

Take caution when administering oxygen. In certain atmospheres chemical reactions could produce catastrophic results.

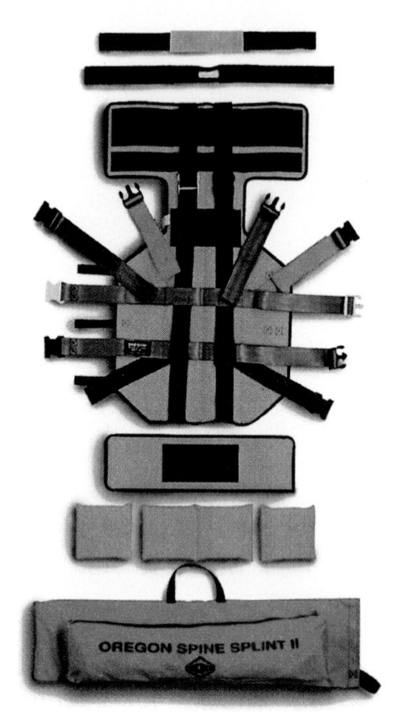

Figure 9.4 Short spine immobilizer

Breathing air equipment is one example of protective equipment, protective clothing, etc. you might use to stabilize a patient. Whatever the type of adjunct equipment, you must secure it as part of the patient's packaging. Technical rescue applications require that all equipment be rigged securely to the rescue system. Falling equipment can be a problem. A falling air or oxygen cylinder is dangerous (see Figure 9.5). It can dislodge the patient's face piece, thereby exposing him or her to bad air. Also, the cylinder valve could strike the ground or some other object, possibly causing the cylinder to take off like a rocket. This is obviously dangerous!

If you use fresh-air breathing apparatus with a sealed mask on a patient, be sure to turn on the air.

Angulated Extremities

Every day, EMTs and paramedics encounter and deal with severely angulated fractures or dislocations. When they involve the patient's extremities, packaging can be very difficult for industrial rescue. The following scenarios illustrate the difference.

In the first case, an EMS crew responds to a call at a ball park. It appears that a male patient was going for a fly ball when he ran into the outfield fence with both arms up. The patient is now writhing on the ground in pain and appears to have possibly dislocated both of his arms at the shoulders. The arms project to each side at a right angle to the body. Fortunately, the EMS unit has a center mount stretcher that can adapt to these protruding extremities. Padded board splints on each side can provide additional support.

Figure 9.5 Falling SCBA backpack and cylinder.

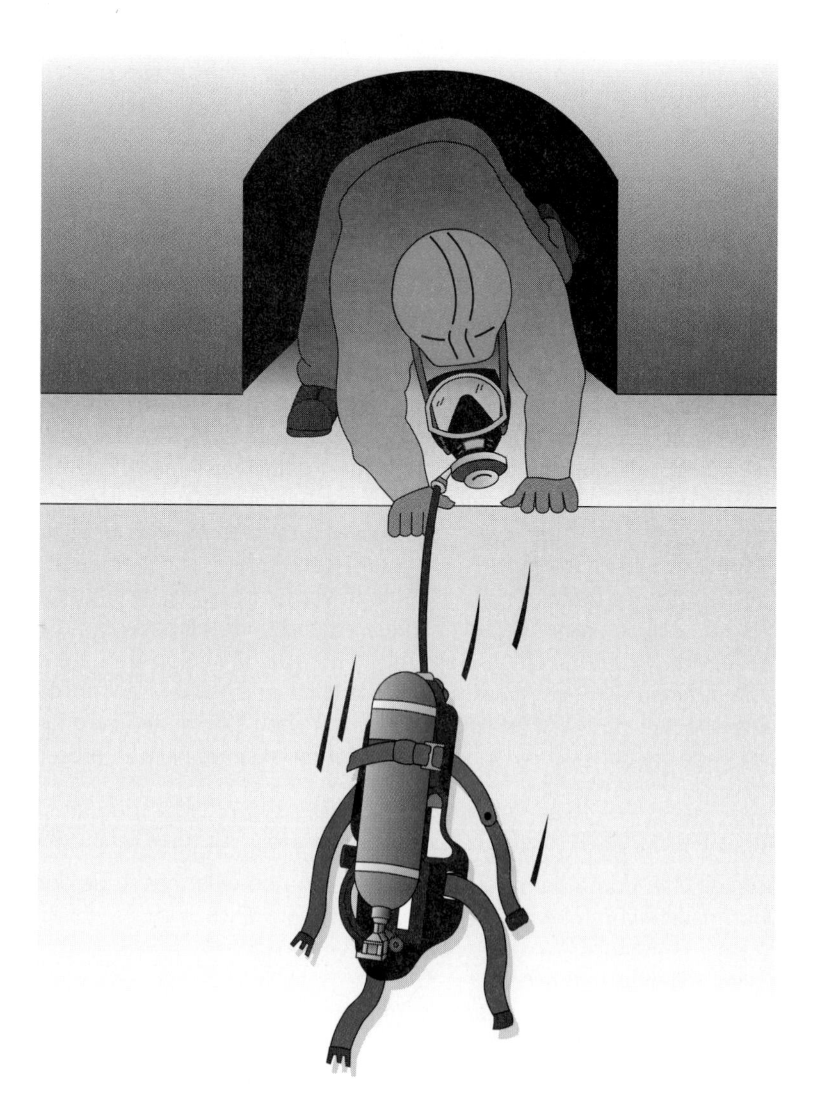

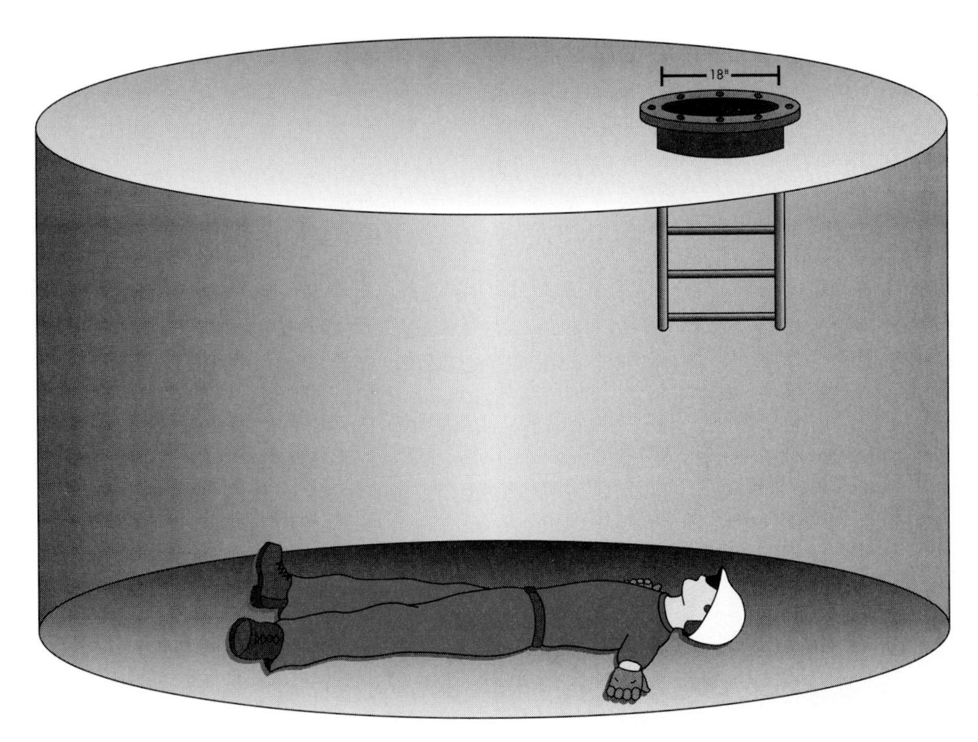

Figure 9.6 Patient only a few feet down in a vessel

Remember, angulated extremities should not be straightened in the field. Severe neurological or circulatory problems can result.

In the second case, the same injury occurs in the industrial environment. The patient has fallen into a confined space (see Figure 9.6). He is only a few feet from the 18-inch-diameter opening at the top of the vessel. It appears to be the only exit and rescuers must get him through it to get to the hospital.

The possibility of spinal injury is very likely because the patient fell several feet into the vessel, dislocating both arms and banging his head. The best thing might be to cut open the vessel. But this could easily take as long as 2 hours. And cutting through the vessel could possibly cause the residual product inside to explode. (In fact, this very event occurred in a large, southwestern city several years ago and resulted in the loss of a rescuer's life.)

Things happen in rescue that require other than a standard approach to patient packaging. Rescuers must preplan for incidents like this. They should have good communication and cooperation with whomever is responsible for EMS and their medical control. These emergencies should be part of a team's training curriculum and conducted in cooperation with the appropriate responsible EMS agency. It is always best to anticipate the worst. An adage that rings true is, "Fail to Prepare . . . Prepare to Fail."

Monitoring the Patient

With any type of packaging, a rescuer must constantly monitor the patient. He or she should frequently check the patient's vital signs and neurological status. The packaging associated with technical rescues often causes significant discomfort to the patient. It sometimes results in injury. In addition, as the rescue becomes more difficult, rescuers tend to pay less attention to the patient.

Never forget the patient! The patient's body will shift in the litter. The rigging will loosen or tighten. Things move around. Injuries can be aggravated or multiplied if a rescuer does not constantly monitor the patient. For example, when improperly lashed into a litter, the patient can be strangled by the lashing should he or she shift during the rescue. Patients can catch on a beam or on the underside of an opening as they are being hauled by the rescue team; this can cause spinal injury (see Figure 9.7).

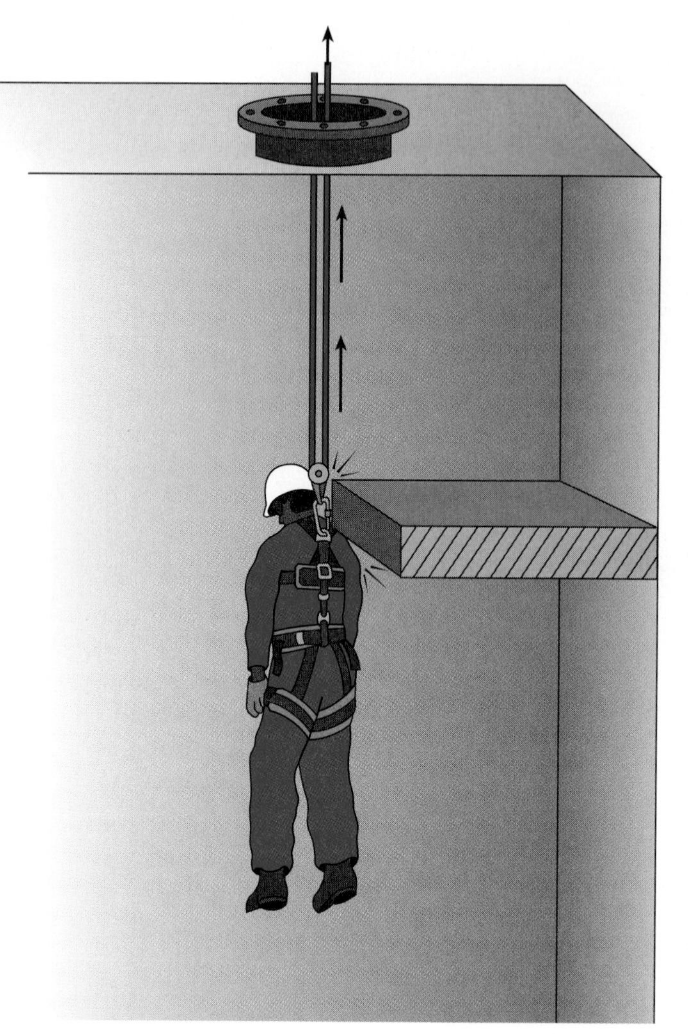

Figure 9.7 Patient caught on projection

To monitor a patient, the rescuer should be familiar with the normal vital signs and neurological checks. The constant changes in patient condition require a hands-on approach to monitoring. This means checking the patient constantly by sight, and touch, when applicable.

A rescuer will not always hear from the patient when there is a problem. The patient might be unconscious, disoriented, numb, or have a facefull of breathing apparatus. Any of these could make it difficult to communicate a problem.

The following scenario is realistic. Rescuers have securely lashed the patient into a litter for vertical extraction from a confined space with a hazardous atmosphere. They have secured him so well that he cannot even move his hands. A rescuer has placed a supplied-air respirator (SAR) on the patient and now double-checks to make sure the face piece is secure. About halfway up, the patient appears to panic. The rescuer attempts to calm this poor soul who is obviously claustrophobic. The rescuers successfully remove the patient from the hazardous atmosphere. Then they remove the face piece and find him dead from acute asphyxiation. Apparently something happened to the patient's air supply during transport. If not operating properly, the victim will not get any air. Obviously, this type of thing should never happen if everyone is paying attention and the breathing apparatus is functioning properly.

Any time patients are in your care, you must carefully and constantly monitor them and their equipment. You must keep your eyes open constantly. Do not let the pressure of the rescue procedure distract you from your primary consideration—*the patient.*

Tied Full Body Harnesses

Harnesses are suited for patients who are conscious and without potential for spinal injury. While this is the general rule, there may be exceptions based on the circumstances surrounding the incident. Because of their superior comfort and integrity, in most situations prefabricated full-body harnesses are preferred to tied full-body harnesses. However, these harnesses can sometimes be slow and difficult to apply. In a real hurry, a tied full-body harness might be more appropriate. This section focuses on the techniques for construction and application of tied rather than prefabricated harnesses.

WARNING

When using a prefabricated harness or any prefabricated rescue equipment, you must consult the specific manufacturer's recommendations for proper application and use.

Harness Applications

Rescuers use a litter to rescue an unconscious person, unless there are overriding considerations such as an immediate threat to life. In these circumstances and situations where there is no suspected spinal injury, rescuers use a full-body harness for the rescue. This type of harness offers both lower- and upper-body support as one unit. These harnesses are also ideal for replacement of a prefabricated harness that has been compromised by a fall or some other incident.

Although there are many excellent tied full-body harnesses, it is impossible to explain all of them here. Instead, the focus is on several methods for one type of tied harness that is both quick and simple to apply and requires minimal equipment and effort. The harness is created using a 20- to 24-foot piece of 1-inch tubular webbing tied in a loop (see Figure 9.8). A water knot (synonymous with tape knot or ribbon knot) is the knot of choice for joining the two loose ends of webbing to form the loop. Rescuers can apply the harness to a patient who is standing, sitting, or lying down. They can apply it facing the patient or facing away. It can even be applied by a rescuer who is suspended upside down on a rope system (see Figure 9.11). Three methods for tying this harness depend on the position of the patient and the disposition of the rescuer. The beauty of this harness is that, with just a little practice, the average person can tie it in less than 15 seconds. Of course, it is more difficult if forced to tie it while hanging upside down.

Although it is a good system, there are disadvantages to the tied full-body harness:

- Once applied, it requires constant upward tension on the attachment points to keep it properly intact. If you lose the tension, you may lose the harness. This is only a problem before the harness is loaded.
- If the webbing is completely severed at any point, the entire harness loses its integrity and may fail.

Rescuers only use this type of harness in extreme emergencies when speed is critical. If time is available, rescuers should apply a prefabricated harness. Here are three methods of application for the tied full-body harness:

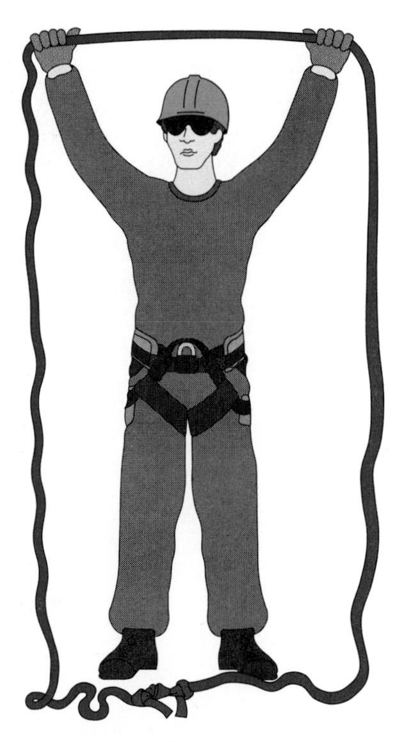

Figure 9.8 Rescuer ready to use a 24-foot section of webbing tied into a loop for a tied full-body harness.

Method 1—Standing Patient

1. Begin this method (see Figure 9.9) by draping a loop of webbing (near the knot) over your shoulder or securing the webbing by other means. Although it could be unsanitary, holding the loop in your teeth actually works well.
2. Find the opposite side of the loop of webbing and form a bight with it. Grasp this bight with your dominant hand.
3. Pass this bight between the patient's legs and upward toward his or her back.
4. With your nondominant hand reach around behind the patient. Grab one side of the bight of webbing while you release it with the stronger hand.
5. Remove your dominant hand from between the patient's legs. Reach around the opposite side of the patient's body toward the back. Grasp the other side of the bight of webbing while continuing to hold on with the nondominant hand.
6. With both hands on the webbing, slide your hands around the patient's body toward you to form two loops of webbing at the patient's chest.
7. Let each of your hands pass through their respective webbing loops from the outside (lateral) toward the inside (medial).
8. With each hand, grab one side of the bight of webbing laying on the rescuer's shoulder or being held in your teeth. While keeping both hands on the webbing, slide your hands apart, creating loops of webbing as they are pulled through the webbing loops created earlier at the chest.
9. Fully extend your arms while pulling the two webbing loops as far apart as possible.
10. Complete the harness by bringing these loops upward and toward the patient's head while constantly maintaining tension.
11. If you attach this harness while facing the patient, it will be possible to pull upward on the single piece of webbing traversing the patient's chest. This should form a third loop of webbing. This may help to alleviate some pressure that might otherwise be placed on the patient's chest. You may attach these three loops to a carabiner while holding tension upward.
12. To use this same method on a patient facing away from you, simply reverse the references to the patient's chest and back.

Method 2—Sitting or Prone Patient

You can use a modification of method 1 to tie the same harness on a patient who is sitting or lying down (see Figure 9.10).

1. Drape the loop of webbing around the patient's body with the knot at the bottom of the loop near the patient's feet. This is sometimes called "circling the wagons."

Text continued on p. 161

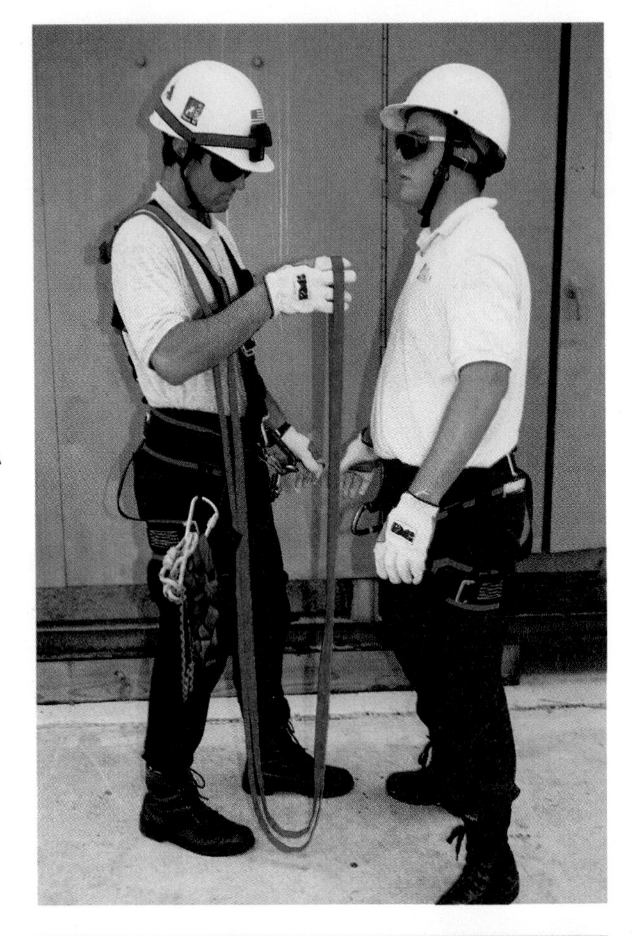

A

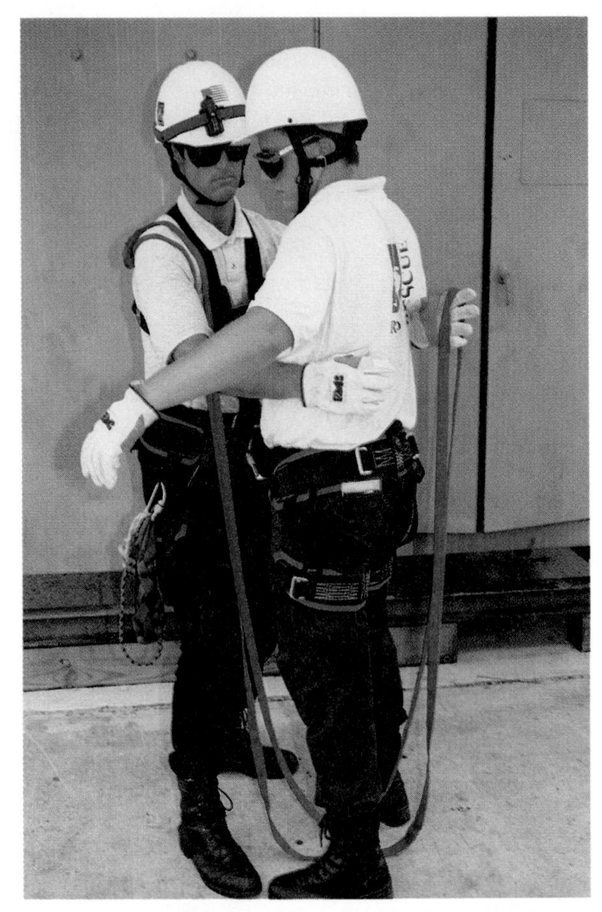

B

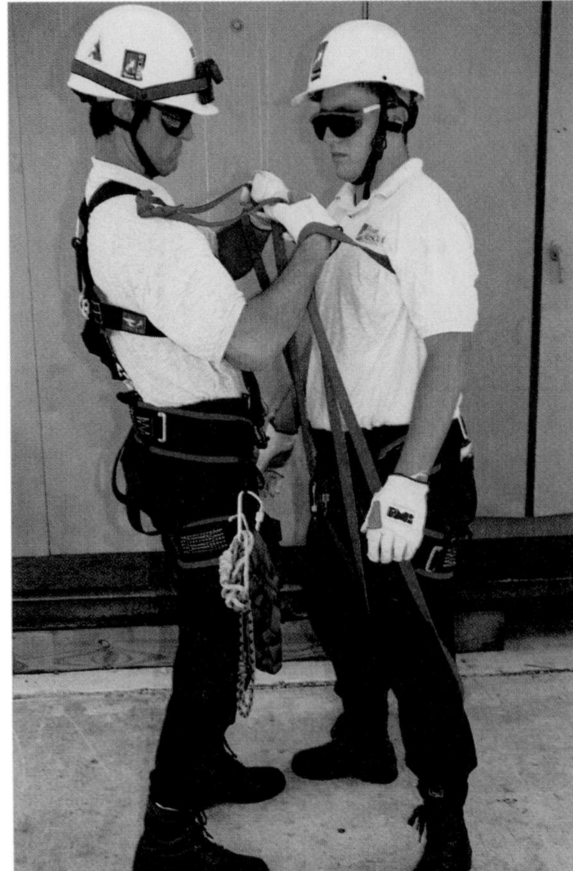

C

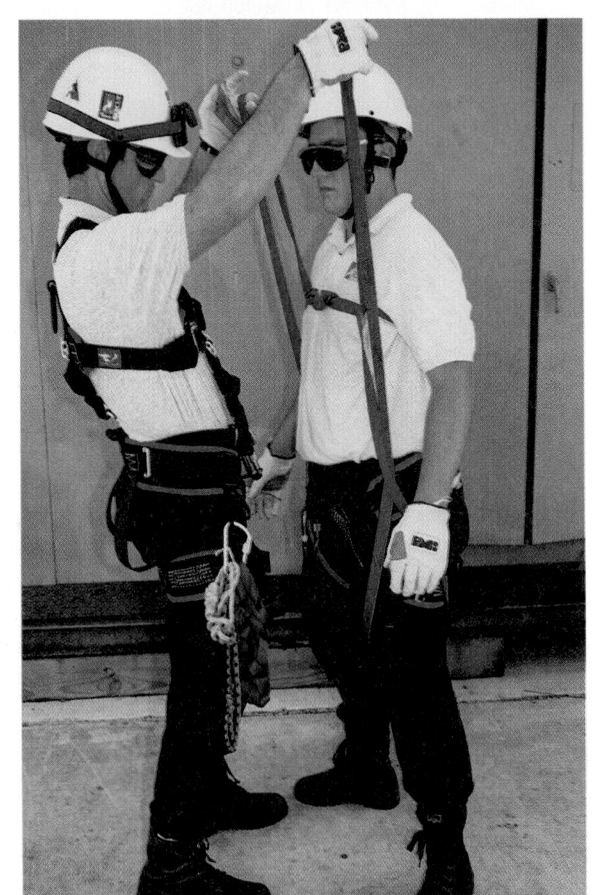

D

Figure 9.9 A–G Tying full-body harness on standing patient

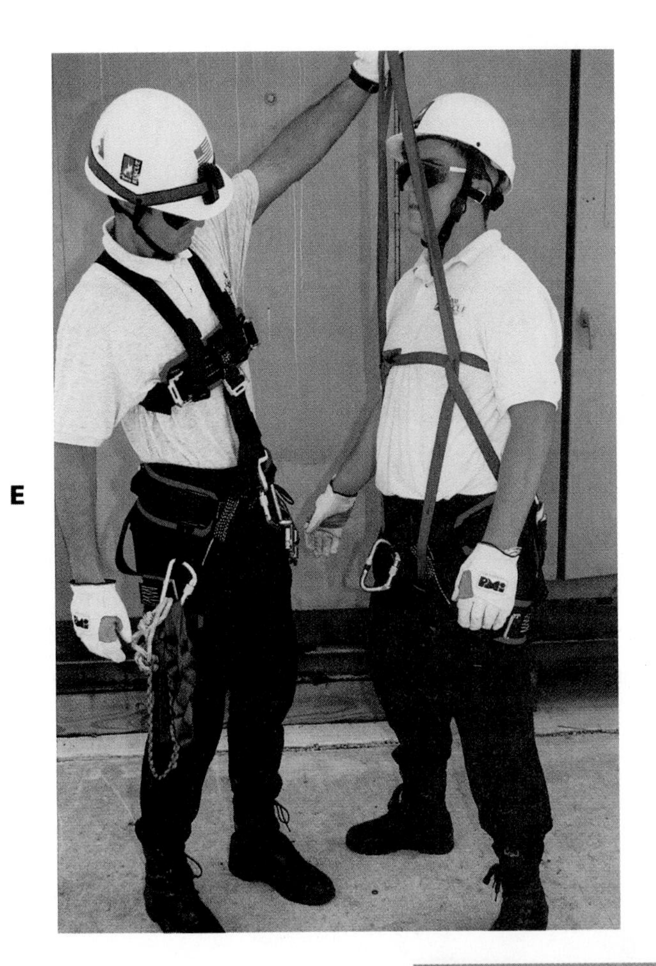

E

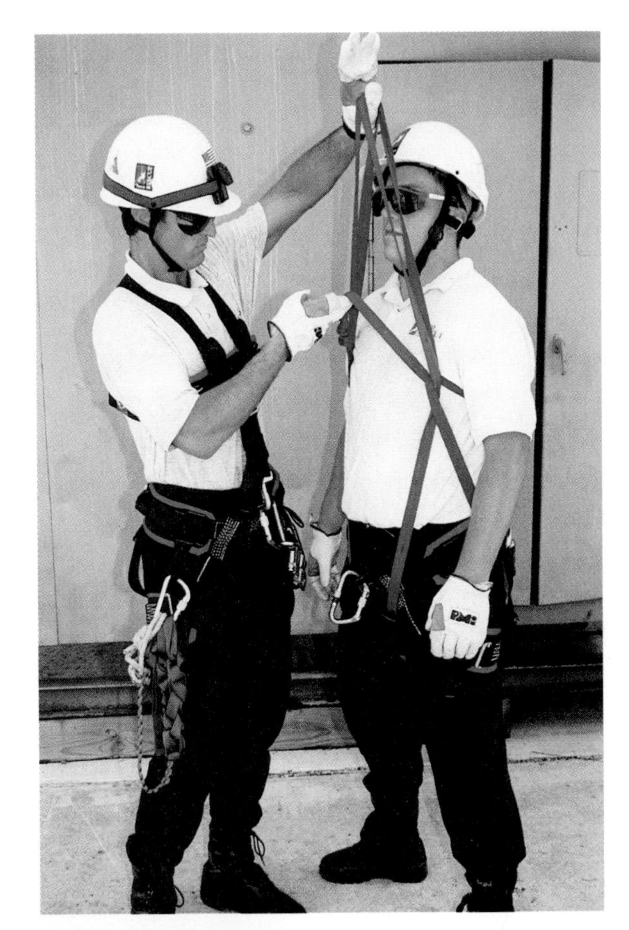

F

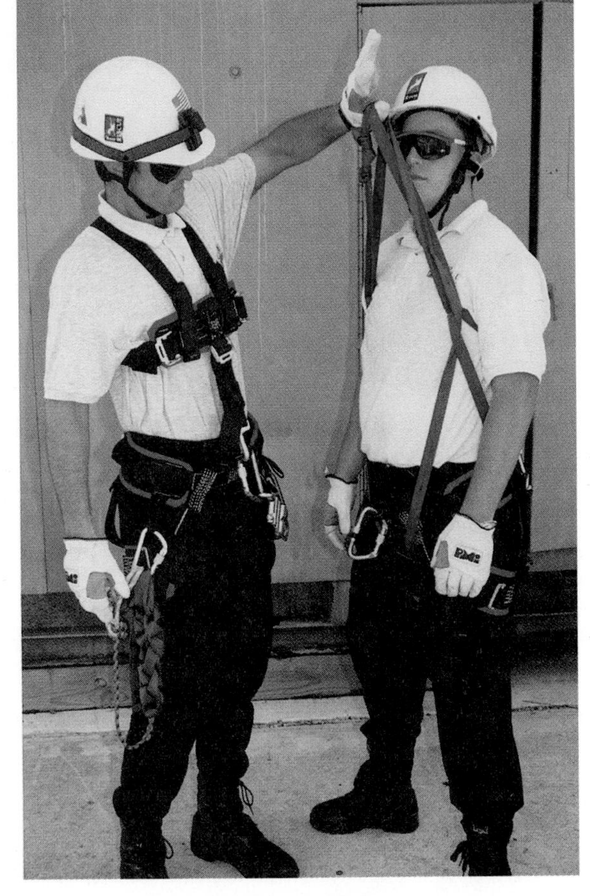

G

Figure 9.9, cont'd.

Figure 9.10 A–E Tying full-body harness on supine patient

A

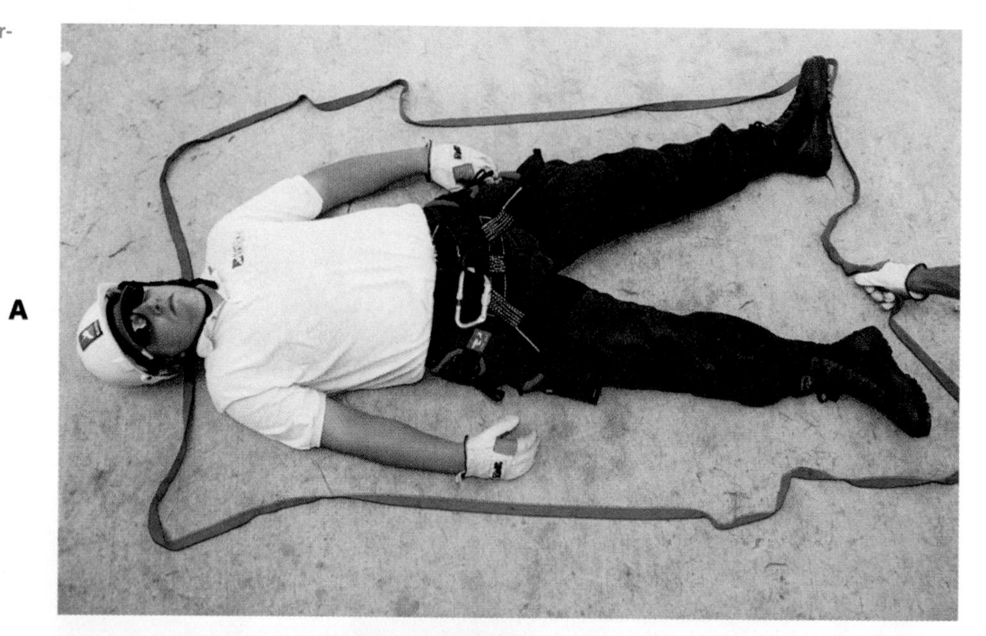

B

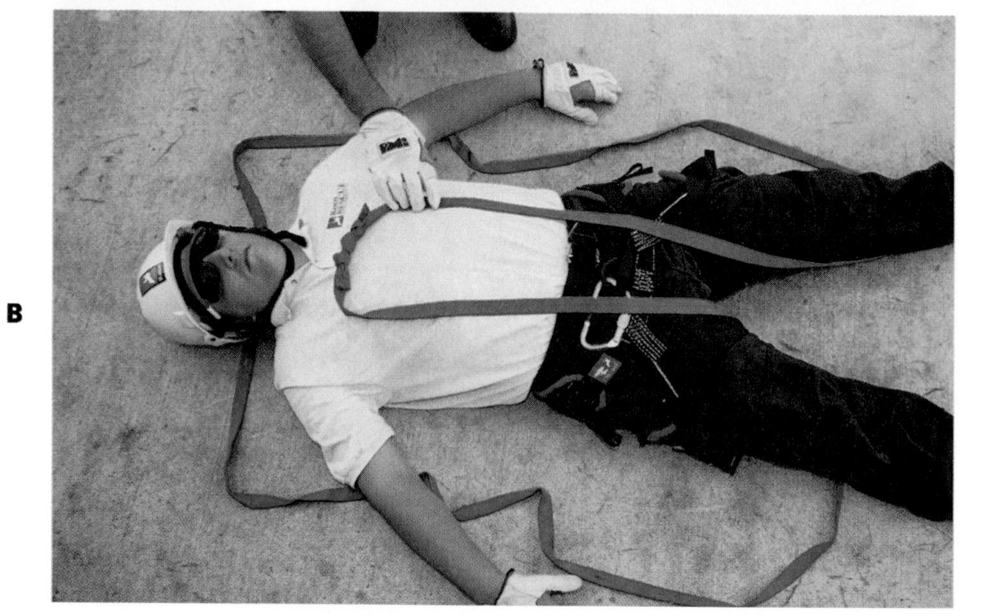

C

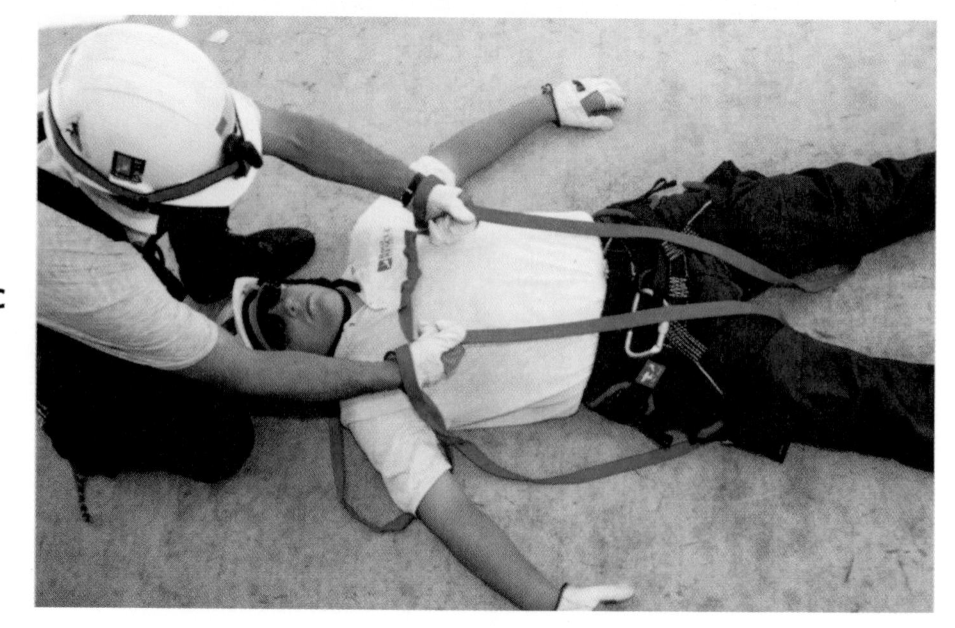

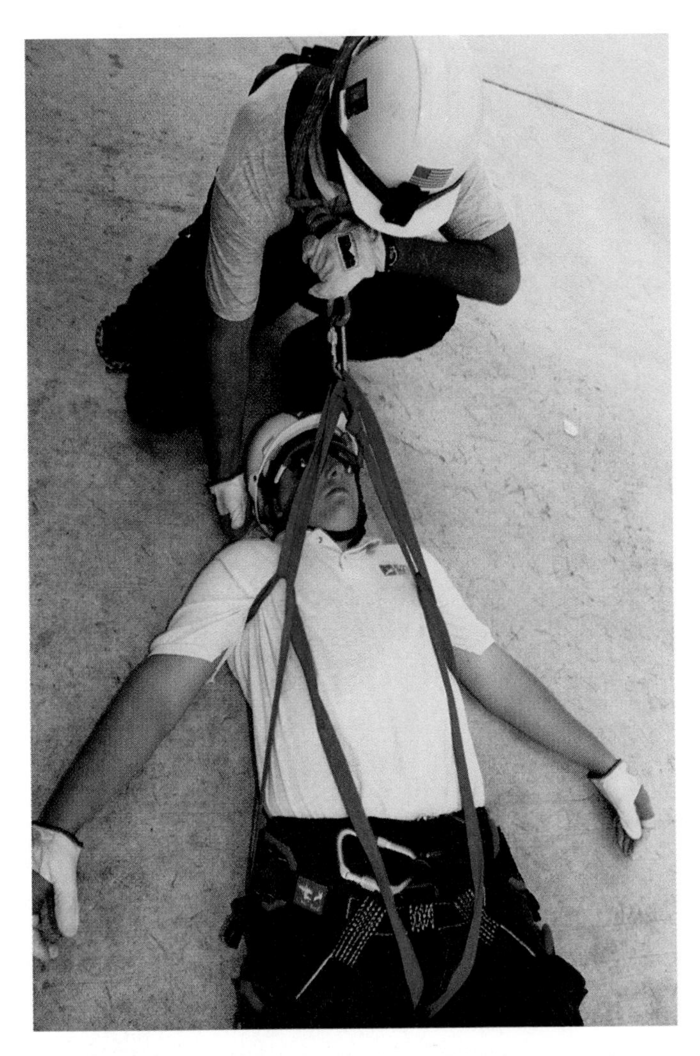
D

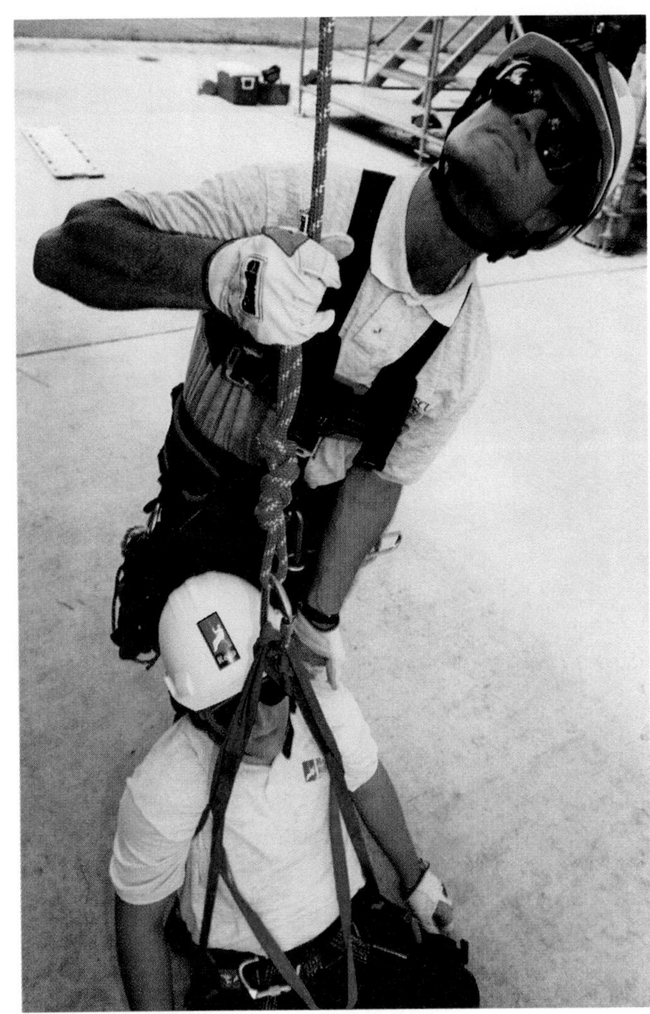
E

Figure 9.10, cont'd.

Pull the webbing behind the patient's head (depending on whether the patient is supine or prone) to the level of the shoulders. Make sure the arms are laying on top of the webbing and not beneath it.

2. Grab the knot and pull it upward, between the patient's legs, to the chest. Lay this loop of webbing on the center of the subject's chest.
3. Find the single piece of webbing running along each side of the patient's body just below the level of the armpits. With one hand on each side of the patient, reach underneath and through these pieces of webbing (lateral to medial). Grasp each of the two sides of the webbing loop at the patient's chest.
4. Pull outward on the sides of this loop, causing two loops to be formed as they pull through the webbing pieces on each side of the patient.
5. Pull these two loops as far apart as possible.
6. Bring the loops toward the patient's head just as with method 1.
7. All other instructions are the same as for method 1.

Method 3—Inverted Rescuer

This method is very similar to method 1 that involves a standing or suspended victim. It requires some preparation and much composure to perform properly. With a little practice, you should be able to tie this harness in less than 30 seconds.

1. Stay well above the patient. Start in the same way as in method 1. By holding a bight with opposite sides of the webbing loop, form a sling that resembles a jump rope.
2. Invert so that you can reach the level of the patient's chest.

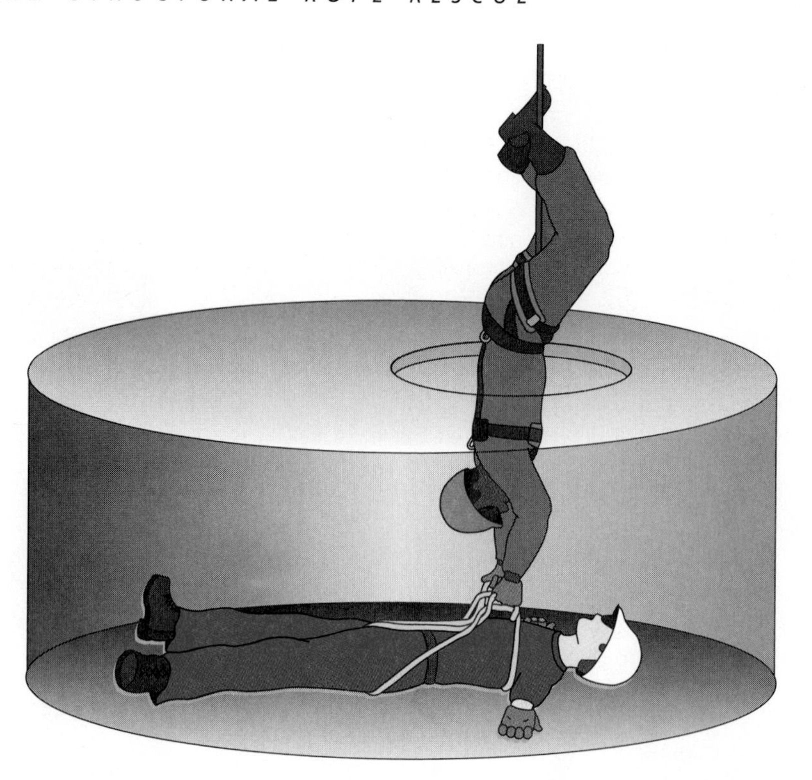

Figure 9.11 Suspended rescuer tying harness

3. Lower the "jump rope" sling down one side of the patient's body near his or her feet.
4. Tell the patient to step over the sling so that it travels from the front of the body, through the legs, and up the patient's back.
5. Hold the bight of webbing in front of the patient's body (assuming the patient is facing the rescuer) under your chin or in your teeth. Remember that it will be difficult to communicate with the patient if the webbing is in your mouth.
6. Reach one hand under each of the patient's armpits and around the back to grasp each side of the bight of webbing. You should have one side of the bight in each hand.
7. Without releasing the webbing, slide both hands around the patient to a point near his or her chest. This forms two loops at the patient's chest.
8. Let your hands pass through their respective webbing loops from the outside (lateral) toward the inside (medial).
9. Grab one side of the bight of webbing that is under your chin or in your mouth with each hand. While keeping both hands on the webbing, slide the hands apart to create loops of webbing as they are pulled through the webbing loops created at the chest earlier.
10. Fully extend your arms while pulling the two webbing loops as far apart as possible.
11. Complete the harness by bringing these loops upward, toward the patient's head while constantly maintaining tension.
12. Bring the third loop up if needed and fasten all three loops together with a carabiner.
13. Reinvert while maintaining upward tension on the loops. Make the attachment to the main systems.

With all three methods, it is important to keep tension on the webbing to prevent it from becoming loose and unworkable. If the patient is left alone after the harness has been tied, the rescuer may wish to have the patient hold tension on the harness.

An alternative method to holding tension involves tying the two loops of webbing together with a square knot to keep the harness intact while the rescuer is performing other work details (see Figure 9.12).

In most situations, full-body harnesses should not be used for patients with suspected spinal injuries. However, extreme situations may require their use.

Spinal Immobilization

Persons with potential spinal injuries require full spinal immobilization. Unless extreme circumstances prevent it, spine immobilization starts at the head and ends at the feet. Spinal immobilization usually involves a long spine board, a means of securing the patient to the board, and some type of cervical immobilizer for the head and neck. Many patients require proper spinal immobilization before being placed in a litter. It is important for every rescuer to know the basic techniques for immobilization.

Even if the patient's spine is not compromised, certain litters require a full spine immobilizer to provide rigidity. This section focuses on some common devices and the techniques for proper spinal immobilization. These procedures and concepts are subject to local interpretation and should not be adopted without the direction of local medical authority.

It is also important to note that most spinal immobilization procedures are ideally performed with three rescuers, though two experienced people are commonly used on ambulance calls. Although two persons can be considered marginal for proper spinal immobilization, a single rescuer may be forced to perform it in an area where only one person can get to the patient. This is sometimes the case in confined spaces. This possibility makes it wise to be ready with Plan A (three rescuers), Plan B (two rescuers), and even Plan C (one rescuer) to perform rescues from tight spots.

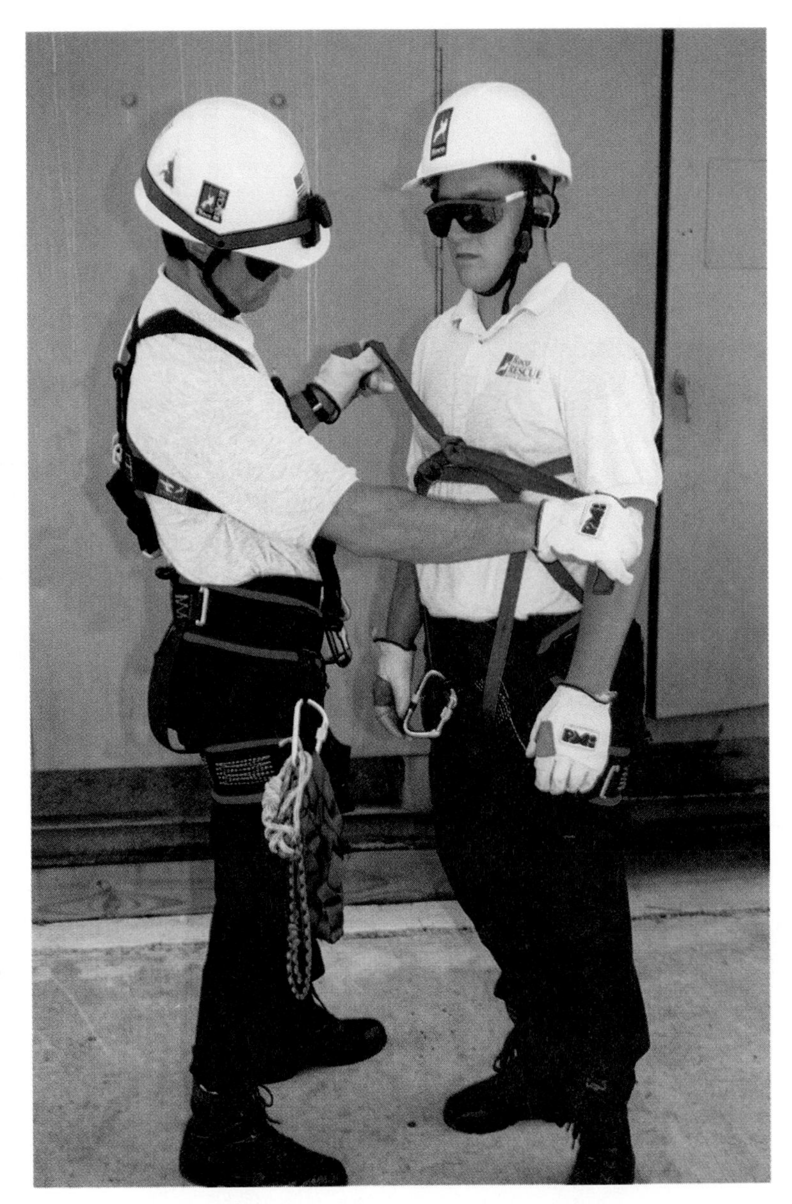

Figure 9.12 Using square knot to keep tied harness intact

Immobilization of the Head and Neck

Cervical spine (c-spine) immobilization involves splinting the head in relationship to the body to prevent movement of the neck. The c-spine, while extremely durable, is the part of the spine most subject to damage from trauma. Ignoring the c-spine can have very serious results. When the bones surrounding the spinal cord are fractured, they can put pressure on the cord or even cut it. Manipulation of a damaged c-spine can result in paralysis of arms, legs, and muscles used for breathing, and even death.

Rigid cervical collars are often used to assist the rescuer with immobilization. But these c-collars are mistakenly applied and left unattended to provide immobilization by themselves. THEY DON'T! Ideally, the first rescuer to access the patient with possible spinal trauma should go directly to the head and maintain immediate manual immobilization of the c-spine (see Figure 9.13) until the head can be secured completely in a cervical spine immobilization device. This means literally holding the patient's head in alignment with your hands (not pulling traction) even after a rigid c-collar has been applied. Someone should keep hands on the patient's head, holding it in a neutral position, until complete immobilization of the c-spine has occurred (this means at least two rescuers).

As a training exercise, rescuers can put a rigid c-collar on and try moving their heads. They quickly see that these collars only assist the rescuer in maintaining the head in proper position. The collar certainly does not immobilize the head. And applying a c-collar to someone wearing a breathing apparatus face piece is very difficult to do. Even collars designed to fit patients with shorter necks ("No Neck" sizes) do not fit well when a face piece is in place. Rescuers must be ready to provide c-spine immobilization with or without the face piece.

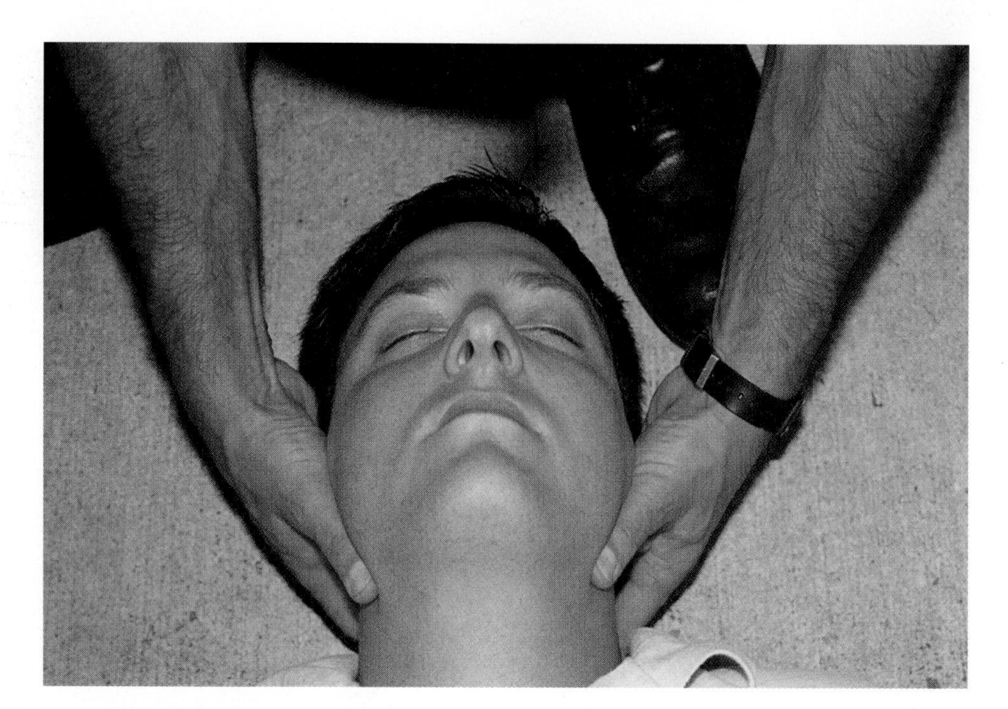

Figure 9.13 Manual immobilization of C-Spine

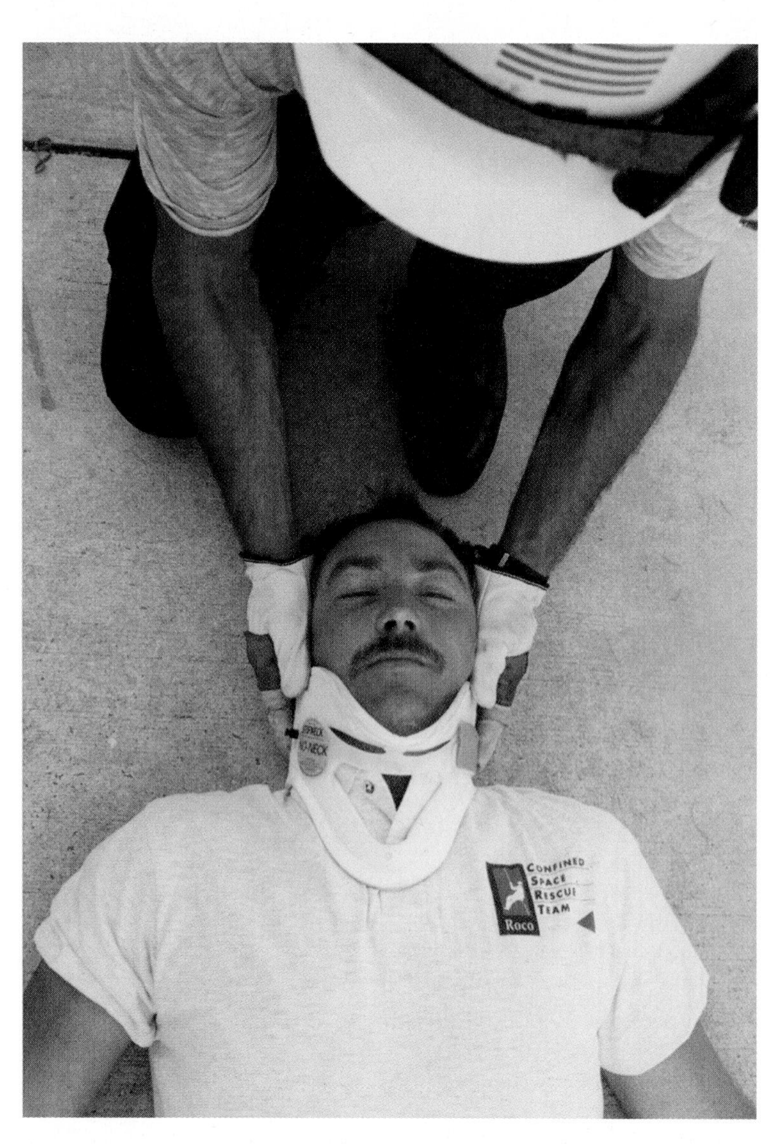

Figure 9.14 C-collar applied and still manual immobilization

There are many methods of cervical immobilization. Rescuers always start with manual immobilization followed as quickly as possible with application of a rigid c-collar (still maintaining manual) immobilization (see Figure 9.14). Then, complete immobilization is obtained, together with a short or full spinal immobilization device. Most short spine immobilizers are constructed to incorporate the c-spine unit as part of the device (see Figure 9.15). Some long spine devices incorporate a c-spine immobilizer, though separate units are most often used in combination.

Cervical immobilization devices can be as simple as a blanket roll positioned around the head and secured with sturdy tape. More sophisticated units can be attached to a long-spine board with dense foam head pads with straps to hold them in place. There are even disposable cardboard c-spine immobilizers on the market.

A rescue team should try several designs to find what works best for team members and their environment. The team and its medical authority should decide which method works best for them, keeping in mind the rescue environment in which they will use them.

For general industry, rescuers use a device that provides good immobilization (even with the application of fresh-air breathing apparatus), is compact enough to make it through narrow passages, and sturdy enough not to be destroyed while doing so.

There are rare exceptions to the normal procedure for managing the c-spine in a neutral position. If the head or neck is in an angulated position and the patient complains of severe pain on any attempt to straighten it, immobilize it in the position

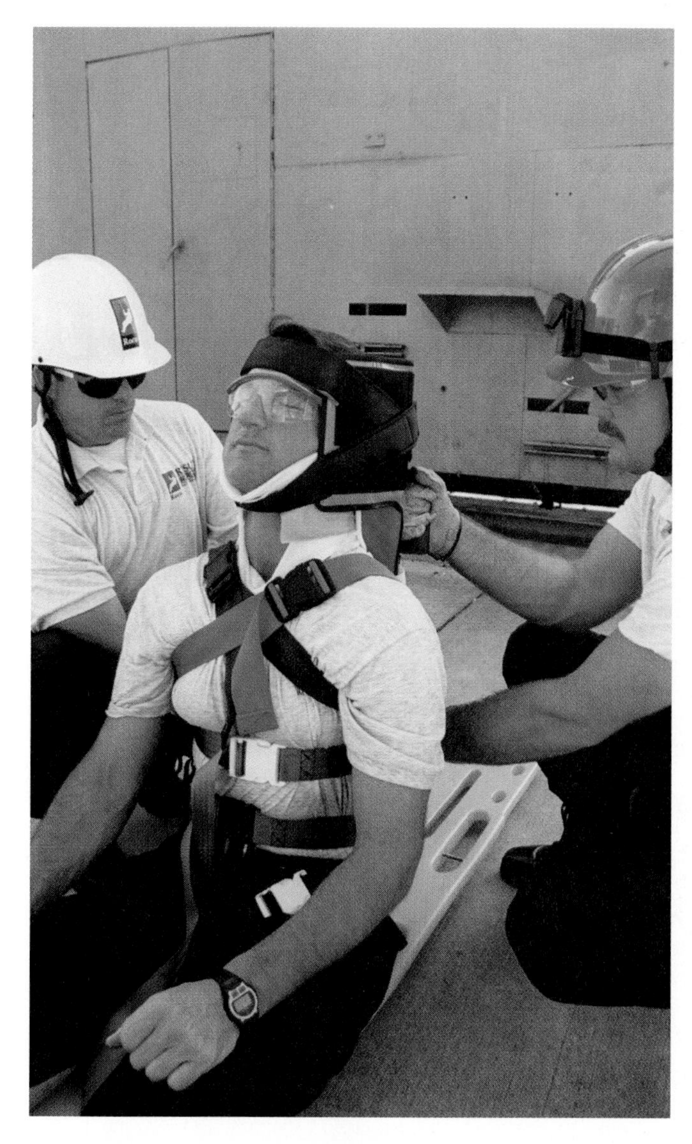

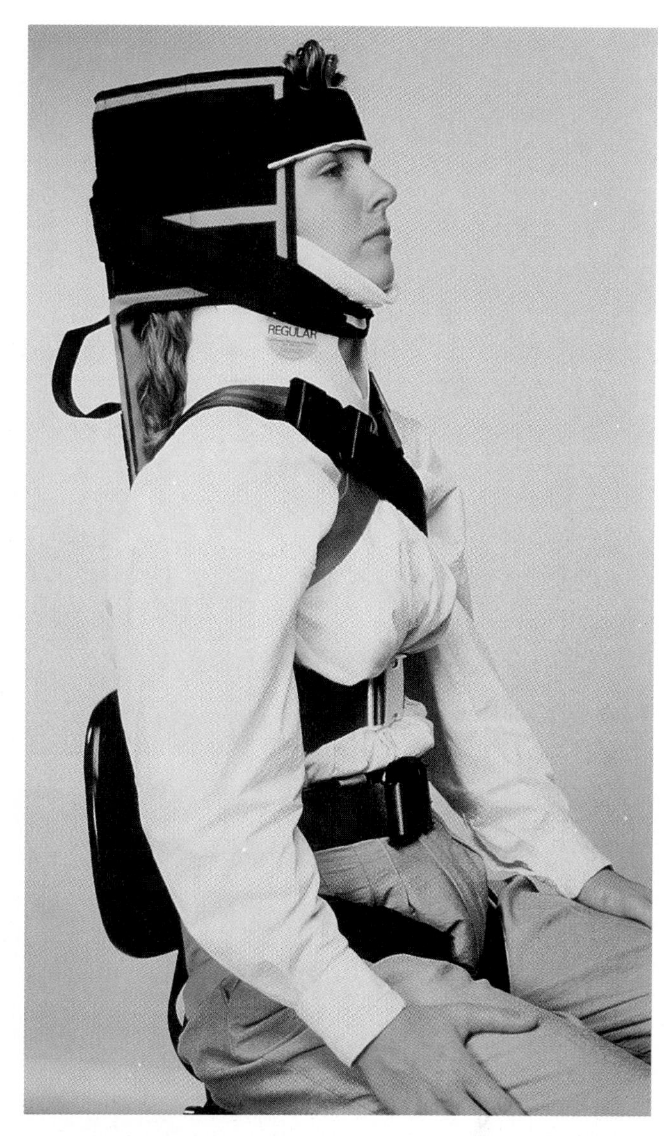

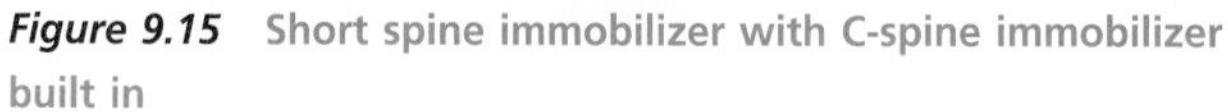

Figure 9.15 **Short spine immobilizer with C-spine immobilizer built in**

Figure 9.16 **Oregon Spine Splint II**

found. The same is true of the unconscious patient whose head or neck is in an angulated position and does not easily straighten with gentle traction. In these cases, you must use blanket rolls, padding, or anything at your disposal to immobilize the head in the position found. Cervical collars and commercial immobilizers probably will not work because they require moving the head to straighten it on the neck before they can be applied.

Short Spine Immobilization

Short spine immobilizers are used commonly in rescues involving spinal trauma (see Figure 9.16), such as at the scene of an auto accident. They are primarily designed to provide a temporary splint while removing a patient from a tight area (such as a crunched automobile or other confined space) to a full spine immobilizer. Although rescuers resort to short spine immobilizers alone for certain industrial rescues, they should not be used routinely by themselves. They are used when full spine immobilizers will not fit, and only until rescuers transfer the patient to a full spine immobilizer (as soon as possible).

If rescuers haul patients in a short spine immobilizer, they must make certain the method for attachment to the rope system is approved by the manufacturer. The fabric lifting handles on many of these units are there to help move the patient around a

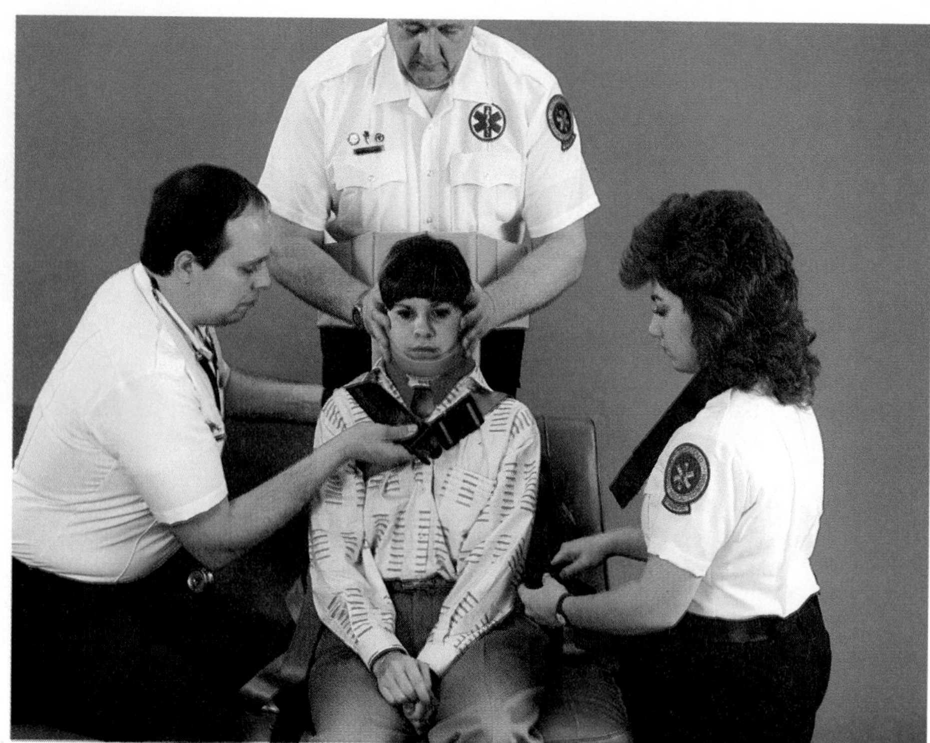

Figure 9.17 Fastening shoulder straps

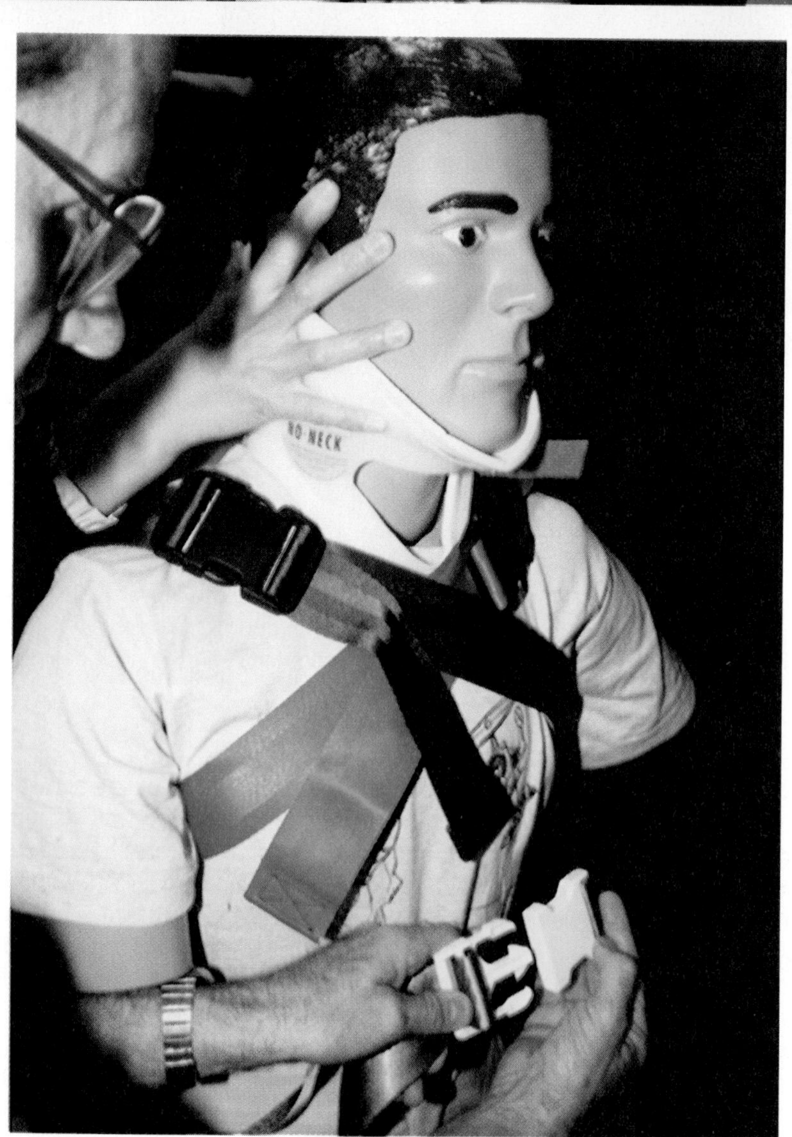

Figure 9.18 Loosely fasten straps on OSS II while positioning

little while placing him or her on a full-spine immobilizer. They are not designed for vertical hauls.

One manufacturer has approved its device, the Skedco Oregon Spine Splint II, for use with a full-body harness. To keep spinal manipulation to a minimum while lifting, rescuers place the harness around both the patient and the short-spine immobilizer. Other devices have a built-in full-body harness for attachment to a hauling system. One example of this is actually a parachute-type full-body harness with V-rings built in for lifting. It has a removable rigid plate and cervical immobilizer incorporated into the device. Rescuers should reserve such units for technical rescue applications. They are constructed primarily of nylon. This material can degrade both from normal use and from the decontamination agents used against bloodborne pathogens. Whatever the short immobilizer, most manufacturers (even those that allow vertical hauling of their devices) do not recommend short-spine immobilizers for vertically lifting patients with potential spinal injuries.

The techniques for applying short-spine immobilizers vary greatly among manufacturers. However, certain basic concepts seem to hold true for most:

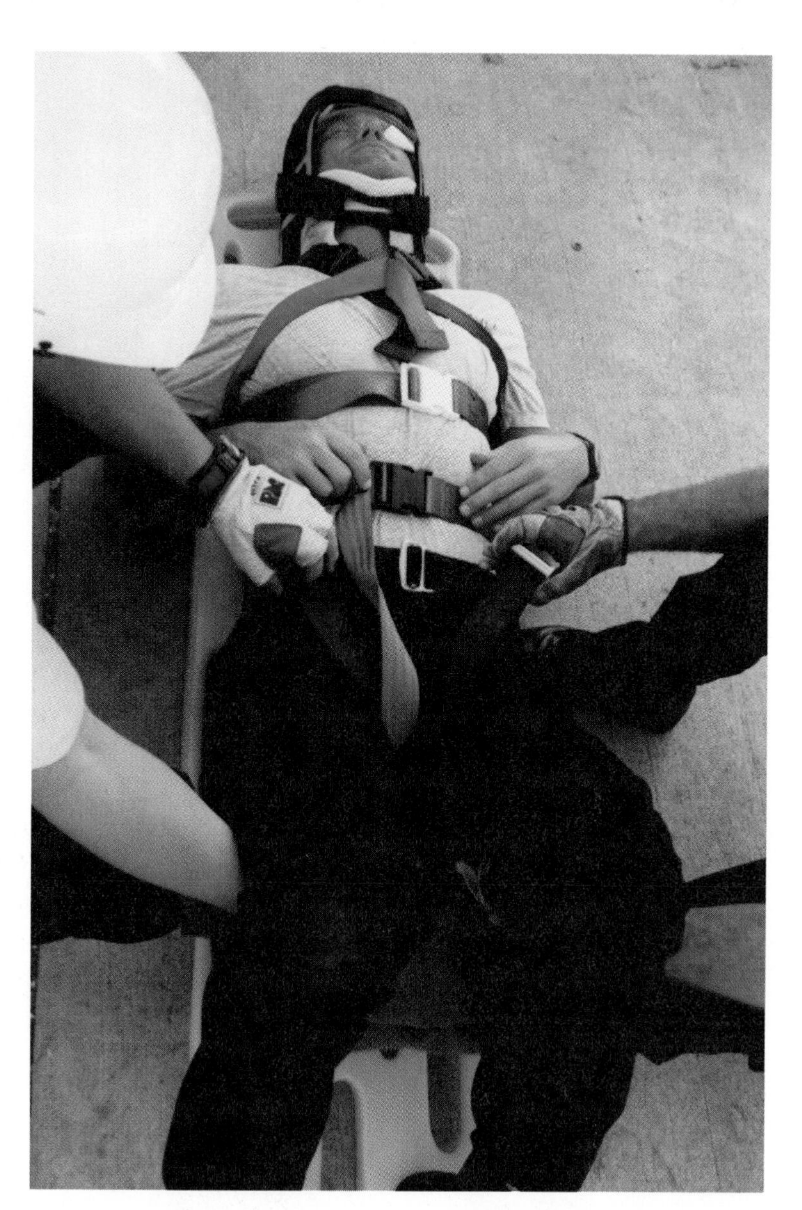

Figure 9.19 Releasing leg straps after patient is on full spine immobilizer

- Straps may or may not be present at the shoulder area. If present, they are intended to help keep the device in the proper position while providing additional stabilization. Shoulder straps are usually fastened and adjusted before torso straps (see Figure 9.17).
- These devices often require the user to loosely fasten straps across the torso while positioning the unit in the proper location (see Figure 9.18). This "proper" position varies with the device.
- Leg straps are secured next and tightened to provide the finishing touches on the torso immobilization. Some of these devices cause quite a bit of discomfort in the patient's groin area when the leg straps are tight. As soon as the patient is transferred to a full-spine immobilizer, release the leg straps to relieve this pressure (see Figure 9.19).
- The head should be the last item to be secured using the c-spine immobilizer incorporated into the device. Some of these c-spine immobilizers do not work well when secured only with the manufacturer's head straps. You may wish to reinforce the securement with roller gauze properly wrapped around the patient's head and the device (see Figure 9.20). If the device has a chin cup, do not place it on the patient's chin. This could cause the patient to aspirate should he or she vomit.

Rescuers should follow the manufacturer's recommendation when applying a short-spine immobilizer, and always follow accepted practice concerning the proper immobilization of the spine.

Full Spine Immobilization

Many techniques for full spine immobilization are available. The method should secure the patient so well to the device that he or she can be positioned on the side or stood up without undue manipulation of the spine. Of course, the cervical spine should be taken care of right away in this immobilization process of patients with a potential for spinal injury. This section focuses on the use of the long spine board as the basis of

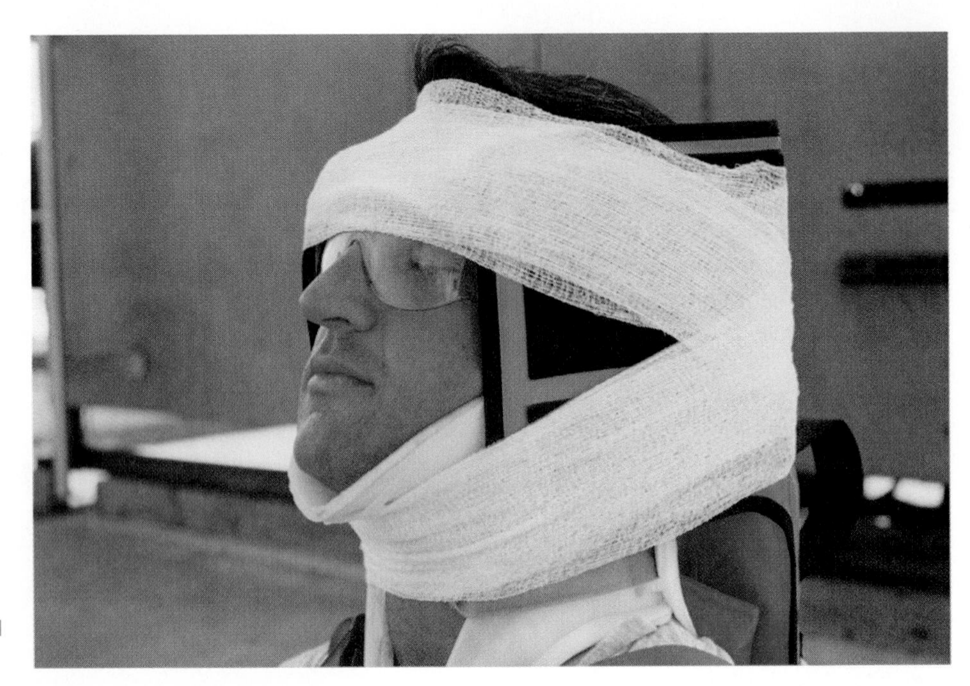

Figure 9.20 Wrapping gauze around head and device

full spinal immobilization. It is an effective, relatively inexpensive, and very common device used throughout the rescue world.

Rescuers must use most long spine boards with strapping or some other means of patient securement and a c-spine immobilizer. Some prefabricated full spine immobilizers incorporate the securement straps and cervical immobilization device into the unit. One such device is the Miller full body splint manufactured by Life Safety Products (LSP) (see Figure 9.21). It is made of high-impact plastic, is only 14 inches wide, and has a split-leg design that will fit into most basket litters with or without leg dividers. Although the common long spine board will provide immobilization, applying it may take a considerably longer time than a full body splint. The full spine immobilizer is more expensive than a common spine board but may speed the rescue operation in industrial applications. Efficiency means streamlining the operation.

Figure 9.21 Miller full-body splint

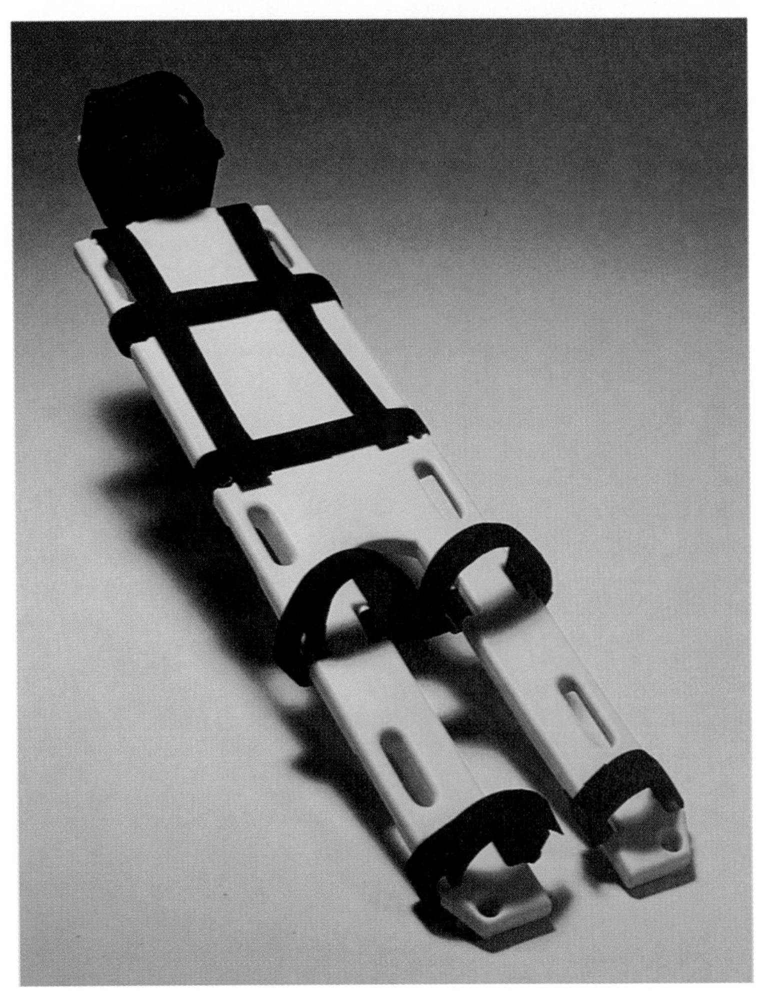

Positioning the Patient

With a long spine board, it is necessary to maintain manual immobilization throughout the process of moving the patient onto the board for complete securement. The methods to make this transition are common to EMS and are standard practice. Log rolls and straddle slides are among the procedures used to place the patient on the long spine board.

If due to cramped space you cannot use one of these recognized methods to place the patient on the spine board, consider short spine immobilizer. This can provide the immobilization needed to transfer the patient onto the board. Some response agencies even practice securement of the patient on a long spine board while standing. This technique is only needed when the patient is conscious and standing, and might have spinal injury.

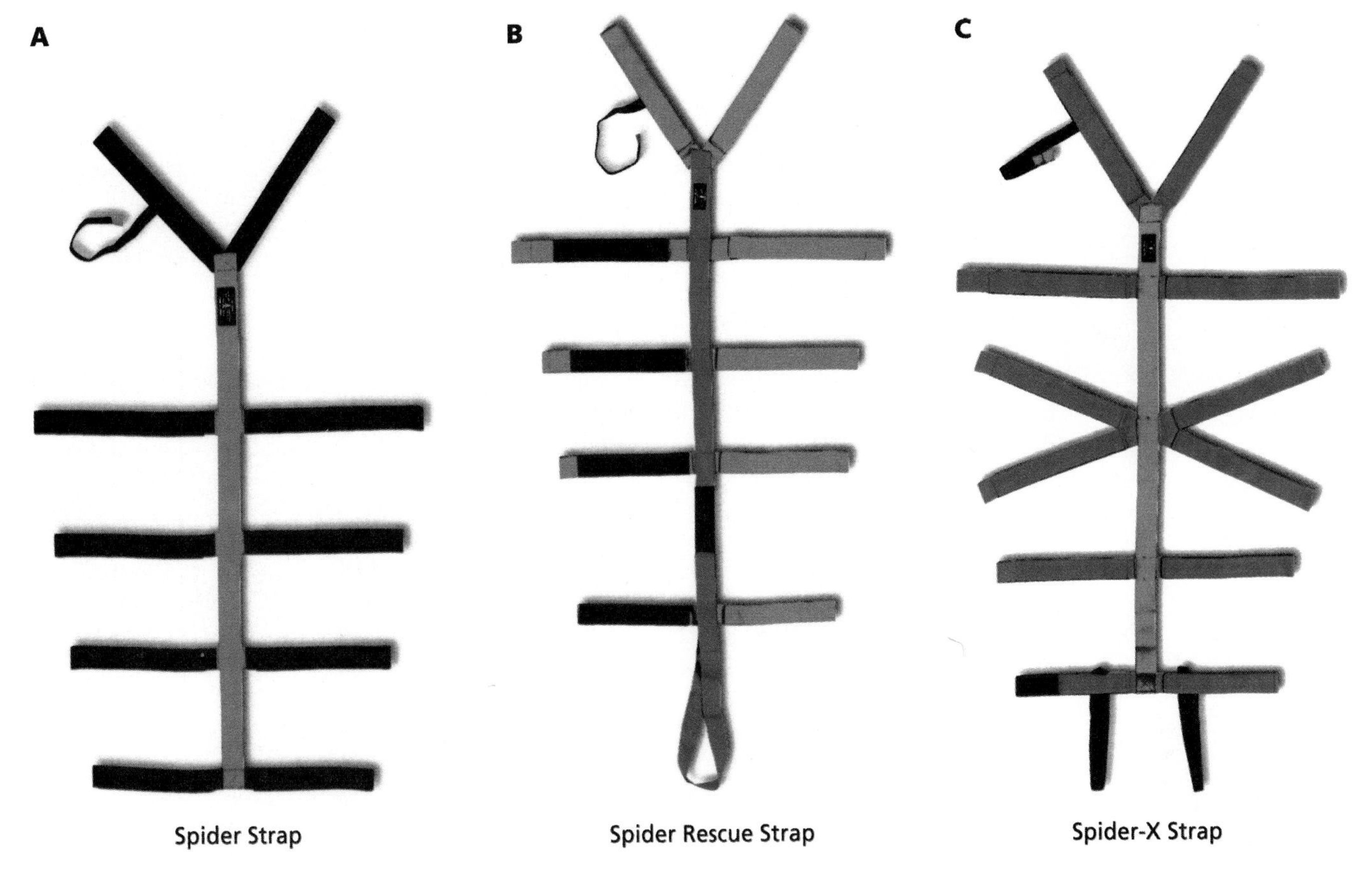

Figure 9.22 A–C Spider layouts

Rescuers should be able to immobilize and transfer the patient to the board whether he or she is standing, sitting, or lying on the ground. Unless the patient is in extreme danger where he or she is, try not to manipulate the spine by moving the patient around or to another location for placement on an immobilization device. Splint the patient where he or she lies. Once placed on the long spine board, the patient must be secured to it.

Securing the Patient

Any method is acceptable that holds the patient so securely that he or she can be turned on the side to vomit or positioned vertically to make it through a narrow opening without causing undue manipulation of the spine. There are probably as many methods and configurations of spine board securement as are stars in the sky. It is not possible to cover them all here.

Most methods involve seat belt–type flat webbing with rescue-grade buckles or tubular webbing woven through openings cut into the spine board in various configurations. There are also prefabricated strapping assemblies such as "spiders" or "quick-clip straps" (see Figure 9.22). These can be used with most spine boards (pin-type spine boards are needed for quick-clip straps) for faster patient securement. Rescuers must be cautious when using push button–release seat belt buckles on any straps used in technical rescue. As the description implies, it takes only the push of a button to release these buckles. They can be purchased with guards that cover the button to prevent release. At the very least, rescuers should turn the push button inward, toward the patient, to prevent objects from bumping and releasing them. Again, rescuers must evaluate various methods and decide on a standard mode of practice with the medical control.

Any software or hardware used for patient securement should be of a grade suitable for technical rope rescue. Do not make the mistake of using the nylon software EMS uses on the street every day. The use and whereabouts of this equipment is usually not well monitored and might have been cleaned with a bleach solution as part of standard decontamination practices. These procedures can seriously damage nylon. Isolate equipment intended for technical rope rescues to technical rope rescues and training only.

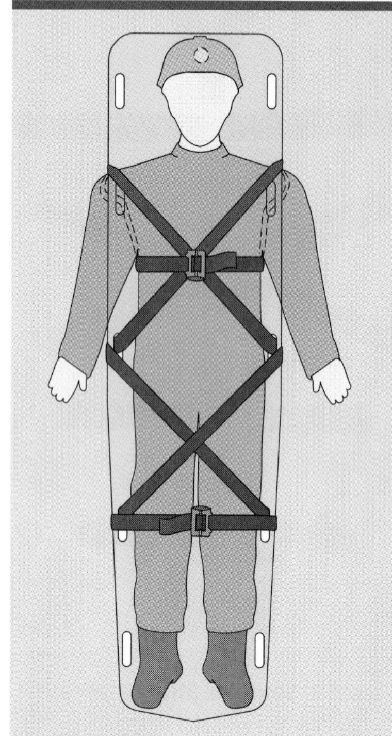

Figure 9.23 The Figure-8 weave

Applying the Figure-8 Weave

1. Lace the loose webbing end of one of the straps through a hole somewhere in the board just above the patient's shoulder on one side.
2. Feed the webbing through the hole from the top, traveling underneath the board on the same side to a hole in the board near the patient's waist.
3. Feed the loose end back up through this hole and pass it diagonally to the hole above the patient's shoulder on the opposite side of the board.
4. Feed the loose end of the webbing downward through this hole and along the underside of the backboard to the hole near the patient's waist. The end should be directly opposite the one previously used on the other side.
5. Bring the loose end back up through this hole and pass it diagonally across the patient's torso and attach it to the buckle at the other end of the strap. This forms a figure-8 with the webbing and secures the torso.
6. Be careful to pad the buckle area to prevent discomfort to the patient.
7. Tighten the webbing enough to prevent the patient's movement but not to restrict breathing.
8. Repeat this process with another strap starting from the holes just above the ones previously used near the patient's waist, or even the same holes if necessary. Overlapping these straps will provide better securement.
9. Use the same technique to work your way down to the holes near the patient's mid thigh. Two or three straps should be woven in place to completely secure the patient's body.

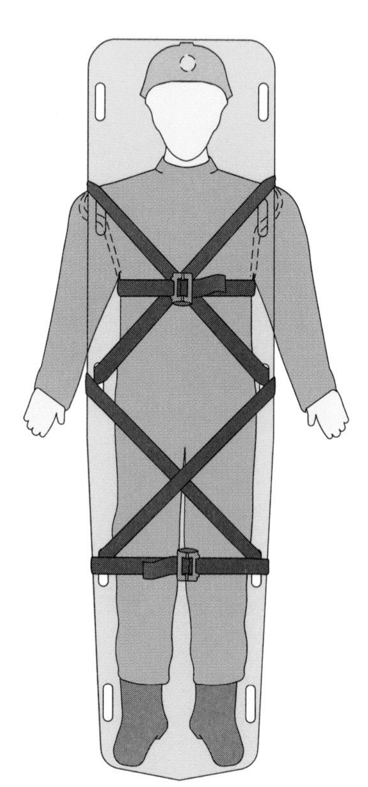

Figure 9.24 The BTLS strapping technique.

Figure-8 Weave One simple method to use with most long spine boards, depending on the number and location of the holes in the board, is sometimes called the "Figure-8 Weave." Two rescuers can usually apply it in less than one minute. The weave requires at least two 12- to 14-foot nylon straps (usually flat-weave webbing nearly 2 inches wide with a minimum breaking strength of 6,000 force pounds) with rescue-grade buckles at one end of each strap (see Figure 9.23).

Different backboards have different handholds. As a result, some boards do not have a hole above the patient's shoulder level. If the nearest available hole is below shoulder level and the webbing is passed up and over the patient's shoulder, dangerous compression of the shoulders can occur when the straps are tightened. In this case it may be necessary to pass the webbing underneath the patient's armpit rather than over the shoulder to form the diagonals. Do not let these diagonal pieces of

The BTLS Strapping Technique

1. After completing proper c-spine immobilization, lace the two straps through the top two lateral holes of the spine board. Apply them so that they connect across the chest below the armpits.
2. Bring the other ends of the straps over the shoulders and across the patient's chest.
3. Lace the straps through the lateral holes at the level of the pelvis.
4. Bring the straps back across the lower pelvis and upper legs, then lace through the lateral holes and connect below the knees. The straps must be tight enough to prevent movement of the patient despite the positioning of the spine board.

webbing apply pressure to the patient's diaphragm (below the arch of the rib cage), which can cause difficulty in breathing.

BTLS Strapping Another method similar to the Figure-8 weave has no known name, but it is commonly taught in BTLS (Basic Trauma Life Support) courses. Therefore, we'll just call it the BTLS method. It requires two 12- to 14-foot straps. It is a simple procedure. With practice, you can do it quickly (see Figure 9.24).

Whatever technique you use, make certain it is adaptable for the patient's injuries and allows access to injured parts. Always place securement straps around the torso and legs of the patient, and avoid the arms. Enclosing the arms in these straps can allow significant movement of the patient's body when the spine board is moved. Secure the patient's hands with wide tape, a webbing strap, or some other wide material to prevent them from falling off the board or grabbing things while being moved around. Some litters provide such sturdy lashing that the patient's hands are secured without tape or webbing.

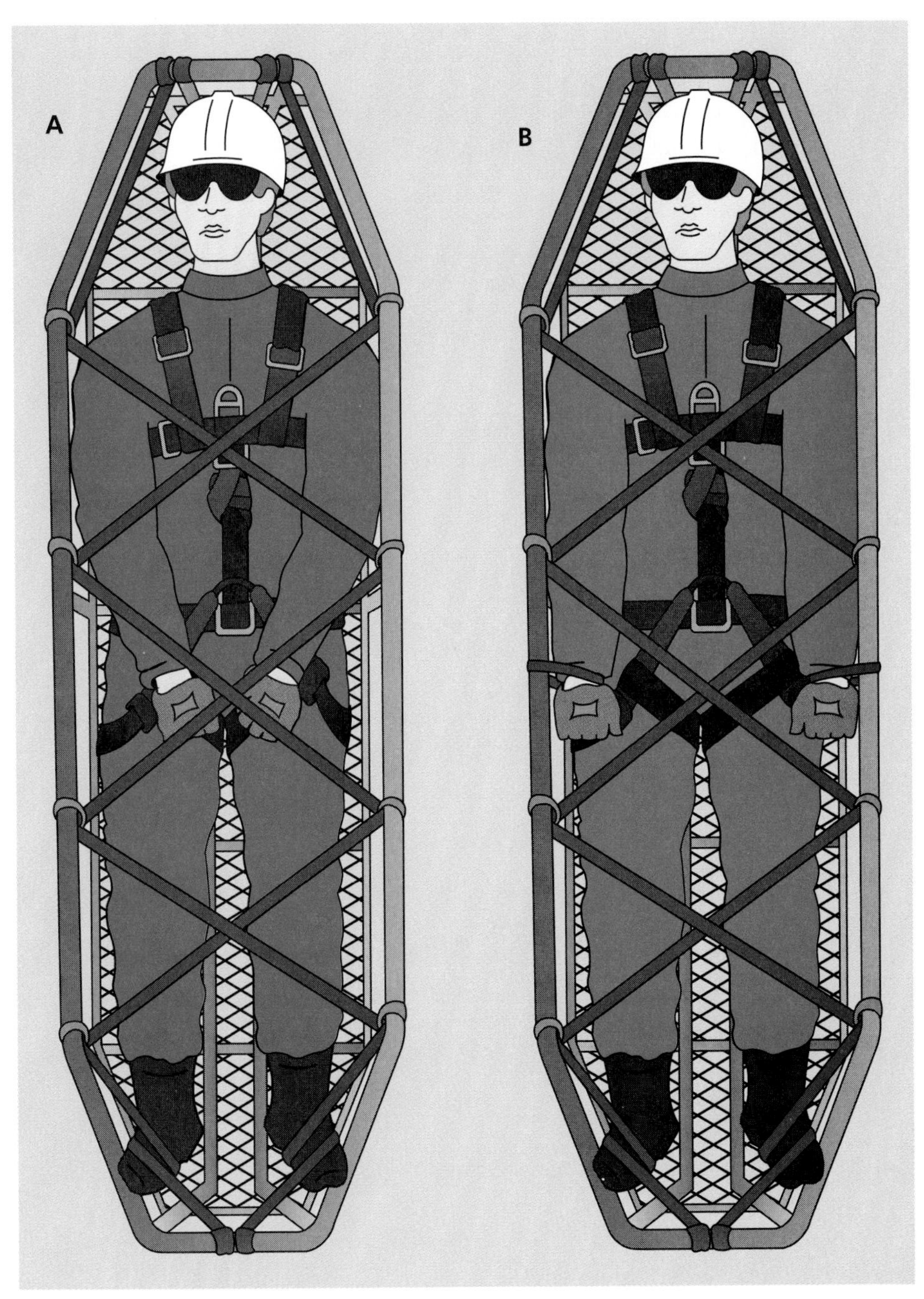

Figure 9.25 Alternatives for securing patient's hands

Summary

There is much more to patient packaging for technical rescues than bandaging and splinting. Changing circumstances cause changes in priorities, requiring alterations in packaging. Package the patient appropriately for the situation at hand and be prepared for changing circumstances. Always attempt to use ideal methods. However, be ready with plan B, C, or even D. Be sure you have approval from your medical authority before performing any procedure that strays significantly from your set protocol. Remember your priorities!

CHAPTER 10

Litter Rigging Techniques

The information in this chapter is provided as a basis for continued training. Each rescuer should consult with his or her own team leader for the correct SOGs for the team. Topics covered in thic chapter include:

- Types of Litters
- Medical Considerations
- Lashing Methods
- Bridles
- Basket Litters
- The Sked Litter
- Tag Lines

Introduction

Rescuers often need to lower subjects or haul them to a safe area for more definitive care and transportation to a medical facility. Whatever rope rescue system they use, rescuers must somehow attach them to the patient to complete the removal.

This chapter explores a few methods to ultimately attach the patient to the rope system for rescue. It emphasizes litters as a transport vehicle, although there are other ways to transport patients. It is important to recognize that there are many methods of litter packaging and rigging. This chapter reviews only a very few of the techniques available.

Some litter systems can cost the rescue team considerable time and effort because they are not streamlined to industrial and structural applications. For example, litter lashing and bridles intended for wilderness applications may not work well in the industrial/structural environment.

To make the rope system connect with the patient usually involves two specific types of rigging:

1. The patient must be placed in the litter so securely that he or she cannot fall out despite the position (sideways, upside down, etc.). If the patient has a spinal or other injury, you must package him or her appropriately in the litter. The method to secure the patient to the litter varies according to the patient's injuries.
2. You must safely and efficiently attach the litter to the rope system. This too can vary with the patient's condition and surroundings.

Rescuers must secure the patient in the litter and the litter to the rope system. Usually these are two separate and distinct functions. They may merge when rescuers use certain specialized litters designed to incorporate both the patient's lashing and the litter's bridle rigging.

Types of Litters

There are two types of litters commonly used in industrial and structural environments. The first type is the "basket litter." It is also called "wire" or "Stokes basket." The litter structures are of various types and strengths. Traditional basket litters are con-

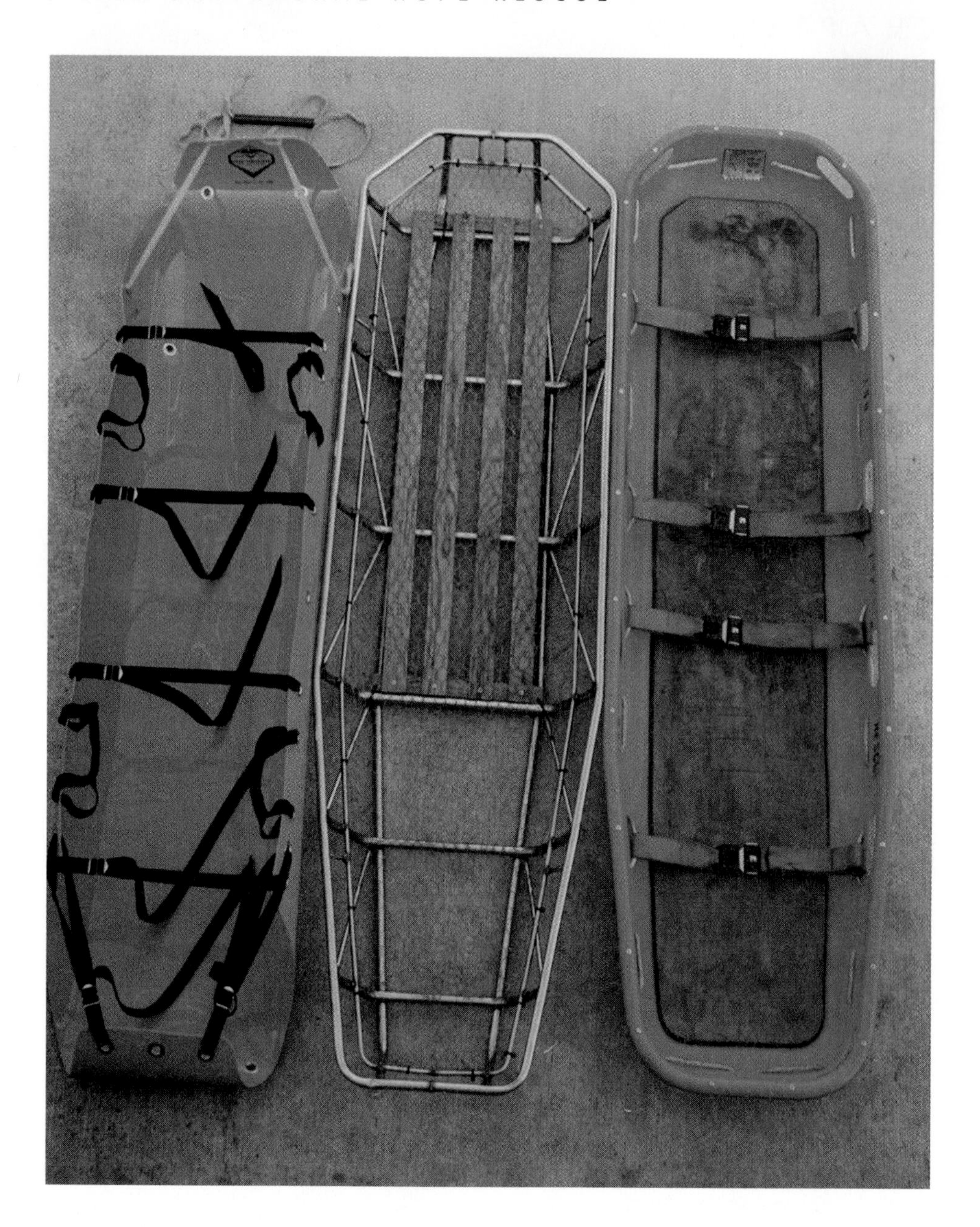

Figure 10.1 Sked, Wire Mesh Stokes, and Plastic Stokes

structed of metal support frames, usually combined with a wire mesh lining. Other basket litters have metal frames and high-impact plastic liners (see Figure 10.1).

Many basket litters should not be used for rescue. This is particularly true of older litters and ones that have been given harsh use. Rescuers must carefully inspect any litter for damage or instability before using it for rescue. Rust, cracks, severe discoloration, and bent frames are all signs of damage. Plastic litters can be damaged by exposure to prolonged sunlight and to corrosive material. Always follow the manufacturer's recommendations on care, maintenance, and retirement of a litter. If in doubt, throw it out.

The other type of litter is the "flexible litter." A flexible litter has no rigid structure of its own. These devices are made of synthetic materials that require some type of spinal immobilizer to provide rigidity. Because they are flexible, they work well to move patients through narrow passageways. They wrap around the patient, like a taco, so the litter is little more than the circumference of the patient's body. This makes it easier to get the patient through small openings. Flexible litters have been used successfully with openings as small as an 11-inch by 14-inch oval (Sked Litter). This obviously depends on the size of the patient.

Flexible litters also have the distinct advantage of being usable with a variety of patient sizes, where a basket litter is very restricted. These litters usually can open at the head and foot to provide room for very tall patients. Rescuers can even rig two of them together to effectively move huge patients. In one well-documented case, rescuers evacuated an 807-pound patient using Sked litters.

As mentioned, one widely used flexible litter worldwide is the "Sked" litter manufactured by Skedco in Oregon (see Figure 10.1). It is a well-known, tried and proven flexible litter. The Sked is ideally suited for many industrial applications, particularly confined space rescue.

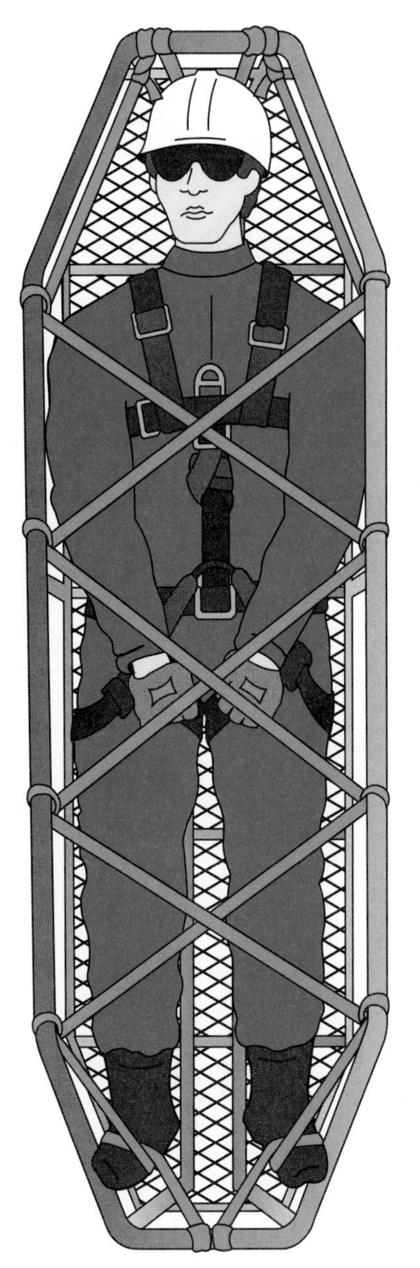

Figure 10.2(a) Diamond lashing of patient in litter

Medical Considerations

Before litter rigging, rescuers review medical considerations that might qualify a patient for litter use. The methods chosen to package a patient should be based on his or her condition and physical surroundings. For example, it would be better to package a person who is conscious and extremely apprehensive in a horizontally positioned litter than in a vertically positioned one. The horizontal litter would prevent the patient from seeing the ground. However, a vertical litter might be necessary to get the patient through a narrow vertical opening.

Because of potential spinal manipulation, it is better to package a possible spinal injury in a litter rather than in a full-body harness. However, rescuers do have to use a harness in certain extreme circumstances such as an immediate threat to life.

Obviously, rescuers may have to take many actions to protect a patient and prevent further injury. Even small things such as lining the bottom of a litter with blankets make it more comfortable. Rescuers should also shield the patient's face and eyes to protect them from falling debris. All rescuers should have competent and qualified training in techniques of patient packaging before attempting to use them in technical rope rescues.

Of course, before placing a patient with a potential spinal injury in any litter, a rescuer must properly immobilize him or her. Then it is time to complete the patient's packaging by securing him or her in a litter for hauling or lowering with a rope system.

Basket Litters

Basket litters are generally very strong and versatile. However, they are not well suited for confined space rescue. Their dimensions limit the area through which they can be passed. More recently, some newer basket-type litter devices have been constructed that are much narrower or designed to operate in confined areas. These devices sometimes sacrifice the patient's protection by reducing the traditional size or configuration of the rigid basket. If the litter cannot make it through very narrow openings with room to spare, rescuers should consider using a flexible litter.

As previously discussed, there are two general considerations when packaging someone in any litter:

1. You must secure (lash) the patient in the litter well enough to allow him or her to be placed in almost any position without falling out.
2. You must securely attach the litter to the rope rescue system.

Lashing Methods

There are several methods for lashing a patient into a basket litter. One method of patient lashing is called the "diamond cross." It uses a 30-foot piece of 1-inch tubular webbing (see Figure 10.2).

The Diamond Cross

1. Start by finding the center of the webbing.
2. Secure it to the bottom rail of the litter using a girth hitch.
3. Split the webbing into two legs.

ALTERNATIVE METHOD

An alternative to this simple wrap is an ankle hitch that encompasses both the ankle and instep of the foot. The ankle hitch also starts with the webbing on the medial (inside) aspect of the sole of the foot near the instep. The webbing wraps over the top of the foot and toward the back of the ankle. It continues around the entire ankle to wrap back across the top of the foot in a diagonal pattern toward the lateral (outside) aspect. Wrap this webbing back underneath and completely around the foot to complete the ankle hitch.

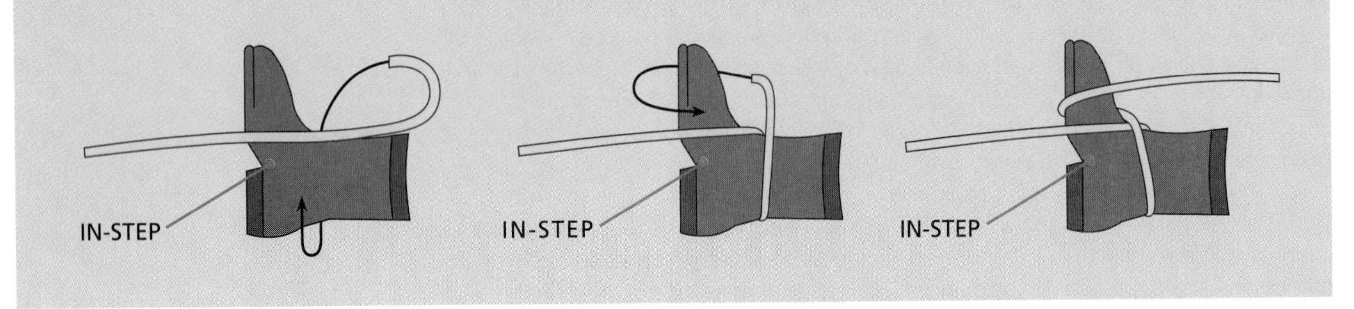

4. Take a wrap around each of the patient's feet with each leg of webbing. The wraps should start on the inside of the foot.
5. Wrap around the foot low on the instep, and end up on the inside again.

   NOTE: It is critical to keep the footwrap within the instep of the foot. If the wrap is too high up on the ball of the foot, the patient can easily wriggle a foot out of the wrap.

Either of these wraps helps prevent the patient from sliding vertically in the basket.

6. Continue the lashing by crisscrossing each leg of webbing, moving upward toward the patient's head.
7. Be certain to wrap the webbing around the vertical support members of the basket frame and not the top rail. You can easily detect the structural members of most basket litters by looking at their path (see Figure 10.4). A structural member travels completely around the underside of the litter; a stop post does not. The stop posts are designed to prevent a knot or carabiner from sliding very far in either direction when attached to the top rail. Keeping webbing off the top rail prevents dangerous abrasion if the webbing were to be rubbed between a wall or other surface and the litter rail.

   NOTE: This is not possible when lashing a patient to most plastic litters since the top rail is the only structural member of the frame (see Figure 10.5). Run the webbing around the top rail in this case.
8. When you have completed the lashing to the level of the upper chest, tighten each leg securely (from bottom to top), one at a time, and finish with a clove hitch attached to the top rail of the basket. The clove hitch should be on the inside of the vertical support member or may split the vertical support member to prevent the knot from sliding down the rail and loosening. NEVER lash the webbing horizontally across the upper chest near the neck. This could strangle the subject if he or she slid down in the litter.

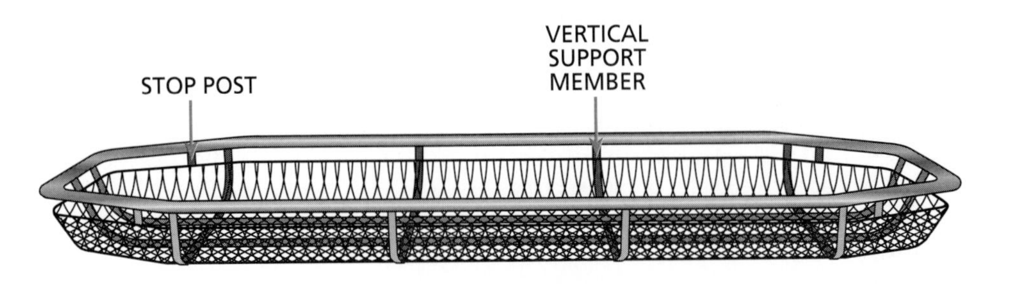

Figure 10.4 Typical basket litter

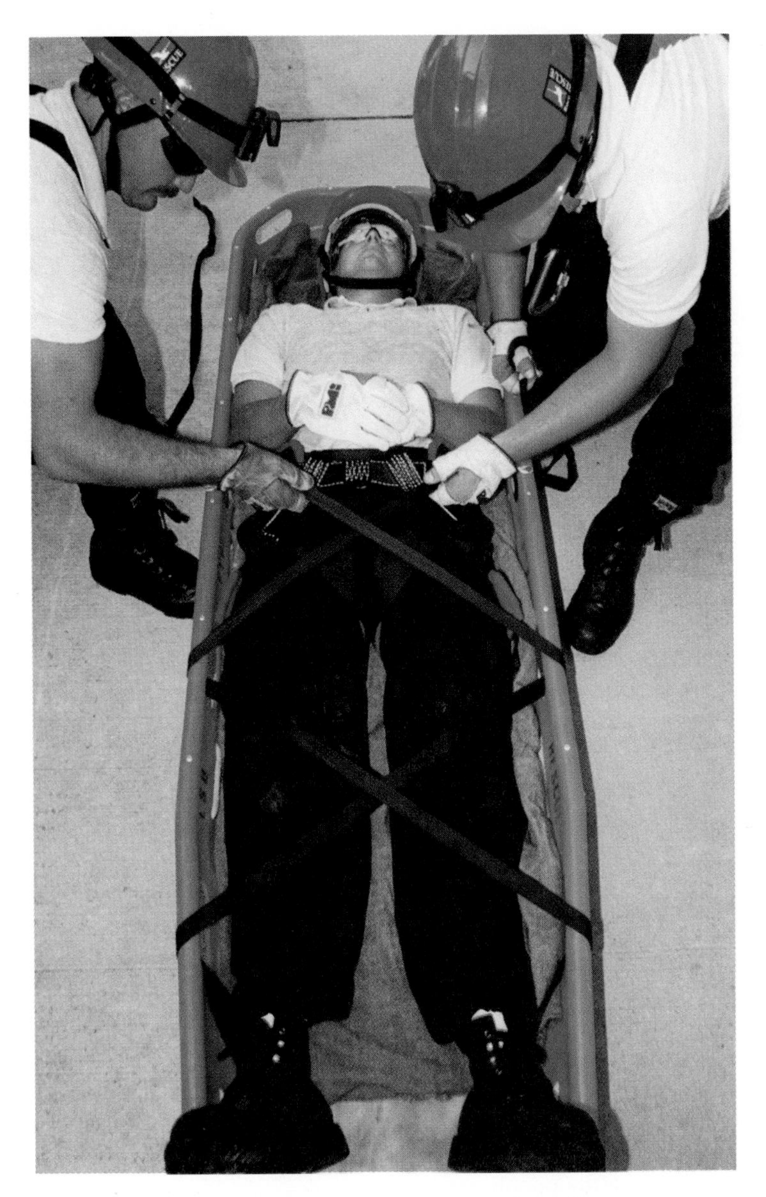

Figure 10.5 Webbing around top rail on Plastic litter

If the patient's injuries cause problems when using this lashing method, rescuers should consider leaving open areas in the diamond weave to expose the injuries as needed. They must be prepared to modify lashing based on the patient's injuries. Trauma to a lower extremity often requires modifications in the diamond weave lashing. If the patient has a leg injury (as patients frequently do), a rescuer cannot very well make a wrap around the foot or tie an ankle hitch to prevent vertical movement in the litter. One way to avoid vertical downward shifting, which would put unwelcome weight on the injured leg, is to create a "sling harness" within the stretcher. Do this with an additional 10-foot piece of 1-inch tubular webbing to be tied onto the patient prior to applying the diamond lashing:

1. If the patient has not been "back-boarded" for spinal immobilization, slip the middle of the piece of webbing underneath the legs perpendicular to the basket in which the patient has been placed. Slide the webbing up to the patient's crotch.
2. Reach between the patient's legs to grab the webbing and pull up a small bend in the webbing.
3. Thread each end of the webbing through the bend coming up in the direction of foot-to-head.

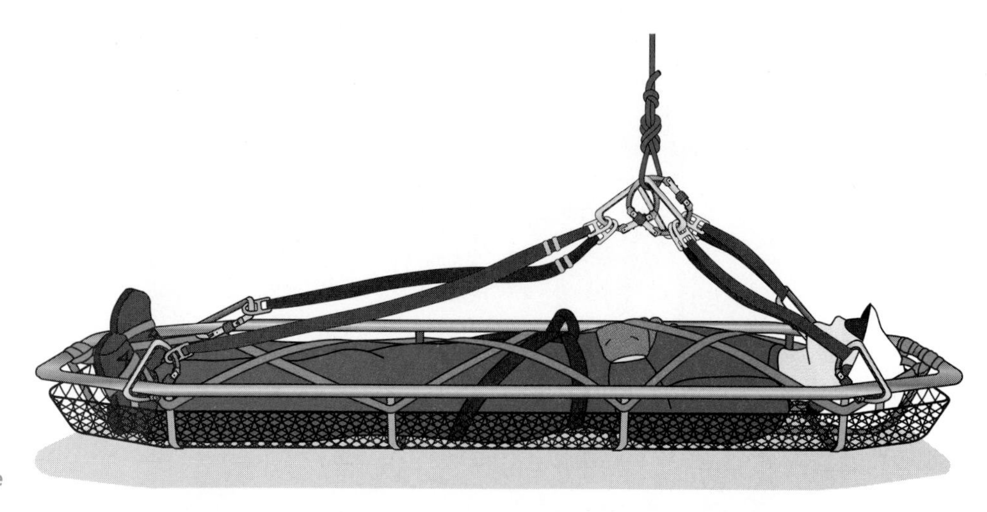

Figure 10.7 Single point litter bridle

4. After snugging the harness around the patient, bring both ends of the webbing straight up over the head of the prone patient. Secure the ends with two clove hitches to the support rail of the basket.

In case the basket is placed in a vertical position, the patient will now hang in the sling harness rather then shifting downward onto injured lower extremities. It is important to point out that the sling harness is not a lashing method in itself and must be used in conjunction with accepted lashing.

Bridles

There are probably ten or more types of bridles and configurations available for all types of uses. The choice of a specific bridle depends on the desired positioning of the litter (vertical or horizontal) and the environment in which it will be used. In the industrial setting, it is important to rig the bridle very close to the litter. Long litter bridles (such as those used in wilderness applications) make it more difficult to get the litter over an edge or to haul it up over an edge or from a passageway with low anchor points. Usually, every inch counts when making the attachment to the litter. Compact knots and a short bridle are important when rigging litters for industrial applications.

Other concerns with litters relate to streamlining the industrial rescue. Most industrial rescues do not require extremely versatile bridles. This is because most vertical rescues take place within 30 feet or closer (rescuer to patient).

In industrial rescue the priorities are to:

1. rig the litter quickly, and then
2. lower or haul quickly (but under control) to get the patient to more definitive care in a controlled environment.

Figure 10.8 Two-point litter bridle

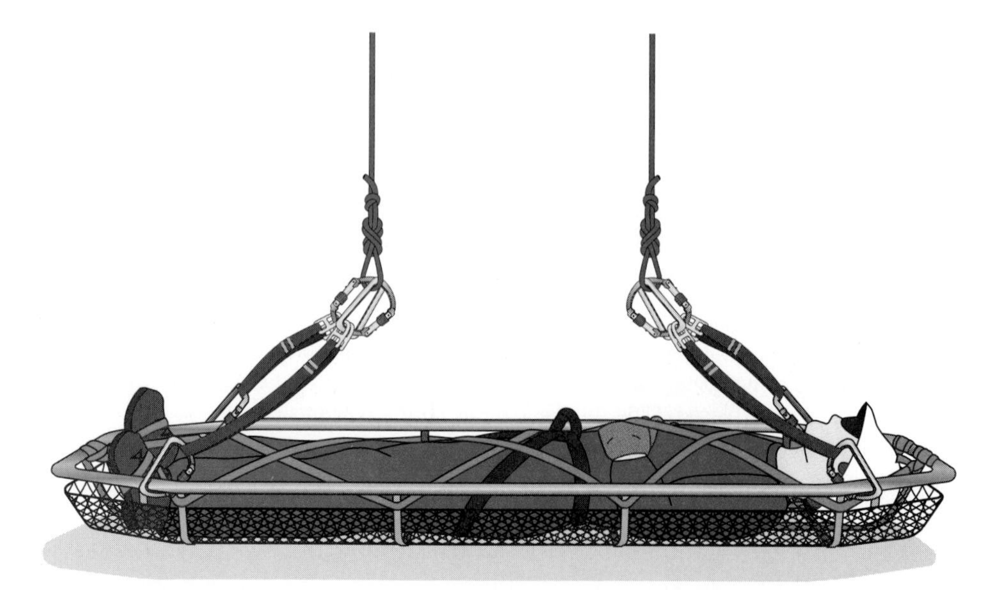

This section discusses methods of providing an adjustable litter bridle for both single-point and two-point applications.

- Single-point bridles bring all the connections to one point and are generally used for single-line lowers or hauls (see Figure 10.7). They use only one main load line.
- Two-point bridles separate the connections to the head and foot of the litter (see Figure 10.8). They usually work well for double-line litter lowers or hauls in industrial rescue.

This chapter describes both a webbing bridle using utility belts and a rope bridle using short sections of $\frac{1}{2}$-inch rope with Prusik loops for adjustment. Both designs can be used for single- and double-line horizontal litter operations. A simple-rope bridle for single-line vertical litter operations is presented.

There are a few prefabricated fully adjustable litter bridles on the market, though most are used in wilderness/mountain applications. The bridles presented here are constructed of materials that can be used for a variety of rope systems. They are both streamlined and appropriate for industrial and structural applications.

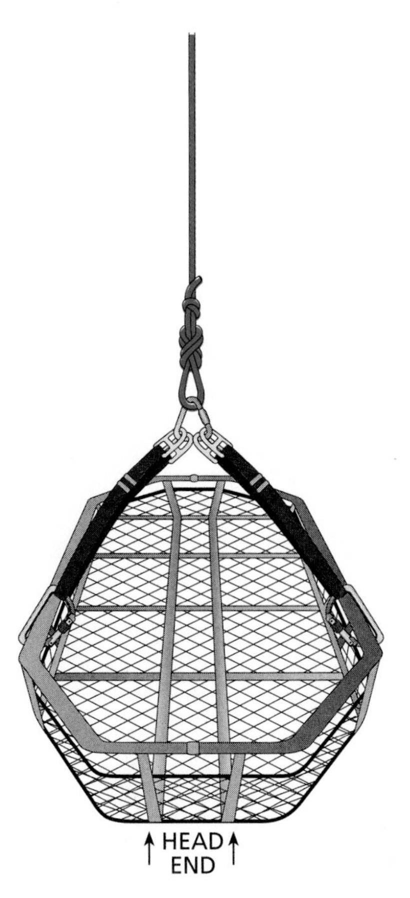

Figure 10.9 Using screw link to attach belts to knot

Figure 10.10 Using carabiners to attach belts to knot

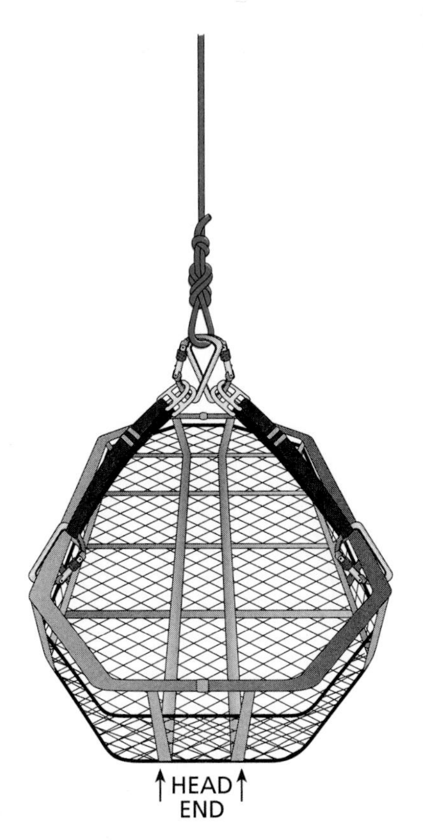

Horizontal Basket Litters

Horizontally configured litters are appropriate for packaging apprehensive patients or those with possible spinal injuries or lower-extremity injuries. In a horizontal basket, an apprehensive patient cannot see the ground below. What the patient does see is blue sky (or dirty ceiling) above that does not show the height of the litter. Patients in horizontally configured litters often feel very secure once they are being moved. For injured patients, the horizontal litter is usually more comfortable for patients complaining of pain in their lower extremities or back.

Utility Belt Single-Point Bridle

Using Utility Belts Rescuers can form a single-point bridle on a basket litter with four adjustable utility belts or anchor straps. They use two at the head and two at the foot (see Figure 10.7). They can form the same style of bridle with loops of tubular webbing, though it is not as easy to apply. Rescuers should fully shorten and double the utility belts used at the patient's head. It is preferable that the D-rings be placed toward the top rather than the bottom. This makes it easier to see what is happening when one knot attaches all utility belts. Things look much cleaner with D-rings than with a bunch of webbing. Rescuers should fully shorten and single the two utility belts (D-rings will be at either end) used at the patient's feet.

The "head" straps are short and the "foot" straps are long because most of a person's weight is in the upper body. If all of the bridle straps were the same length, the patient would hang head down. Most conscious patients are uncomfortable in this position. Unless they are suffering from hypovolemic shock, it is not a good idea. When the head straps are shorter, the patient assumes a slightly head-up attitude when the litter is loaded on the line. Of course, since the belts are all adjustable, a rescuer can position the litter just about any way based on the patient's condition and the physical surroundings.

To create a utility belt single-point bridle:

1. You need 4 utility belts and 8 locking carabiners.
2. You can use 2 carabiners with each of the 4 utility belts.
3. Use one to attach the bottom end of the belt to the top rail of the basket.
4. Use the other to attach the top end(s) of the belt(s) to the primary rope system.

Industrial litter bridles must be tight against the litter. Long bridles do not work well. Because the head portion of this bridle is so tight to the basket, using only one carabiner to attach the two belts to the main line knot may actually load the carabiner in three directions rather than along its long axis. A triangular screw link can connect the belts to the knot, but can be slow and difficult because of the size of the screw gate (see Figure 10.9). Or a separate carabiner can connect each belt to the knot (see Figure 10.10). Since the belts used to form the foot part of this bridle are much longer, a rescuer can probably use a single carabiner to attach both belts to the main line knot without creating a side load. The reason for the two carabiners is to allow a prerigged litter to be converted easily from a single-point to a two-point bridle.

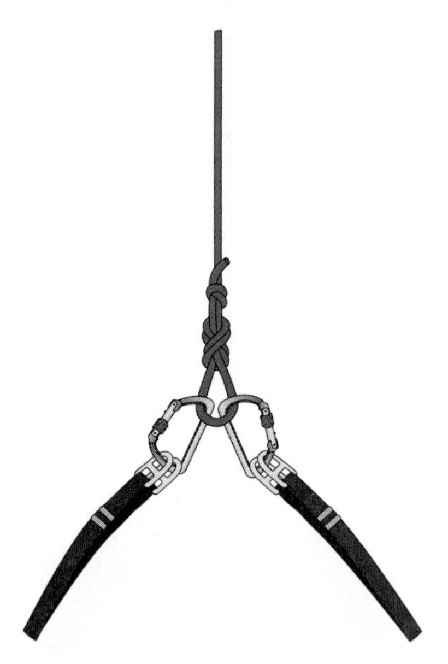

Figure 10.11 Reversed and opposed carabiners at top of litter bridle

Attaching Carabiners

There are at least two reasons for using carabiners to attach the belts to the top rail of a litter instead of just wrapping belts around the rail:

1. You can make the attachment faster with carabiners. You can fasten a prerigged utility belt in place in just seconds. Wrapping the belt around the railing requires more steps and more time.
2. Using carabiners helps prevent webbing abrasion. Abrasion might occur if the belts were simply doubled around the litter rail. They could be rubbed between a wall or other surface and the litter rail. This is a legitimate concern only on litter lowers or raises next to a wall or other structural surface that the litter might drag across. Even then, it only affects the side of the litter exposed to this surface. With this single-point bridle, the only real concern would be on the head end of the wall side of the litter, if the utility belt were wrapped around the top rail rather than being attached with a carabiner. The foot utility belts are not doubled and must be attached with carabiners anyway.

In short, to save carabiners with this bridle, rescuers simply use one carabiner to attach the two foot utility belts to the main line knot. They eliminate the carabiner used for the head utility belt/side rail connection on the outside (away from the wall) of the litter.

Rescuers make certain the gates of the carabiners attached to the top litter rail of the litter are facing inward. This helps prevent accidental unlocking should they contact a ledge or other type of projection. Some trainers also teach that at least two of the carabiner gates at the top of the litter bridle be reversed and opposed (see Figure 10.11). This is intended to prevent accidental opening of all the carabiners if their gates were to be pressed simultaneously against a ledge or projection. Although this is not a bad idea, it is based on an old practice involving nonlocking carabiners. Rescuers used nonlocking carabiners in pairs, with the gates reversed and opposed, to prevent accidental opening. They no longer use carabiners in pairs because they no longer use nonlocking carabiners for rescue. Locking gates are designed to protect accidental opening if the carabiners are bumped. Although it might be possible, it is improbable that more than one carabiner could become unlocked and accidentally opened simultaneously.

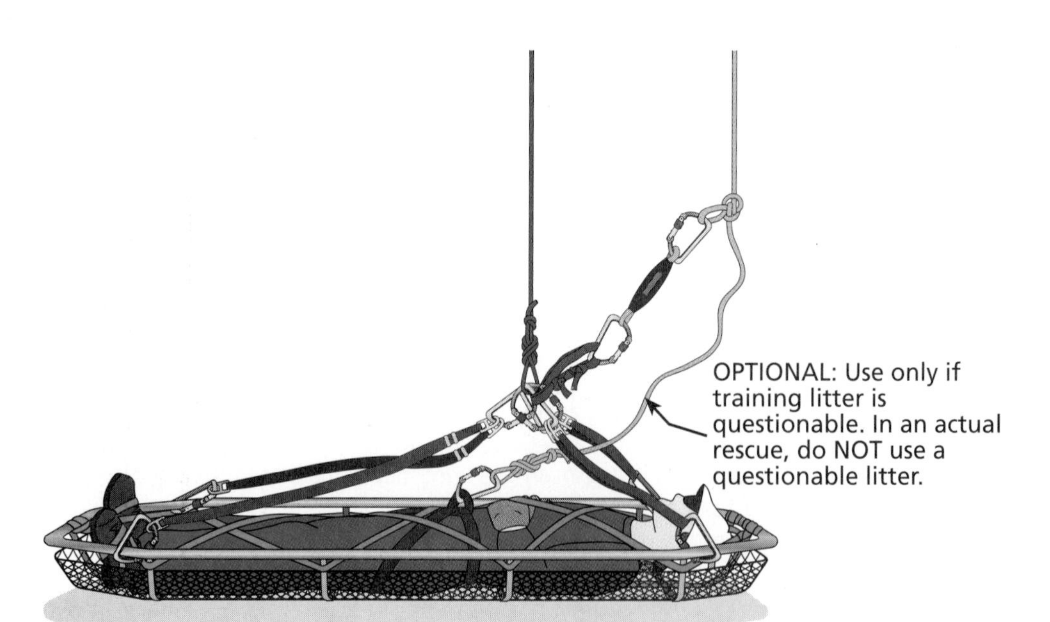

Figure 10.12 Safety line belay system attached to bridle

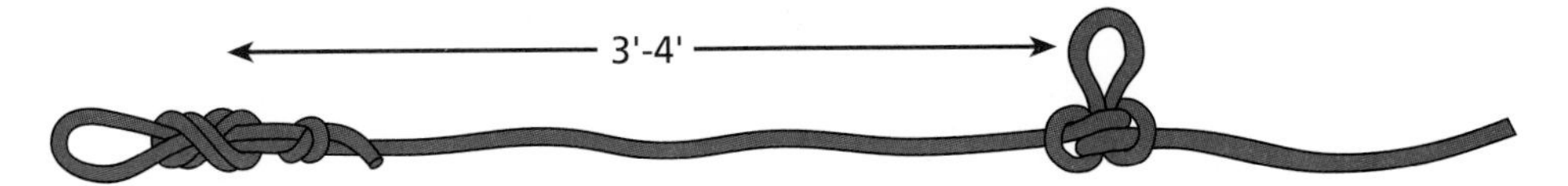

Figure 10.13 To training patient safety line To litter bridle via a shock absorber

Attaching the Safety Line Belay System

When using the litter in training with a single-point bridle, rescuers should attach an additional safety line belay system. Attach the safety line both to the bridle and to the student patient's harness (see Figure 10.12) if the litter is questionable in any way. This rigging is time consuming, and unnecessary for litters not in question.

Bear this in mind: The term "questionable" as used in this text does not imply that the litter is "bad." Litters known to be bad should be destroyed. Instead, it refers to common litters that, in extreme circumstances, might sustain damage or fail. It can also refer to the times when, for any reason, you lack confidence in the litter. Never use a litter you know to be damaged or bad. If not absolutely sure about the litter's integrity, even if there are no physical signs of damage, consider it questionable and back it up.

If the primary rope system fails, being attached to the complete litter bridle will probably provide the least catastrophic effect. If the litter falls apart, the patient is attached to the same rope by his or her harness. You can quickly make these two connections by tying a midline knot, like the butterfly knot. Tie it 3 to 4 feet from the knot in the end of the safety belay line (see Figure 10.13). The distance placed between these two knots is to compensate for the extra length needed to place a shock absorber in-line between the midline knot and the bridle attachment. If the shock absorber activates, it will extend lengthwise. The spacing between these two safety line knots will also help compensate for this extension. Ultimately, there should be no more than 18 inches of slack in the safety line between the bridle attachment and the patient. Attach the midline knot to all three or four carabiners connecting the utility belts to the main line. You can do this by wrapping a short loop of tubular webbing through the bridle carabiners and making the attachment with an additional carabiner (see Figure 10.14). Another method involves attaching the safety line directly to the lowering line knot (see Figure 10.17). Attach the knot at the end of the safety line to the patient's harness.

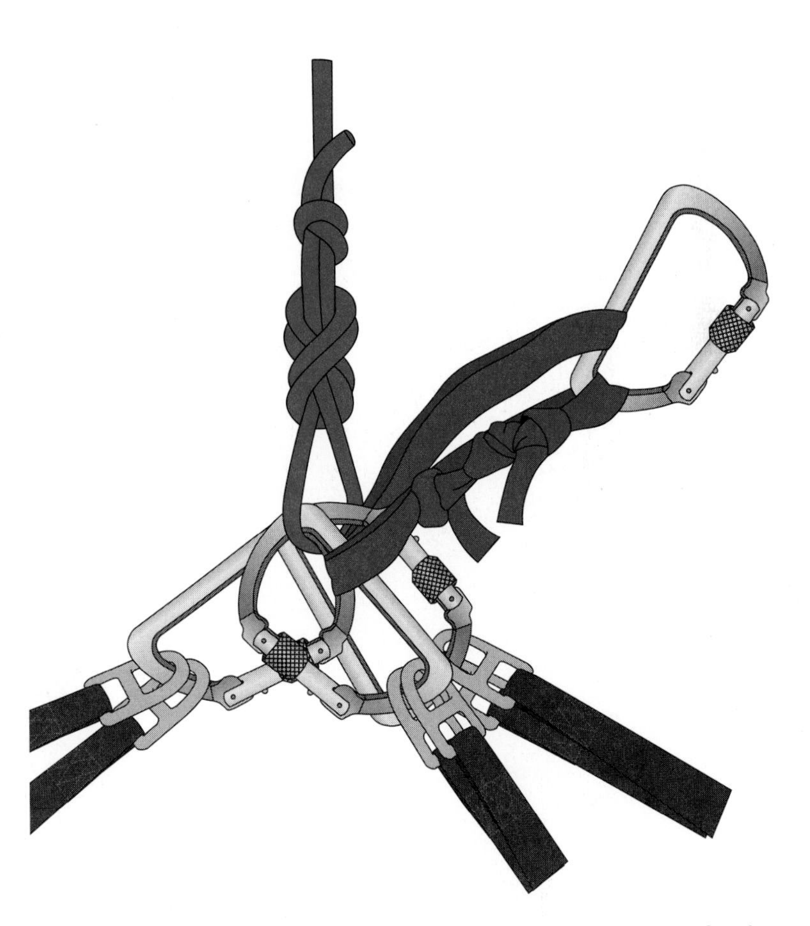

Figure 10.14 Optional Loop of webbing used to attach midline knot to litter bridle (may attach directly to knot loop; see Figure 10.17)

Placing Shock Absorbers

The placement of the shock absorber in this system provides some relief from the impact load that might be created by any drop. The device is placed in-line between the litter bridle and the rope system because this will be the first place to see the impact load (see Figure 10.12). Because there is no shock absorber attached to the patient's harness, if the litter falls apart the patient will receive quite a shock. That is why it is very important to limit slack in the rope between the bridle and the patient to a maximum of 18 inches. This attachment is a last-ditch effort in case of nearly impossible failure. You should only worry about this in training or if using a questionable litter. If you have a second shock absorber you should certainly place it in-line between

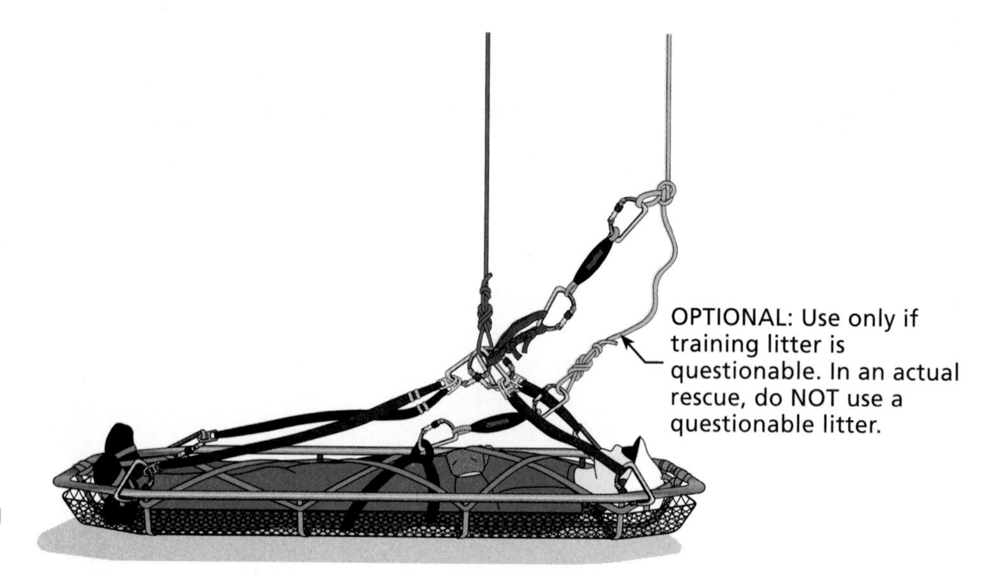

Figure 10.15 Using a second shock absorber in-line between patient and safety line

Figure 10.16 Single-point bridle using two 18 ft. sections of rope

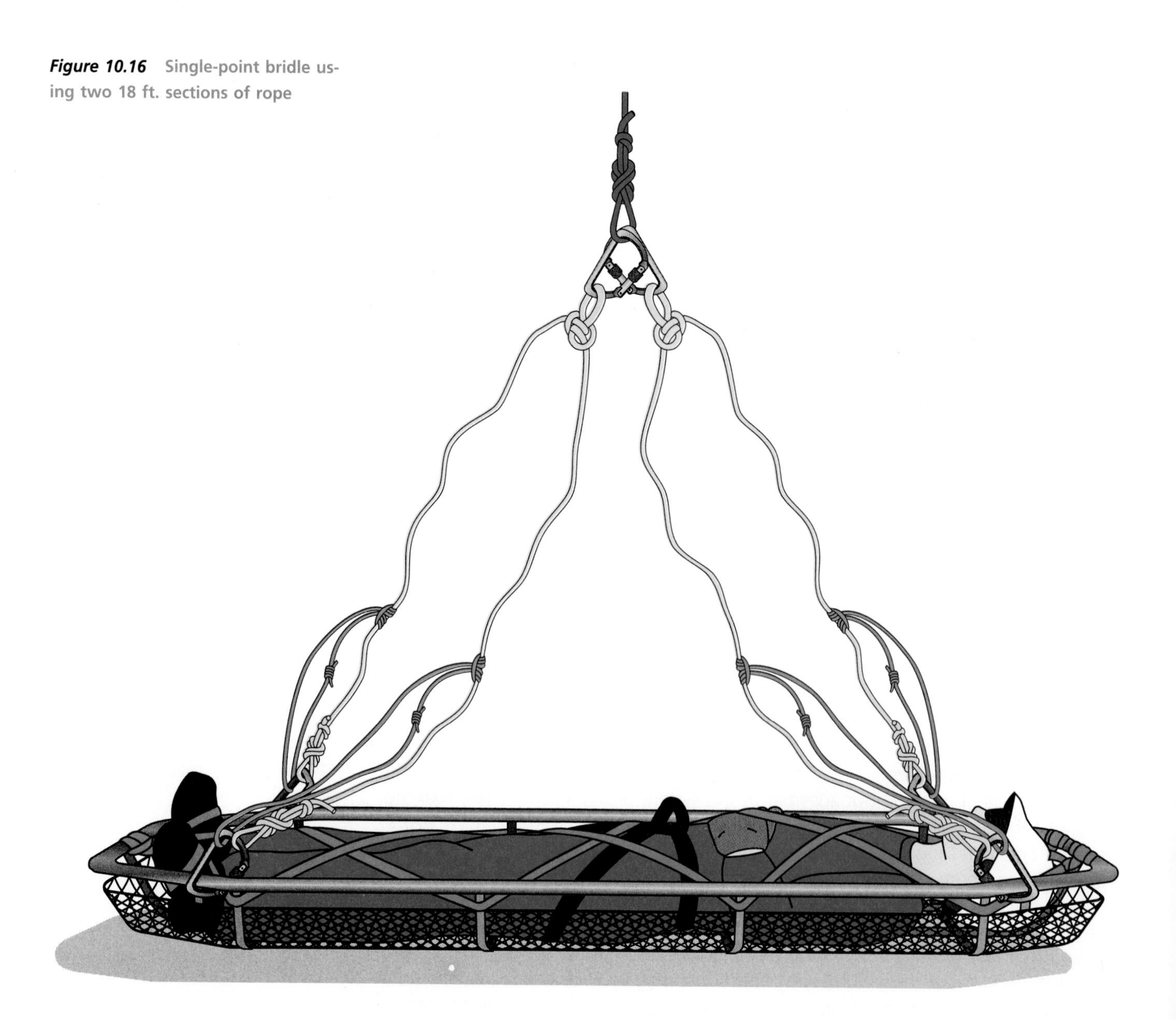

the patient and the safety belay line (see Figure 10.15). If you do not, you should place it at the attachment to the litter. The most likely failure will be of the primary rope system due to adverse conditions and the shock hits there first.

Rope Single-Point Bridles

The use of a couple of short ½-inch rescue ropes (each about 18 feet long) works well with four 8-millimeter accessory cords (about 6½ feet long) (see Figure 10.16). This will form a two-piece bridle with adjustable legs from 1 to 5 feet long.

Tying the rope

1. Tie a compact anchor knot in both ends of each rope. A figure-8 on a bight works well for this application.
2. When the end knots are tied, find the exact middle of each rope and tie a butterfly knot. The butterfly knot is used in case of a tight angle in the bridle, creating a three-directional pull. This completes the main part of the bridle, one rope for each end of the basket litter.
3. Using carabiners, attach the end knots of each rope to lateral points on the side rails of the litter. Attach one near the head and the other near the foot.
4. Now bring the two butterfly knots together. Attach them with one or two carabiners to the primary rope system, depending on whether the two knots will load properly (on the long axis) with just one carabiner. A triangular screw link can be used instead of carabiners at the butterflies, if needed to eliminate problems with multidirectional loading. This makes a single-point bridle with two legs at the foot and two at the head.

Adjusting the Legs

Unfortunately, these legs are much too long for most industrial applications. You can easily make them adjustable by using four nylon kernmantle accessory cords 8-millimeter in diameter and approximately 6½ feet long. The 8-millimeter cord is recommended for ½-inch rescue rope to provide maximum strength and durability while still being small enough to cinch up and grip the rope when loaded. The bigger the diameter cord in relationship to the rescue rope, the easier it will slip.

1. Tie each of these cords into a Prusik loop using a double fisherman's knot.
2. Now tie a double- or triple-wrap Prusik knot to each leg of the bridle with the Prusik loops.
3. Attach the loops issuing from the Prusik knots at each bridle leg to the corresponding carabiners used to connect the bridle legs to the top rail of the litter.
4. Lock all the carabiners.

This assembly allows you to move the Prusik knots up or down the bridle legs independently, providing length adjustment from approximately 1 to 5 feet. Since the ½-inch rescue rope is also attached to the top rail of the litter, the connection of the bridle will not be compromised if a Prusik loop fails for some reason. Normally, you should adjust the head bridle legs so they are shorter than the ones at the foot, although you can adjust them as required based on the situation.

Adding the Safety Line Belay System

Attach this rope bridle to the primary and safety belay systems in the same way as the utility belt bridle (see Figure 10.17). You can pretie this bridle (leave the knots unloaded when in storage for long periods of time) and deploy them quickly in case of a rescue. It requires only five or six carabiners and is inexpensive compared with the utility belt bridle. However, it is not as durable as the utility belt bridle and may require frequent replacement. Inspect both the ½-inch rope and accessory cord carefully after each use.

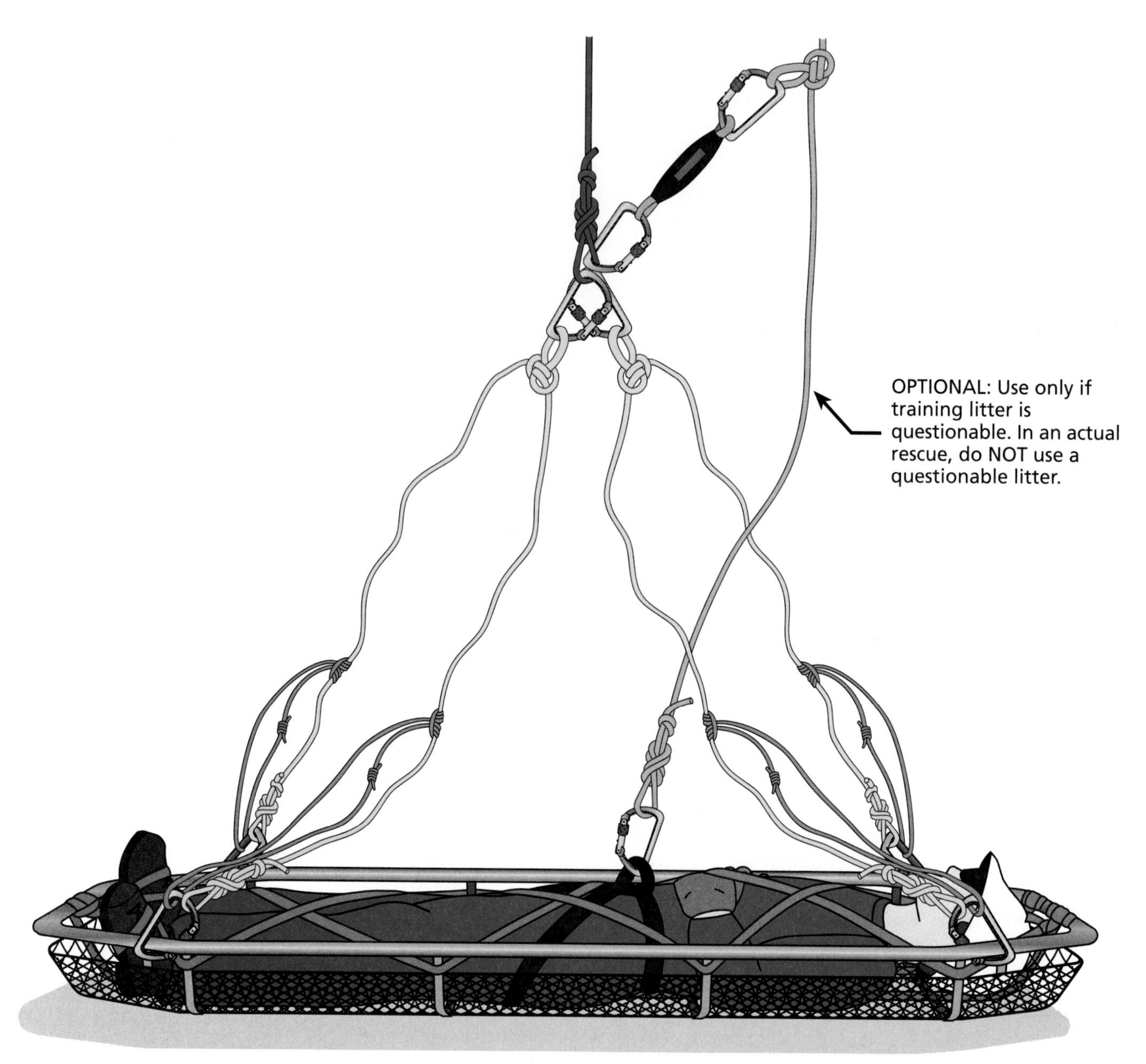

Figure 10.17 **Attachment of rope litter bridle to main line**

Two-Point Bridles

Rope Two-Point Bridle

Both two-point litter bridles presented here are similar to the single-point systems previously covered. The rope bridle is basically the same whether used with a one- or two-rope system.

For two points of attachment, simply split the two butterfly knots, one at the head and one at the foot of the litter (see Figure 10.18). Fully shorten each of the bridle legs. This is because a double-line rope system can adjust the position of the litter without the aid of adjustable bridle legs.

Utility Belt Two-Point Bridle

To adapt the bridle from a single-line to a double-line system (see Figure 10.19):

1. Double the utility belts at the foot end. Keep them fully shortened with the D-rings up.
2. Attach the two head utility belts directly to the head lowering line.

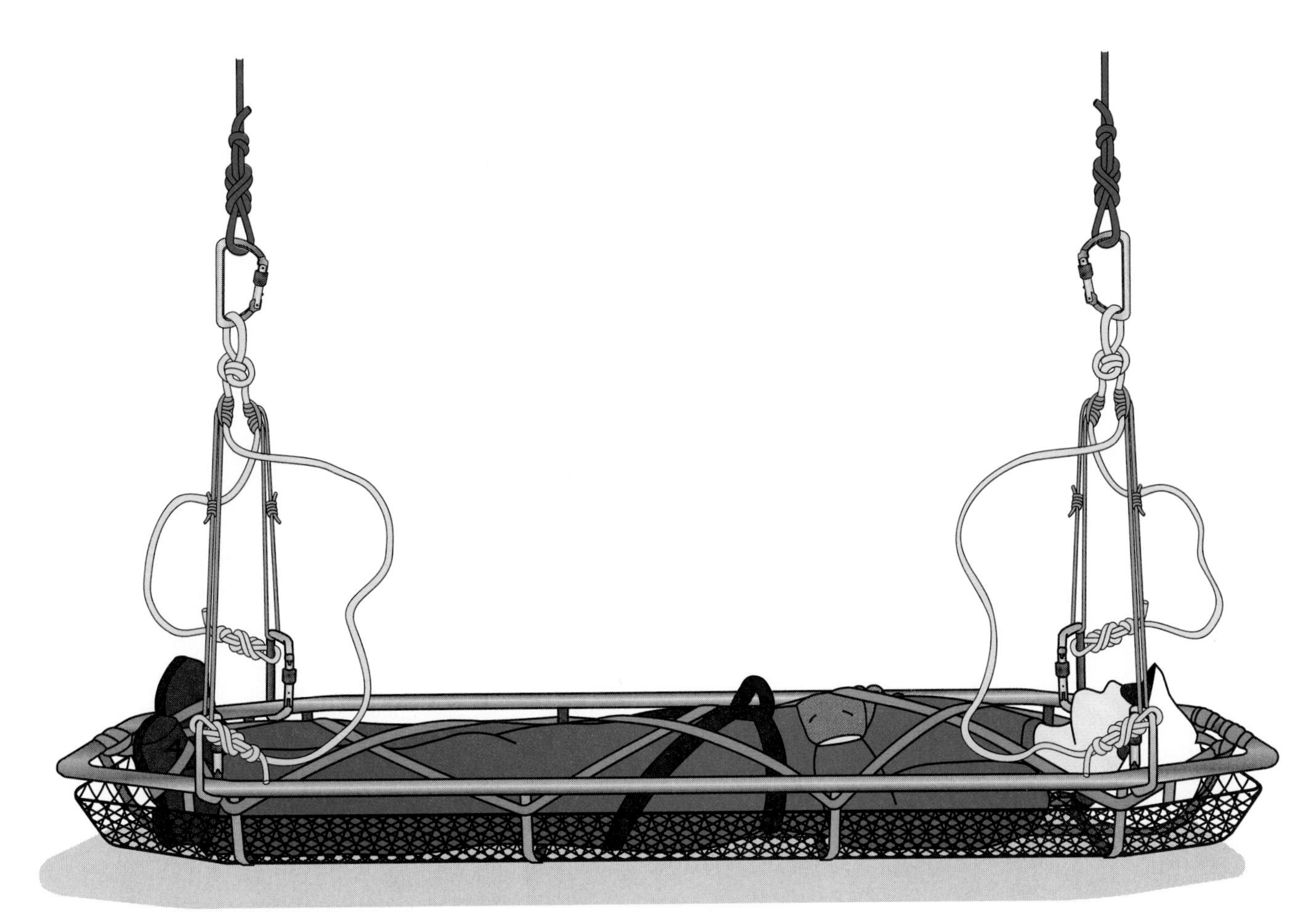

Figure 10.18 **Splitting butterfly knots for two attachment points**

3. Attach the two foot utility belts to the foot lowering line.
4. The angles of both the head and foot portion of the bridle are tight in relation to the litter. To avoid improper loading, use a separate carabiner (four together) to attach each utility belt to the head and foot knots of the rope system. You can also use a triangular screw link instead of carabiners at these attachment points to adapt to the multidirectional pull.

If needed, you can eliminate two of the carabiners required to make this bridle. Just wrap both outside utility belts (those away from the wall) around the top rail of the litter rather than attaching them to the top rail with carabiners (see Figure 10.19). This side of the litter is usually not affected by abrasion from the wall or other structural surface, so carabiners are not required.

Safety Line Belay with Two-Point Bridles

Most double-line rope systems do not use an additional safety line belay. This is because each rope is supposed to back up the other. If you need an additional safety belay line, attach it to both bridle attachment points for best results in case of primary system failure. This can be done in several ways. One quick method uses a double-loop figure-8 knot (see Figure 10.20). Tie it large enough for the loops to be split and attached to each point of the bridle. The loops should be large enough that they are not pulled between the two bridle attachment points during normal operations.

Any other safe anchor rigging is acceptable for making this connection. Most double-line rope systems do not incorporate shock absorbers. Because both lines are constantly under tension, the potential for impact loading is not quite as great.

Safety with Two-Point Bridles

As with single-point bridles, rescuers must secure the patient to the rope system when using questionable litters and in training. This provides a backup in case of litter failure, but not a rope system failure. Rescuers can use any safe rigging capable of sup-

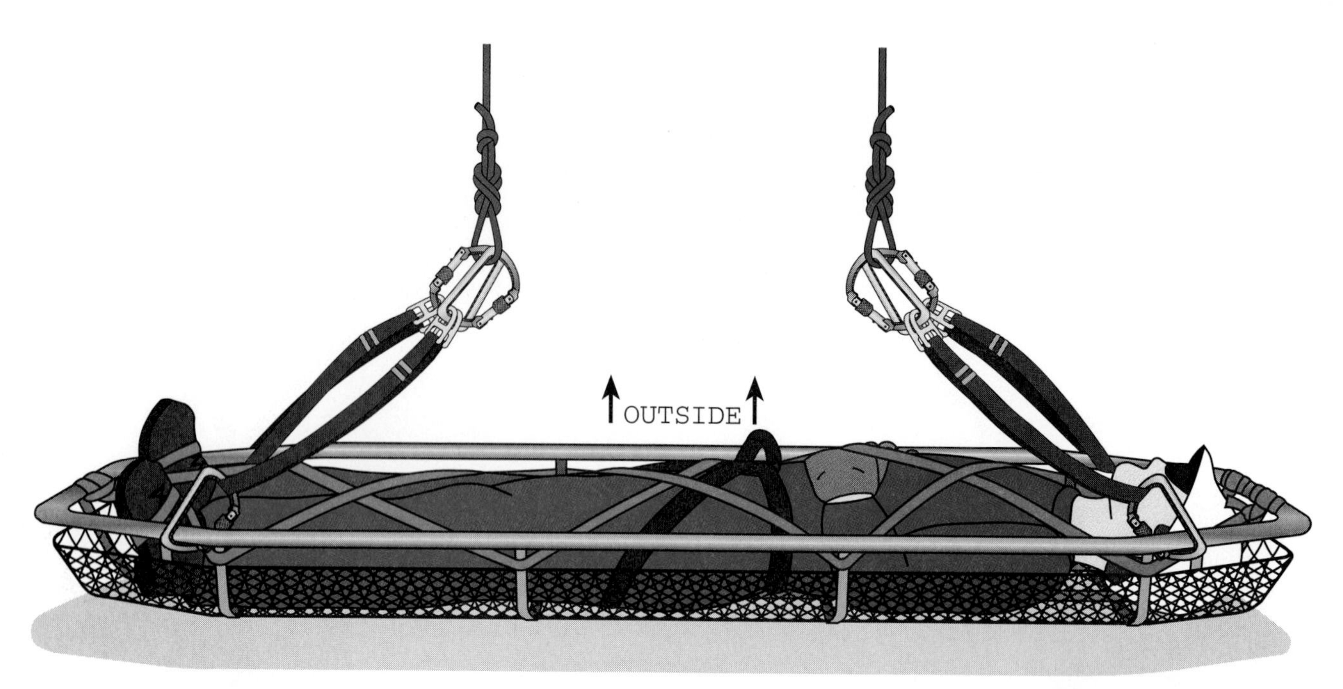

Figure 10.19 **Eliminating two carabiners from litter bridle**

porting a one-person load to attach the patient's harness to one of the two ropes in the rescue system. Some rescue trainers recommend the foot line to attach a patient. This advice is the result of a nonscientific test that suggested that a patient might be more susceptible to traumatic injury with a head-end rope attachment. This "backyard" test involved the use of a tight bridle such as the ones presented here with a double-line litter lower system. An articulated dummy played the role of the patient and actually lost its head when the basket was dropped, causing the dummy to swing forward into the remaining head end bridle assembly. A foot end attachment did not yield the same results. Although these tests were nonscientific and the results not consistently repeatable, it was impressive enough for those at the scene of the test. In any case, there should be some attachment. Rescuers make their own choices about which line will work best.

Figure 10.20 **Safety line belay using double-loop figure-8 knot**

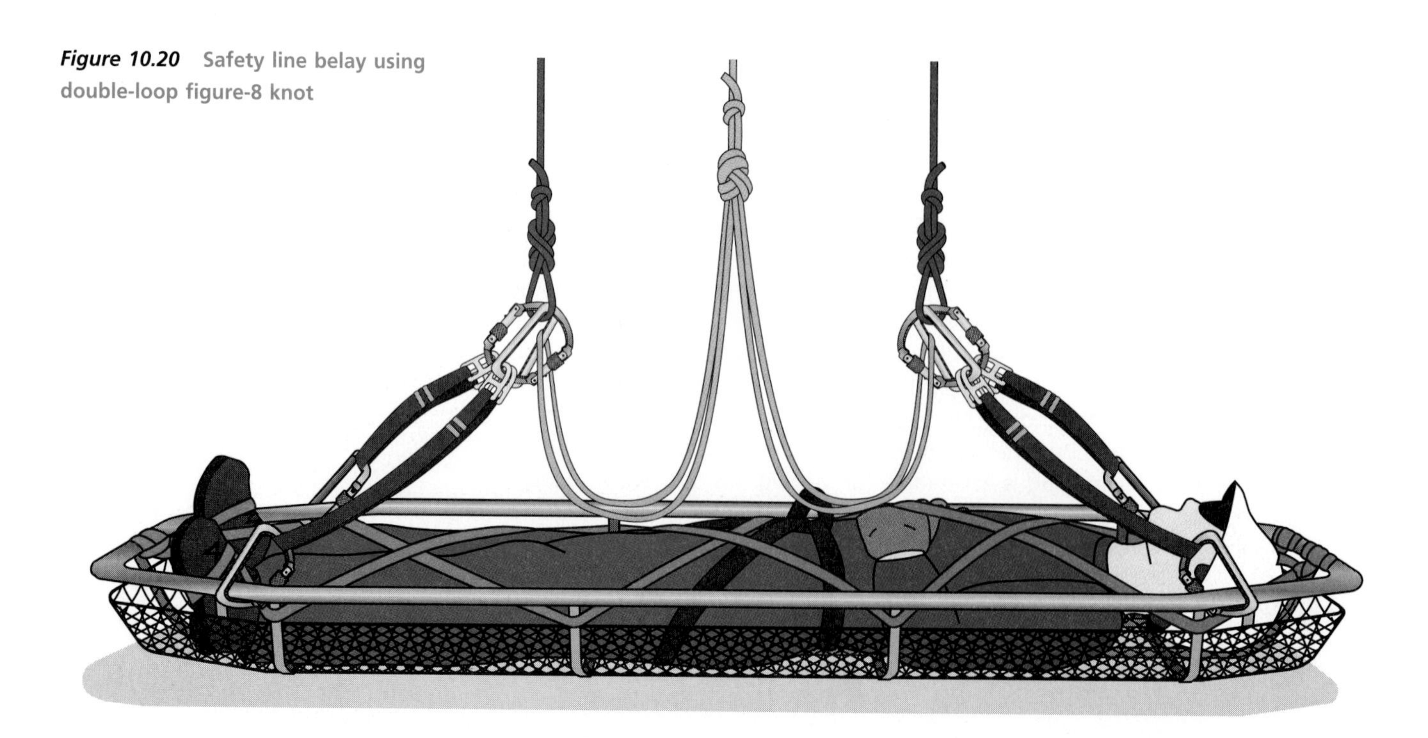

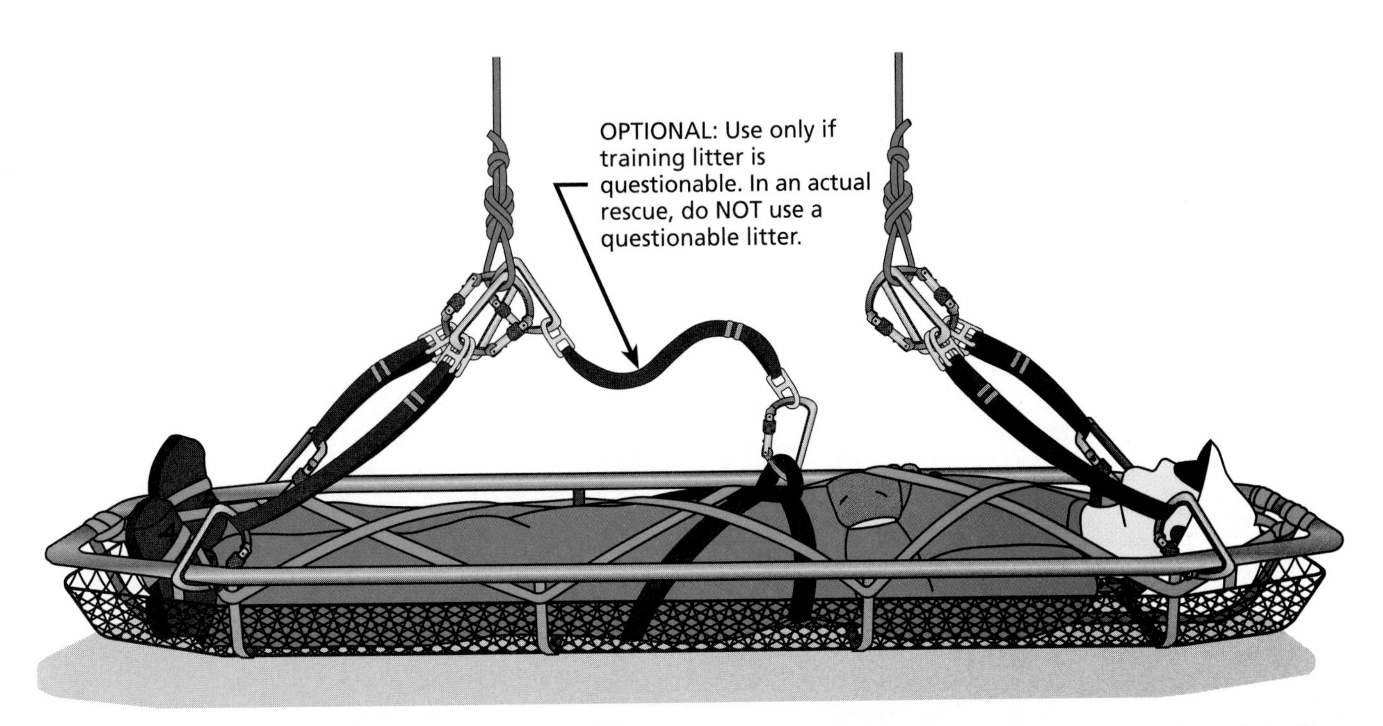

One method uses a fully extended and singled utility belt with a carabiner at each end to make the connection from patient's harness to the FOOT of the rope system (see Figure 10.21).

Figure 10.21 Fully extended utility belt connects patient to main line

Patient Safety

Another method simply leaves a long tail on one of the rescue system ropes for attachment to the patient's harness with a knot (see Figure 10.22). This is similar to the attachment of a safety belay line to the litter bridle and patient in a single-rope system. This rigging should be long enough to prevent tightening at the patient's harness should the other rope fail.

Figure 10.22 Long tail on foot end attaches to patient's harness

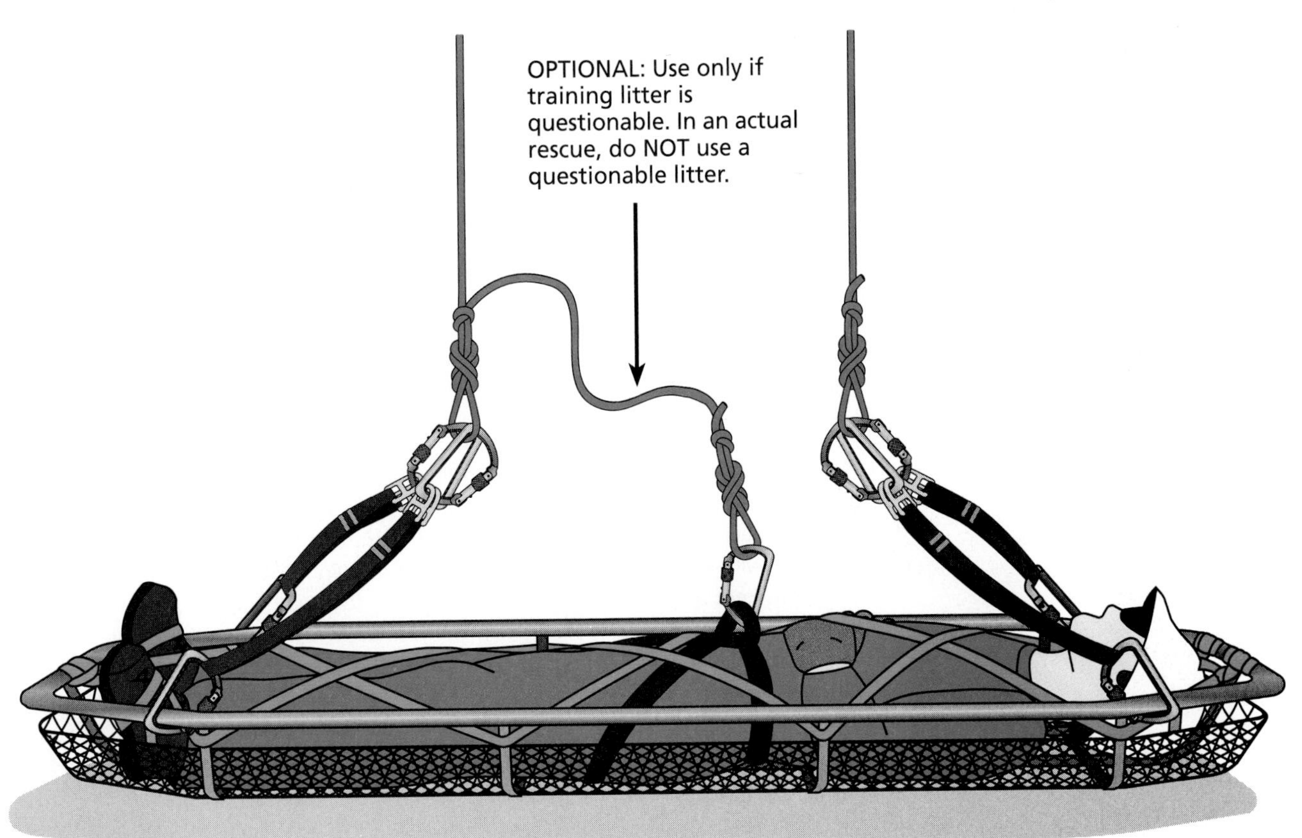

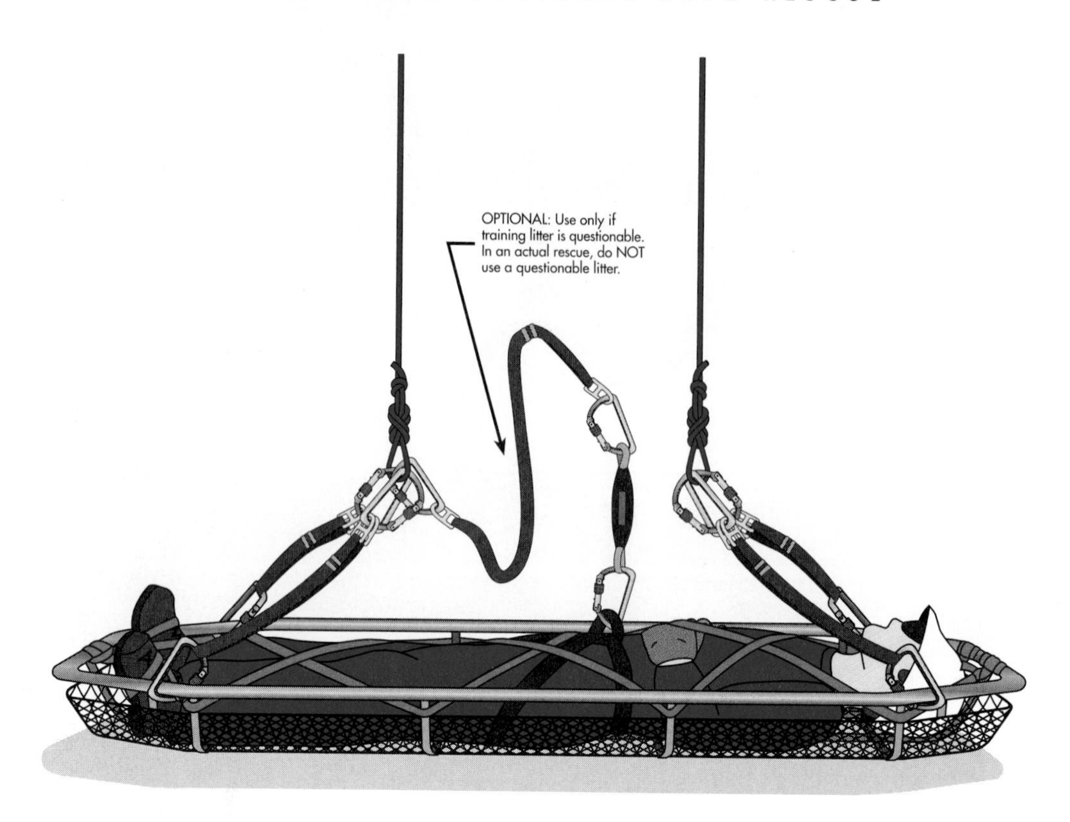

Figure 10.23 **Shock absorber between patient and tail of rope on main safety line**

Shock absorbers are not usually incorporated into double-line rope systems. If the integrity of the litter is in question, however, a rescuer may wish to use a shock absorber in-line between the patient and the safety rigging (see Figure 10.23). This will alleviate some impact load otherwise felt by the patient in case of litter failure.

Vertical Basket Litter

To lower or raise a litter through a narrow opening, rescuers configure it vertically. Vertical bridles use only a single point of attachment to the rope rescue system. Only one method of building a vertical bridle is covered here because it is extremely quick and efficient. The goal with a vertical bridle is to grab as much load-bearing litter surface as is possible. The more contact the bridle has with the structural members of the litter, the stronger the system.

Avoid attaching a rope or webbing bridle to one spot at the ends of the litter rail. Some litters have a butt weld in the rail at each end. This is a structural weak point and could fail under the weight of the load. Whatever type of basket litter you use, always have the bridle make a great deal of contact with the structural members.

1. Take a 25- to 30-foot piece of static kernmantle life safety rope that is suitable for one-person loads ($\frac{3}{8}$-inch or greater) (see figure 10.24).
2. Tie a compact anchor knot (such as a double-loop figure-8) in the middle of this rope. This knot will serve as the attachment point to the primary rope system.
3. Wrap this knot around the top rail of the litter at the head end. Wrap it once or twice to start. If the knot will not pass under the top rail, wrap each of the two legs of rope extending from the knot around the top rail of the litter at the head end several times. Keep the knot as tight as possible against the top rail. This may cause the bridle legs to exceed the maximum 120 degree angle initially. However, it will stretch under load, bringing it to an acceptable position. Remember, every inch can count in industrial applications.

4. Continue to wrap the ropes around the railing in the same direction, moving downward toward the feet. On a wire basket litter, pass the rope ends through the slots created between the vertical structural members and the stop bars, as you wrap the top rail. Pass through the handholds, which are on most plastic basket litters.
5. Stop wrapping the top rail somewhere just above the level of the patient's knees. At this point, there should be one rope wrapped down and around the railing on each side of the litter.
6. Finish the bridle by making several full wraps (at least three) with the loose ends of the rope around the top railing at lateral points just above the patient's knees.
7. Tie the loose ends with a square knot to easily remove all slack.
8. Tie off both loose ends issuing from the square knot with safety knots. As noted before, do not use square knots to tie two ropes together for direct life loads. However, in this application, the square knot does not directly take the weight of the load. Wrapping the rope around the railing several times creates somewhat of a tensionless hitch and keeps most of the weight of the load on the litter railing and off the finish knot. As an additional precaution, tie off the loose ends from the square knot with safety knots. Instead of the square knot, you could try to tie the two rope ends with a figure-8 bend or a double fisherman's knot. If you do try this, it will be very difficult to remove all the slack. Once the bridle is loaded, this slack will probably work its way up, creating an attachment point 2 or 3 feet above the top of the litter. Many rescuers agree that the square knot is safe when used in this application.

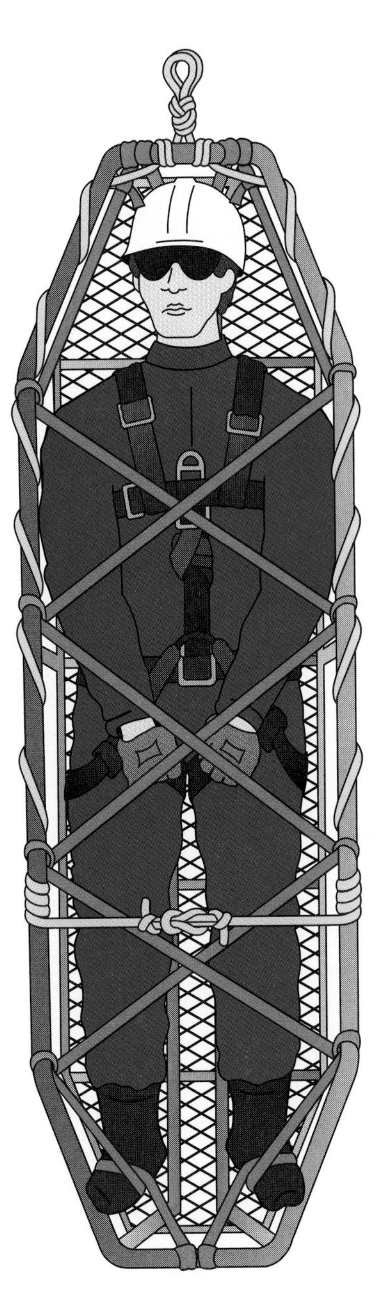

Figure 10.24 **Vertical Bridle**

The Sked Litter

The Sked litter, a type of flexible litter, is ideal for many structural and industrial rescue applications (see Figure 10.1). It is made of a high-tech plastic that is very resistant to chemical exposure and extreme temperature. Stored in its bag, it is very compact. It is lightweight and easy to maneuver through small openings. When properly applied, the flexible litter conforms to the patient's body, reducing its size and making it easier to pass through a narrow opening. Just as with the basket litter, rescuers can use the flexible litter in vertical or horizontal configurations.

Rescuers should use a full spine immobilizer, usually a long spine board, with the Sked to provide rigid support for the unit (see Figure 10.25). However, situations arise where the Sked must pass through a way too narrow to allow passage with a long spine board. In these cases, rescuers can modify the configuration by substituting a short spine immobilizer in place of the full spine board (see Figure 10.26). This type of immobilizer provides rigid support while conforming to the patient's body.

Other minor adaptations of standard methods are necessary if the patient will not fit through a narrow passage. For instance, with extremely narrow openings, the patient's arms should be secured over head when being packaged in the Sked (see Figure 10.27). This reduces the patient's circumference and makes it easier to get him or her through the tight opening. Do this only in extreme circumstances.

The following instructions for the various applications of the Sked have been approved by the manufacturer. Some of these methods are modifications of the original manufacturer's instructions made by the authors and based on industrial/structural considerations. Rescuers should never use the Sked or any commercial rescue equipment in a way that is not recommended by the manufacturer.

Unpacking the Sked

Keep the Sked rolled and stored in its nylon bag. When removed from the bag, the plastic has a memory and retains the rolled shape until straightened. To straighten the Sked:

1. Remove the Sked from its bag and place it on the ground.
2. Unfasten the retaining straps and step on the foot end of the Sked. The foot is the end with two black 1-inch straps attached to two grommets. The head end has a yellow (or green) ½-inch webbing pull handle attached to it.

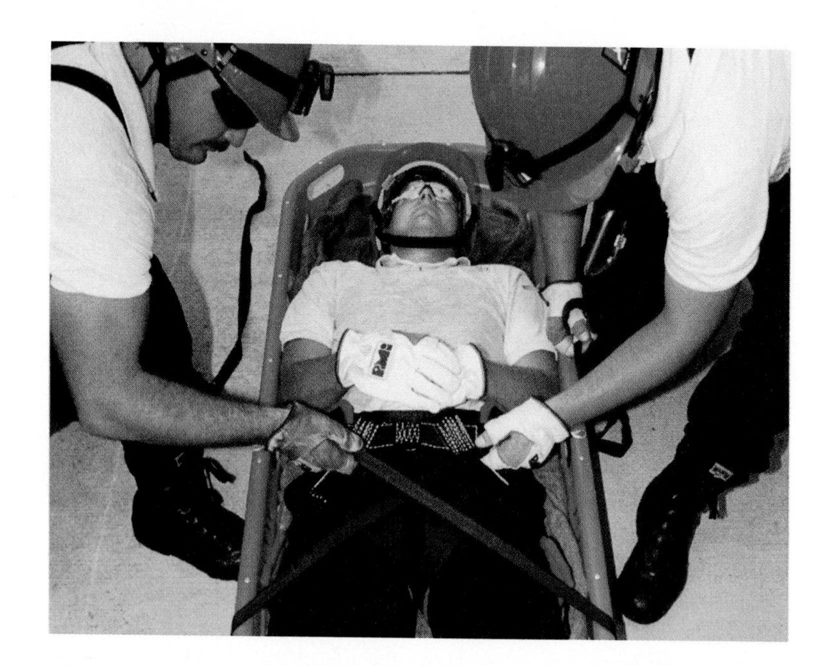

Figure 10.25 Long spineboard in Sked

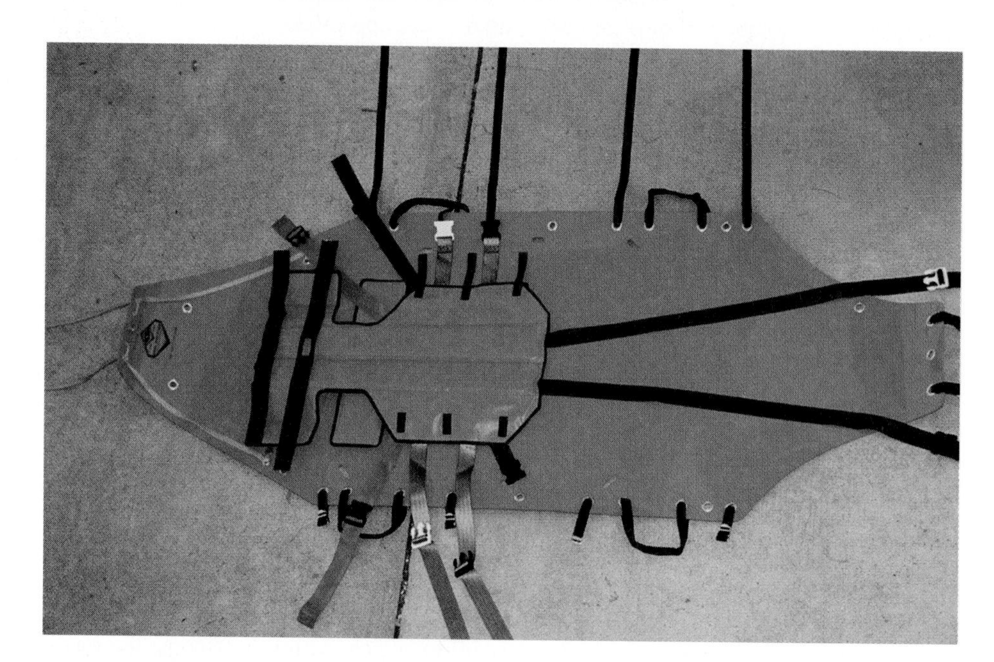

Figure 10.26 OSS II in Sked

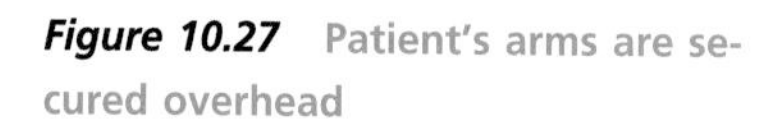

Figure 10.27 Patient's arms are secured overhead

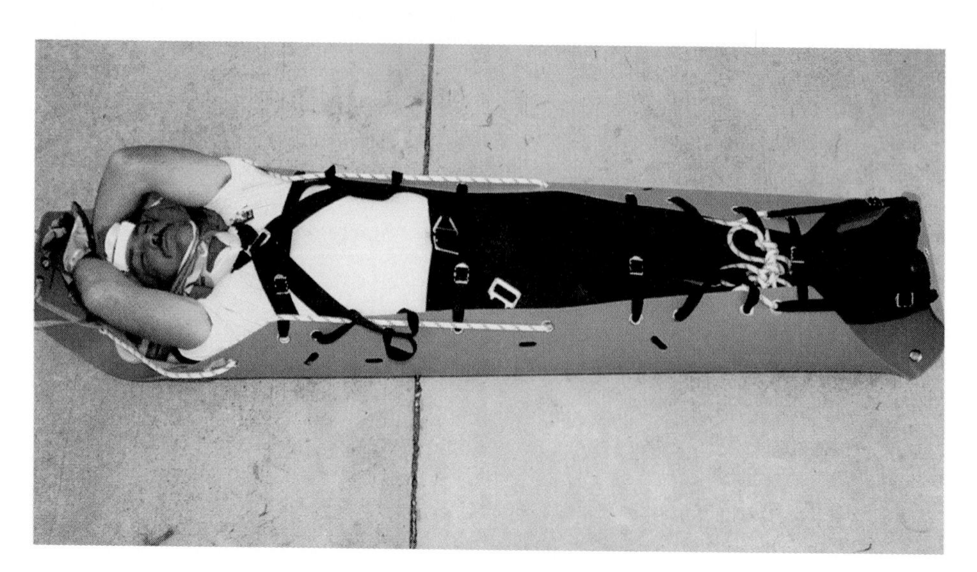

3. Unroll the Sked completely to the opposite end.
4. Bend one half of the Sked over backwards and back roll it.
5. Repeat this procedure with the opposite end of the litter. The Sked should now lie flat.

Lashing Patients to a Sked Litter

The Sked has built-in lashing straps (see Figure 10.28). These straps are designed to hold the patient securely. There are four black straps crossing the patient's body at approximately the chest, waist, thighs, and lower legs. There are two black straps located at the bottom of the litter. These are designed to roll up the foot end of the device to make it more streamlined and protect the patient's feet. Secure all straps by weaving them through the metal buckles that are also attached to the Sked.

If spinal injury is suspected, a rescuer should properly immobilize the patient (see Chapter 9, Patient Packaging) with immobilization technique that allows repositioning the patient without manipulating the spine. Even if there is no suspected spinal problem, the patient should still be placed on a full spine (or short spine in some cases) immobilizer. These devices provide rigidity and support the litter whatever the patient's condition.

To lash the patient in the Sked litter:

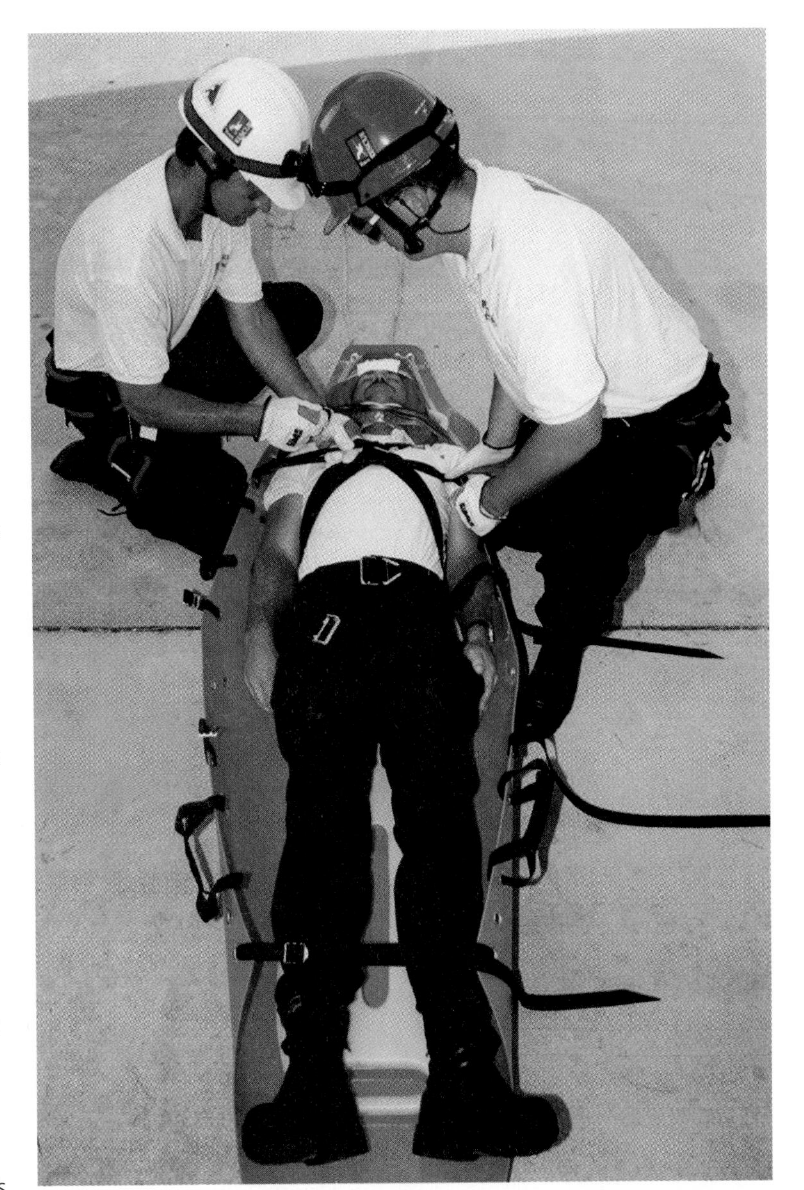

Figure 10.28 Sked being lashed

1. Unroll the Sked using the described "reverse roll" technique and lay it flat.
2. Position the immobilized patient on the Sked.
3. When fastened, the upper cross strap should fall at a point on the patient's chest just below the shoulders. **Never allow this strap to cross near the patient's neck.**
4. Center the patient horizontally.
5. Position the patient's arms at his or her side. This will keep the hands and arms secured inside the litter once the lashing is completed.

   NOTE: *For training exercises, you may wish to allow the mock patient's hands to cross in the front at waist level. This will allow the patient to use his or her hands to help in case of a problem. For comfort, pad the forearms where they contact the edge of the plastic.*
6. Bring the four black straps from the side of the Sked across the patient's body.
7. Fasten each strap to the buckles on the opposite side.
8. Feed the foot straps through the unused grommets at the foot end of the Sked (from the bottom upward).
9. Bring the loose ends back to the buckles for securement.
10. For most applications, position the patient's feet between these two foot straps (together with toes pointing forward [anterior]).

Horizontal Sked Bridles

The Sked is often seen in a single-line vertical rescue system. This is because it is well suited to narrow openings often associated with industrial vessel extraction. However, rescuers can easily rig the Sked horizontally in either a single- or double-line rescue system. The following section presents methods for both the single-point and two-point horizontal litter bridle. Both methods are approved by the manufacturer of the Sked. All of the patient packaging considerations previously mentioned for the hori-

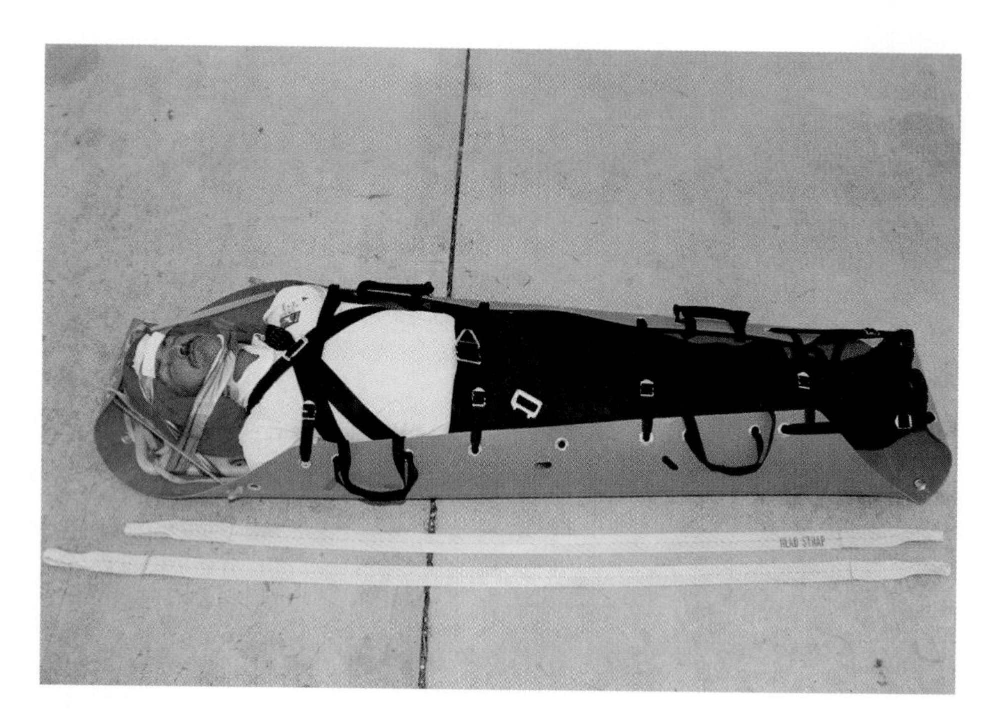

Figure 10.29 Two yellow Sked straps used for horizontal rigging

Figure 10.30 Positioning head strap under slot

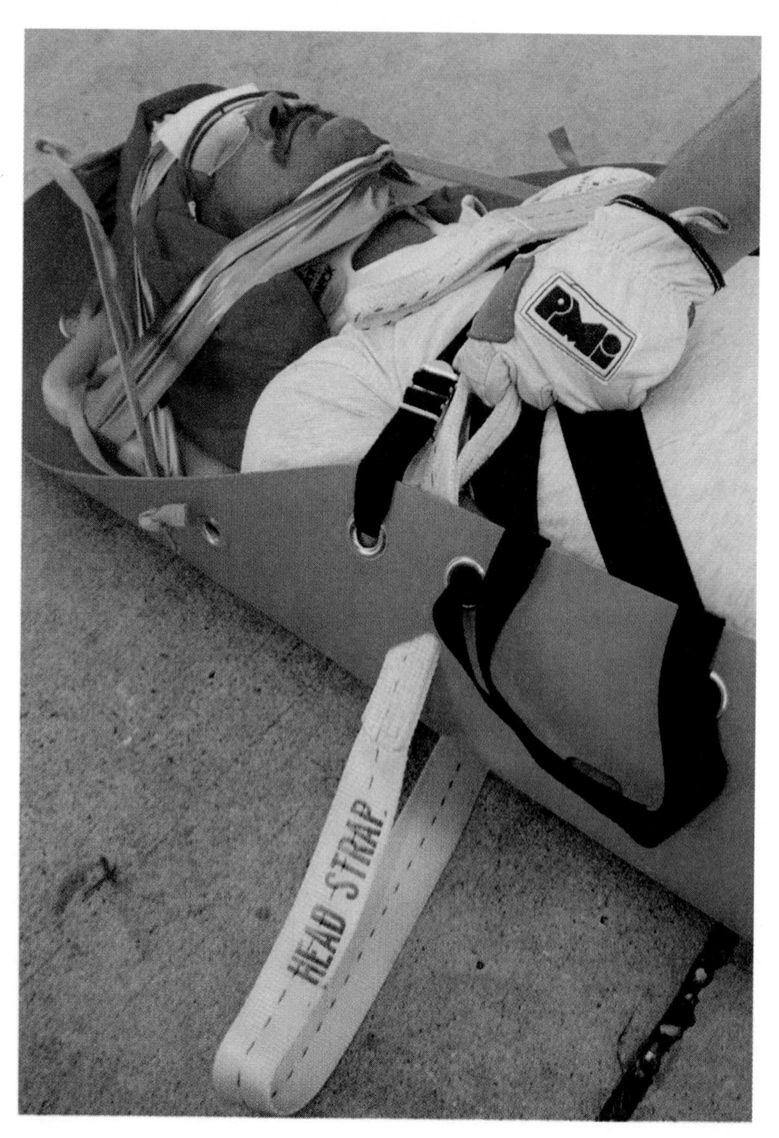

zontal basket litter also apply to the horizontal Sked.

Horizontal Single-Point Bridle

Two yellow nylon webbing straps rated at 3,800 pounds each (end to end) are used for horizontal lifting or lowering of the Sked (see Figure 10.29). One strap is 6 inches shorter than the other and is designed for use at the head end of the litter. This is an important factor when using a single-point bridle because most of the patient's weight is in the torso. The shorter strap at the head will help maintain the litter in a level or slightly head-up position. This head strap can be shortened even more to provide a more significant litter angle (discussed later in this section). With double-line systems, the strap length does not affect the positioning of the litter. The head and foot bridle attachments are controlled independently of one another.

1. Start by laying the head strap under the Sked. This strap should be perpendicular to the litter and in line with the diagonal openings near the head. These diagonal openings are the lift slots.
2. Insert the loose ends (loops) of the head strap through the lift slots on each side from the outside inward (see Figure 10.30).
3. Equalize the straps and bring the presewn loops together above the Sked.
4. Attach both of these loops to the rope system with a single carabiner. Normally, the angle created by the legs of the bridle strap is not very wide. Since side loading is not a factor, you only need one carabiner.

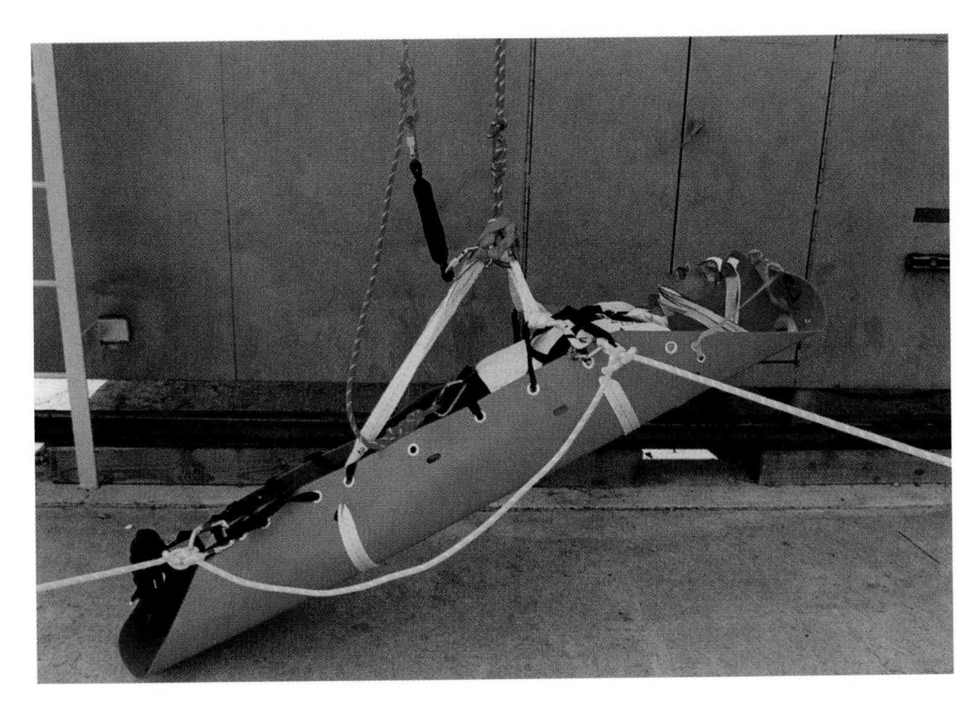

Figure 10.31 **Wrapping handles to shorten head strap**

5. At times you must shorten the bridle legs for a more heads-up litter position. Since this widens the angle of the bridle legs, you may need a carabiner in each loop to prevent improper loading. If needed, use a tri-link instead of two carabiners. To shorten the bridle straps (see Figure 10.31):
   A. Wrap the looped ends of the bridle straps around the webbing handles on each side of the Sked.
   B. Three to four wraps will place the patient at approximately a 45-degree heads up position.
6. Repeat steps 1 through 3 with the other bridle strap at the foot of the Sked. Shortening the foot strap is not usually appropriate, however, it can be done if a slightly head-down position is needed. This might be the case with a patient in hypovolemic shock. This head-down (Trendelenburg) position might help shunt blood to the vital organs, providing needed oxygen.
7. Attach the foot and head carabiners to the main line of the rope system. Consider reversing and opposing at least two of the carabiner gates to make accidental opening very difficult.
8. You can use a safety line belay system to back up both the primary rope system and a questionable litter. The Sked litter is not considered questionable, but circumstances surrounding the incident might make it prudent to back it up. The attachment of the safety line and litter backup is identical to that used for a basket litter with a single-point bridle. Shock absorber placement is also the same.

Horizontal Two-Point Bridle

A horizontal bridle for a double-line system is almost identical to that of a single-line system (see Figure 10.32). The straps for a two-point bridle attach to the Sked in the same way. One goes to the head, the other to the foot. There is only one difference. With the two-point bridle, there is no need to shorten the bridle straps. Control litter positioning by the operation of the rope system, not the bridle configuration. Therefore, you only need one carabiner for the loops at the head and foot bridle straps for attachment to their respective system ropes. If circumstances require shortening of the bridle legs, they can be adjusted by the method previously described for the single-point bridle.

Double rope systems can provide a built-in backup. If you need an additional backup for the primary rope system, try the same method presented earlier for the two-point basket litter bridle (see Figure 10.20). You can also back up a questionable Sked litter in the same way as a basket litter.

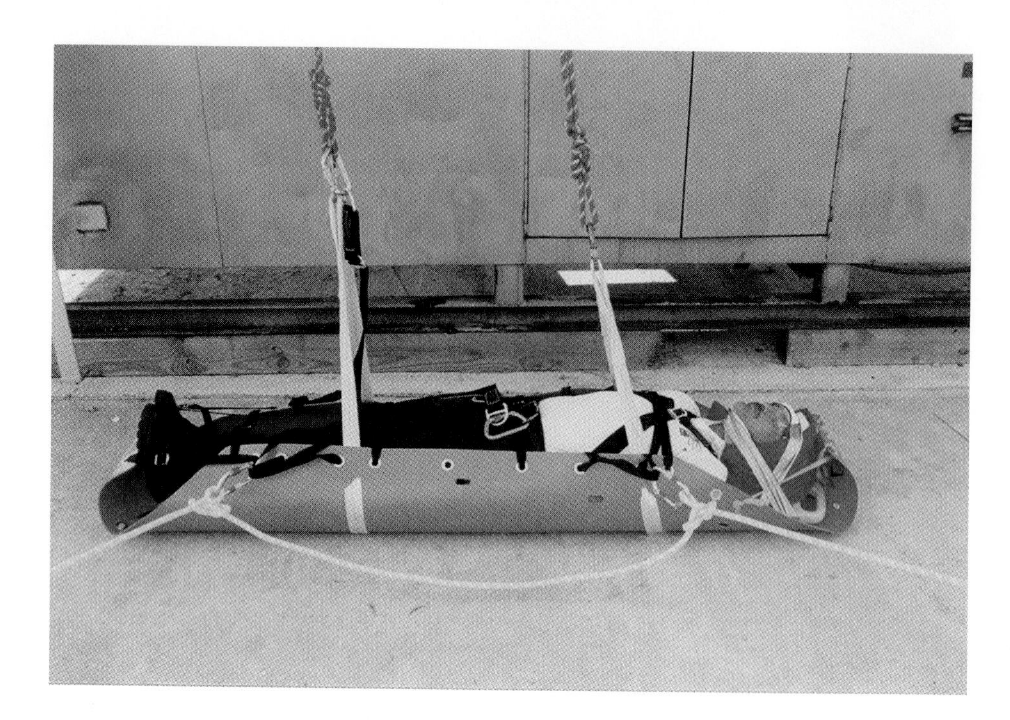

Figure 10.32 Sked two point litter bridle

Vertical Sked Bridles

One of the greatest advantages of the Sked is its ability to be passed through very narrow openings. This is often the case when rescuers have to haul or lower patients through obstructions or manways. Rescuers can use the Sked in a vertical configuration to make the best of these tight situations.

This section presents two methods of creating vertical single-point Sked bridles. The first method is similar to the one listed in the manufacturer's instruction book. The second method is a modification designed to adapt to certain patient injuries. The modification is a little slower to rig, but more comfortable for patients with lower-extremity injuries. Both methods are tailored to the industrial environment and have been approved by Skedco.

Figure 10.33 Vertical Sked without immobilizer

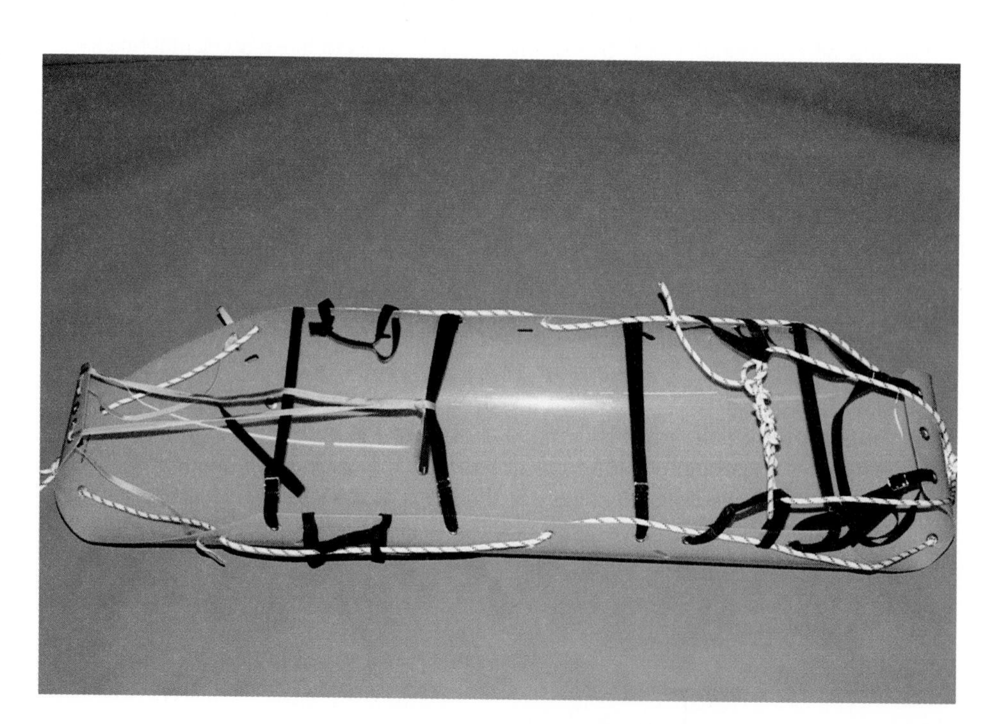

Standard Method

To create the vertical Sked bridle (see Figure 10.33):

1. Securely lash the patient in the Sked before starting this procedure. Make sure you tighten the foot panel against the patient's feet. This will keep the patient from sliding downward when you load the Sked vertically.
2. Use the 30-foot length of $\frac{3}{8}$-inch low-stretch rope that comes with the Sked. Tie an anchor knot in the middle of the 30-foot rope. The knots approved by the manufacturer include the figure-8 on a bight, the double-loop figure-8, or the butterfly knot.
3. Pass each end of the rope through the grommets at the head end of the litter (from the back to the front). For industrial applications, keep the knot centered and pull out all of the rope slack. This will keep the knot tight against the top of the litter. As with the vertical basket litter, this wide angle narrows when the bridle is loaded.
4. Continue feeding the rope through the next set of unused grommets (from the outside to the inside). Keep the slack out of the rope as you go. If the ropes contact the patient's shoulder area, place padding between the patient and ropes.
5. Pass the rope over the first lashing cross strap and through the center of the first set of webbing handles.
6. Repeat steps 4 and 5 for the next set of grommets and webbing handles.
7. Pass the ends of the rope around the sides and through the empty grommets at the base of the Sked (from inside to the outside).
8. Remove all the slack from both ropes and tie them together at the base of the Sked with a square knot. Remember, a square knot is not used for tying together load-bearing ropes. However, a square knot makes it easier to get all of that slack out of the bridle rope. Since the manufacturer chose to use the square knot here, extra precautions will be taken to make sure it is secure.
9. Now bring the ends of the rope up and over the end of the Sked.
10. Pass the rope ends through the lower webbing handles and pull the ropes tight.
11. Secure the loose ends with another square knot. With the loose ends, tie safety knots on each side of the square knot. The bridle is finished.
12. Attach the safety belay system, shock absorber, and litter backup (if needed) in the same way as for a vertical basket litter.

Alternative Method—Long-Spine Immobilizer

This alternative method alleviates pressure on the patient's lower extremities. It does this by eliminating the need for tightening the foot panel. Instead, the patient is securely fastened to a spinal immobilization device. The device is then attached to the bridle assembly well enough to prevent vertical movement. This method does not rely on the bottom foot panel to hold the patient in the litter.

Start by properly immobilizing and positioning the patient in the litter. Fasten the Sked lashing straps to their respective buckles, leaving them loose. Create the vertical bridle as follows (see Figure 10.34):

1. Take the 30-foot length of $\frac{3}{8}$-inch static kernmantle rope supplied with the Sked and tie an appropriate anchor knot in the middle of it.
2. Pass each end of the rope through the grommets at the head of the stretcher (from the back to the front).
3. Center the knot between the grommets and remove the slack between the knot and the grommets.
4. If using a long-spine immobilizer, repeat steps 4 and 5 of the standard method to create a vertical Sked bridle.
5. To attach the rope bridle to the long spine immobilization device, start by passing the rope ends through the next set of empty gromets on each side of the sked.
6. To secure the long-spine immobilizer:
   A. Find a carrying handle on each side of the spine board (or other long-spine immobilizer) below the level of the gromets just used.
   B. Pass the ropes around the carrying handles on each side of the spine board. Wrap the rope around each handle a minimum of 2 times. This wrap will form

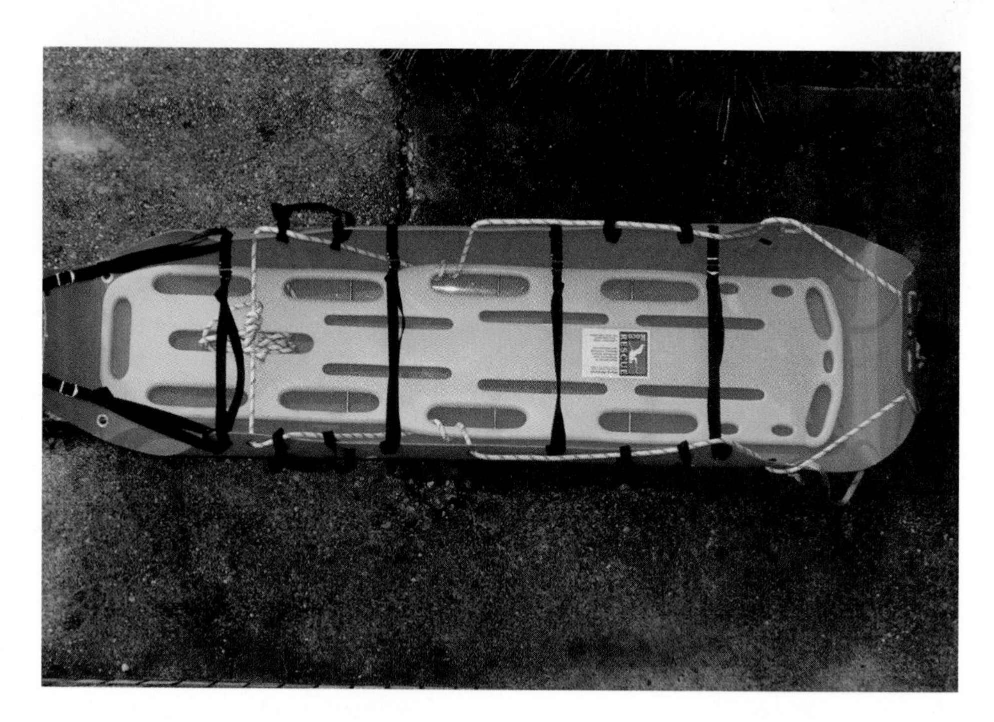

Figure 10.34 Vertical Sked with immobilizer

the load-bearing attachment to the immobilizer. It is very similar to the tensionless anchor presented in chapter 4.

C. Bring the rope ends under the third patient-lashing cross strap. Proceed to step 7.

7. Tighten the top two lashing straps while pulling all the slack out of the bridle rope and through the double-wrapped spine board handles. THIS IS EXTREMELY IMPORTANT! It ensures that there will be little or no slippage of the immobilization device in the Sked when the litter is loaded vertically. Be sure to keep the anchor knot at the top of the Sked centered.
8. Continue to bring the rope through the next set of handles and through the grommet used for securing the foot straps of the Sked.
9. Tie the two ends of the rope together with a loose square knot over the patient's lower legs. Avoid placing the knot directly across his or her knees. If this cannot be avoided, pad the knee area.
10. Before tightening the square knot, fully tighten all black lashing cross straps. Remove all remaining slack in the bridle rope.
11. Now tighten the square knot and safety each side with an appropriate knot. The square knot will not see the patient's load due to the double friction wrap on the handles of the immobilization device.
12. Attach the safety belay system, shock absorber, and litter backup (if needed) in the same way as for a vertical basket litter.

WARNING

Never suspend the Sked litter by a single grommet. The grommets pull out between 350 and 500 force pounds. They are not individually designed to suspend the weight of a patient. Use the rope and webbing bridles in the manner for which they are provided. Potential rescuers should practice and familiarize themselves with the Sked before using it on an actual rescue. This text is no substitute for hands-on training by a competent person.

Alternative Method—Short-Spine Immobilizer

If the opening to be negotiated is very narrow, a semirigid short-spine immobilizer may be necessary when using the Sked. This will conform better to the patient's body, making it easier to pass through the tight space. There is a slight difference between using a short- and a long-spine immobilizer with this alternative vertical Sked bridle.

To attach the rope bridle using a short immobilizer (see Figure 10.35):

1. Apply a seat harness (prefabricated or tied) around both the patient and the immobilization device. Do this before lashing the patient. Attach a tri-link to the harness if there is no D-ring.
2. Securely lash the patient in the Sked before starting this procedure. Make sure all lashing straps are tight.
3. Follow the same initial alternative method procedures but stop after passing the ropes through the first set of webbing handles.
4. Bring the rope ends through the gromets housing the lower end of the first set of webbing handles (outside to inside) and downward to the patient's waist.

5. Wrap the D-ring or tri-link with each rope once. This will provide somewhat of a friction wrap.
6. Bring the rope ends back through the empty grommets housing the second patient-lashing cross strap inside to outside. Be sure the rope ends return to the side from which they originally came.
7. Pass the rope ends through the next set of empty gromets from outside to inside. Remove all rope slack before proceeding.
8. Steps 8 through 12 of the alternative method previously described for a long-spine immobilizer are identical.

Other Sked Packaging

Other alterations in the Sked packaging may be required when passing the patient through extremely narrow passageways. The patient's shoulders are the widest part of the body. Rescuers can reduce shoulder width by placing a patient's arms above the head. They can alter Sked packaging to allow this. Simply place the patient's arms above his or her head (see Figure 10.27). Flex both arms back and secure the patient's hands behind or beside the head. When using this procedure, be careful to avoid manipulation of the spine.

No further modification is needed to pass the Sked through a narrow horizontal opening. However, negotiating narrow vertical passages requires slight alteration with either of the vertical bridles presented here. The rope bridle must begin at the shoulder-level grommets rather than the top grommets normally used. Rescuers can then leave the top panel of the Sked loose enough to allow appropriate arm placement.

Figure 10.35 Vertical Sked with short spine immobilizer

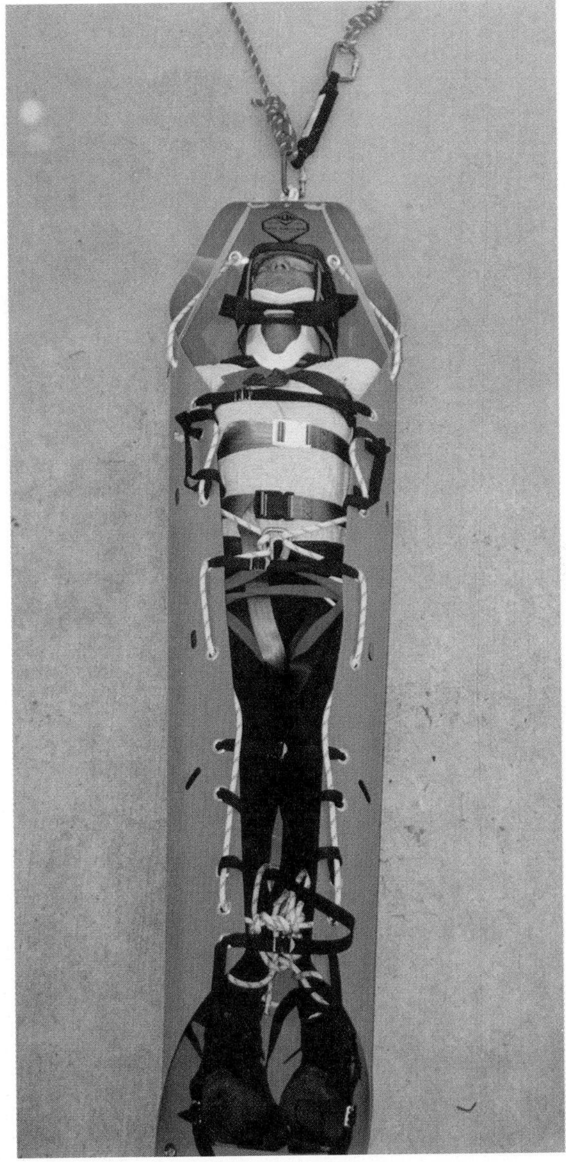

Rolling up and Repacking the Sked

An additional webbing strap comes with the Sked. This "retainer strap" is ideal for keeping the litter roll secure.

1. Start by laying the litter out flat.
2. Place the retainer strap, buckle side down, under the foot of the Sked.
3. Fold all the patient securement cross straps on top of the litter. Leave the foot straps free.
4. Starting at the head, roll up the Sked as tight as possible. Roll up the plastic drag handle (located at the head) inside the Sked (see Figure 10.36).
5. Continue to roll the Sked, using your knee to keep it from unrolling.
6. Fasten the preplaced retainer strap to the buckle and place the Sked roll in the back pack bag. Store the Sked in the cordura pack, since prolonged exposure to sunlight (UV rays) can damage all plastics.

Tag Lines

Tag lines are ropes attached to a litter or other object. Rescuers use them to pull the object away or around obstacles that might otherwise cause it to "hang up." When used with single-point bridles, tag lines can also prevent a litter from rotating accidentally. Rescuers should use two tag lines, with attachment points separated as much as possible, with vertical or horizontal litters. This provides maximum capability when negotiating obstructions and prevents accidental rotation.

The attachment points of the tag lines vary with the litter configuration. With vertical litters, attach tag lines to either side, near the base (foot). With a litter basket, this means the top rails on each side (see Figure 10.37). When using the Sked, the lower webbing handles make excellent attachment points (see Figure 10.38).

On horizontally configured litters, attach the tag lines to the outside (the side away from the wall or structure). The top rail is again

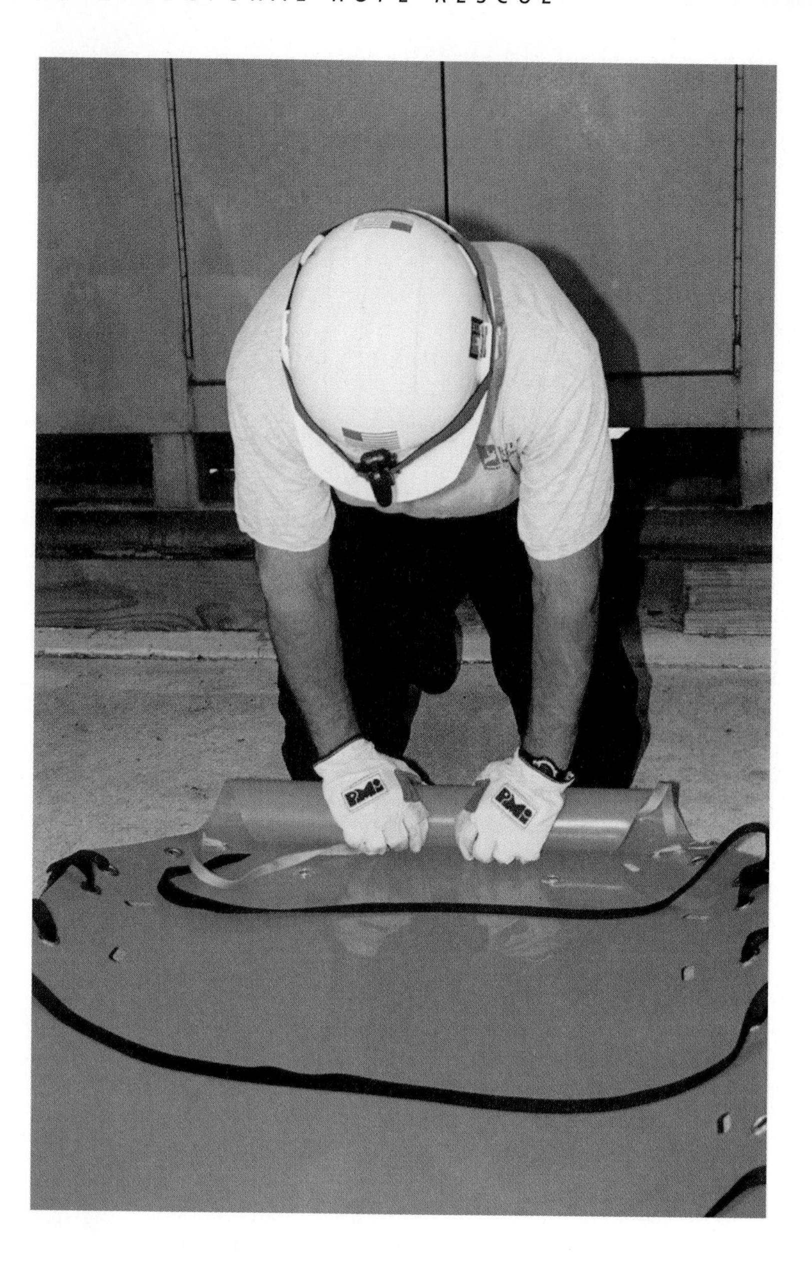

Figure 10.36 Rolling up Sked

the attachment point of choice for basket litters (see Figure 10.39). Attach one tag line near the head and one near the foot. Be sure to attach the lines to one of the smaller openings created by the litter frame. This will prevent the tag line from sliding more than a few inches on the railing. Attach tag lines to the outside legs of the Sked's yellow bridle straps (side away from the wall or structure) (see Figure 10.40).

Rescuers can either tie the tag lines directly to the litter or attach them with carabiners. Just about any knot works for attachment, but anchor knots seem to work best. Proper use of tag lines will be discussed in detail in the next chapter on lowering systems.

Summary

In general, a basket litter is quick and easy to rig for a vertical application. However, it is often not the litter of choice because it is too wide. A Sked litter is usually quicker and easier for a horizontal application because the vertical bridle is not required. However, the Sked is not rigid and may not provide the patient much protection against ledges or projections.

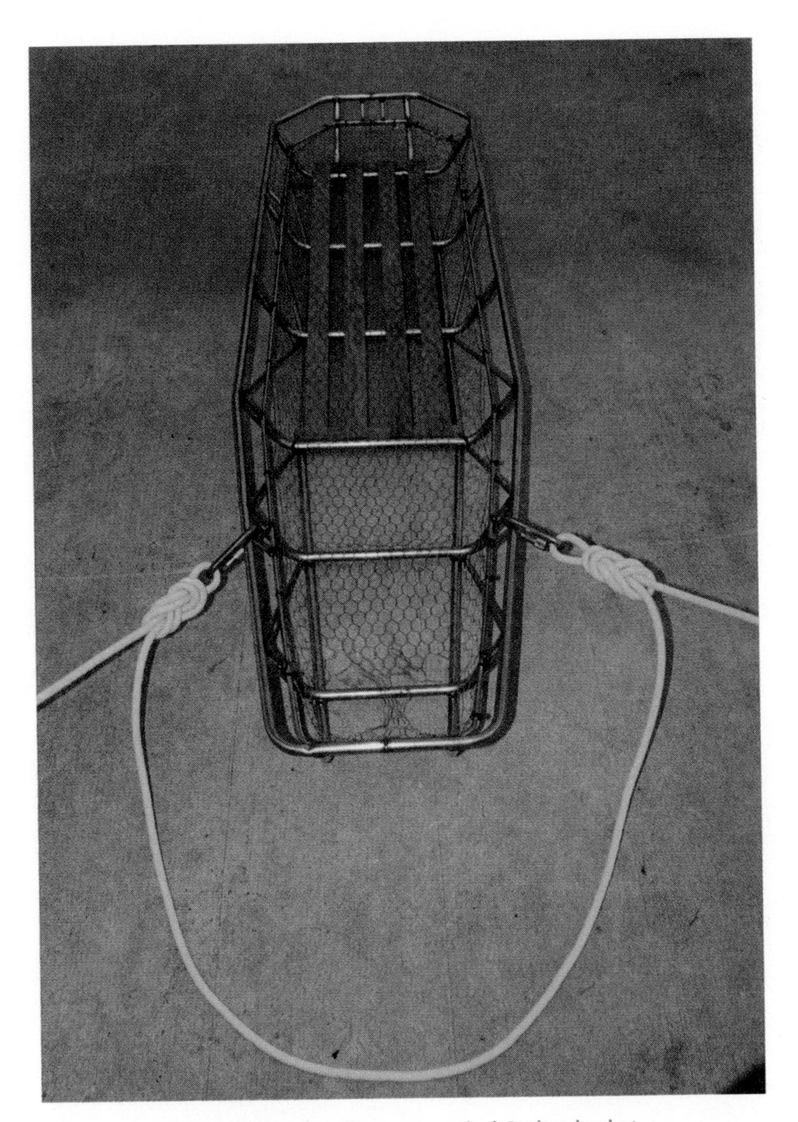

Figure 10.37 Tag lines on vertical Stokes basket

Figure 10.38 Tag lines on vertical Sked

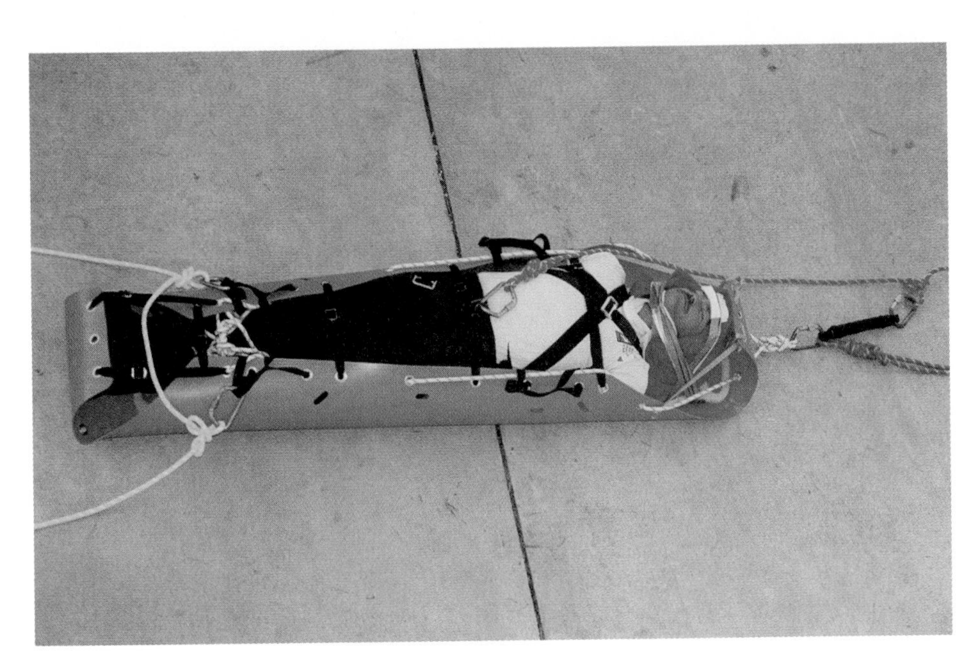

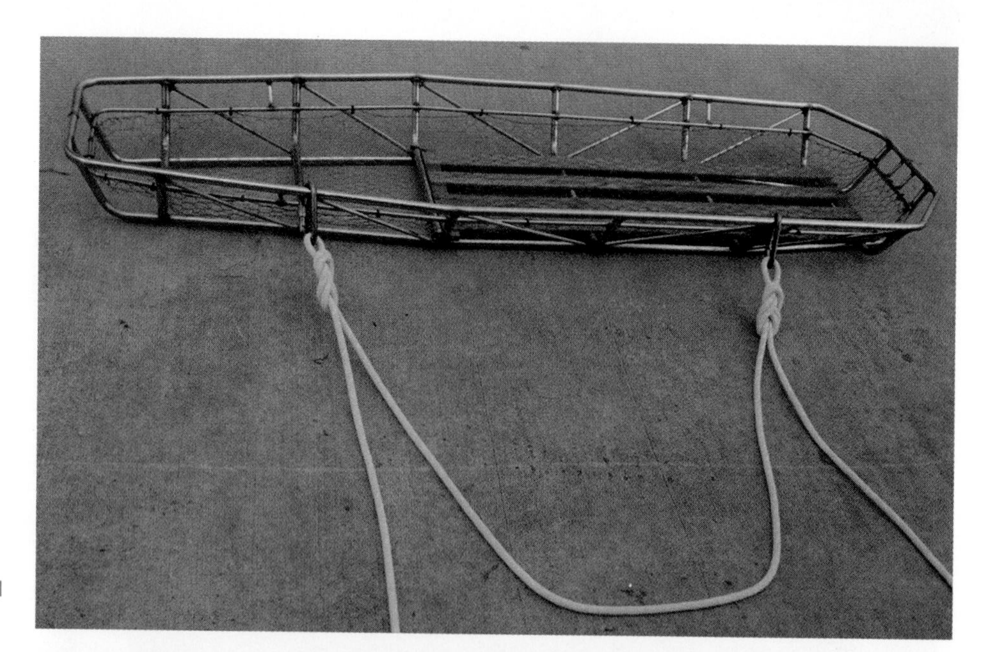

Figure 10.39 Tag lines on horizontal Stokes basket

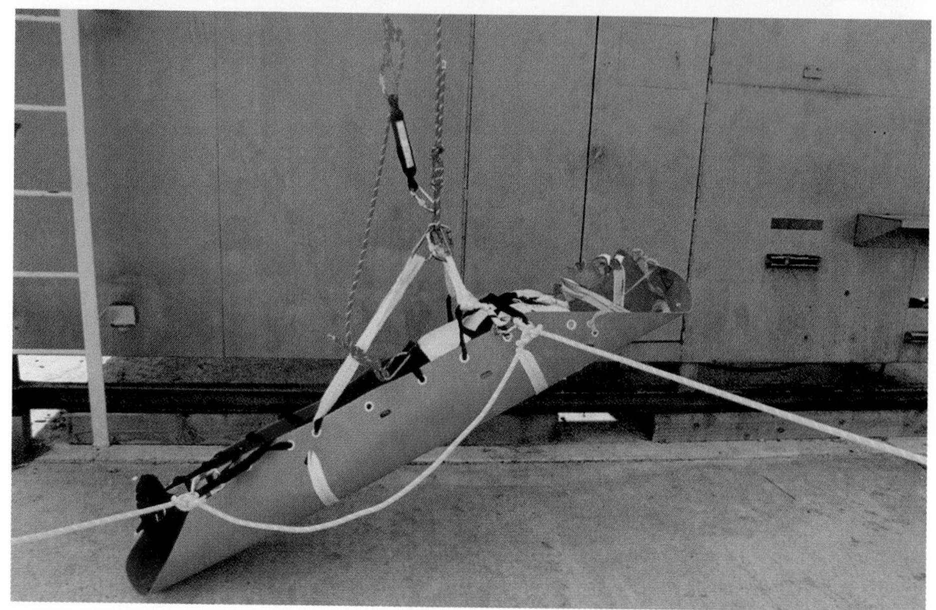

Figure 10.40 Tag lines on horizontal Sked

Rescuers use litters in a variety of ways. The type and configuration must be based on the same factors discussed in chapter 9 on packaging. The patient's condition and physical surroundings mean everything when choosing the methods and techniques of rescue. There are many packaging devices in existence that are not presented in this chapter. Some of these include rescue litters and special immobilization equipment.

It is necessary for the competent rescuer to receive specific training on these items based on the manufacturer's recommendations. The information presented here is not intended to supplant competent hands-on rescue training.

CHAPTER 11

Lowering Systems

The information in this chapter is provided as a basis for continued education. Each rescuer should consult with his or her own team leader for the correct SOGs for the team. Topics covered in this chapter include:

- Overcoming Edge Problems
- Victim Safety
- Single and Double Line Litter Lowers
- Litter Attendants

Introduction

This chapter describes one method of transporting the victim in a high-angle rope rescue environment. Lowering systems can be attached to harnesses or litters. They can involve single- or double-line systems. Rescuers choose to place attendants on some litter lowers to help negotiate obstacles or care for the patient. As with packaging, the type of lowering system depends largely on the type of rescue.

The lowering systems described in this chapter can be seen as rappel systems in reverse. With a rappel system, a rescuer moves down a fixed line using a descent control device (see Figure 11.1). In a lowering system, the descent control device is fixed (anchored) and the rope travels through it as the person is lowered (see Figure 11.2). Both take about the same number of personnel, though their operational assignments differ slightly. Even the problems are similar.

One of the greatest difficulties for a rappeller can be the negotiation of edges, ledges, projections, and other obstructions. The same applies to a rescuer using a lowering system. In fact, the challenge of negotiating an edge is very likely the most common to both.

Overcoming Edge Problems

Lowering systems are basically the same regardless of their anchors. However, certain considerations play a big part in how well those systems function. Rescuers must modify the operations to make negotiation of the edge as simple as possible. The location of the edge in relation to the path of the lowering line has a big effect on edge negotiation. In most cases, a litter can be placed smoothly over an edge if the lowering line runs from a point well above that edge (see Figure 11.3). If the lowering line must run directly over the railing (with no high point of attachment), rescuers must decide how to keep the litter from dropping and shock loading the rope when it is placed over the edge (see Figure 11.4). Again, this is very similar to rappelling. If the rappel rope is anchored well above the edge, it is much easier for the rappeller to negotiate. He or she simply attaches as high as possible on the rappel line and steps over the edge (refer to Chapter 7, "Rappelling and Self-Rescue"). If the rope is anchored at a point level with or below the edge, the rappeller must carefully calculate the correct attachment of the descent control device to the line. If this "plumb point" is not measured properly and the rappeller climbs over the edge, he or she may drop quite a distance before finally loading the rope (refer to Chapter 7, "Rappelling and Self-Rescue").

In general, the higher the rope's path can be directed above the edge to be negotiated, the easier it will be to get the patient over that edge. One way to accomplish this is by rigging the descent control device from a point above the level of the patient. A rescuer can then lift the patient or litter while removing all slack in rope between them and the descent control device. This usually allows the patient to be placed gently and easily over the edge. While this might solve the problem of negotiating the edge, it might also hinder the operation by interfering with communications. Unless rescuers are using some type of radio communications, working on different levels makes hand or verbal signals much less effective.

There is another way of getting the transport vehicle above the edge without compromising communications. By running the lowering line through a pulley or other device anchored high above the edge, the descent control device can be rigged and operated at the same level (see Figure 11.5). This principle can be applied anywhere in a rope system to redirect the rope's path for convenience. Either way, a high point of attachment has been established to help make the edge negotiation easier.

Sometimes the edge or opening to be negotiated helps determine the configuration and type of transport vehicle to be used for the lower. For example, a vertically configured litter would need to be lifted higher than one with a horizontal attitude to get it above the edge to be negotiated (see Figure 11.6). A full-body harness or a flexible litter may be required in order to fit the patient through

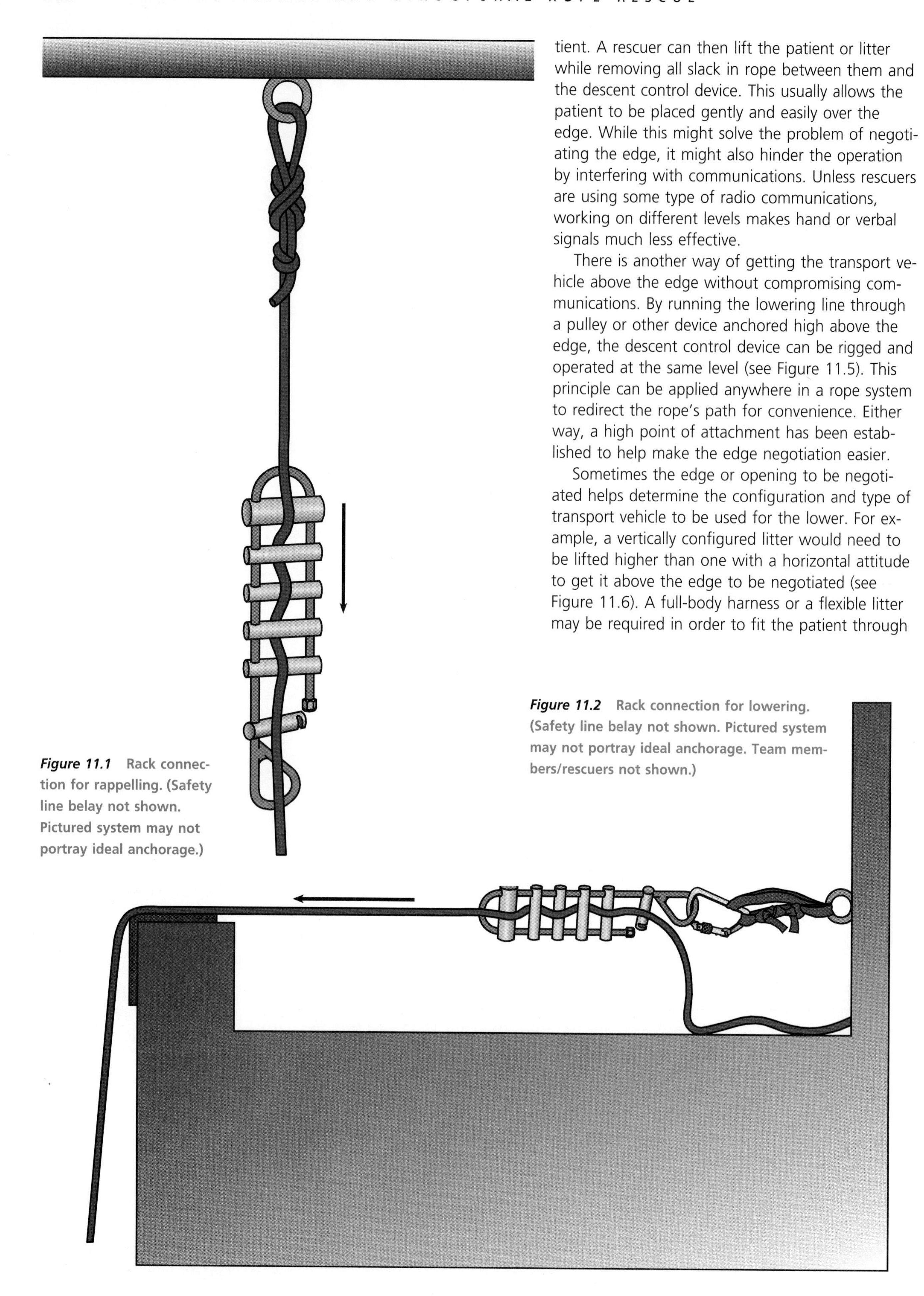

Figure 11.1 **Rack connection for rappelling. (Safety line belay not shown. Pictured system may not portray ideal anchorage.)**

Figure 11.2 **Rack connection for lowering. (Safety line belay not shown. Pictured system may not portray ideal anchorage. Team members/rescuers not shown.)**

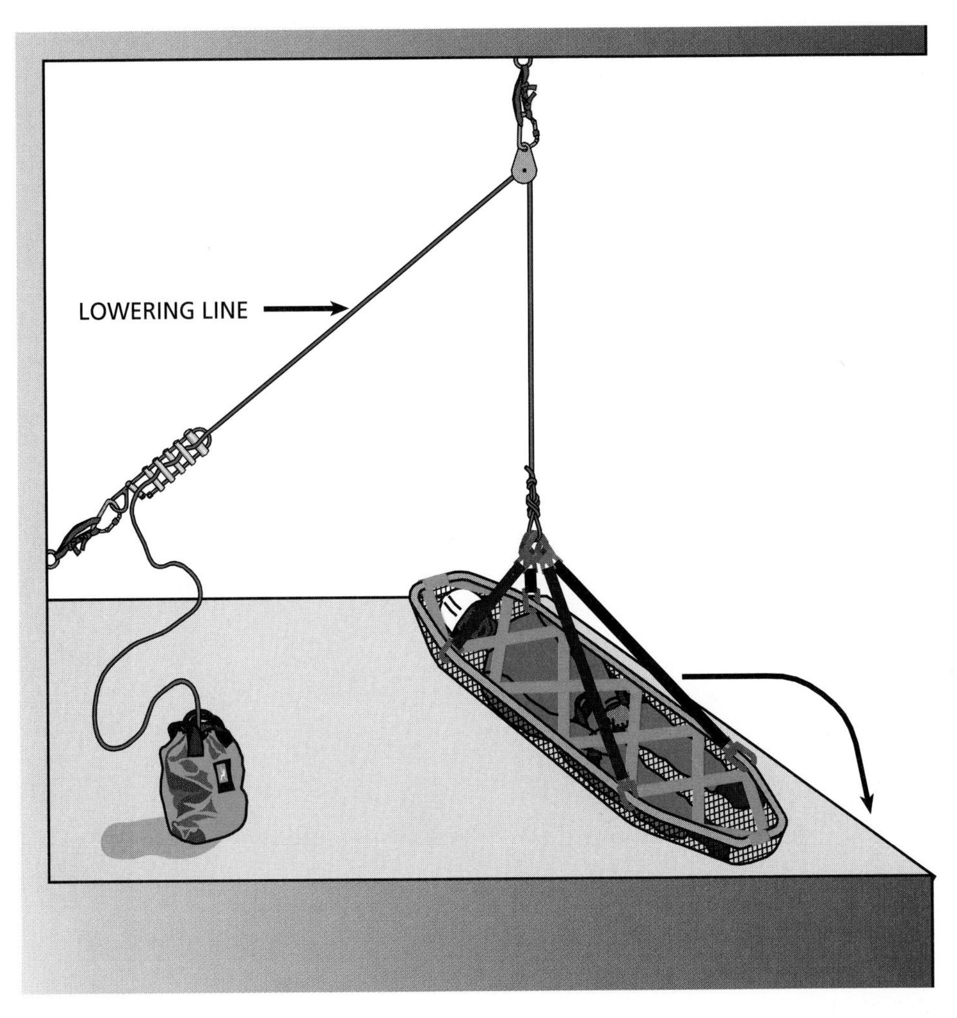

Figure 11.3 Lowering system with high-point directional. (Safety line belay not shown. Pictured system may not portray ideal anchorage. Team members/rescuers not shown.)

Figure 11.4 Lowering system with low-point anchor. (Safety line belay not shown. Pictured system may not portray ideal anchorage. Team members/rescuers not shown.)

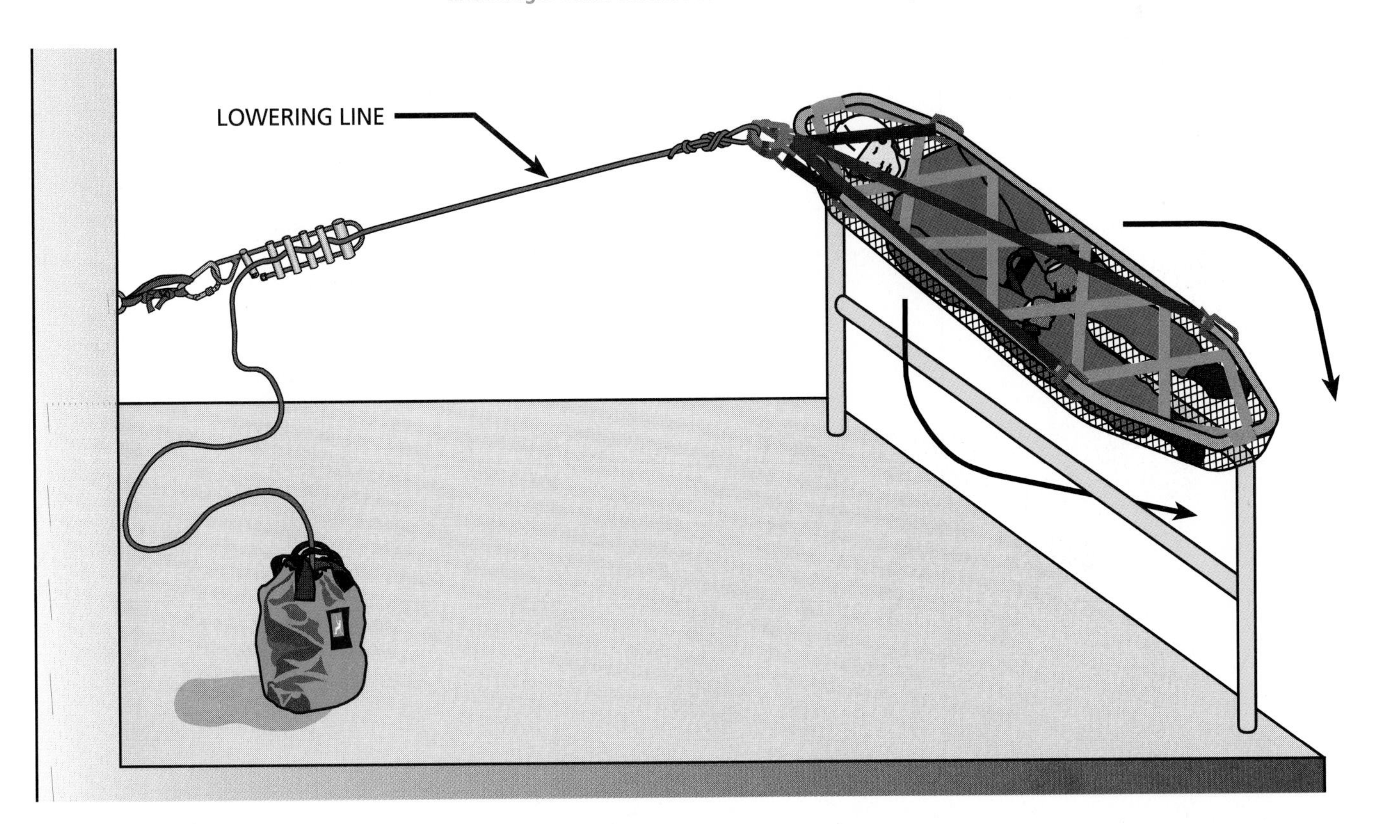

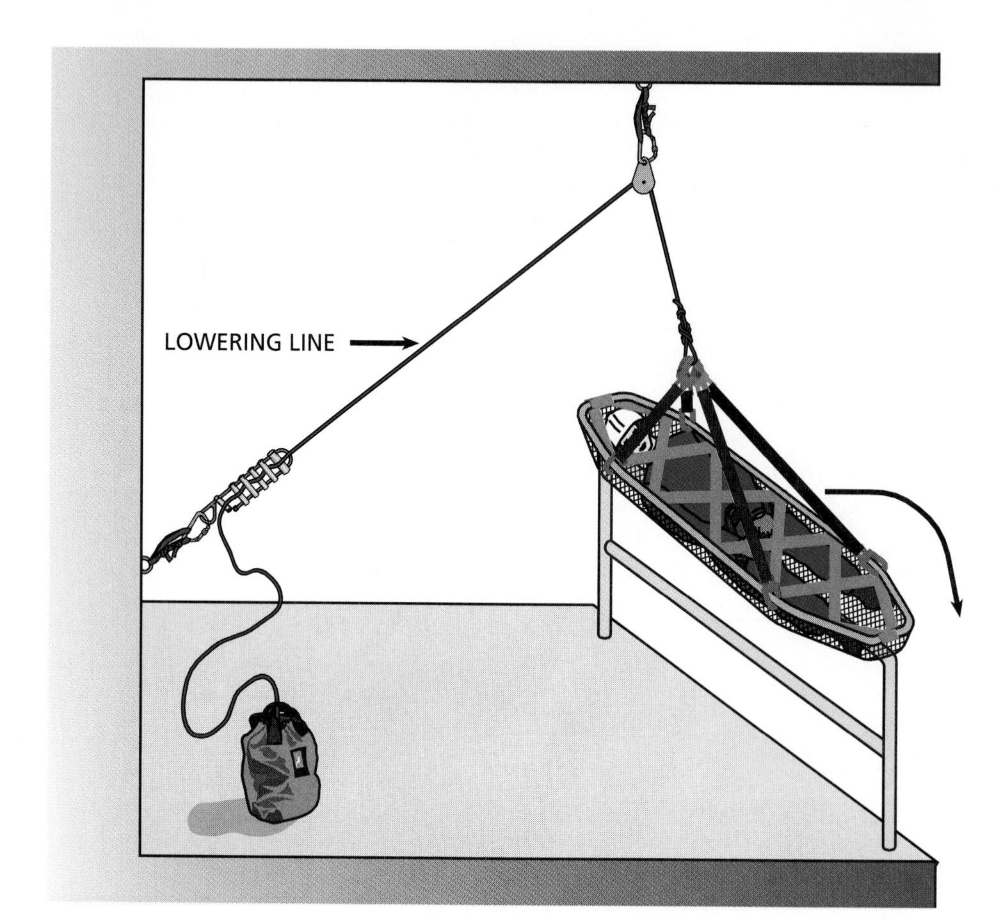

Figure 11.5 Lowering system with high edge (Safety line belay not shown. Pictured system may not portray ideal anchorage. Team members/rescuers not shown.)

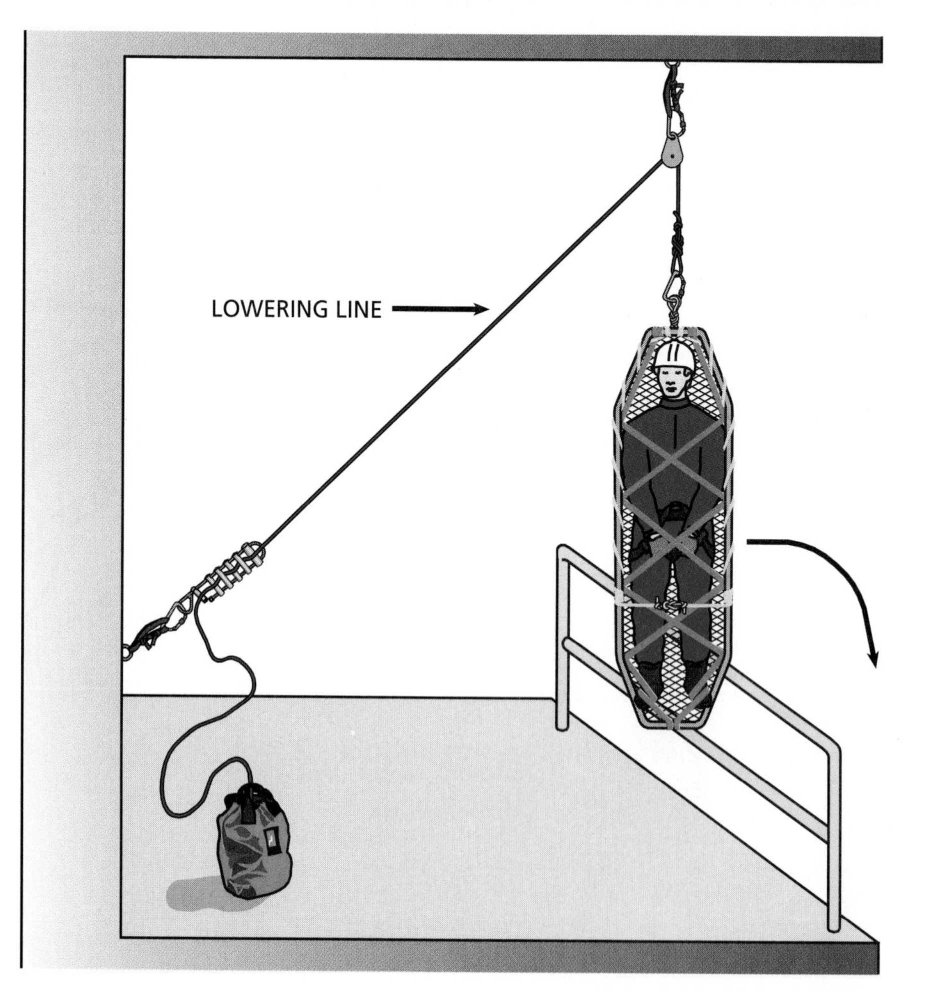

Figure 11.6 Lowering system with vertically configured litter (Safety line belay not shown. Pictured system may not portray ideal anchorage. Team members/rescuers not shown.)

a narrow opening. It may be easier to place a vertically configured litter through a narrow window opening with a low point of attachment rather than attempting to establish a high point of attachment above the window frame (see Figure 11.7). These examples represent only a few considerations necessary to determine the methods for lowering. Because there are many ways to accomplish the same task, rescuers evaluate each situation to determine the safest and most efficient method for the job at hand.

Single-Line Litter Lowers

Single-line lowering systems involve using one main rope for lowering the patient. This rope is attached directly to the litter or patient's harness and is controlled by a descent device such as a rappel rack or figure-8. The addition of a safety line belay system is highly recommended for protection against failures of primary system components. Tag lines also help steady the load, keep it from spinning, and guide it away from obstacles during lowering operations.

Although single-line lowering systems can be attached directly to a patient's harness or a litter, traumatic injuries are usually better stabilized with litters. Lowering patients in litters is more difficult than lowering patients in full-body harnesses. Therefore, litter lowers generally represent the worst-case scenario. The litters can be bulky and rigid, making it difficult to negotiate edges and narrow openings. All of the single-line systems discussed here can be attached easily to a full-body harness for lowering. This is often the method of choice for patients who are calm or have no injuries.

Unfortunately, many of the rescues in the industrial environment involve traumatic injuries and/or apprehensive patients. For this reason, this chapter concentrates on the use of litters in lowering systems. It reviews two litter configurations used with single-line lowering systems—horizontally configured and vertically configured. Although the lowering system is the same for both configurations, the negotiation of edges and projections may require slightly different techniques. Many times, there is no overhead anchor from which to rig the lowering line. In this case, the litter must be placed directly over the edge. Low-point anchors are usually considered the most difficult.

Horizontal Litter Lower with Low-Point Anchor

The first single-line lowering system uses the example of a horizontally configured basket litter as a transport vehicle. This litter was chosen based on a specific scenario and may not be the litter of choice in others. The techniques for lowering a horizontal litter with a low-point anchor are generally the same regardless of the type of litter.

Safety Check

Before movement of the litter begins, double-check that all major elements of the lowering system are in place and prepared. These elements include:

- The patient has been medically assessed, stabilized and treated, and his or her condition is being monitored.
- The lowering and safety belay ropes have been properly attached to the litter.
- Secure anchors have been set and appropriate lowering (braking) and belaying devices are attached to them.
- The lowering rope is properly attached to the braking device and locked off.
- The brake person has the rope in hand and is ready to operate the brake.
- The belayer is ready to tend the belay (safety line) system.
- An optional line tender can be used to hold the loose end of the lowering line and feed it to the brake person to prevent tangling.

This check is the primary responsibility of the rescue master, but each team member should inspect the system as well. If problems are discovered, they should be corrected before continuing. When all points are verified, the rescue master directs the litter team to lift the litter for placement over the edge.

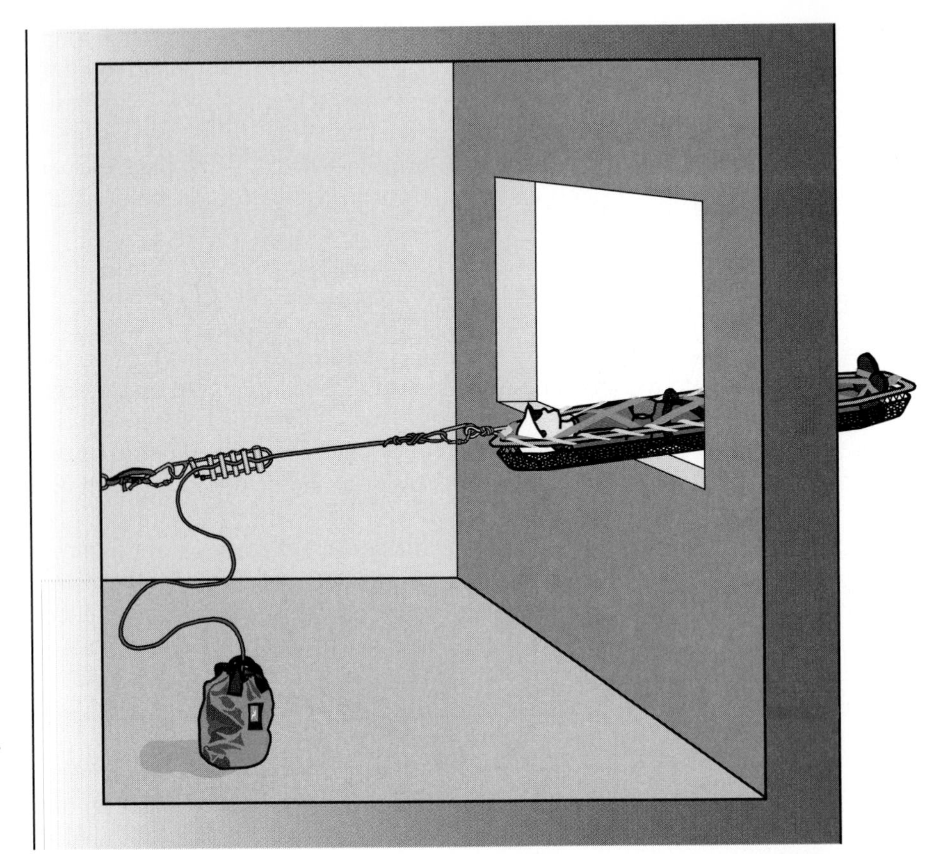

Figure 11.7a Low-point anchors are sometimes easier when placing vertically configured litters through small widows or doorways. (Safety line belay not shown. Pictured systems may not portray ideal anchorage. Team members/rescuers not shown.)

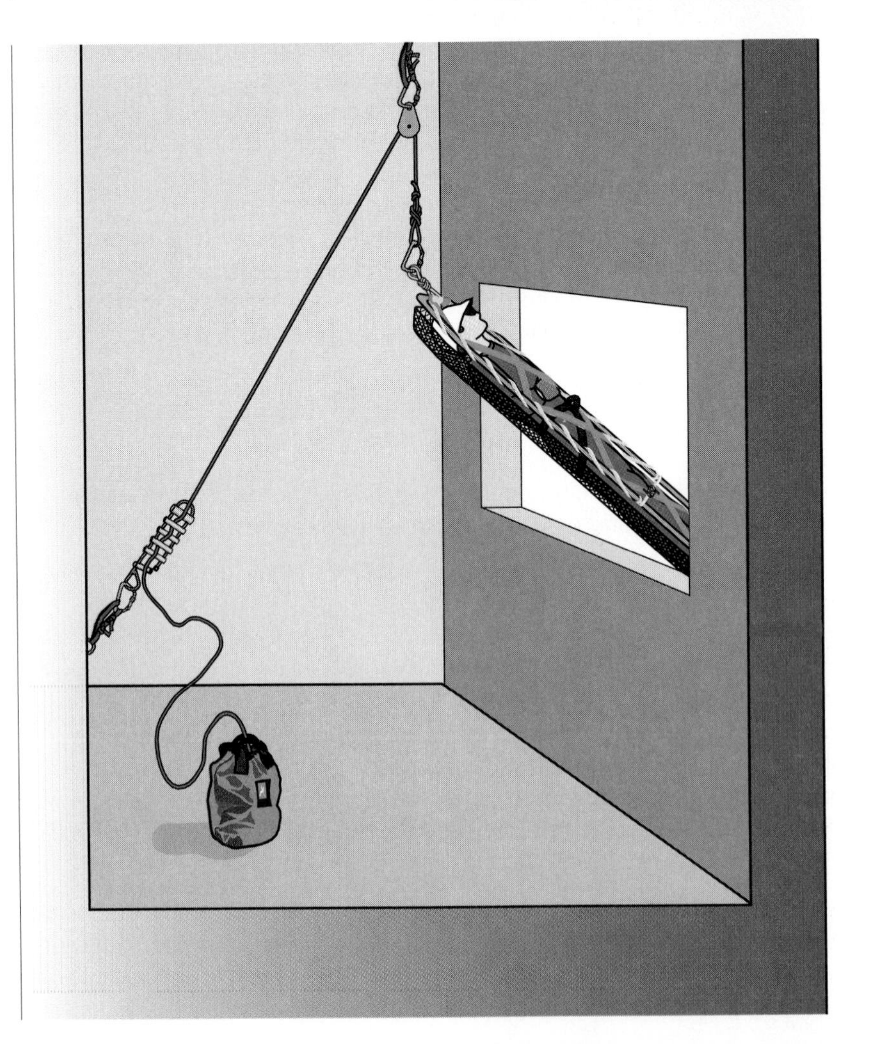

Figure 11.7b High-point directional anchors sometimes make it more difficult to place litter through windows or doorways. (Safety line belay not shown. Pictured systems may not portray ideal anchorage. Team members/rescuers not shown.)

Measuring the Rope

1. Make certain that both the lowering and the safety line belay ropes are long enough to reach the designated landing zone.
2. When everything is ready, carefully measure the knot end of the lowering line (intended for attachment to the litter) from the descent control (brake) device to the edge over which the litter will be lowered. Do this to prevent having too much or too little slack in the line. Place the knot just over the edge (approximately 1 inch). This is referred to as a "plumb point" and serves the same purpose as the plumb point in a low-point rappel system. Remember that the litter bridle will add 1 to 2 feet of length to the system.
3. Take all of the slack out of the brake device. In this example, a rappel rack is the brake device.
4. With the right hand the brakeman drops off three bars of a six bar rack, then pulls all the slack from the lowering line while holding the top bar of the rack away from the anchor point with the left hand.
5. He or she then adds 3 bars to make a total of six bars, weaving the rope around them for additional friction.
6. The brakeman then holds the loose end of the rope forward, toward the tip of the rack, and prepares to lower on command.
7. Attach the knot end of the lowering line to the litter bridle.
8. If you are using a safety line belay system, the belay (or safety) person attaches the safety belay rope to the belay device. The belay rope always has about 18 inches of slack in it and will be tensioned only in an emergency to catch a falling load.
9. Attach the knot end of the safety belay rope to the litter bridle, as detailed in a previous chapter. You can also attach this line to the patient, which backs up both the lowering line and the litter in the event of a failure of either.
10. If you use a shock absorber, place it inline between the safety line and the litter bridle.

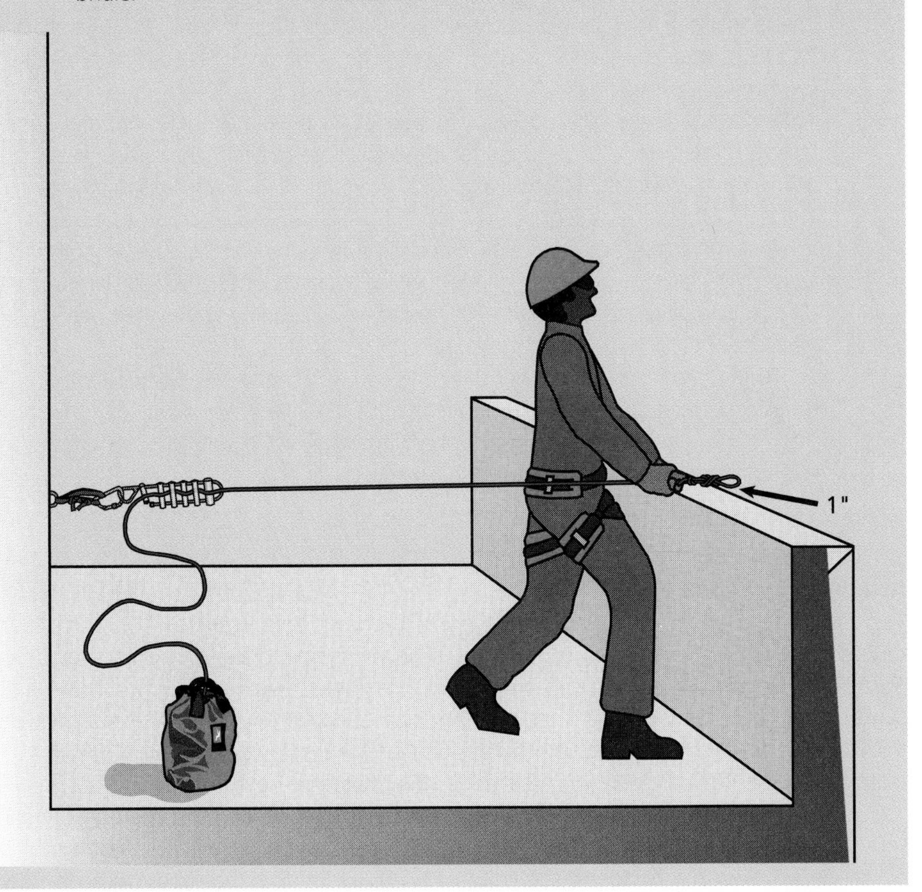

WARNING

Avoid removing slack from the lowering device in a single-line lowering system after the litter has been placed near the edge. If the litter were to fall over the edge, the system might be unable to catch it.

WARNING

If anything is available to catch on the railing of the litter as you attempt to place it over the edge, IT WILL! Be very observant during this operation. If you see something that might stop the litter and later drop it, stop the operation until the obstruction is cleared. Any drop of the litter might cause psychological trauma for the patient.

Lifting the Litter

1. Usually three or four rescuers comprise the lift team (see Figure 11.9). They should position themselves on the same side of the litter, farthest from the edge over which they will place it. If it is possible for a rescuer to stumble and fall over the edge during the operation, he or she should first be tied securely to anchor systems. Members of the lift team should position themselves at the head, chest, hips, and thighs of the patient. It is usually a good idea to position the stronger lift team personnel at the torso to bear the greater portion of the patient's weight.
2. When the rescue master has given the okay to lower, the lift team member at the head should give the commands for lifting the litter. Many command sequences can be used but the simple "prepare to lift" and "lift" commands represent work well.
3. The members of the lift team should lift with their legs, not their backs. They should place one hand on the inside rail and the other on the outside rail when lifting. It does not matter which hand they use for which rail, but all members of the team use the same pattern.
4. The member at the head then gives the signal to lift. The litter is lifted and rolled at a 45 degree (or smaller) angle into their bodies with the outside rail up.
5. The lift team positions the inside rail of the litter on the edge. In this manner, the litter "rests" on the lip. This allows the edge to take the load while rescuers prepare to place the litter over the side. Let the tool do the work. Let the edge hold the load.
6. Keeping the litter angled toward them, each lift crew member places the heel of one hand on the inside rail, then they ease the basket out over the edge, inside rail first. BE CAREFUL! It is easy to catch a finger between the basket rail and the edge when you are pushing the bottom rail out.
7. To ease the rail over the edge, the lift team uses open palms (fingers up).
8. Placing one end of the litter over the edge at a time makes a smooth transition. The foot of the litter should be placed over the edge first, followed by the head. This helps keep the patient's apprehension to a minimum by keeping the feet below the level of the head.
9. As rescuers ease the litter out over the edge, they must maintain supportive contact with the outside rail of the litter. If rescuers are not fully supporting the litter at this point, when the litter is eased over the edge, it will drop several inches. This can distress the patient or even pinch the skin, or cause some other trauma. Whenever possible, rescuers try to make the transition over the edge smooth.
10. Once over the edge, the litter should then be rotated outward to the flat horizontal position (90 degrees from the lift team member's body) and loaded onto the main line.
11. To aid in lowering the litter over the edge, rescuers sometimes place a loop of tubular webbing at both the head and foot of the litter. This allows members of the lift crew to apply tension to the webbing loops and gently ease the litter over the edge until the lowering line is fully loaded.

WARNING

Do not attempt to grab a falling litter. This mistake can quickly pull you over the edge. If you are not secured to an anchor, it can mean severe injury or death.

Attaching Tag Lines

Tag lines can be attached to the outside rail of the litter (see Figure 11.10). This allows tagmen to pull on the ropes to guide the litter away from ledges, projections, or other obstructions that might be encountered during the lower. Because the rope is at an acute angle near the edge, tag lines might not be effective for the first several feet of a lower. It is often desirable to use the designated tagmen as assistants on the lift team. Once the litter is safely over the edge, they can go to and attend the tag lines.

After the lift team has placed the litter over the edge, the tagmen position themselves to operate the tag lines. Each of two tagmen should wrap a tag line around his or her body below the buttocks (see Figure 11.11). By holding the ropes on each side

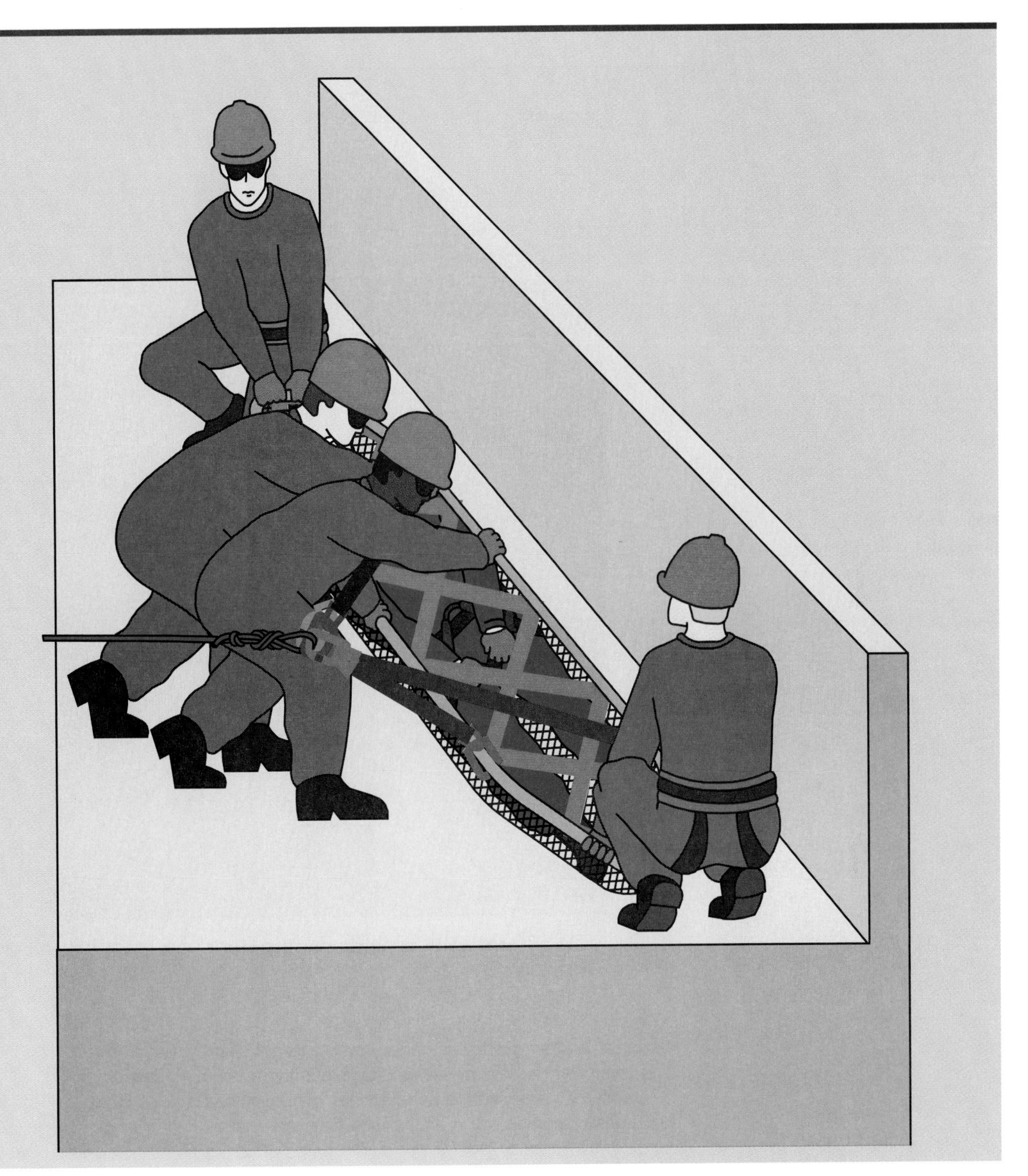

Figure 11.9 Lifting the litter

of their bodies, they can now give or take up slack by walking toward or away from the structure. This positioning of the rope around the lower torso places the stress of the pull on the upper legs and not the lower back. This helps prevent back injury due to strain. Tagmen keep the litter clear of obstructions and should concentrate on smooth pulls to prevent a rough ride for the patient. The way the litter is tagged can mean the difference between a smooth ride or a roller coaster for the patient.

Communication

The brakeman should have all six bars on the rack while the litter is being placed over the edge. Once over the edge and upon the rescue master's command, "prepare to

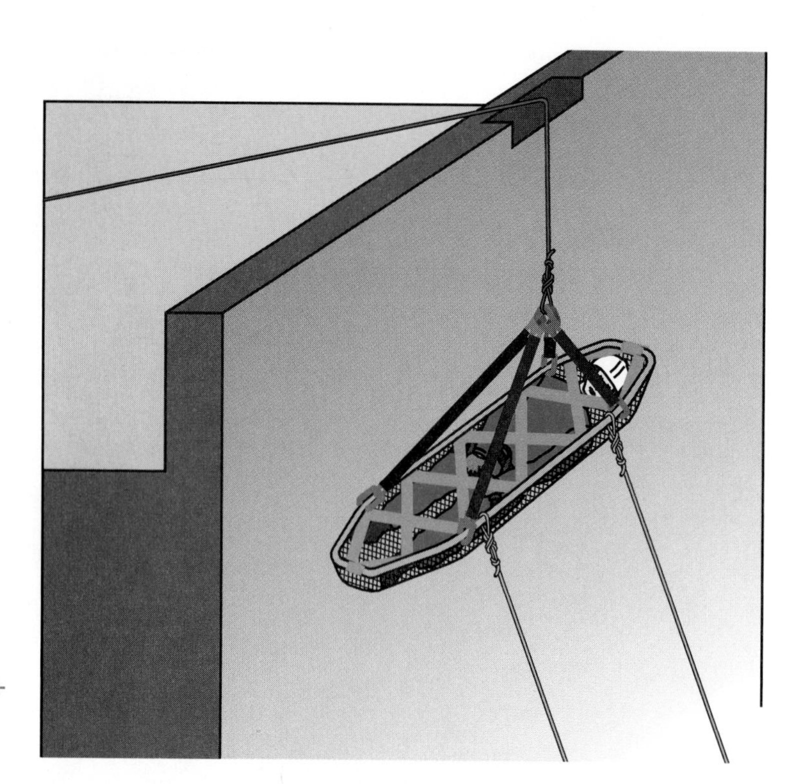

Figure 11.10 Tag lines should be attached to the outside of the litter. (Safety line belay not shown.)

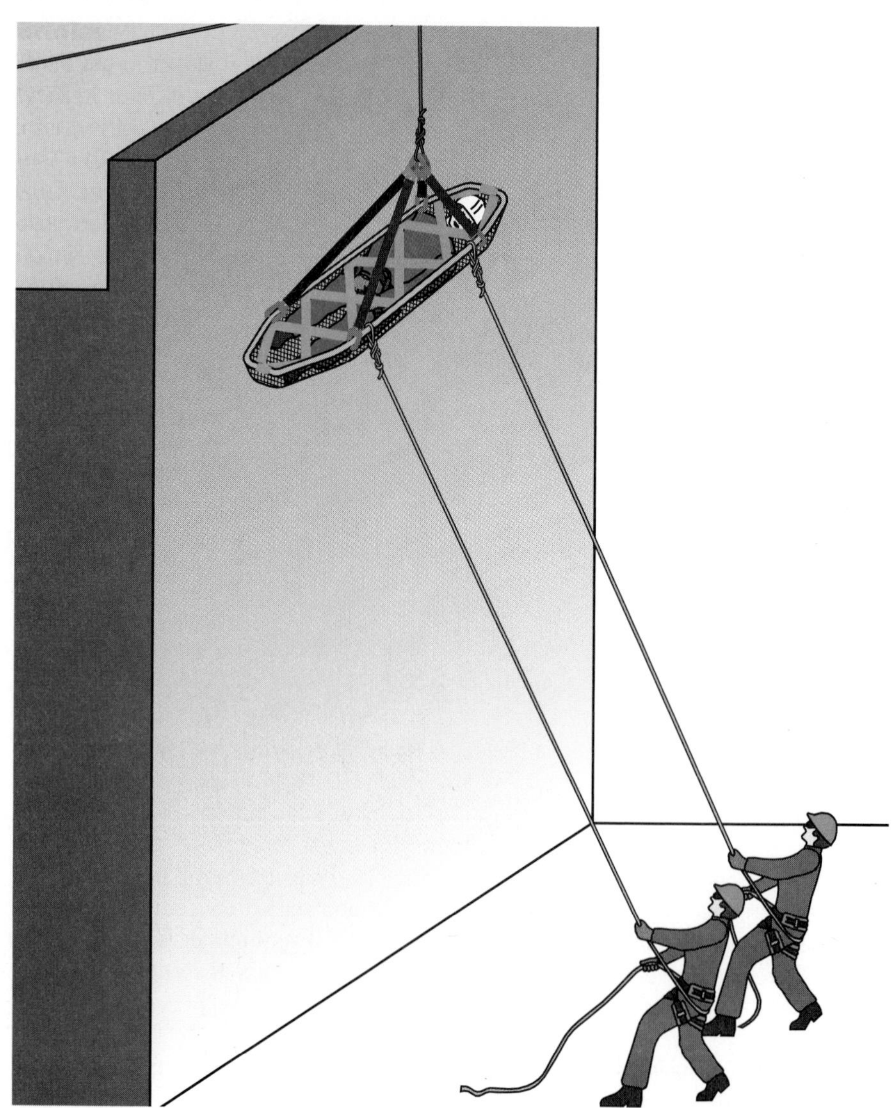

Figure 11.11 Tag lines should be wrapped around each tag man's body below the buttocks. (Safety line belay not shown.)

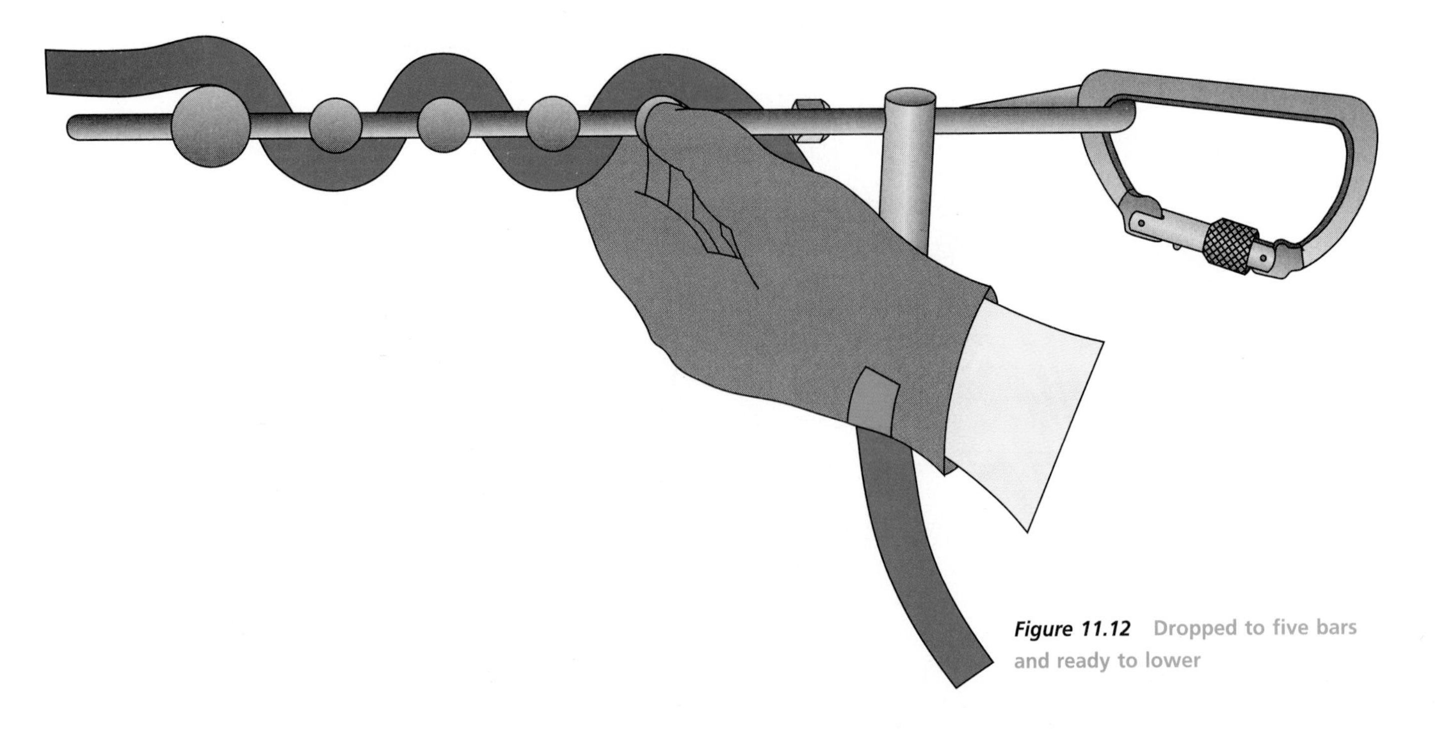

Figure 11.12 Dropped to five bars and ready to lower

lower," the brakeman may drop to five bars and be ready to lower (see Figure 11.12). The rescue master issues commands to the brake person for lowering:

- "Lower" means to reduce the friction on the rack to allow the rope to slide through. The rescue master may designate slow or fast.
- "Stop" means to immediately halt lowering until given another signal. If using a brake bar rack, the brake person should immediately wrap the loose end of the lowering rope up toward the tip of the rack, hold the two ropes together, and wait for further orders from the rescue master (see Figure 11.13).
- "On the ground" means that the litter has reached the ground and the brakeman should give slack on the lowering rope.

Hand signals are often necessary in noisy environments. Many methods for signaling can be used. A team should use whatever methods work best for the environ-

Figure 11.13 Holding two ropes together awaiting further commands from the rescue master (defined as a "wrap-up" vs. a "lock-off")

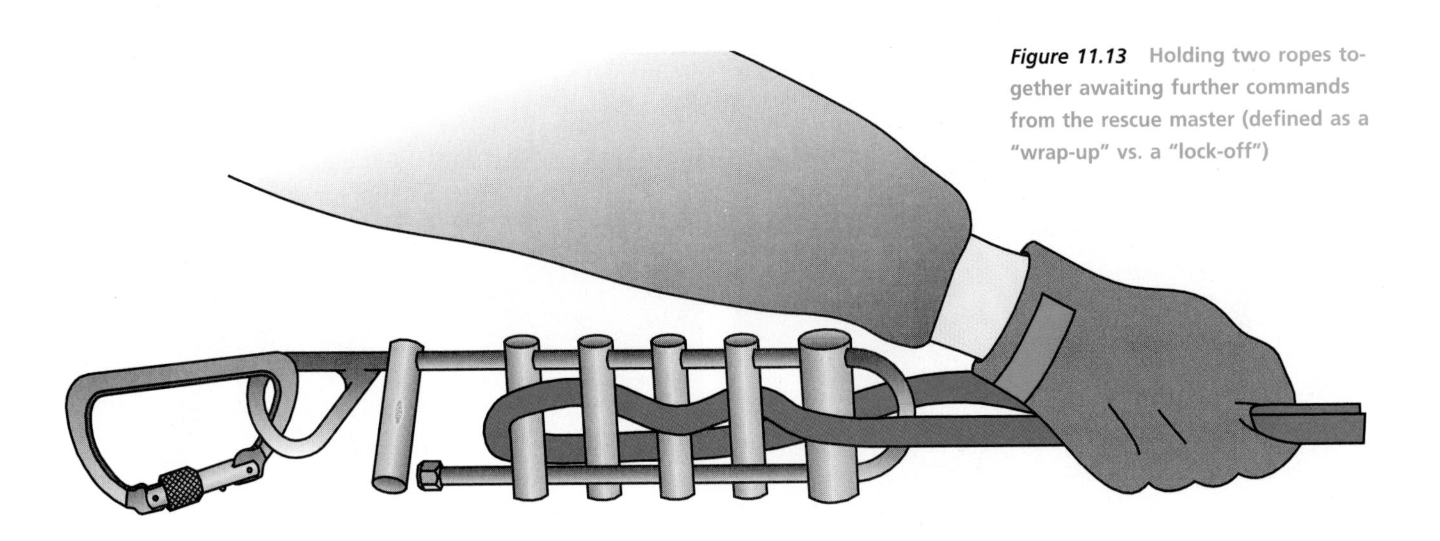

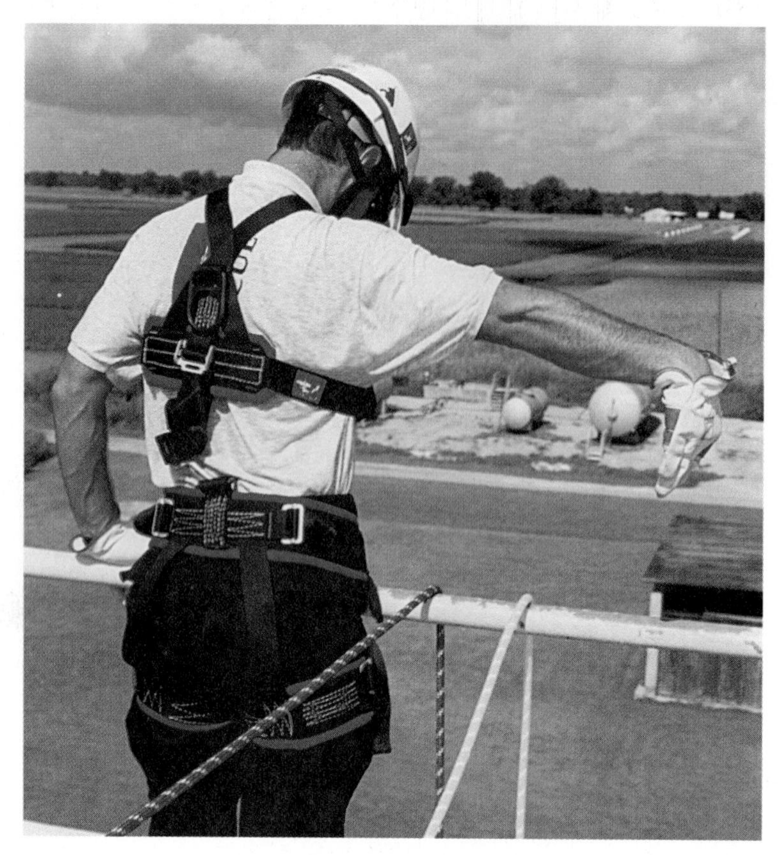

Figure 11.14 Hand signal for "Lower"

ment. Whatever the signals, they should be simple and easy to see and understand. The following series of lowering signals are performed with one hand and are easily seen and understood even when the signaling rescuer is wearing gloves. The rescue master can give these signals while looking at the progress of the lower over the edge and without having to worry about being heard. The brakeman simply watches the rescue master's hands.

- Keeping the hand flat (open palm) and bending 90 degrees at the wrist corresponds to the verbal command "lower" (see Figure 11.14).
- Keeping the hand flat and holding it straight up in line with the forearm corresponds to the verbal command "stop" (see Figure 11.15). This resembles the stop signal used by traffic officers.
- Holding a clenched fist high in the air corresponds to the verbal command "on the ground" (see Figure 11.16).

Again, any workable signaling method can be used as long as the entire team uses the same one. Using many types of signals to communicate the

Figure 11.15 Hand signal for "Stop"

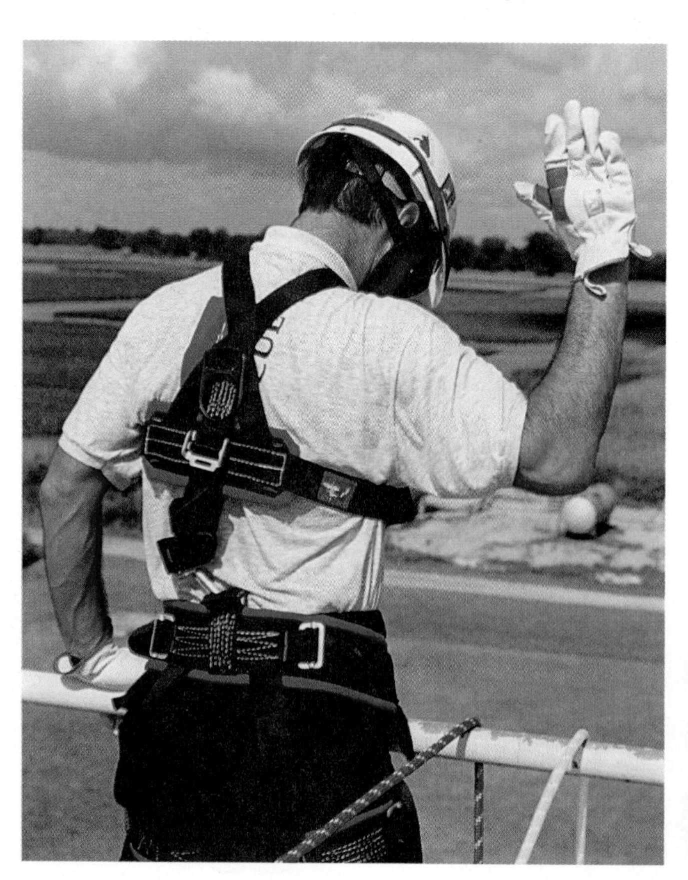

Figure 11.16 Hand signal for "On the ground"

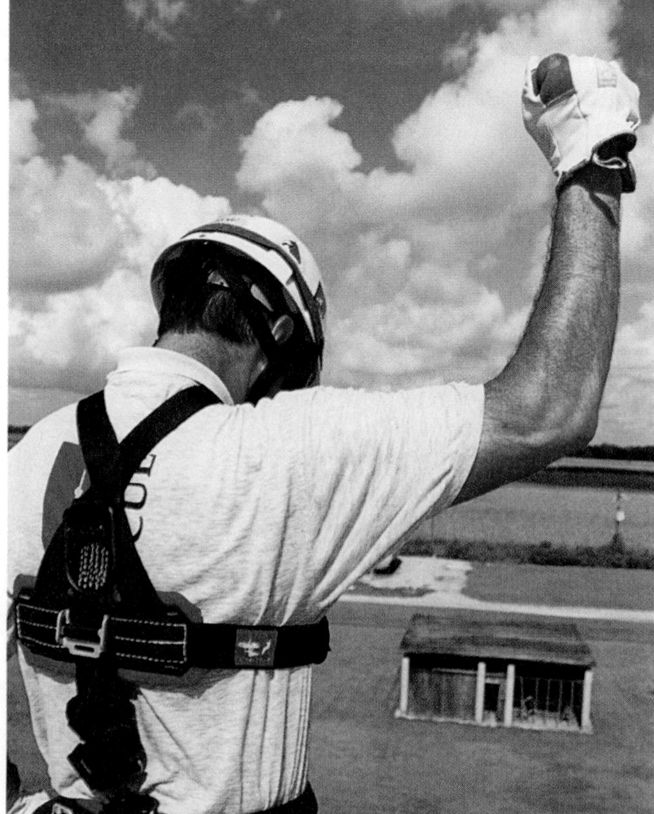

same thing can be quite confusing. There are already enough difficulties to contend with on the emergency scene without compounding the problem with poor signals. Be clear, concise, and uniform. (More signals are discussed later in this chapter.)

Reaching the Ground

Once the litter has reached the ground, the tagmen should immediately pull the litter out and away from the structure to prevent falling debris or equipment from striking the patient (see Figure 11.17). Care of the patient should be transferred to a qualified emergency medical staff.

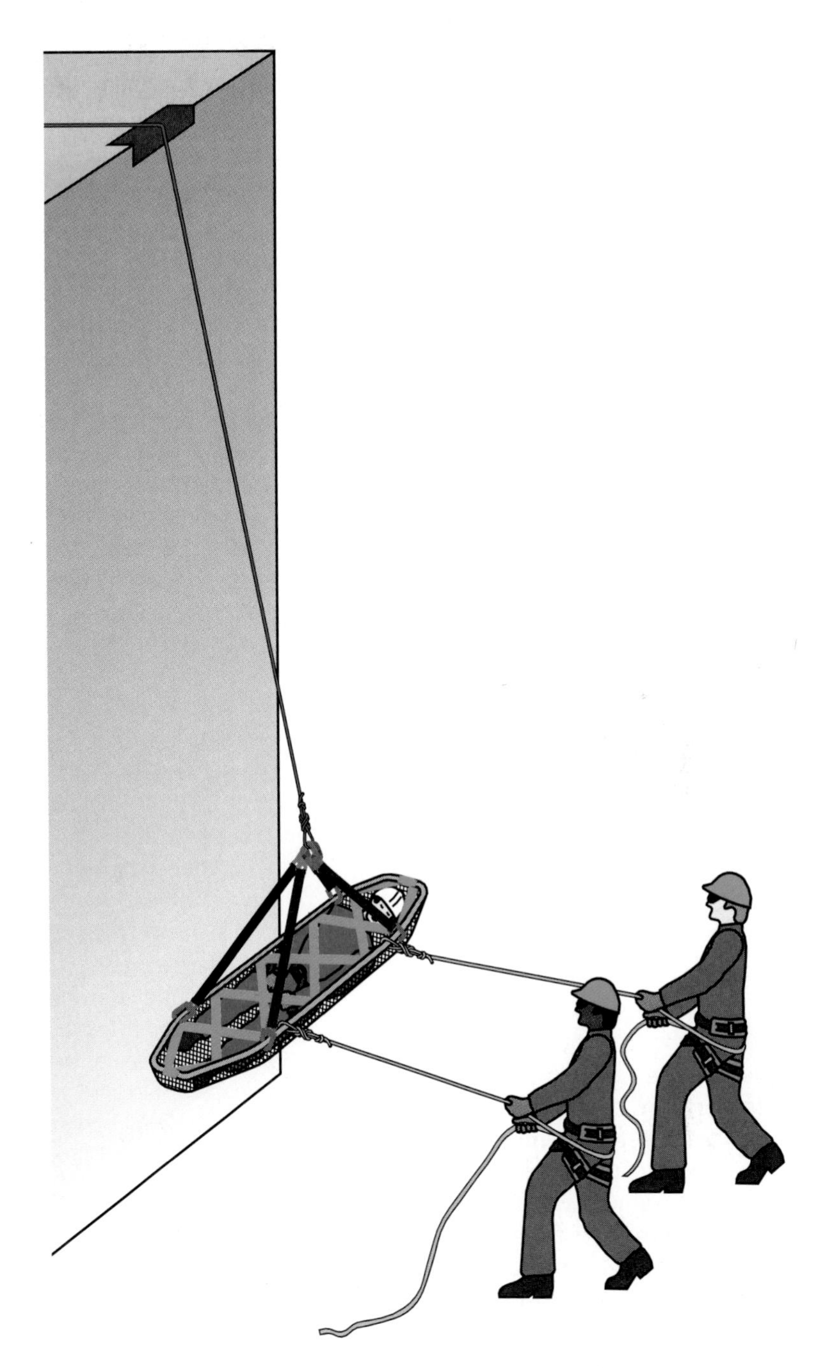

Figure 11.17 **Once near the ground, tag men should pull the litter away from the fall zone (safety line belay not shown.)**

Vertical Single-Line Litter Lower with Low-Point Anchors

A litter can be lowered vertically instead of horizontally. Vertically configured litter lowers may, however, be more traumatic for extremely apprehensive patients. The fact that patients cannot see the ground during horizontal lowers adds much to their comfort. The opposite is true of patients in vertically configured litters. If conscious, they can see everything around and below them. The vertically configured lower is also less desirable for a patient with spinal injury. This is largely because of compression of the spine due to gravity when the patient is in a standing position. Sometimes, however, it is unavoidable.

Although a horizontal lower generally seems better for the patient, many situations require a vertically configured litter. Confined spaces often have narrow or limited openings through which the litter must fit. Structures with a multitude of obstructions or narrow windows can be negotiated more easily with a vertical litter. The following lowering system assumes that a vertical litter must be used and there is no high-point anchor.

Nearly the entire operation for lowering the vertical litter is identical to that for lowering a horizontal litter. The greatest difference lies in the way the litter is placed over the edge. The safety belay and lowering lines are attached in the same manner as with the horizontal litter lower. Two tag lines are attached near the bottom of the litter on opposite sides (as far apart as possible) rather than on the same side of the litter.

Narrow Opening Procedure

The plumb point must be measured and secured before starting this operation. All lines should be attached to the proper points. All parts of the rescue system must be checked and double checked. Once this has been done, the patient is ready to be placed over the edge.

Lowering a Vertical Litter through Narrow Opening

1. If the opening to be negotiated is narrow, such as a window, the litter must be eased out. It is important to make the following preparations prior to placing the litter through the opening.
   —Loop a piece of tubular webbing, 24 to 30 feet long, around the side rails near the bottom of the litter (see Figure 11.18). This will be used to prevent the foot of the litter from slipping over the side. The webbing is tensioned and slowly released to allow the litter to cantilever over the side under control. If desired, two pieces of webbing can be used, one on each side. If tag lines are used for the lower, they can be used in place of the webbing.
   —The rescue master should check and double-check all rigging. This should be done for all rope rescues prior to life loading the system.
   —The brakeman should have the descent control device locked off or rigged for maximum friction (six bars if using a rappel rack) to secure it while placing the litter over the edge. The brakeman should be positioned in an appropriate and secure manner and ready to operate the device. The plumb point must be set properly.
   —The belayman should be on the safety-line belay system with slack out, ready to operate it.
   —A four-man lift team is desired, two on each side of the litter near the head and foot.
2. When the rescue master gives the okay, the lift team should lift the litter and walk it, feet first, toward the opening. As with all rescue operations, if a team member is close enough to an edge to fall, he or she should be rigged securely to an anchor system.
3. The two lift team members at the foot of the litter should approach the opening while each holds one of the webbing loops or tag lines attached to the foot of the litter.
4. Place the foot end of the litter through the opening.
5. While the two lift team members at the head continue to ease the litter through the opening, the two at the foot release the litter and grasp the webbing loops or tag lines with both hands and bend the webbing over the nearest edge to create friction.
6. As the litter is eased through the opening, the foot of the litter begins to slip. The webbing loops or tag lines use friction to create a cantilever and prevent the foot of the litter from dropping.
7. The team members continue to lower the litter through the opening until the lowering line is taut and the webbing loops are loose. This should be done in one quick and fluid motion, taking no more than seconds to complete. Moving too slowly with certain flexible litters can prolong pressure on some of the components. This can cause minor damage to the litter.
8. Once the litter is loaded on the lowering line, the two lift team members at the foot can release one end of their webbing loop and pull the other end, removing it from the litter in preparation for lowering. If the tag lines instead of webbing loops were used to assist, be sure the area below the litter is clear before dropping them. This may prevent injury to workers or bystanders who are in a position to be struck by the falling rope.
9. The tagmen, if used as part of the lift team, can now take their tag line stations.
10. The rescue master gives the command, "prepare to lower" and checks to make sure the belay and brakemen are ready. Continue the lower as with the horizontal litter lower.
11. The tagmen should spread out and slightly away from the structure to prevent the litter from spinning. If the lower is in a tight area that would not allow the tagmen to spread out, they should pull straight down on the tag lines to stabilize the litter and prevent spinning.

WARNING

As with a horizontal lower, when using a wire basket litter, you must watch carefully to prevent hanging its horizontal members on an edge or projection. This could create a significant drop and shock load if the litter suddenly becomes free.

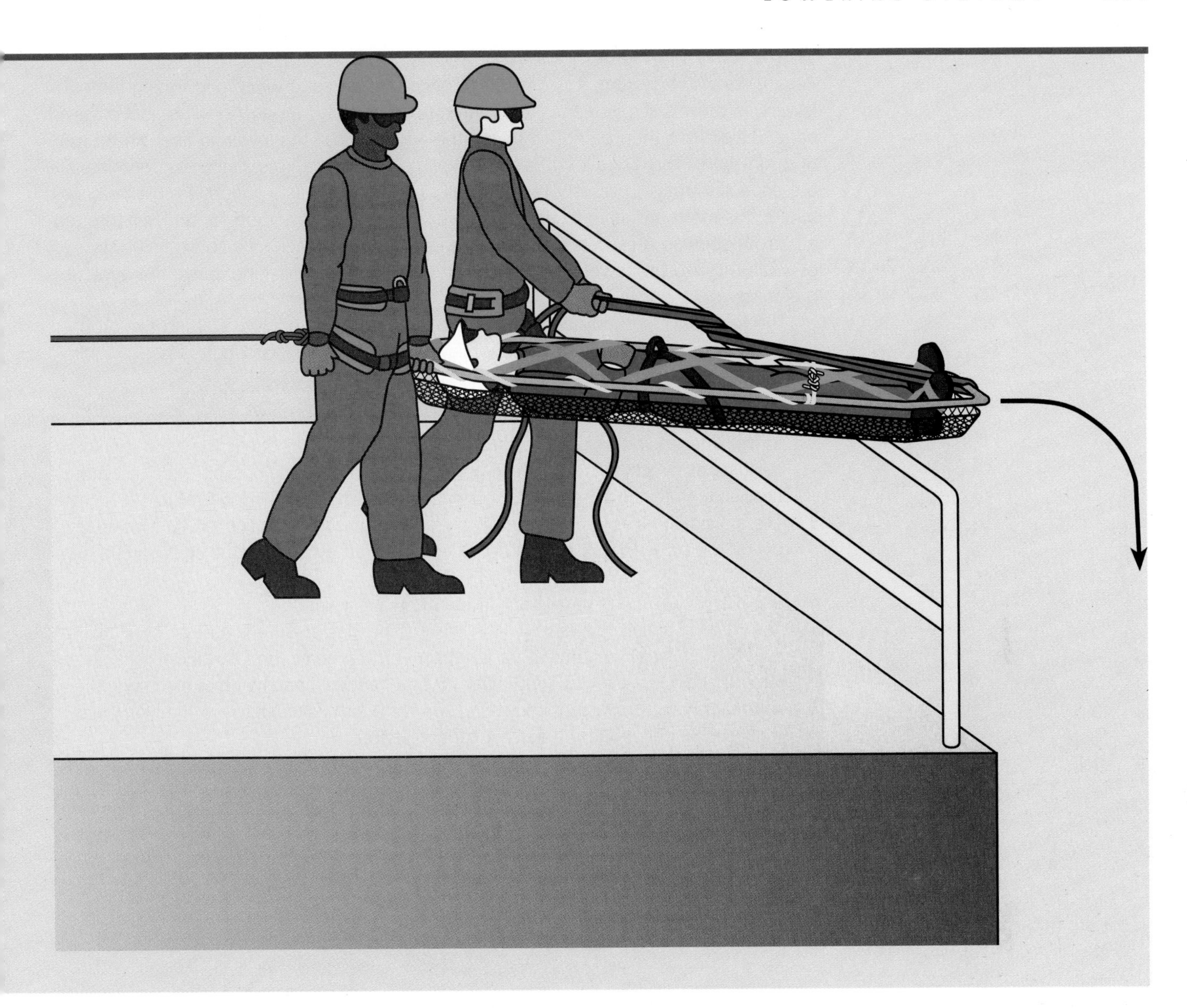

Figure 11.18 Wrapping webbing around litter rail for friction.

Large Openings Procedure

If a vertical litter lower is indicated and the opening is large and unrestricted (the length of the litter), rescuers can use a different procedure to place the litter over the edge. Before starting this procedure, they must secure the plumb point and take all of the precautions previously mentioned for vertical lowers with narrow openings.

1. The lift team members position themselves on the same side of the litter, as if performing a horizontal lower, and place the litter lengthwise on the edge.
2. The lift team member at the foot holds a single loop of webbing, which has been wrapped around the foot of the litter, and wraps it over the edge to create friction. This webbing loop is used in much the same manner as for a lower through a narrow opening. It is used to lower the foot of the litter into a plumb position. If rescuers use tag lines with the lower, one tag line can be used instead of a webbing loop to serve the same function.
3. The team then eases the foot of the litter off the edge, allowing the webbing loop or tag line to lower the foot slowly until it reaches a plumb position. A rescuer can then remove the webbing loop from the litter and the team can complete the lower. Remember to be cautious when releasing a tag line to prevent injury to persons below.

Single-Line High-Point Lowers

Regardless of the system, it is difficult to negotiate an edge when performing litter lowers. In most cases, a team should attempt to establish an anchor high above the edge. Pulleys can then be rigged above the edge so that the lowering line can be run through them. This will allow the rescue team to raise the litter higher to negotiate the edge smoothly. In cases where a small opening (such as a window) must be negotiated, it is more desirable to use the previously described method for a lower through a narrow opening. Rescuers must judge based on their experience and training. In general, running the lowering line through directional pulleys high above the edge is preferred.

The following method does not require a plumb point prior to starting the procedure. Instead, the litter will be lifted while slack is removed (see Figure 11.19).

1. The rescue master commands the brakeman to prepare to take up slack.
2. After receiving an okay from the rescue master, the lift team uses proper techniques to lift the litter to waist or even chest height (the higher, the better). The team should be standing as directly under the high-point directional pulley as possible without being near enough to the edge to drop the patient over the side. THIS IS CRITICAL!
3. The brakeman takes up ALL slack and returns to maximum friction (six-bars on a rappel rack) on the descent control device and locks off (wrap the rope up if using a rappel rack).
4. The belayer also takes up all slack in the safety belay line.
5. The lift team simply releases the litter, now suspended in air, and eases it over the edge. Often, small amounts of slack remain in the system. The following technique can remove additional slack to get the litter over a handrail or some other high edge.
   —A team member grasps the lowering line with both hands between the high-point directional pulley and the descent control device.
   —He or she then pulls downward with his or her body weight to lift the litter an additional few inches. This sounds like a minor adjustment but can have a major effect on the edge negotiation.
6. The lower continues as previously described.

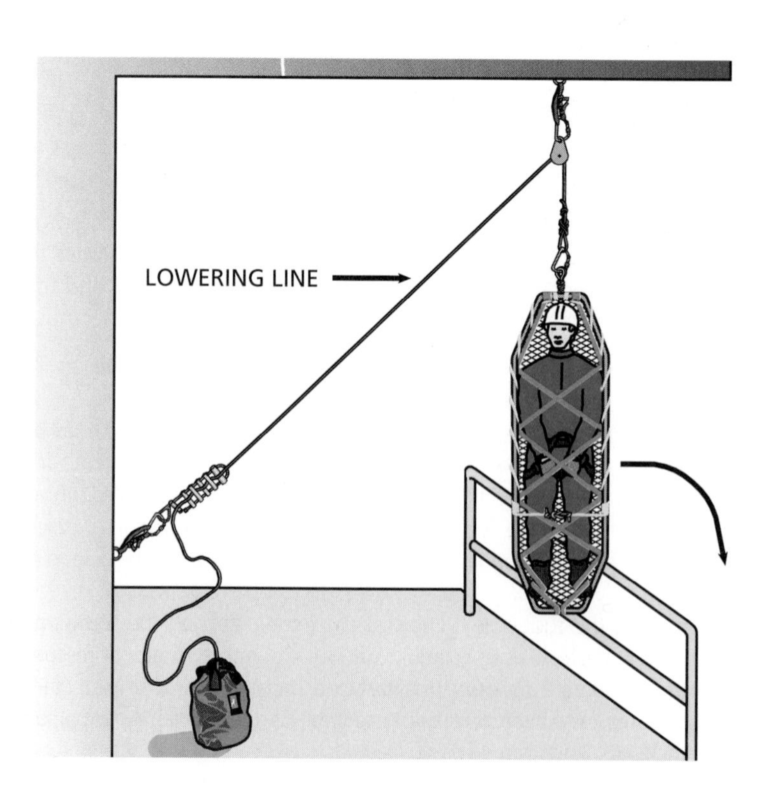

Figure 11.19 Single-line high-point lowering (Safety line belay not shown. Pictured systems may not portray ideal anchorages. Team members/rescuers not shown.)

Stairwell Lower

The stairwell lowering system uses the same basic technique as a horizontally configured single-line litter lower.

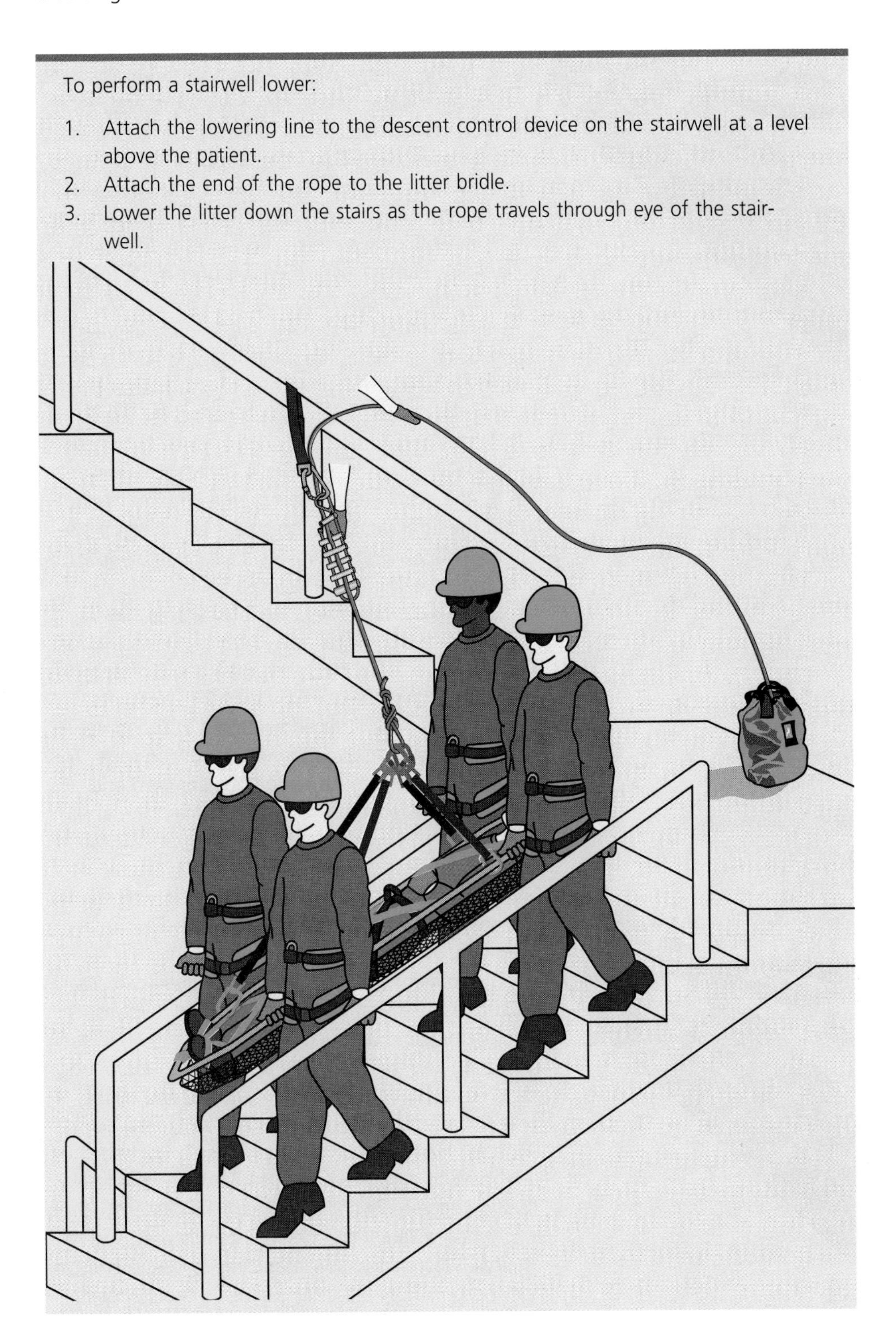

To perform a stairwell lower:

1. Attach the lowering line to the descent control device on the stairwell at a level above the patient.
2. Attach the end of the rope to the litter bridle.
3. Lower the litter down the stairs as the rope travels through eye of the stairwell.

The "well eye," or "well hole," is a narrow space between the center beams of most continuous scissor-type stairwells that runs from the top of the stairway to the bottom. This is not the case for all designs and configurations of stairs. Stairwell lowers work well on most fire escapes and interior stairwells. Many split-level stair configurations found in industrial process units are not conducive to this type of lowering system because they lack a continuous well eye.

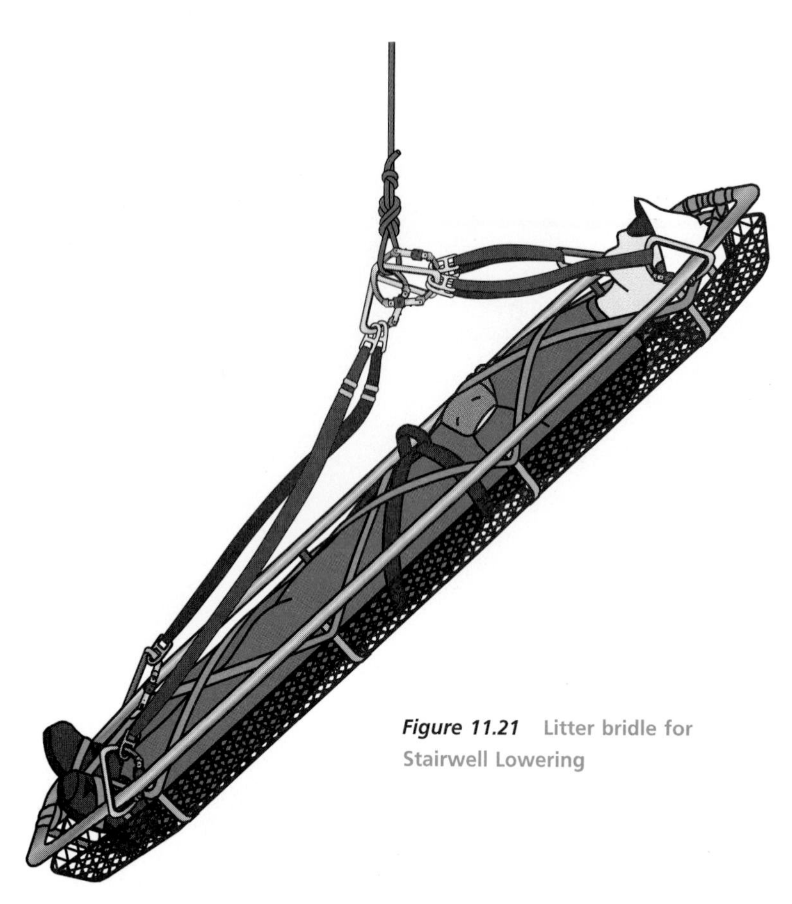

Figure 11.21 Litter bridle for Stairwell Lowering

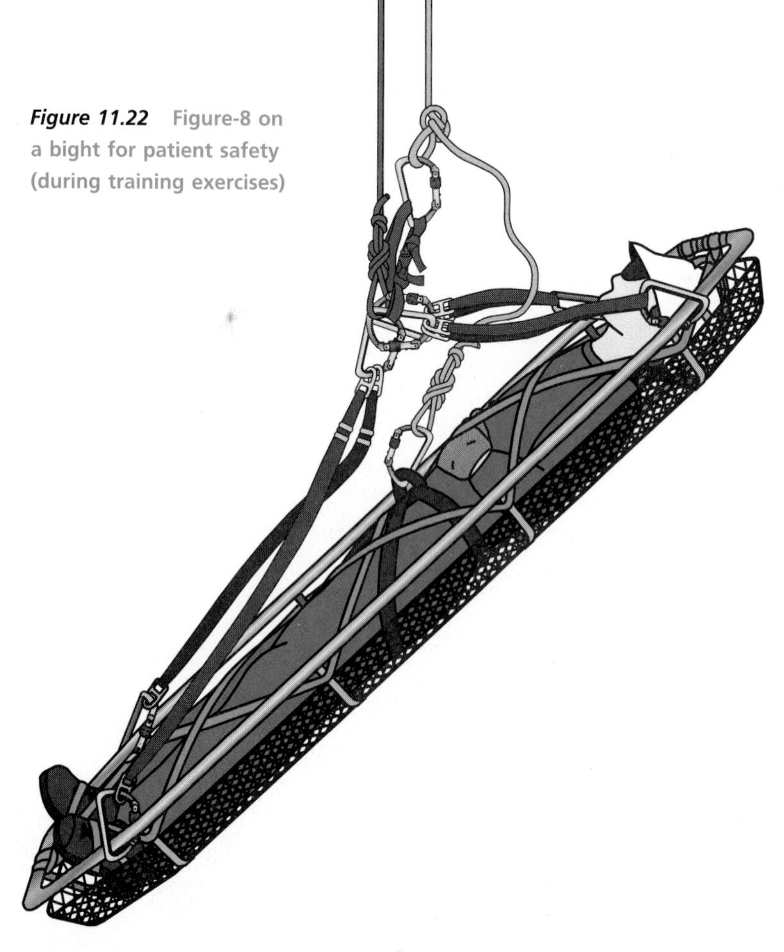

Figure 11.22 Figure-8 on a bight for patient safety (during training exercises)

If feasible, this method of lowering can be a very practical and frequent application of rope rescue. Rescuers commonly carry sick or injured persons down stairwells. This poses the dangerous potential both for back strain and for dropping the patient. Employing an evacuation method that quickly and safely takes the load off the rescuer yet accomplishes the goal clearly saves time and effort.

For the stairwell lower, a basket or flexible litter can be used. A flexible litter works better in very narrow stairwells such as an exterior fire escape.

A safety line belay system is not usually required for stairwell lowers. This is because the lift team maintains contact with the litter during the lower and acts as the safety to hold it in place should the lowering line fail. However, line failure is always a possibility, so the optimum lift crew for this type of rescue is two at the head and two at the foot of the litter to walk down with it during the lower. This crew should be positioned and ready to hold the litter in place if a line fails. If for some reason (e.g., the stairs are too steep), the lift crew cannot hold the litter well enough to act as a backup system while walking down the stairs, a safety line belay system is the logical backup.

For a stairwell lower, the litter should have a single-point horizontal bridle, which allows the feet to ride lower than the head at an angle of approximately 45 degrees (see Figure 11.21). Rescuers should lower the litter and rotate it 180 degrees at each stair level to avoid pendulum of the rope. This pendulum could cause dangerous abrasion and could cut the rope if allowed to contact the abrasive metal of concrete edges on the underside of most stairs. Prior to the lower, rescuers should always inspect the stairwell beams at the well eye to identify abrasion that can be eliminated with padding.

If a patient safety is desired, rescuers can create it in one of several ways. One method involves using an in-line knot (such as a butterfly knot) in the lowering line for the bridle attachment, and a loop (such as a figure-8 on a bight) at the end of the line for attachment to the patient's harness (see Figure 11.22). Rescuers can also use a utility belt or webbing to create a safety link between the litter bridle and the patient (see Figure 11.23).

When a safety line belay system is used with a stairwell lower, twisting it and the lowering line can be a problem as the litter rotates in the stairwell. To alleviate this problem, rescuers can attach a rescue-grade swivel device between the two ropes and the litter bridle (see Figure 11.24). This device allows the litter to rotate completely without lines twisting. One type of swivel allows attachment of three large carabiners on one end and only one on the other. The litter bridle carabiners could be attached to a triangular screw link, which can then

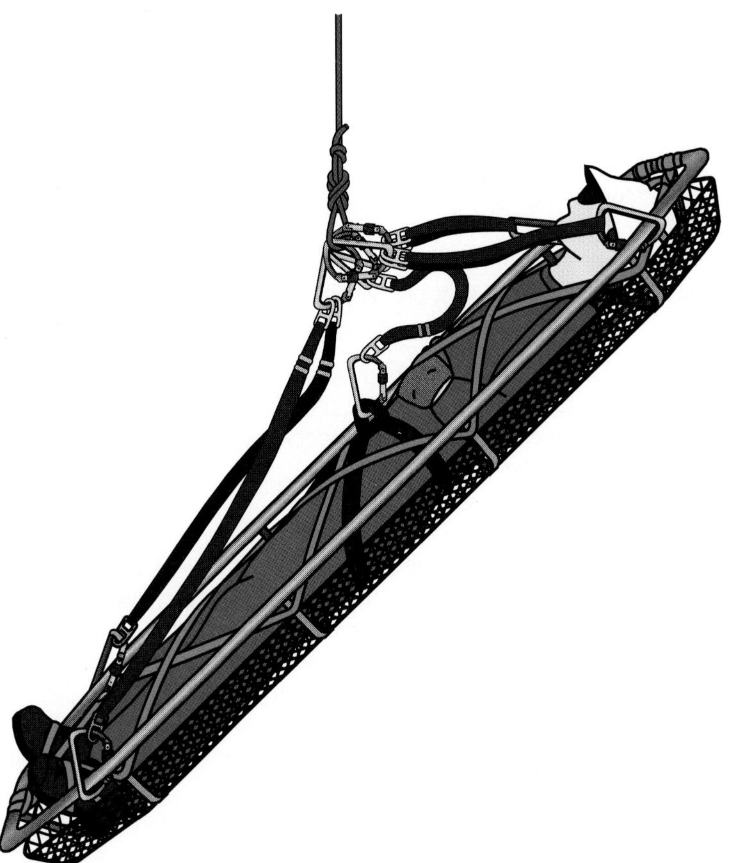

Figure 11.23 Utility belt for patient safety

WARNING

Be aware that reaction times can be slowed considerably with this type of communication. Try to anticipate these problems and relay communications immediately.

Figure 11.24 Litter bridle carabiners attached to the main line with a swivel

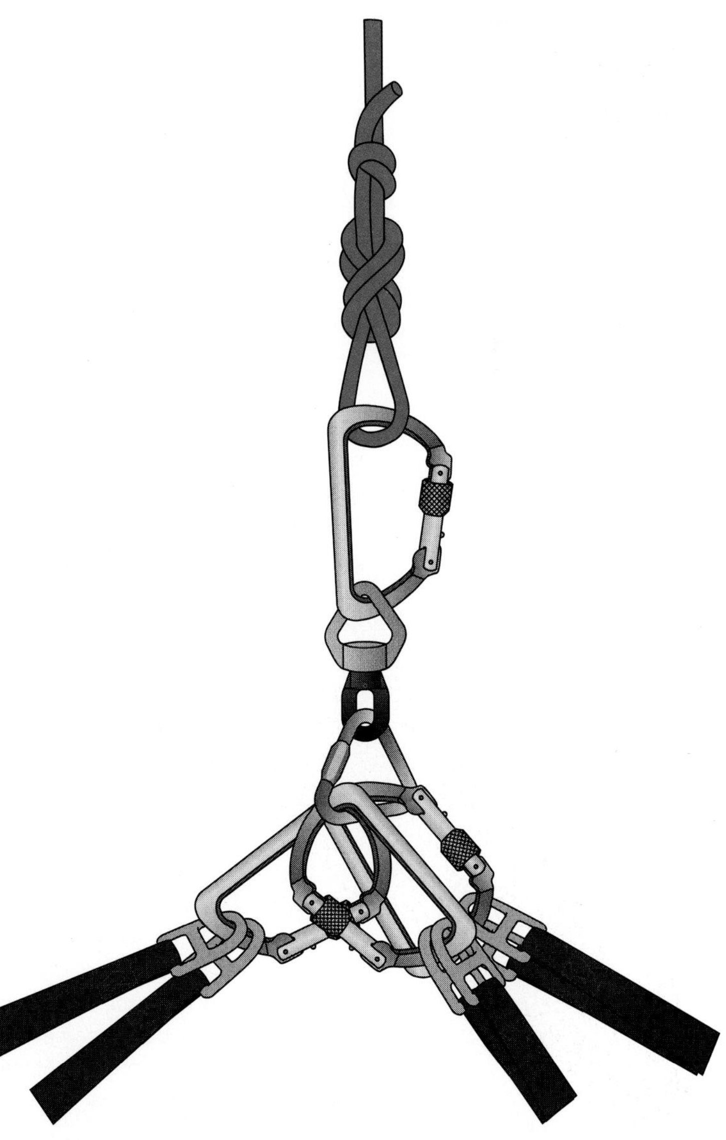

be attached by a carabiner to the bottom connection of the swivel.

As the litter is lowered through the well eye, rescuers turn it into the stairwell at each landing, being careful not to swing back and forth. Pendulum can damage the rope very quickly if it makes contact with a sharp or abrasive edge.

Depending on the height of the stairwell, communications between the lift crew and brakeman can be difficult. In these cases, portable radios provide one of the most desirable means of communication. If radios are not available, it is wise to place personnel at intermediate points (every few landing levels). One person on the lift crew should be designated to communicate to the brakeman. Commands should be relayed from the lift crew to the brakeman through the intermediate contacts.

Double-Line Litter Lowering

As the name implies, double-line systems differ from single-line systems by using two ropes attached to the litter. Some rescuers use a single descent control device for both ropes. However, two devices, one for each rope, are recommended because they make operation of the lowering lines safer. Also, double-line systems allow the lowering lines to be operated independently of each other to change the angle of the litter if necessary. This system has at least two advantages over single-line systems:

- The double lines create a built-in back-up system. Each rope backs up the other in the event of a failure. In most situations, there is no need for a separate safety line belay system.
- Rescuers can change the position of the litter easily by stopping the lower on one line while continuing it on the other. This is helpful when negotiating obstacles or attempting to clear a patient's airway if he or she vomits.

The double-line system also has certain disadvantages. It requires an increase in both personnel and equipment to set up and operate properly. Double-line systems require a rescue master, two brakemen, a three- or four-person lifting crew (four preferred), two tagmen, and a line tender.

Procedure

This section reviews a double-line system that requires two independent descent control devices, one for each lowering line. Although certain brake devices allow both lines to run through the same device, it may be more difficult to control each line independently. Two devices also have the distinct advantage of an inherent backup in the lowering system. Should one line fail, the other will be maintained independently. The failure will still be traumatic to the patient, but perhaps the additional line will prevent injury or death, which is otherwise certain.

One procedure for operating a two-device double-line litter lower with low-point anchors is described below:

1. First lash the patient into the litter and attach the lowering lines to the double-line litter bridle.
2. Attach one line to the head and the other to the foot of the litter.
3. If using a low-point anchor, establish an approximate plumb point for the end of each rope. An exact measurement is not critical with a double-line system because slack can be adjusted in the lines, one rope at a time. This means that at least one rope is always attached and secured to a descent control device during the process. If the litter accidently slips over the edge, although it may be traumatic, the patient will not fall to the ground.
4. Attach and secure the lowering lines to the litter and the descent control devices. Since the load is being distributed between two descent control devices, the friction setting normally used with a single-line system would probably create excessive friction in a double-line system. For example, it is recommended that a rappel rack for a single-line system (with a one-person load) be placed on six bars while rescuers negotiate the edge and on a minimum of five bars while they lower a litter. If five bars are used for lowering on each rappel rack in a double-line system, the combination may provide too much friction (the equivalent of ten bars), depending on the load distribution. With rappel racks, at least four bars on each descent control device are recommended when rescuers are placing over the edge or lowering a one-person load. Regardless of the descent control device, rescuers should consider and compensate for this factor for load distribution.
5. Both brakemen should be in the appropriate positions, in complete control of their respective devices, and ready to lower.
6. Lay out or bag excess rope behind the descent control devices and place a person in position (if available) to monitor the ropes as they feed into the devices. The optional team member in this position is a "line tender." His or her job is

to prevent tangling or knotting of the ropes, which might hinder the operation of the descent control devices.

7. The lift crew lifts and rolls the litter at a 45-degree angle toward their bodies with the outside rail up.
8. With the litter in this position, rescuers place the inside rail on the edge. This is identical to the procedure described for the single-line horizontal litter lower with a low-point anchor.
9. The brakemen then take up the slack one at a time. The brakeman at the foot is designated "foot," the brakeman at the head is designated "head." The rescue master designates which brakeman is to remove slack (i.e., "Take up slack on head"). The other brakeman remains secured with his or her descent control device until commanded to take up slack by the rescue master. To take up slack on a rappel rack:
   A. Go to three bars (including the top bar).
   B. Hold the sides of the top bar with the thumb and forefinger of one hand pulling the rack away from the anchor and in line with the rope's path.
   C. With the other hand, pull all of the slack rope through the rack.
   D. Wrap the rope up around the second bar and continue to wrap in bars until four bars have been wrapped securely.
   E. Advise the rescue master of your readiness (i.e., "Ready on foot!").
10. After both brakemen have removed all slack in their lines, the lift crew eases the litter out over the edge as previously described in the section on single-line horizontal lowers. The brakemen remain on four bars minimum during the lower.
11. The tagmen can then go to the ground. Tagmen fulfill the same objectives with any lower: keep the litter away from obstacles and guide it around projections and obstructions.

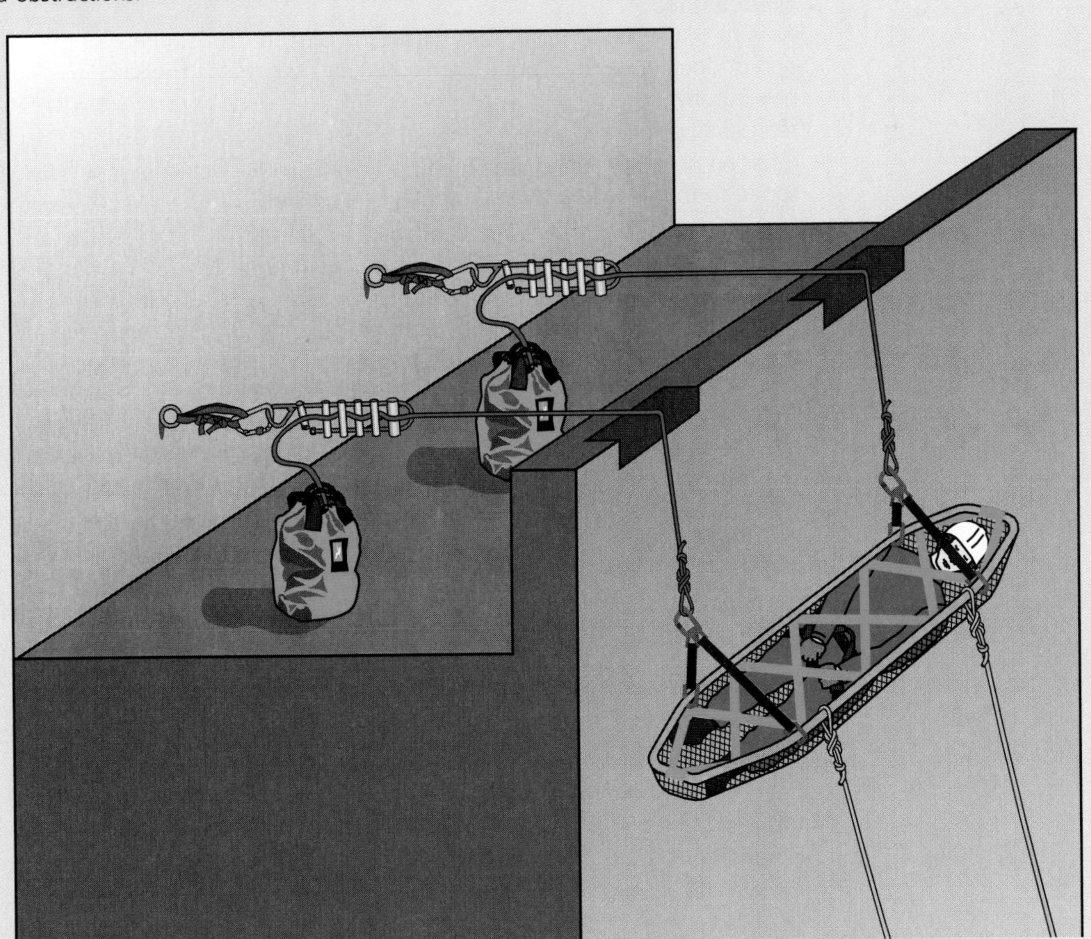

Communication

The rescue master gives signals for the lower. As already discussed, proper signals are important during a lowering operation with a single-line system. These signals are even more crucial when coordinating the movement of two lowering lines. If lowering does not take place in a coordinated manner, the patient's position is acutely affected.

The signals presented here for double-line systems are only slight modifications of those covered previously. The difference is that rescuers use both hands. Each hand coordinates the movements of one lowering line.

Verbal Signals

Because two lines are involved, an identifier must be used in verbal signals to designate the action of the foot and head lines. The following verbal signals represent coordinated movements of each of the lowering lines to accomplish a specific litter position:

- "Head"—This command indicates lowering on the head line and stopping on the foot line. It is used to lower the head of the litter.
- "Foot"—This command indicates lowering on the foot line and stopping on the head line. It is used to lower the foot of the litter.
- "Both"—This command indicates lowering of both lines simultaneously. Brakemen make every effort to lower at the same speed. It may be possible for brakemen to see movement of the other lowering line in their peripheral vision well enough to coordinate lowering speed. However, their primary attention should always be directed toward the rescue master.
- "ON THE GROUND"—This command indicates that the litter has reached the ground.

Hand Signals

As with single-line systems, some situations require visual signals for effective operation of double-line lowering system. The hand signals are the same as single-line signals but involve both hands, one for each line. The foot brakeman watches the hand representing the foot lowering line. The head brakeman watches the rescue master's other hand, which represents the head lowering line. The following hand signals correspond to the designated verbal signals (see Figure 11.26):

- Keeping the HEAD hand in the LOWER position and the FOOT hand in the STOP position corresponds to the verbal command "head."
- Keeping the FOOT hand in the LOWER position and the HEAD hand in the STOP position corresponds to the verbal command "foot."
- Keeping both hands in the LOWER position corresponds to the verbal command "both."
- Holding both clenched fists high in the air corresponds to the verbal command "on the ground."

From above, the rescue master often finds it difficult to judge accurately the angle of the litter during the lower. Depth perception becomes more difficult as the litter travels farther away from the rescue master. Thus, it may be difficult to keep the head of the litter in a correct position relative to the foot.

One method of dealing with this problem is to have one person on the ground in a position to see the litter from the side. From a side view this person is usually in a good position to judge the attitude of the litter and can relay this information to the rescue master. One method of signaling the rescue master involves having the groundman hold both arms out to either side (similar to airplane wings) and lean as the litter tips. If the litter is level, the groundman's arms remain level. If the left side of the litter is down, the groundman leans to his or her left, and so forth. This method deals with the difficulty of judging depth in most cases. Many other methods (e.g., radio communications from a tagman) can be effective. Rescuers use whatever works based on resources and the situation.

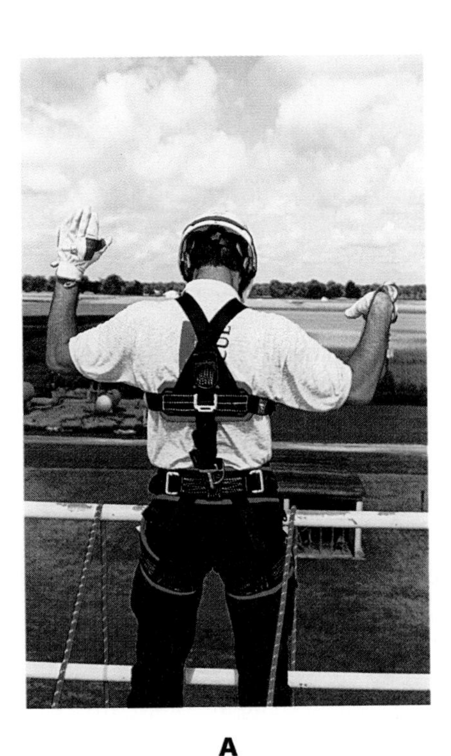

A

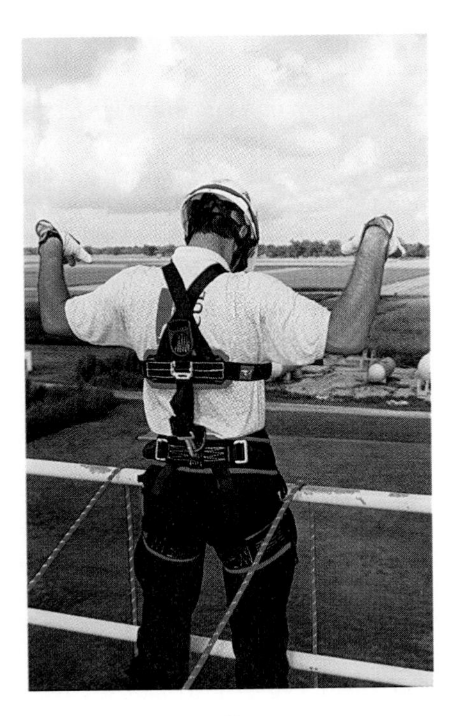

B

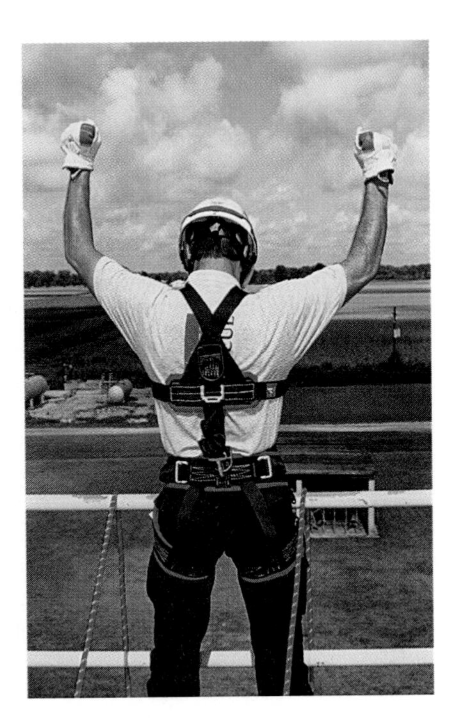

C

Figure 11.26 A–C Hand signals for double-line litter lowering

Litter Attendants

Sometimes it is necessary to attach a person or persons to the litter for a lower. There are usually two reasons for doing so:

- A patient requires constant contact because of apprehension or a need for medical attention.
- Ledges or projections of some type must be negotiated during the course of the lower but tag lines are not possible due to obstructions.

In industrial rescue, there is usually very little critical medical care performed during a lower. This is because most lowers are very short (less than 40 feet) and most teams focus on a strategy of

1. performing definitive patient care right up until time to lower,
2. stopping care followed by immediate and rapid lowering, and
3. resuming definitive care as soon as the patient is within reach of qualified personnel.

In critical situations, rescuers can resume care of the patient within a couple of minutes following cessation. If this cannot be done and/or definitive care is needed, a litter attendant or attendants should be positioned in such a way as to perform the required care. Focus on immediately life-threatening problems while on line.

Rescuers may wish to consider the effectiveness of cardiopulmonary resuscitation (CPR) during a lower. It may be quite time consuming and difficult to set up and perform effective CPR during the ride. It might be better to perform CPR during packaging and until the last minute. Then stop, quickly lower the patient to the ground, and resume CPR. It can be quite difficult to perform effective CPR while riding a litter as an attendant. It is possible but not often expedient in industrial and structural rescues.

Although critical care may not be a reason to use attendants in many rescue situations, relief of a patient's apprehension certainly is. Laypersons are not accustomed to being suspended on a small-diameter rope far above the ground. It tends to make them frightened and agitated. It may even cause deterioration of their already diminished conditions. A litter attendant can do much to help relieve or reduce the patient's apprehension. Just being there, face to face, to comfort the patient can make all the

WARNING

When an attendant is on a vertical litter lower, it is easy for the attendant's rigging to make contact with the patient's face during the lower. Be alert to the positioning of the rigging with relation to the patient's body. Push yourself out and away from or to the side of the litter to prevent further injury or discomfort to the already sick or injured patient. Remember, you are not glued to the litter. You CAN move around. Use it to your and your patient's advantage.

difference in the world. Consider litter attendants with any lower of an apprehensive patient.

The other common reason for litter attendants involves the negotiation or avoidance of obstacles, ledges, or other projections. This is very common in the industrial environment where hot and cold pipes, pipe racks, and other nuisances abound. Although tag lines usually aid negotiation of these obstructions, proper positioning might be impossible due to the proximity of other structures.

Another consideration involves the number of attendants. Although it may seem unnecessary to use more than one litter attendant in most rescues, the situation might legitimately dictate two. When a patient's care (contact) and negotiation of obstacles are both part of the same scenario, the reason is easy to see.

Two litter attendants may sometimes be needed based on the situation. If this is required, a double-line system must be used to provide the appropriate safety factor for system strength.

The methods discussed here involve adjustable anchor straps called utility belts. The attachment methods described for horizontally configured litters assume that a utility belt bridle has been used (as described in chapter 9). There are many other excellent methods for attaching attendants to the litter. They may range from rappelling or lowering a rescuer in unison with the litter lower to attachment with any combination of ropes, webbing, or special-purpose equipment such as etriers (short ladders made of webbing). Many elaborate systems are available that have been derived from the complexities of cave and wilderness rescue. They also work well for the industrial environment. Choose a method streamlined for speed and efficiency that allows a full range of motion to all parts of the litter with your hands or feet. This will prevent attachment of the attendant from slowing the rescue effort while providing the mobility to negotiate obstacles. Attendants should always be supported by the lowering line(s) of the system, not by the litter structure alone.

One Attendant

Single-Line Lowering System

In all operations involving litter attendants, the litter is placed over the edge first. Rescuers lower the litter no farther over the edge than absolutely necessary. The farther the litter is over the edge, the farther the litter attendant must be lowered before loading the system.

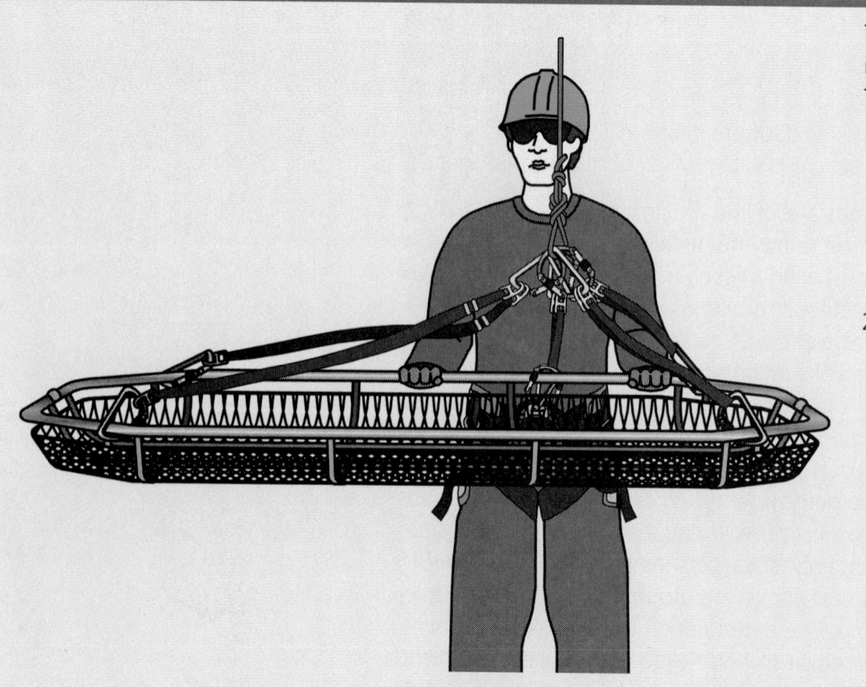

There are many simple methods of placing an attendant on a single-line system. The attendant should be:

1. attached to the lowering line with an adjustable or preadjusted rigging system or rope long enough to allow good mobility and strong enough to adequately support a one-person load, and
2. attached to the litter with rigging to allow the rescuer to pull the litter away from obstacles. This attachment can also be rigged to provide a second point of contact, although attachment to a safety line belay system is more appropriate.

In a horizontal single-line litter lower, the attendant can even be attached to the end of the lowering line itself with a loop (such as a figure-8 knot) while the litter bridle is attached to an in-line knot (such as a butterfly knot) in the same rope a couple of feet from the loop. The attendant could then use a carabiner to attach his or her harness to a structural member of the litter for easy manipulation of the litter during the lower. A safety line belay system could also be attached to the rescuer and/or litter bridle for added safety.

In a vertical single-line litter lower, the attendant could be attached in the same manner. One method involves the use of an adjustable utility belt (adjusted to allow the attendant to touch down just before the litter, making it easier to negotiate obstacles) attached to a knot in the end of the lowering line (see Figure 11.28). This is the same knot used to attach the litter bridle to the lowering line. This belt could be adjusted at any point where the rescuer could rest his or her weight on an object (such as a handrail or beam).

To allow more mobility, the attendant can be attached to the lowering line with a small rope/pulley mechanical advantage (hauling) system. This would allow the attendant to adjust his or her position up or down as needed. If a safety line belay system is used, the attendant can be attached to the end of the line with a knot, after attachment of the safety line to the litter bridle and patient's harness.

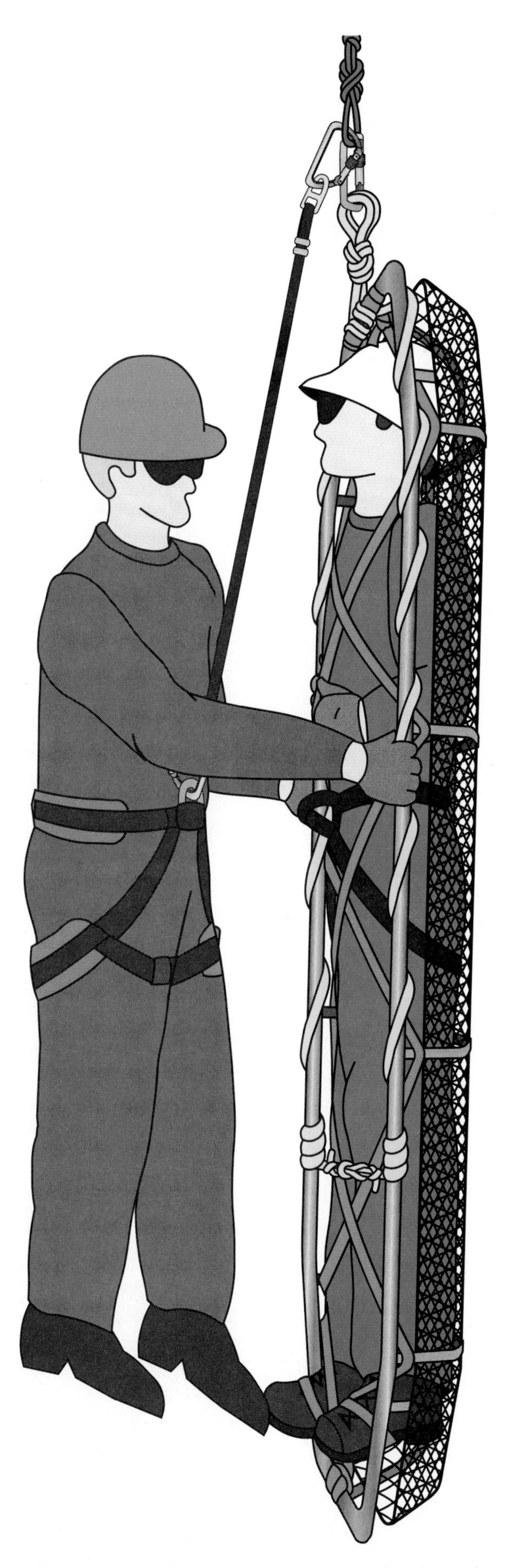

Figure 11.28 Vertical litter lower with one attendant (attendant's feet should be slightly lower than the litter)

Double-Line Lower Method

The following procedure uses a utility belt attachment system. This system allows very little adjustment while suspended online but is prerigged to provide adequate mobility.

1. With a carabiner, attach a utility belt to each lowering line. These belts are usually doubled and must be premeasured to the center point of the outside (side away from the structure from which the litter is lowered) or outside rail of the litter. Some litter structures dictate that the belts be singled (end to end) rather than doubled in order to reach this center point. Make allowances as needed.
2. Take this measurement when the litter is still on the ground, just before placing it over the edge. The goal is for the litter attendant to be attached and suspended at a point near the center of the litter's outside or outside rail and no more than a few inches below the top of it.
3. With a carabiner, attach one end of the doubled utility belts to the head and foot lowering line knots. The ends with the D-rings are preferred to prevent crowding near the top of the litter bridle.
4. Attach the looped ends of the belts to carabiners and allow them to hang loose.
5. Have someone pull the head and foot lowering lines taut (as they would be during a lower) while another rescue team member grasps the carabiners at the lower end of the utility belts and pulls them to a center point on the outside or outside rail of the litter.
6. Adjust the belts to allow the base of the carabiners to meet at a point within an inch or so below the uppermost point of the litter's side or side rail. If this measurement is not taken, the attendant will end up in a position too far above or below the litter to be effective. Allow these utility belts to hang freely in a position easily reached by the attendant once the litter is over the edge.
7. Place the litter over the edge in a horizontal position, as described in the section on single-line horizontal litter lower.
8. With a carabiner, attach the utility belt at the head lowering line to the attendant's harness.
9. During this process, consider a second point of attachment for the attendant. Attachment to a lowering system or safety-line belay system while the attendant is climbing around the edge of the litter attached to the utility belt is a good backup.
10. The attendant climbs over the edge around the head of the litter and positions him- or herself to the side of the patient near the head. Climbing around the head of the patient is important because you must lower the opposite end of the litter in order to reach the carabiner of the second utility belt for attachment to the attendant. If the attendant were to climb around the foot instead, the head of the litter would have to be lowered to make the attendant's second connection. This would place the patient in a heads-down position, which might increase apprehension. Although these points may seem insignificant and do not involve risk of life or limb, they may be key to the patient's psychological well-being and deserve consideration.
11. Now, lower the foot of the litter to allow the attendant access to the utility belt at the foot.
12. With a carabiner, attach the utility belt at the foot of the litter to the attendant's harness.
13. A third attachment can be made with a carabiner to the litter's top rail or lift handles. It will be difficult to place a third carabiner in the attendant's harness attachment point, so attaching in one of the two carabiners already in the harness or a small loop of webbing is acceptable.
14. Lowering should take place using more friction than required for one-person loads. This is due to the increased load of an additional person on the same num-

ber of descent control devices. If using a rappel rack, a minimum of five bars on each of the rappel racks is recommended. For figure-8 descent control devices, a double wrap may be wise.

15. The attendant should have preestablished hand signals for communicating with the rescue master during the descent. The attendant may be able to help the team lower the litter evenly by advising the rescue master of the position of the litter as it is lowered. A radio or hand signals can be effective options.

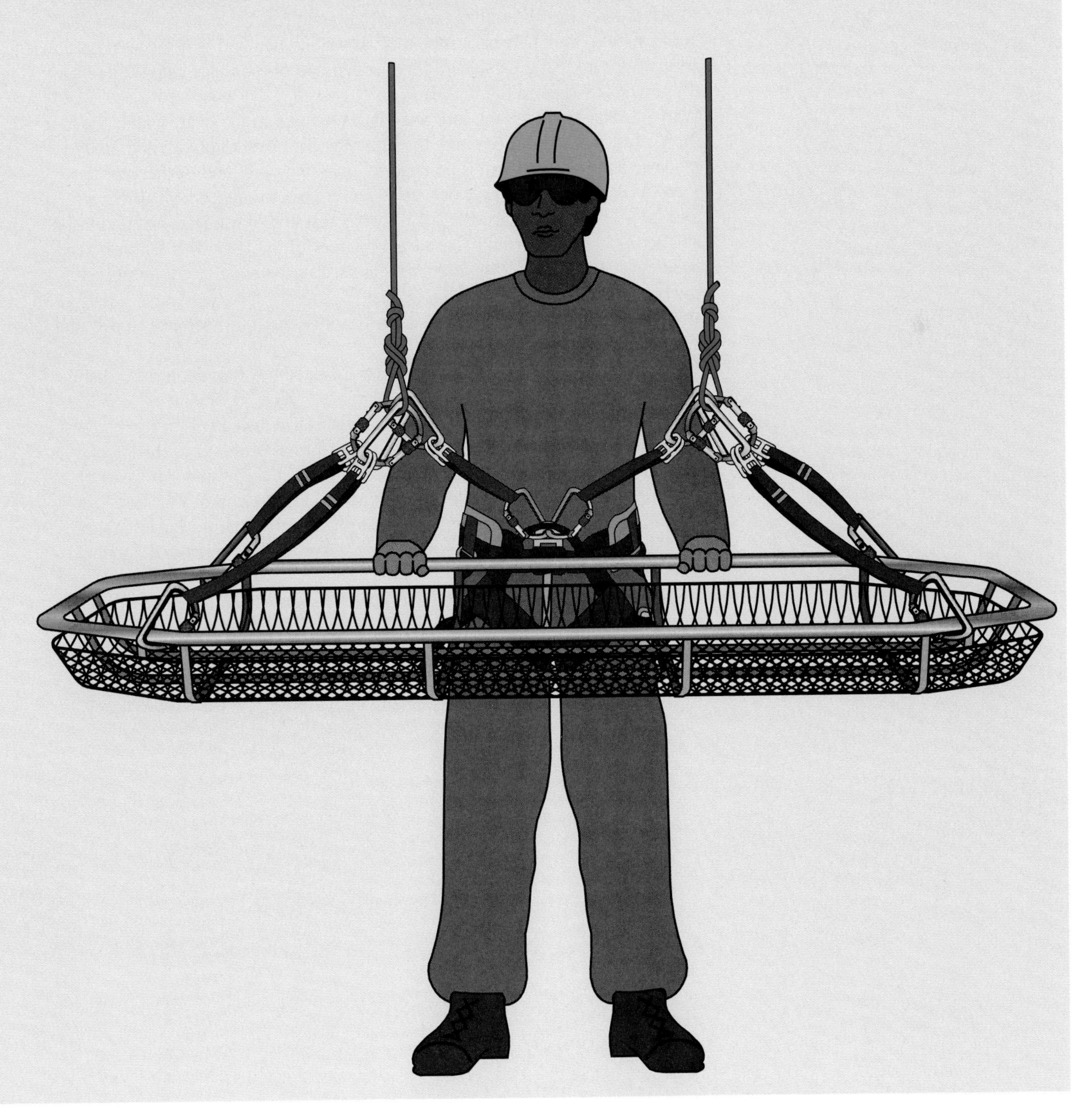

Two Attendants

A lowering rescue that requires two attendants should ***never*** be attempted with a single-line system. The two-attendant system is usually necessary to negotiate a difficult projection or obstruction, or when a patient's care requires it. In this case, the head attendant is usually in a better position to manage the patient while the foot attendant coordinates negotiation of ledges or projections. The foot attendant is also responsible for communicating with the rescue master during the lower.

The following procedure for attachment is similar to the method previously described for one attendant with a double-line system:

1. Attach a utility belt to the head and foot lowering lines.
2. In this system, the utility belts should be fully shortened and doubled, D-rings up. This will ensure that a carabiner in the looped end of the utility belt will be near the top of the litter on the outside.
3. With a carabiner, attach the foot attendant's harness to the utility belt at the foot.
4. With a two-attendant procedure, the foot attendant may climb out and around the litter first because there is no need to lower the other end of the litter to make a connection since only one utility belt is used for attachment. There are also the added advantages of loading the lightest end of the litter first and being able to see and talk to the patient from the foot of the litter. This can help keep a patient calm while the other attendant climbs over the edge to get into position at the head.
5. The foot attendant climbs over the edge after the litter has been placed over the edge.
6. The foot attendant also attaches with a carabiner to the litter's top rail or handholds near the foot.
7. The head attendant then attaches the head-end utility belt to his or her harness and climbs over the edge after the foot attendant has attached to the litter.
8. Some rescuers use a second point of attachment such as a safety line belay or lowering system while each attendant climbs around the end of the litter. This increases safety until the attendant can make the attachment into the litter also.
9. The head attendant also attaches with a carabiner to the top rail or a handhold near the head of the litter.
10. If possible, the friction on the descent control devices should be increased even more due to the additional load of a third person. If using a rappel rack, lowering should take place using a minimum of six bars. Double-wrap figure-8 descent control devices for maximum friction.
11. The head attendant cares for the patient. The foot attendant communicates with the rescue master.

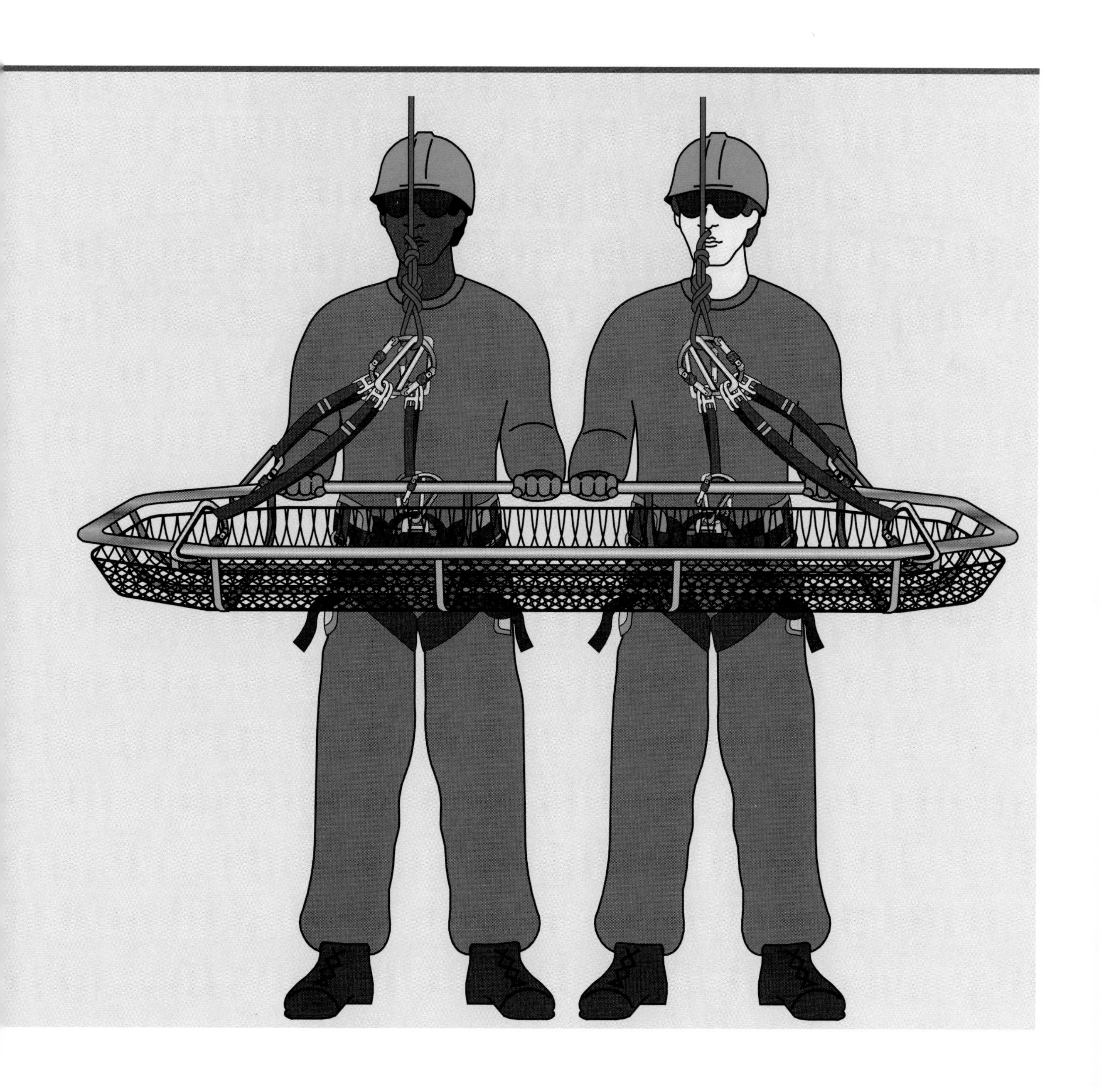

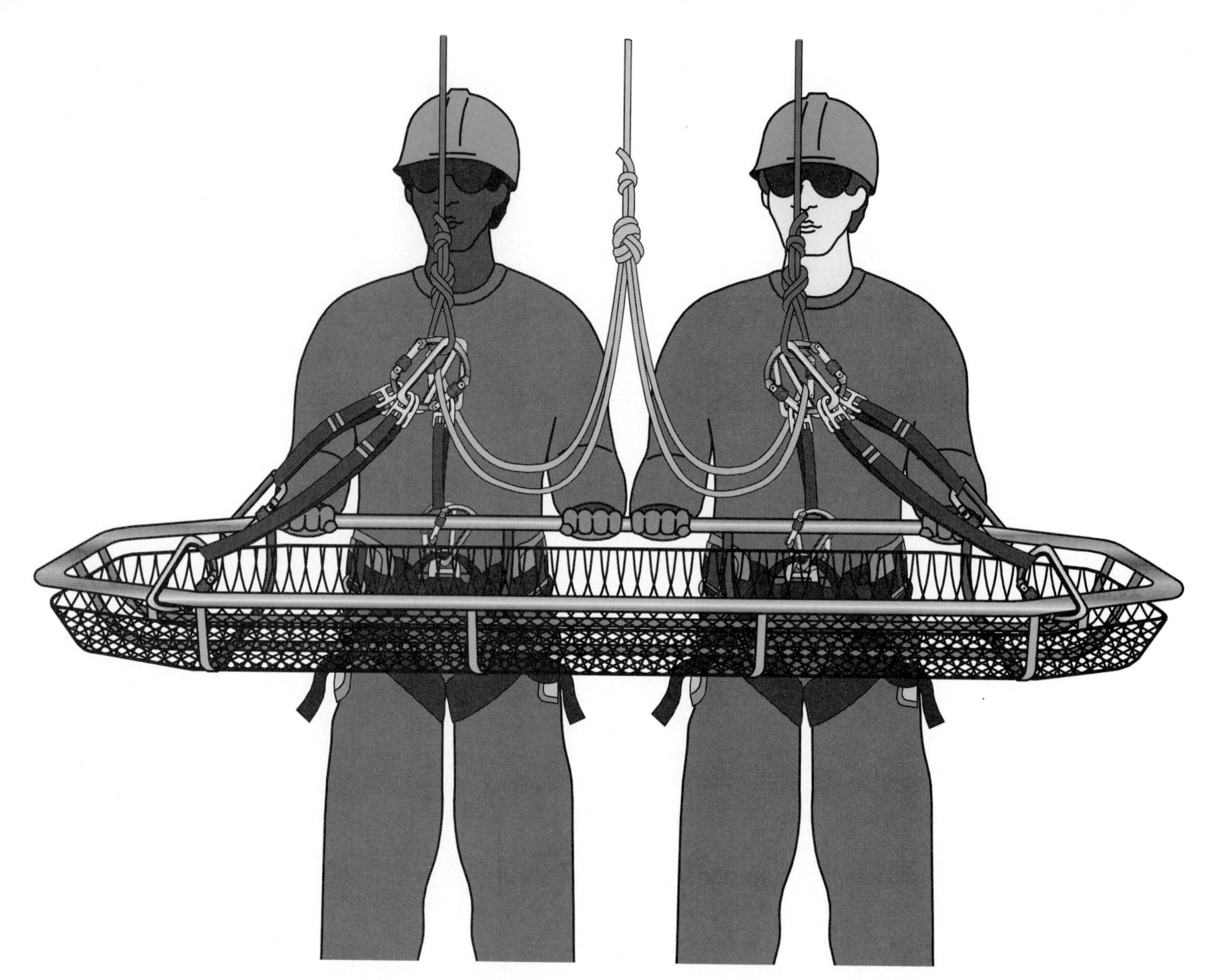

Figure 11.31 Double-line horizontal litter lower with two attendants using safety belay line

If a line fails during a two-attendant litter lower, it can place more than a two-person load on a single line. This is highly unlikely because there is the built-in back-up system provided by a double-line lower. However, rescuers can prevent this by attaching an additional safety line belay system to the litter bridle assembly and both attendant bridles. Rescuers can use a large double-loop figure-8 knot in the end of the safety line with one loop attached to either the head or foot bridles. Attach the other loop attached to the bridle assemblies at the opposite end of the litter (see Figure 11.31). This method reduces the severity of the shock should the failure of one line occur.

Summary

A variety of rope systems can be used to perform a controlled lower of an injured person from an elevation. The techniques discussed in this chapter are not the only safe methods for rescue. The systems presented have been chosen based on proven effectiveness with a high degree of safety. As we have reiterated throughout this text: there is no one right way to accomplish your rescue task. Your team, and in some circumstances, only a few members of your team, have the important job of determining which method to use in getting the patient to safety.

Remember, not just the injured person depends on you to know what you are doing. Your teammates count on you to know how to perform safely and efficiently with the equipment and the team under adverse conditions in stress-filled emergencies. That takes knowledge and practice.

CHAPTER 12

Hauling

The information in this chapter is provided as a basis for continued training. Each rescuer should consult with his or her own team leader for the correct SOGs for the team. Topics covered in this chapter include:

- Pulleys
- Classification of Rope/Pulley Mechanical Advantage Systems
- P-Method

Introduction

Rescuers use hauling systems to lift victims or rescuers vertically (or drag them horizontally in some cases) from in sites such as shafts, vessels, excavations, and below-grade manholes. Rescuers can configure these hauling systems in a variety of ways (vertically, diagonally, or horizontally) as the need arises. These systems rely on the concept of mechanical advantage (M/A) to spread the weight of the load along several ropes and pulleys instead of along a single element (such as one rope). Of course, the more spread out the load (i.e., the greater the M/A), the more time it takes to perform the same work. However, the input force required of the person(s) operating the system is significantly decreased. For example, if you had two 50-pound weights in a big bag and wanted to move them across the room you could choose either to move them all at once or separate the load and make two trips. If you decided to move one weight at a time you would have to travel twice the distance but use only half the force (or energy) for each trip that you would use to pick up both weights at once. This is similar to a 2:1 M/A.

Mechanical advantage is the amount of energy required to move an object. It is stated in a ratio of the weight of the load to the input force required to lift it. Input force is used here to describe the pulling force required of the haul team members. For example, if a 100-pound load can be moved with a rope using 100 pounds of input force, the M/A is 100/100 or 1:1. There is no such thing as a zero mechanical advantage.

If a 100-pound load can be moved with a rope using 50 pounds of input force, the M/A is 100/50 or 2:1. This chapter explains the concepts of creating mechanical advantage with ropes and pulleys. Rescuers need to understand mechanical advantage well enough to create the appropriate hauling system for the situation at hand. They are not limited to two or three specific "hauling system" configurations. With a thorough knowledge of M/A, rescuers have the tools to build virtually any hauling system.

Classification of Rope/Pulley M/A Systems

The three basic classifications for rope/pulley M/A systems are

1. simple M/A
2. compound (or stacked) M/A, and
3. complex M/A.

This chapter concentrates on simple and compound M/A systems. These systems appear to be the most practical for use in the industrial/structural environment. It

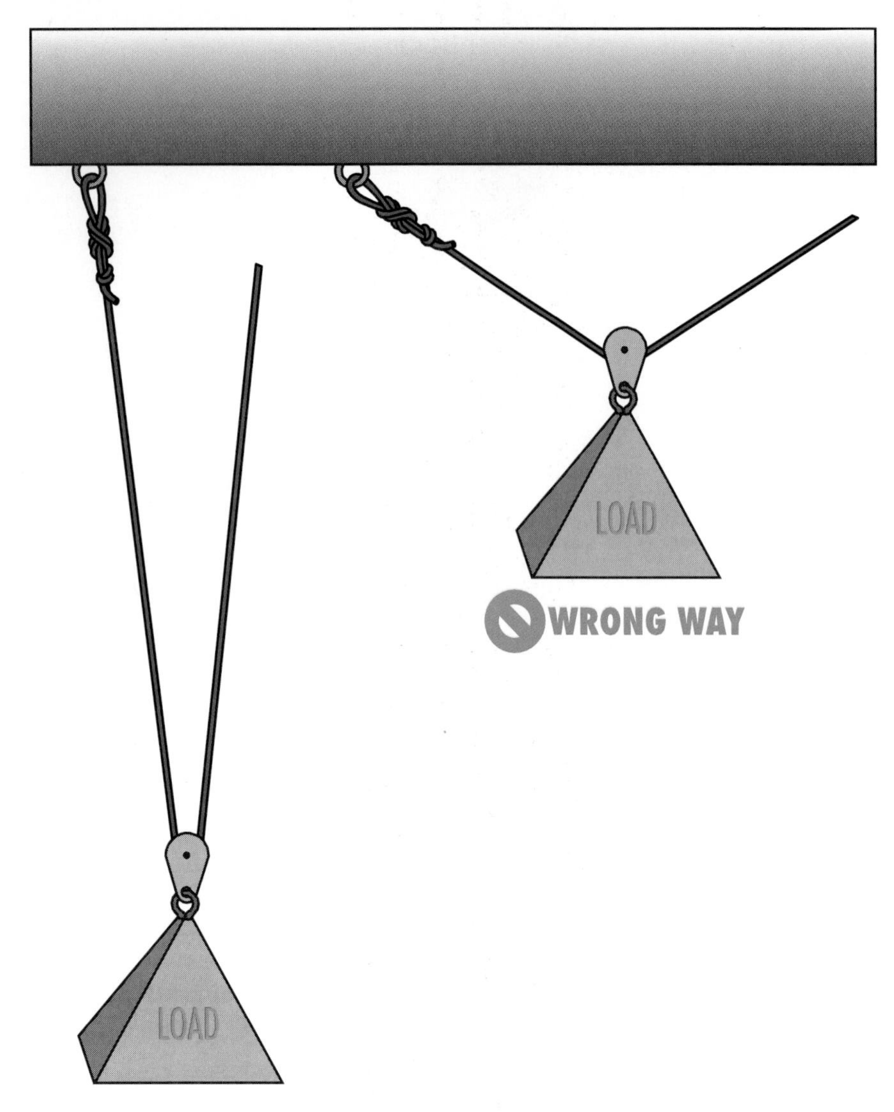

Figure 12.1 Keep the angle between the lines as small as possible

is important to note that, in the following discussion of hauling systems, this book deals only with *theoretical mechanical advantage.* Theoretical M/A discounts any actual loss of efficiency in a hauling system due to friction from pulleys and improper angle of the haul line. *Pulley efficiency* depends on the type and brand of equipment. *Haul line angle* refers to the angle of all the lines in a hauling system. It is optimal when all of the lines are parallel. As you can see in Figure 12.1, if you increase the angle of the haul line (the line you pull on), you decrease the efficiency of the system.

Pulleys

Pulleys are an integral part of any M/A system. A pulley anchored to a non-moving structure is called a "directional pulley" (see Figure 12.2). Directional pulleys simply change the direction of the rope path for convenience. Rescuers can insert as many directional pulleys in a hauling system as they deem necessary to make the system work as they wish. However, for each directional pulley in the system, there is some loss of efficiency. Therefore, the number of directional pulleys in a mechanical advantage system should be kept to a minimum. Usually, rescuers install directionals based on where they want to position the haul team and in which direction they want to pull the haul line.

Pulleys attached to the load move with the load toward a predetermined destination (see Figure 12.3). A pulley that moves during the hauling operation is known as a "traveling pulley" and always creates some M/A in a system. This mechanical advantage is calculated in different ways according to the classification of the rope/pulley M/A system.

Block and Tackle Systems

The most common simple mechanical advantage system is the traditional block and tackle (see Figure 12.4). To build this system, rescuers first have to decide how much mechanical advantage they are going to require. Since a 1:1 system requires too much backbreaking work and the 2:1 is just slightly better, they would normally pick a 3:1, 4:1, or 5:1 system. Some factors to consider in selecting a M/A system are

- available personnel
- work area (space for team to set up may be very limited, e.g., the top of a reactor tower)
- weight of both rescuer and patient
- the distance to be traveled

Simple Mechanical Advantage Systems

Simple mechanical advantage is calculated by adding the total number of lines (not ropes) attached to or leaving the load (see Figure 12.5). A M/A of 1:1 means a single rope (line) is attached to the load. A M/A of 2:1 consists of two lines (although there is only one rope) attached to or leaving the load. Note that in Figure 12.3 one line is anchored and therefore static while the other line moves (or travels) through the pulley attached to the load.

Each line shares an equal portion of the load in the example of a 100-pound load. A 1:1 M/A has one line attached to the load, and therefore, holds 100 pounds. A 2:1 M/A has two lines attached to the load, therefore, each line holds 50 pounds. A 3:1 M/A has three lines attached to the load so each line holds 33 $\frac{1}{3}$ pounds. A 4:1 M/A has four lines attached to the load and each lines holds 25 pounds, and so on.

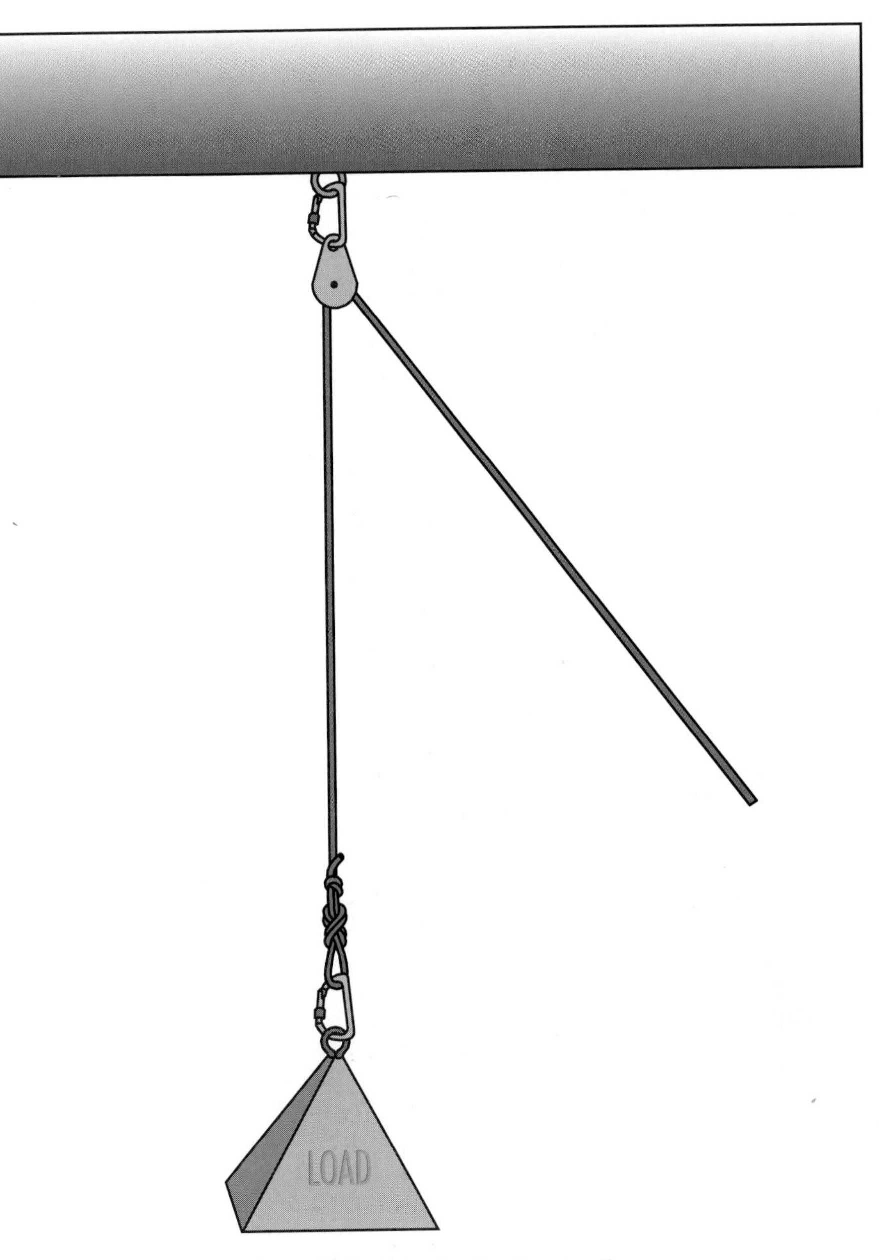

Figure 12.2 Use of a directional pulley

Block and Tackle—Vertical

The first system configuration is a vertical block-and-tackle system. This is an excellent choice when rope length is not a limitation (simple block-and-tackle systems can take lots of rope) and there is a small work area at the opening to the vertical corridor. This system is well suited for vertical shafts or vessels less than 40 feet deep. Some basic principles and considerations to be aware of when using vertical block-and-tackle systems for shaft rescue are:

- For maximum efficiency, anchor these systems to a point high above the opening of the shaft. This will facilitate removal of patients and rescuers.
- As with all unprotected openings, be certain persons working near the top of a vertical shaft are secured with appropriate rigging and fall protection equipment to prevent accidents and injury.
- If the vertical shaft is a confined space, do not attempt to enter without taking necessary monitoring, safety, and personal protective precautions. (See chapter 14 for further information on confined space rescue.)

The more M/A built into a block and tackle system, the more rope needed. Although the M/A decreases the amount of required input force, it increases the distance the ropes have to travel and, therefore, the time required to perform the work. These systems can require an enormous amount of rope to operate. For example, removing a victim from the bottom of a 100-foot shaft using a simple 3:1 block-and-tackle M/A system would require at least 300 feet of rope. Rescuers would have

WARNING

The authors recommend that a safety line belay system be used when working with mechanical advantage (M/A) systems. When used carelessly, M/A systems can create forces that exceed the rated capacity of some of its component parts. There have been cases in which ropes, anchors, hardware, and rigging were pulled to failure because a system was used without proper precautions to handle its strength.

Also, the force exerted over an edge when hauling a load with an M/A system is greater than that produced on the same edge when lowering a load. This is because of the increased forces applied to work against the natural law of gravity. This increased force pushing down on the edge can easily damage edge padding and increase rope abrasion.

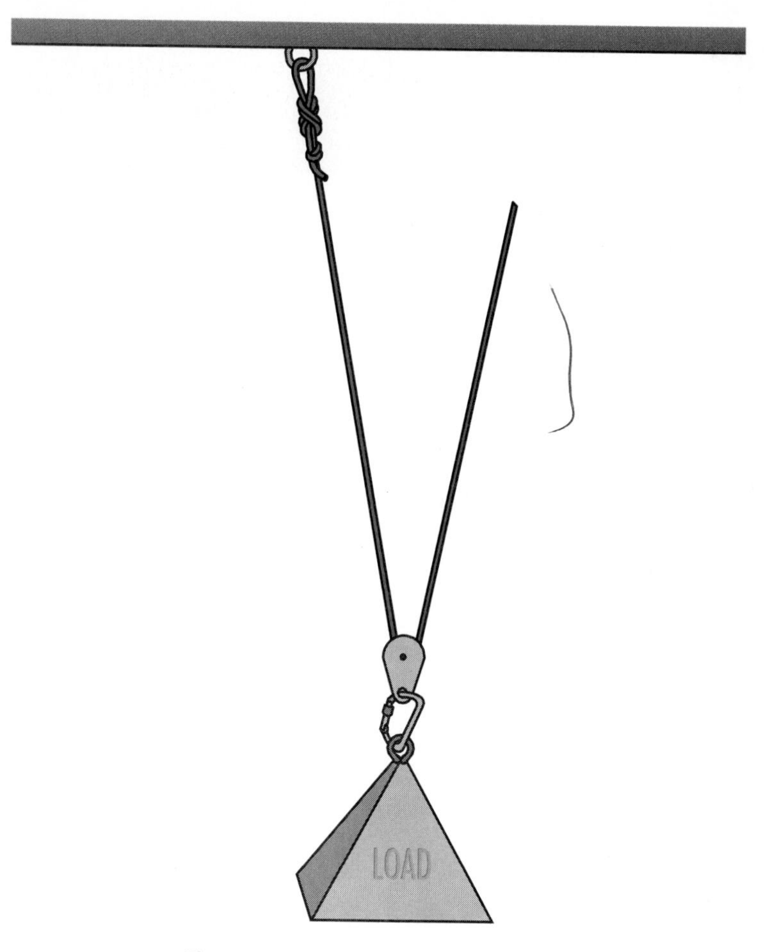

Figure 12.3 Use of a traveling pulley

to haul 3 feet of rope through the system at the haul line in order to move the load a total distance of only 1 foot.

Configuring the Block-and-Tackle System All block-and-tackle rope/pulley M/A systems start with the knotted end of the rope. In a 1:1 simple system, the knotted end of the rope is attached directly to the load. Conversely, the end of the rope on a 2:1 M/A is attached away from the load at the anchor. The anchor knot of the rope for all odd systems (1:1, 3:1, 5:1, etc.) is attached to the load. The anchor knot of the rope of even systems (2:1, 4:1, 6:1, etc.) is attached to the anchor. Knowing where to place this knot (anchor or load) is important when trying to build these systems.

For example, two team members can build a simple 3:1 system quickly by designating one person as the anchor and the other as the load. They can then start the building process by handing the knotted end to the person designated as the load (since a 3:1 M/A is odd) and then wrap the rope through pulleys at both ends until three lines are counted coming from the load. If the two rescuers decided to build a 4:1 system, they would start with the knot at the anchor.

As previously mentioned, simple M/A systems can be configured in a variety of ways. The following sections explore some of the common system configurations.

Equipment for the Block-and-Tackle The equipment required to build a 3:1 simple block-and-tackle M/A system differs only slightly from the equipment required to build a 4:1:

- **One haul line rope.** Remember, a 3:1 block-and-tackle requires a rope at least three times the depth of the shaft or vessel, a 4:1 M/A requires a rope four times the depth.
- **Two pulleys.** The preferred pulleys for a 3:1 system are one single-sheave and one double-sheave, although two single-sheave pulleys can be substituted effectively for a double-sheave if necessary. For a 4:1, two double-sheave pulleys are preferred.

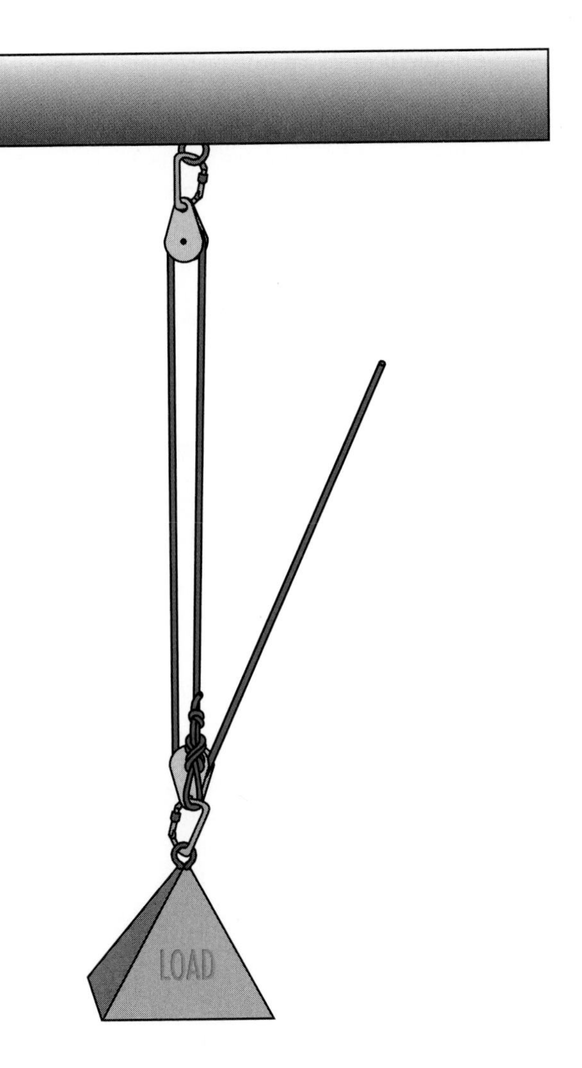

Figure 12.4 3:1 Simple Block-and-Tackle Mechanical Advantage System

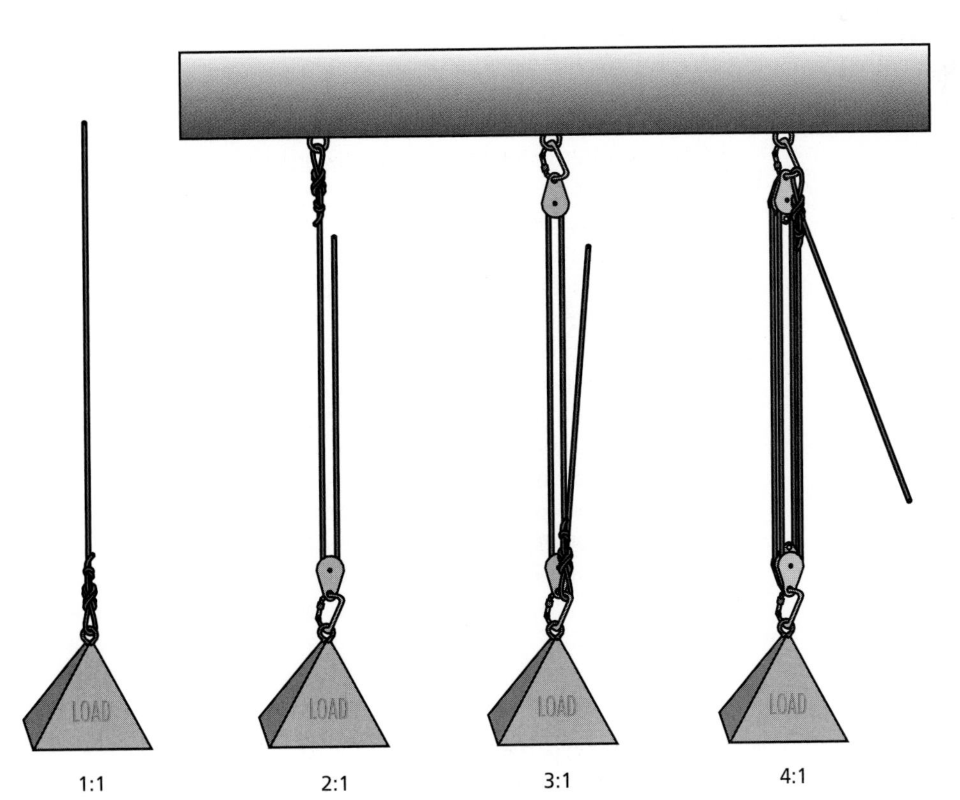

Figure 12.5 Mechanical advantage can be easily determined by counting the number of lines attached to the load

Double-sheave pulleys with beckets are extremely useful in vertical block-and-tackle systems.

- **A mechanical rope grab.** This acts as a progress capture device that will hold the load in place should the need arise to release the haul line. This device is not intended to act as a belay system to catch a falling load. A separate safety line belay system should be in place for this purpose.
- **Carabiners and anchor rigging.** These should meet applicable standards for construction and strength of rescue equipment.
- **A separate safety line belay system.** This is highly recommended for all hauling systems.

Building the Block-and-Tackle

To build a simple block-and-tackle M/A system:

1. Start by tying an anchor knot, such as a figure-8 on a bight, in the end of the rope. This knot should be very compact with a small loop to allow maximum hauling distance.
2. Using a two-member team to build the system, designate one as the anchor and the other as the load.
3. Assemble (lay out) the equipment needed by each member on the ground beside him or her. Have each member kneel on the ground about two feet apart and face each other. By not spreading the rope over a large area, you reduce confusion and the chance of crossing lines during construction of the system.
4. Depending on the system being built, hand the knot to the appropriate person. For an even M/A system, the knot should go to the anchor person. For odd, it should go to the load person.
5. The knot should be held or placed on the ground below any pulley in the system. The pulleys should be held flat with the side plates parallel to the ground. This makes it easy to reeve the rope through the pulleys and minimizes confusion.
6. Loop the rope in concentric circles from the ground up, going from one pulley sheave to the other.
7. When using a double pulley, wind the first bight around the bottom sheave and if there is a second bight, wrap it around the top sheave. Working from the bottom toward the top alleviates confusion during construction of the system.
8. Continue to reeve the rope through the pulleys in this fashion until the proper number of lines are attached to the load. Remember, for simple M/A systems, the number of lines is determined by counting the ropes at the load end of the system.
9. After completion of the system, each member should clip a carabiner through the proper opening in the pulley side plates.
10. The knot is clipped into the same carabiner as the pulley at the applicable end of the system.
11. The system can now be attached to an anchor point.
12. In all block-and-tackle M/A systems, a device should be attached in the system to suspend the load in place in case the need arises to release the haul line during operation. A mechanical rope grab device can serve this purpose.

    This text refers to this device as a "ratchet cam" since most mechanical rope grabs incorporate a cam that presses the rope against the shell or body of the device. The term "ratchet" applies more readily to systems presented later in this chapter as they are used to hold the load in place while the hauling system is reset. The ratchet cam is not necessary to make the block and tackle work and therefore could be considered optional in a haul. However, we

Incorporating the Ratchet Cam The ratchet cam (also known as progress capture device) is not intended to catch a falling load in case of system failure. Its purpose is to hold the load in place so the haul team can release the line if needed. The safety line belay system is in place to catch a falling load in an emergency. Avoid placing a mechanical rope grab in a position to receive a shock load because it can damage the rope.

Because it is possible that the ratchetman might accidentally let go of the rope grab during a lowering operation, it is recommended that the ratchet cam be placed on the line with the greatest load reduction (see Figure 12.6).

When attaching the ratchet cam, the arrow on the cam shell should point towards the load. The one exception to this is described in detail later in this chapter. The cam

suggest its use for convenience in case the hauling team has to stop the haul for some reason after it has been initiated. Simple block-and-tackle systems can also be used for lowering on a load reduction. This will be covered more thoroughly later in this chapter. When the block-and-tackle is being used as a lowering system, the ratchet cam must be held open or disengaged from the rope.

13. Always use an additional safety line belay system with a M/A system. This is the backup device should a system fail or the haul team accidentally drop the rope while operating the system.

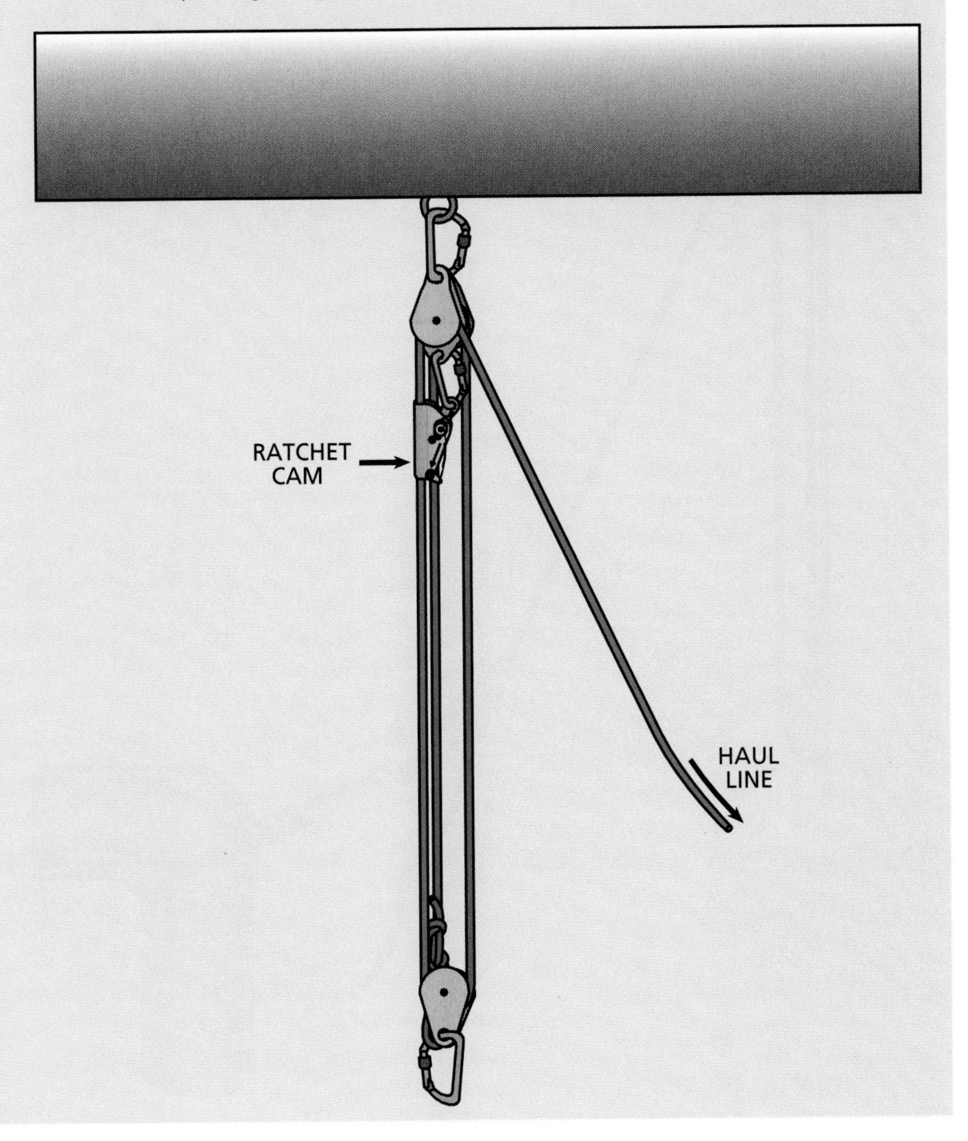

operates properly when attached to any rope moving in an upward direction during hauling. However, the greatest load reduction is achieved by attaching the cam to the upward-moving rope nearest the haul team. In systems with a top directional pulley, this is always the first rope on the other side of the pulley from the haul team. Attach the ratchet cam to the upward moving line nearest the haul team.

The ratchet cam should be anchored in one of the following ways:

- Attach it to the becket of a multisheave pulley with a carabiner (see Figure 12.6), or
- Attach it to a utility belt or doubled webbing loop anchored above the top directional pulley, which allows the cam to hang at the desired level of 1 to 2 inches below the top pulley sheave. Remember, any anchor should be strong enough for structural rescue. When hauling a victim upward, always attempt to establish a high-point anchor well above the top of the shaft to eliminate additional difficulties with removing the victim, or

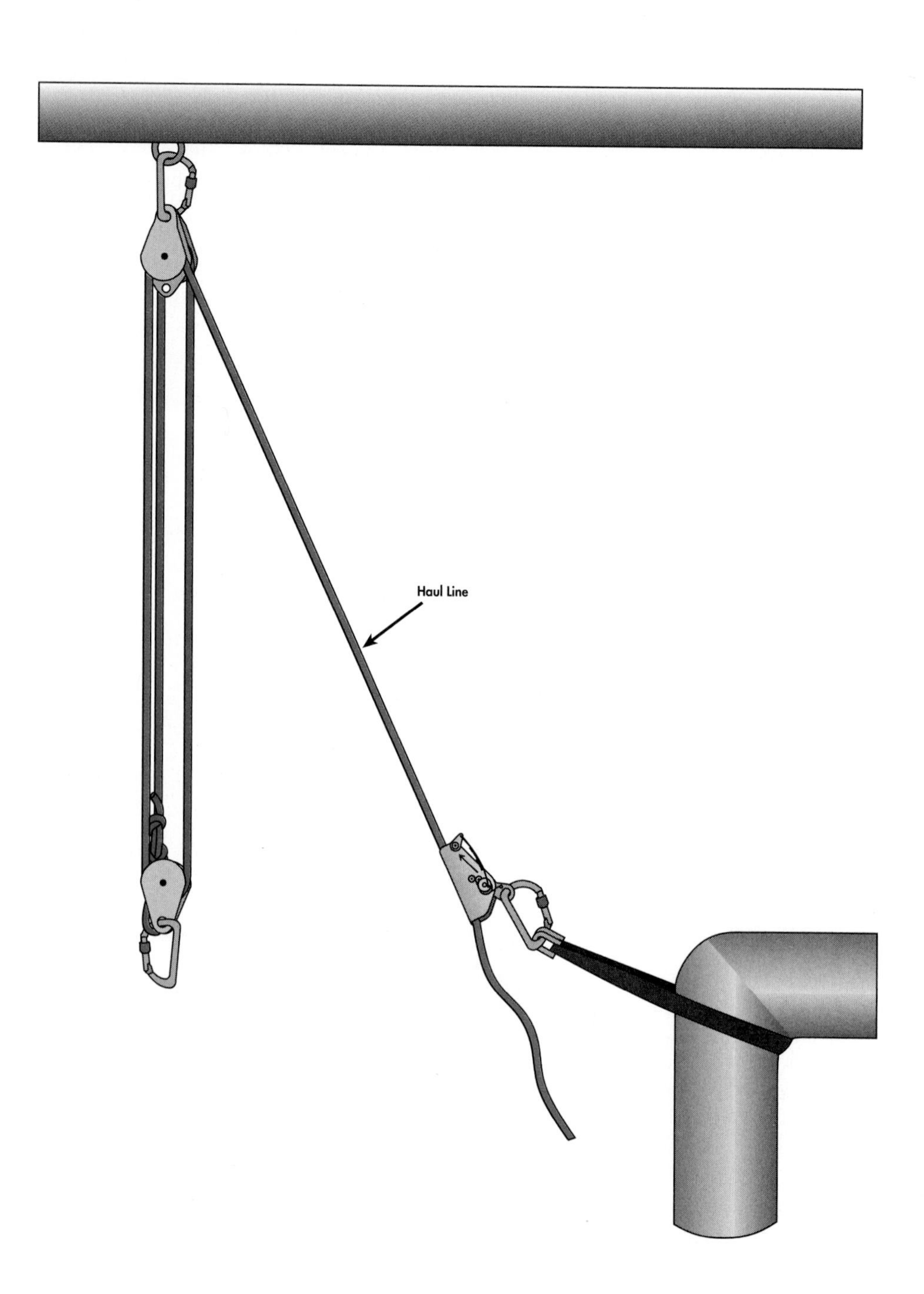

Figure 12.7 3:1 Block-and-tackle with ratchet cam anchored in line with the haul line

- Attach it to the same anchor system as the haul system or to a separate anchor system in line with the haul system. You can also attach the ratchet cam to the haul line at any point to serve the same purpose (see Figure 12.7). If it is attached behind the haul team, the ratchetperson must pull the slack created in the haul line during operation of the M/A system.

Personnel Requirements Along with the equipment, certain personnel are required to operate the system efficiently and safely:

- **Haul/lower team**—The team lifts or lowers a victim, depending on the situation and mode of operation. If the load becomes entangled during hauling, the input force exerted on the end of the haul line is multiplied as it travels through the system. This is the reverse effect of normal M/A systems. As long as the load is traveling freely, the M/A system serves to reduce the weight of the load over multiple ropes and pulleys. When this load is wedged on obstructions or otherwise trapped, tremendous amounts of force can be transmitted to the load and system components. For example, if seven strong haulers are creating an input force of 1000 pounds on the haul line of a 3:1 M/A system, the theoretical force exerted on the entangled load is approximately 3000 pounds. This could damage system components and injure or kill the patient. There are two ways to address this potential for disaster. First, limit the number of haulers to allow them to feel resistance if the load becomes entangled. This number is largely a matter of judgment but a good rule of thumb is to have no more than four haulers for a M/A of 4:1 or less and no more than two haulers for M/A systems greater than 4:1. Just being able to feel resistance does not eliminate the danger to the system components and the load unless the haulers react to the situation and stop when they feel it. If obvious resistance is encountered, DO NOT pull harder. Stop, inspect the system for problems, and continue only after everything has been checked and found to be safe. Remember, these suggested haul team numbers are meant as guidelines and should not override independent judgment based on the strength of the haulers. The second way to prevent this dangerous situation is to assign a rescuer to watch the load.
- **Load watch**—This rescuer carefully watches the load and communicates the position of the load to the rescue master. This team member also alerts the team and stops the operation immediately if the load becomes entangled. The ratchetman may be in a good position to double as the load watch.
- **Ratchetman**—In a simple vertical block-and-tackle M/A system, the ratchet cam usually grabs automatically to hold the load in place whenever the haul line is released. The ratchetman need only hold the cam open or release the pin to allow lowering with the system. Again, the ratchetman may also function as the load watch.
- **Haul captain/rescue master**—This rescuer watches over the operation and gives commands for safe completion of the procedure. Though not recommended, this person could handle the

Figure 12.8 Hauling procedure for simple block and tackle system

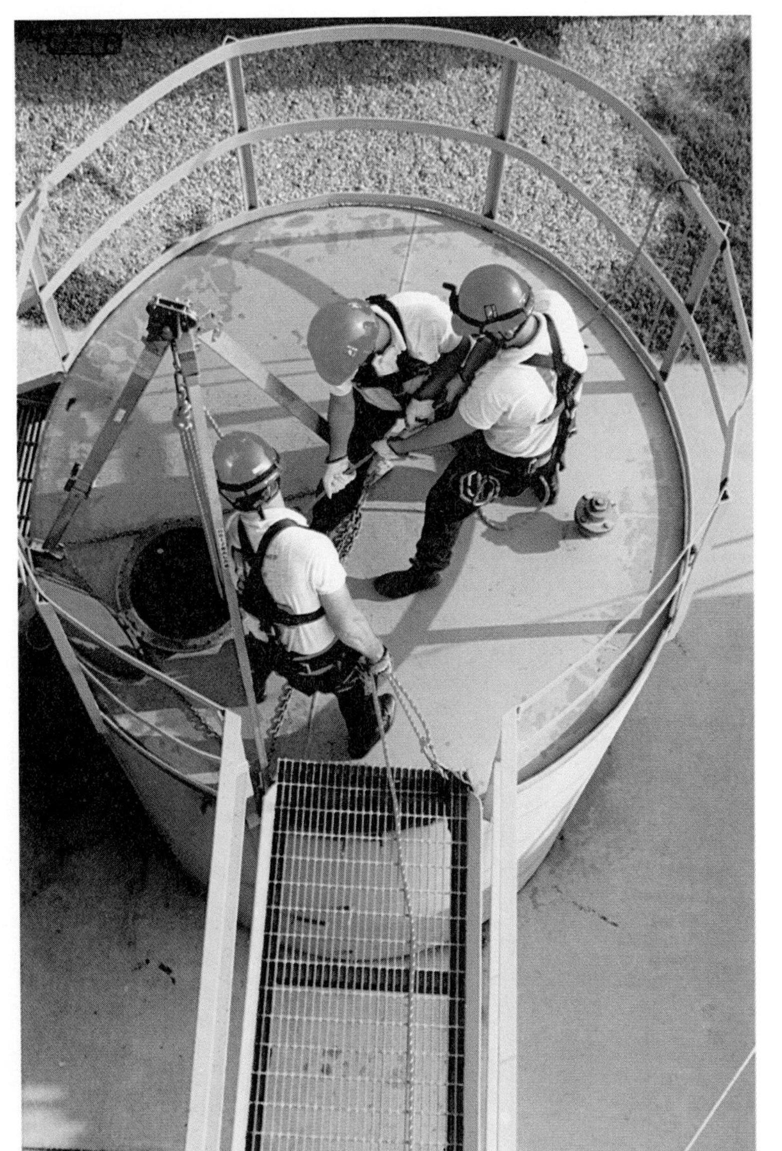

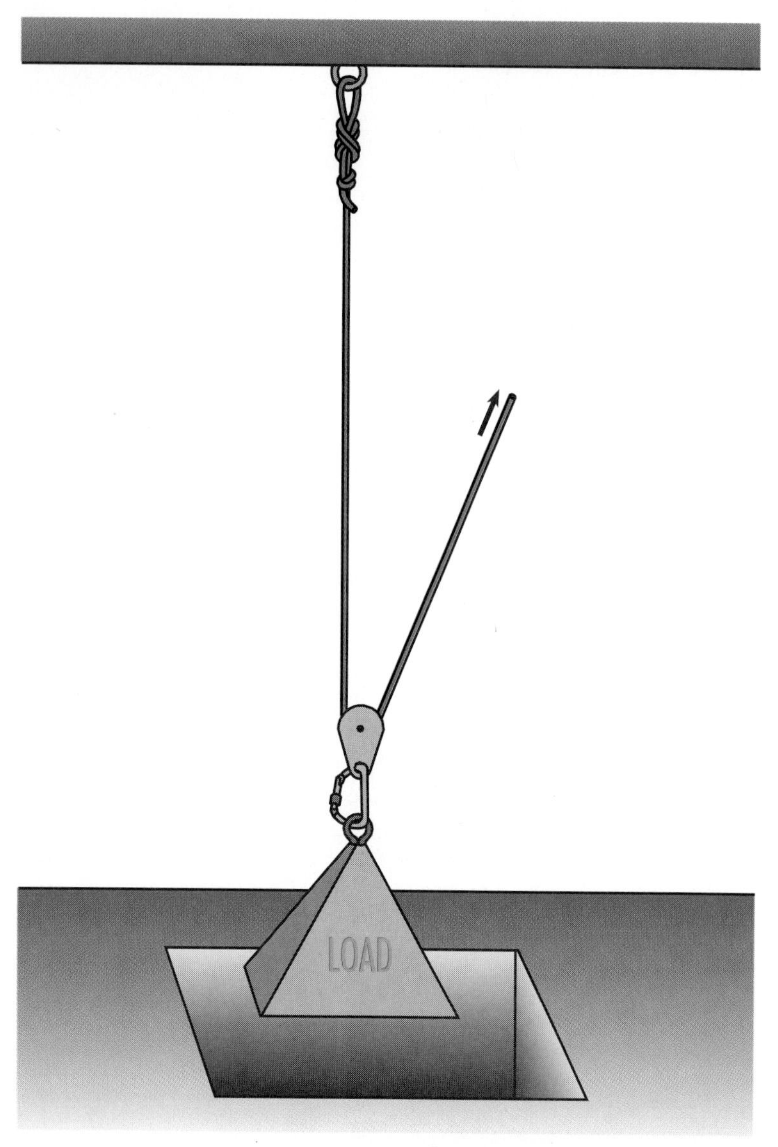

functions of both the load watch and the ratchetman in addition to command duties. Circumstances such as limited personnel or tight working space may require a person to handle multiple jobs.

- **Safety/belayer—**This rescuer operates the safety line belay system.
- **Primary rescuer—**This is the person who accesses and packages the patient. He or she can also serve as a tag person during the haul operation.

Hauling Procedure and Communication The hauling procedure for the simple block-and-tackle M/A system follows (see Figure 12.8):

1. Remove the slack in the system and confirm that the safety and M/A systems are attached to the load.
2. Attempt to position the haul captain with a field of view of both the load or load watch and the haul team. If the captain and/or load watch are near the edge, they should be secured to a safety line.
3. Position the haul team members with the rope in their hands ready to haul.
4. The haul captain gives the verbal commands:

   "Haul"—The haul team begins hauling. If applicable, the ratchetman pulls slack rope through the ratchet cam. The circumstances dictating this need are addressed in the discussion of the next command.

Figure 12.9 Using a small 2:1 to get the load up a short distance and out of the hole

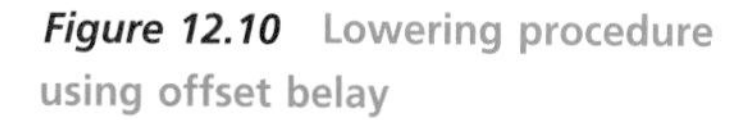

Figure 12.10 Lowering procedure using offset belay

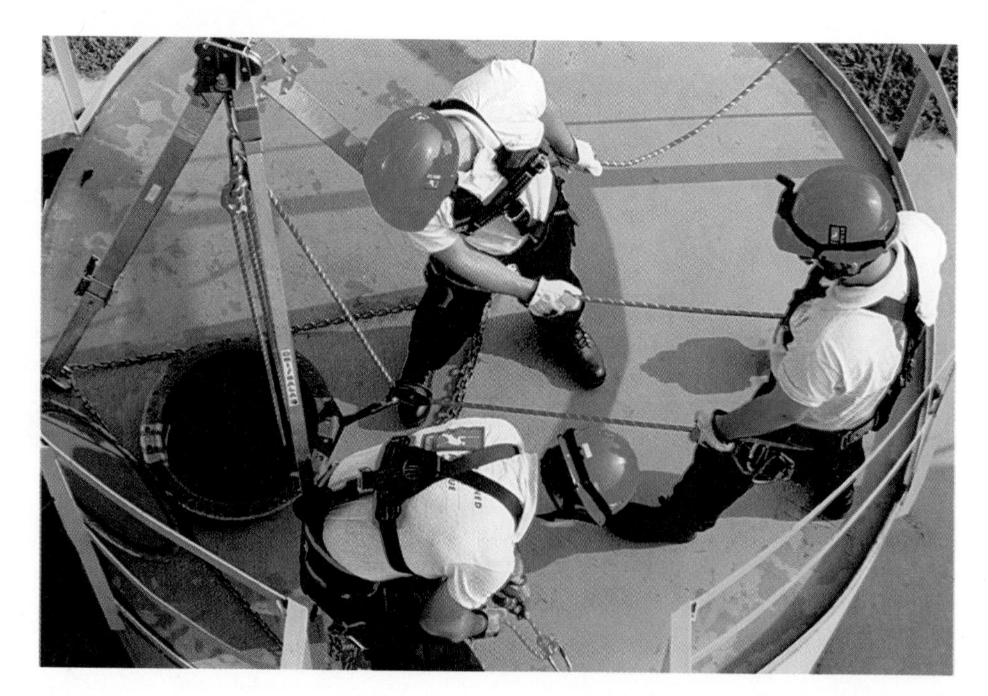

"Set"—The haul team stops hauling and slowly releases the end of the haul line. The ratchetman ensures the rachet cam sets, taking and holding the load in place. The ratchetman then responds to the rescue master by loudly repeating the verbal command, "set." This assures the rescue master that the ratchet cam is in place. This command can be used to suspend the operation for any nonemergency reason.

NOTE: *When the ratchet cam is in front of the haul team, this command is seldom necessary because the rope travels through the device automatically and sets quickly if the team releases the end of the haul line. However, if the rachet cam is located behind the haul team, the ratchetman must pull the haul line through the device to prevent slack from accumulating. This command tells the ratchetman to remove all remaining slack from the system by pulling the haul line through the device until it is taut.*

"Stop"—This command stops the operation immediately and should be used only in situations requiring urgency. It can be issued by any member of the team who sees something wrong. Because M/A systems multiply human strength, they can be dangerous. In general, team members should not speak unless a member of the team spots a problem. Otherwise, the haul captain, ratchetman, and load watch are the only team members who should speak during normal operations. If a team member spots a problem, he or she should loudly say "STOP!" as many times as necessary to cause the haul team to halt. The team must be disciplined enough to observe what is going on around them and simultaneously react to the rescue master's commands.

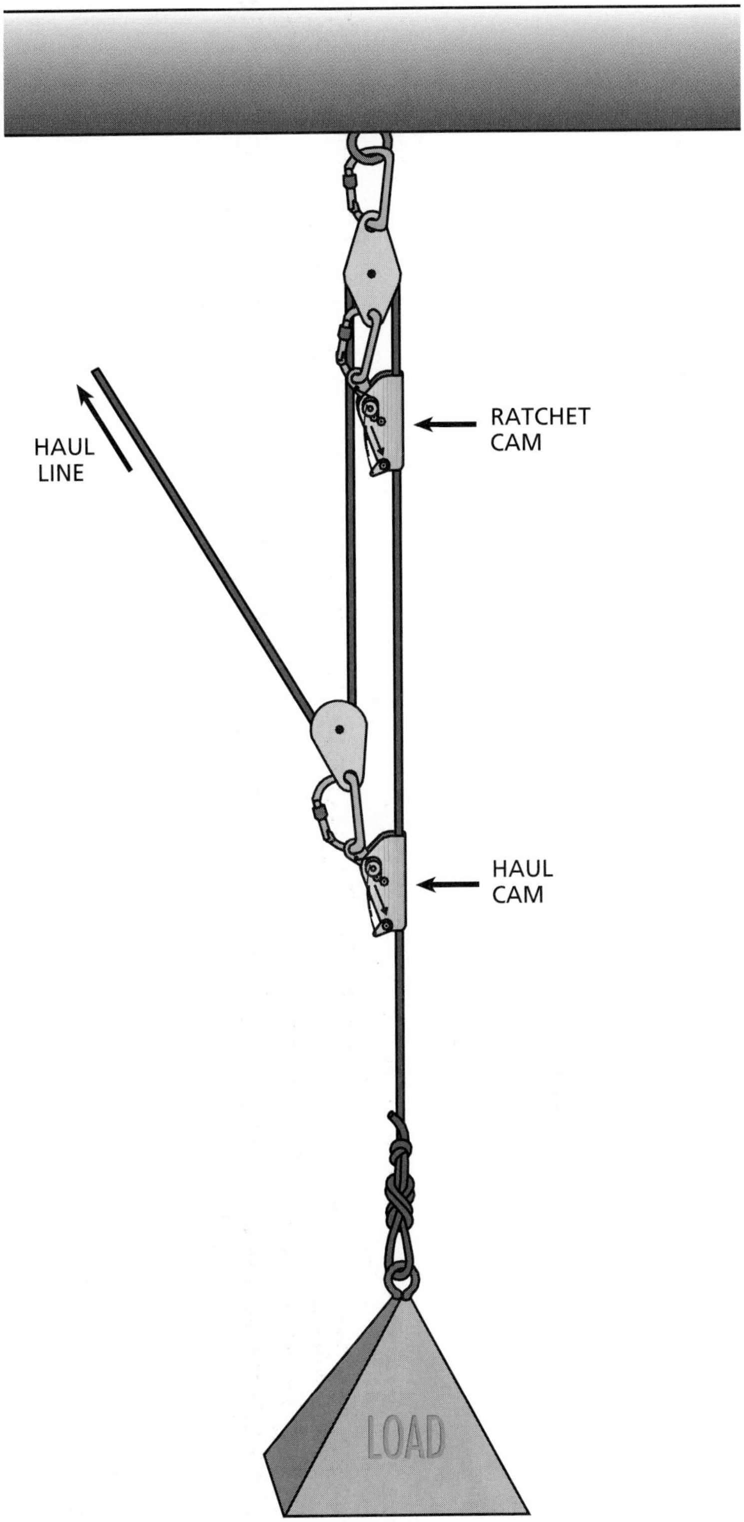

Figure 12.11 Vertical Z-Rig Mechanical Advantage System

When hauling, rescuers might raise the patient to the full extent of the primary system, only to find that more lift is needed to complete removal from the space. This usually occurs when an anchor point of insufficient height has been chosen. In this case, consider tying a separate piece of rope or webbing at one end to a high-point anchor above the patient. This might be the same anchor used for the primary system. Run the other end through a carabiner or pulley attached to a low point on the patient. The loose end of the rope or webbing can now be hauled to create a separate 2:1 simple M/A system (see Figure 12.9). This can help complete the removal of the patient from the shaft.

Lowering Procedure An important and useful feature of the simple vertical block-and-tackle M/A system is that a load, a rescuer for example, can be lowered into a vessel and then raised quickly if a problem occurs, using the same system. The lower can be accomplished with a load reduction in the same way that the M/A reduces the input force required to lift the load.

Only two adjustments change the hauling system to a lowering system (see Figure 12.10):

1. **Open the ratchet cam.** The ratchetman holds open the ratchet cam or completely removes the pin from the cam.
2. **Create an offset belay.**
   A. Two haul team members face each other approximately 4 feet apart.
   B. The individual farthest away from the M/A system faces the system. The second member is in front of the first, facing him or her and slightly off to his or her left or right.
   C. The haul line from the system should come around the body, beneath the buttocks of the team member facing the system in a type of body belay. The loose end leaving the first individual should go to the second member where he or she will also do this type of body belay, offset to that of the first individual. The rope, when using the offset belay, should be the shape of an "S". The "offset belay" is designed to provide enough friction to easily lower the already reduced load with a great margin of safety. It can be used whenever you are lowering someone with a vertical M/A system of 3:1 or greater. Because of significant heat buildup caused by rope friction traveling across the body, potentially causing burns, the rope in the body belay must run under the buttocks and not the armpits as in a normal body belay.
   D. If you have problems trying to lower a load with the offset belay due to the size of the load and/or the number of team members available, you can run the rope through an anchored descent control device such as the rappel rack or figure-8 plate.

Simple Z-Rig System

As noted, the main disadvantage of the simple vertical block-and-tackle M/A system is that creating it may require a lot of rope. For example, a 100-foot haul with a 3:1 system would require a minimum of 300 feet of rope to haul out the patient.

If rescuers only had 150 feet of rope, they could still use a simple system. But instead of a vertical block and tackle, they could set up a vertical or horizontal system capable of being reset. One such system is called a "Z-rig."

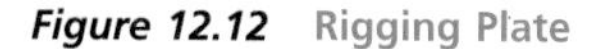

Figure 12.12 Rigging Plate

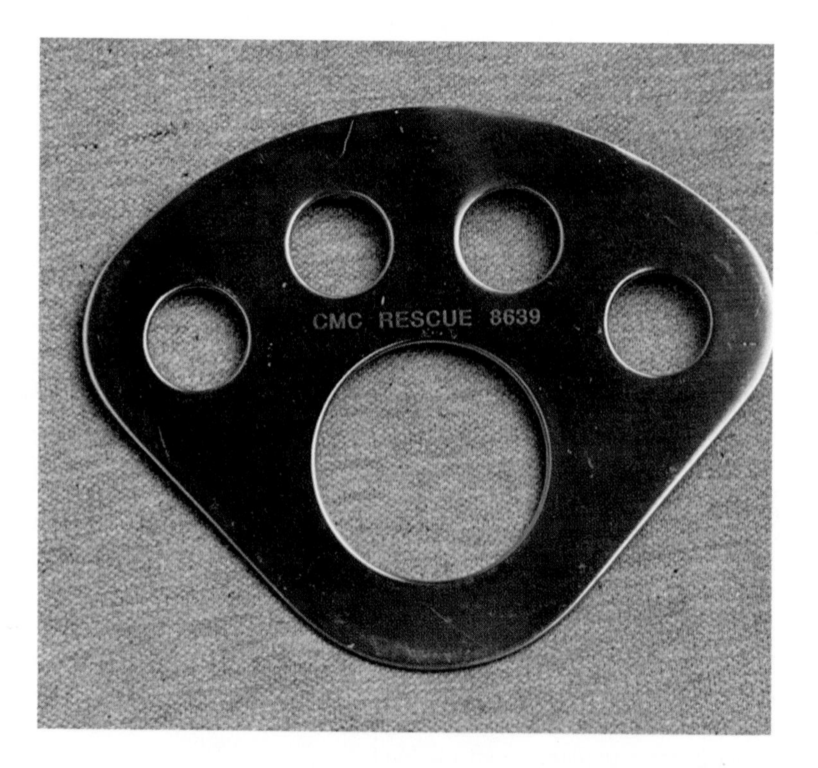

Configuring the Z-Rig A Z-rig is a simple 3:1 M/A system designed to be reset with only one line attached to the load. This system is quick and easy to build and operate. It does not require as much rope to build as other simple systems. The Z-rig works well for hauling, but is not as versatile as the vertical block and tackle for lowering (see Figure 12.11). For this reason, it is not recommended for situations that require a single M/A system to act as both lowering and hauling systems.

Equipment for the Z-Rig The equipment required for the Z-rig system is slightly different from that required for the vertical block-and-tackle M/A system:

- one haul line rope
- two pulleys (one directional and one traveling)
- two mechanical rope grabs (one haul cam and one ratchet cam)
- steel locking carabiners and appropriate anchor rigging
- a separate safety line belay system

There are two names for the rope grabs in this system. The name for the device depends on its placement in the system (see Figure 12.11):

- A "haul cam" is a traveling mechanical rope grab that grabs a load line and pulls it during a haul.
- A "ratchet cam" is an anchored mechanical rope grab that holds the load in place temporarily while the haul cam and traveling pulley are "ratcheted" forward, which resets the system for another haul.

Remember, a ratchet cam is designed to hold the load in place while the haul team resets the system. It is not meant to be a safety device to catch a falling load resulting from a failure of some part of the haul system or operation. **Mechanical rope grabs are not recommended for use as belay devices!** If severely shock loaded, they can cause damage or failure of a rope.

Personnel requirements The personnel requirements for operation of the Z-rig are the same as for the vertical block-and-tackle M/A system but without the lowering personnel.

Building the Z-Rig

1. Start by attaching the knotted end of the rope to the load (odd system) (see Figure 12.11).
2. Lay out the rope in a small Z pattern near the anchor point.
3. Attach a pulley to the bight of rope formed by the back of the Z pattern.
4. Anchor this rear directional pulley to the anchor.
5. Place the haul cam (arrow pointing toward the load) on the rope coming from the rear directional pulley and attached to the load. Move it to a position near the bight of rope formed by the front of the Z pattern.
6. Attach a pulley to the bight of rope formed by the front of the Z pattern.
7. With a carabiner, attach this traveling pulley to the haul cam.

Figure 12.13 Rigging plate with Z-Rig incorporated

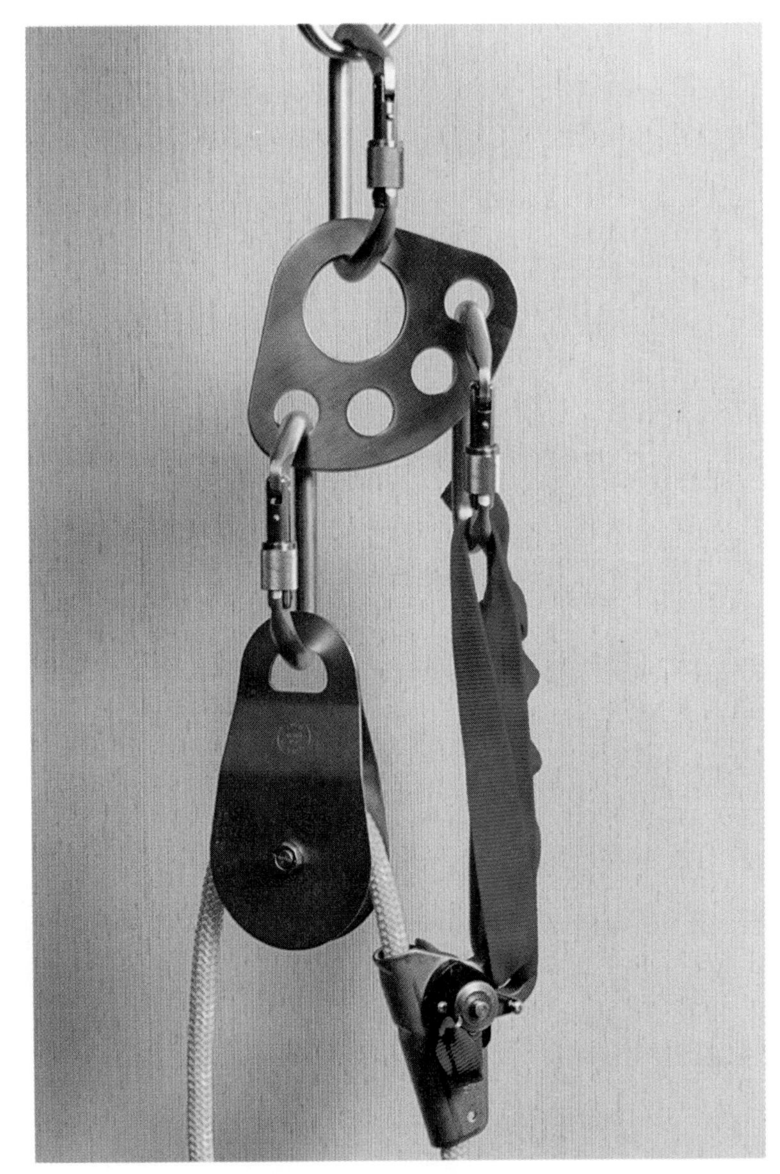

8. Place the ratchet cam (arrow pointing toward the load) behind the haul cam on the same rope. Move it to a position just forward of the rear directional pulley. Anchor the ratchet cam at this position, keeping it directly in line with the anchor rigging for the rear directional pulley.

   NOTE: *A rigging plate is a special piece of general-use auxiliary rescue equipment not specifically addressed by NFPA 1983 standard (see Figure 12.12). A rigging plate can be used to separate the directional pulley and ratchet cam enough to allow easy operation but keep them close enough to be in line with each other (see Figure 12.13). Rigging plates are not presented in the chapter on Related Rescue Equipment since they are often used inappropriately to support several different loaded systems. This is the equivalent of using the same anchor system for support of several different rescue systems. In the case of the Z-rig, the weight of the load is simply being transferred between the rear directional pulley (during hauling) and the ratchet cam (during resetting). It is acceptable to attach both components to the same anchored rigging plate. The rigging plate should be anchored following guidelines presented in Chapter 10.*
9. Rig a separate safety line belay system to back up the primary rescue system.
10. Recheck all connections and prepare to haul.

Teamwork in Constructing Hauling Systems Teamwork is an important aspect of building a rescue system. As with any system, hauling systems can be built efficiently when the process is broken down into several components. The more tasks that can be assigned to individuals to accomplish simultaneously, the faster the system will

Figure 12.14 Short cut for building Z-Rig System

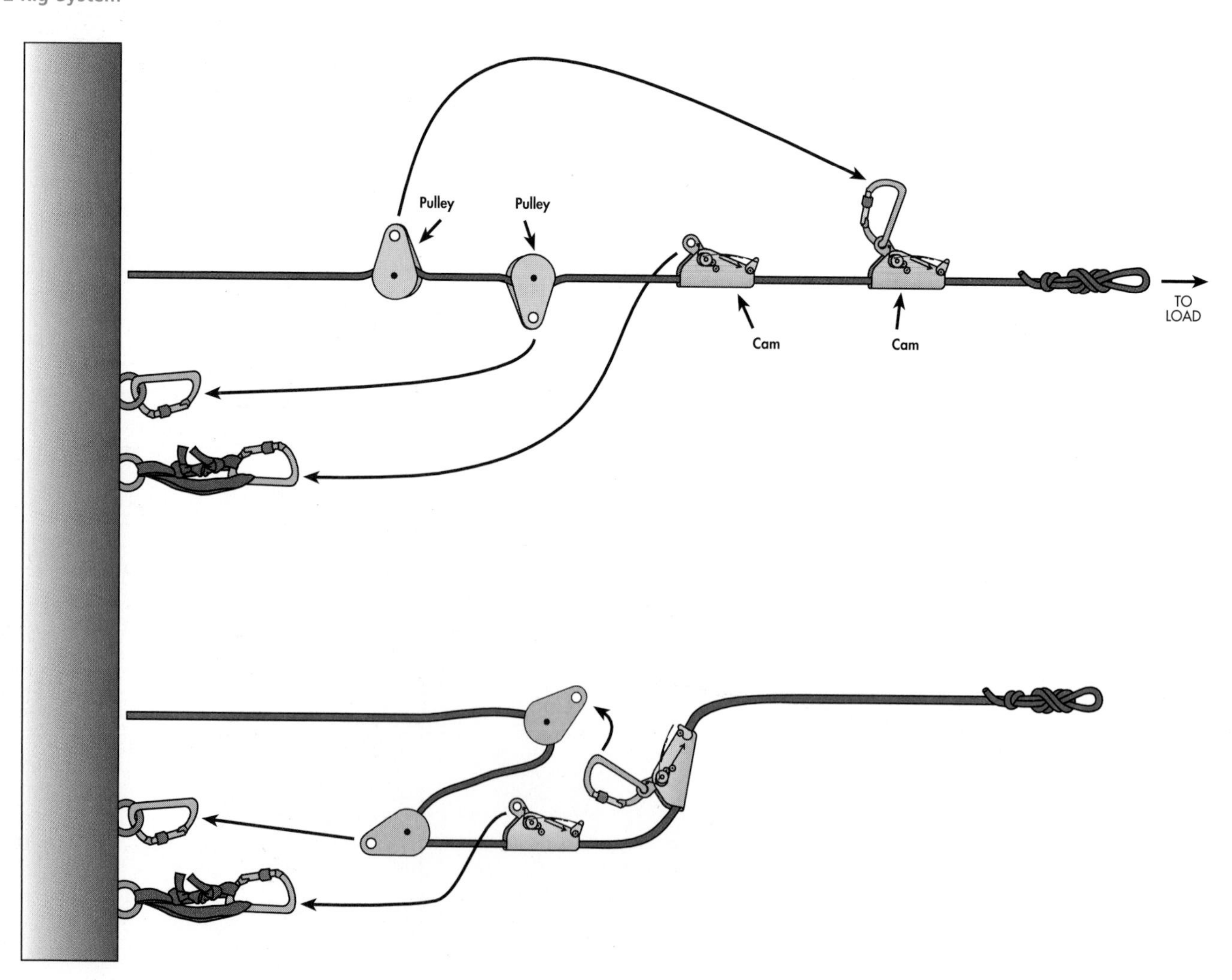

come together. When assigning these tasks, the leader of a rescue team is limited by many variables.

- **Exceeding the span of control**—"span of control" indicates the number of personnel or subteams that a team leader can supervise effectively. The average supervisor can control from three to seven people; the optimum number is five.
- **Lacking personnel**—Having too few team members for the number of tasks to be performed is often a problem for the average rescue team. Regardless of how well a process or rescue system is divided into its component parts, the system can only be built quickly and efficiently if there are enough team members to complete the tasks.
- **Assigning too many tasks to individual**—In general, the more a leader can subdivide the system and the fewer tasks he or she can assign to each team member, the more efficiently the system will be built.

When assigning tasks to teams building the hauling system, the leader should attempt to assign as few components as possible to each team member. Once the team member has completed his or her first task, he or she can be given a second assignment. Having one member or subteam perform too many tasks simultaneously makes it difficult to complete any of them efficiently.

For example, you may wish to assign a single team member to attach a haul cam to a rope rather than assign that person to attach the haul cam and a pulley. This is more efficient than having one team member attempt to do both jobs. Be cautious! It is also possible to assign *too many* people to complete a given task. This can cause congestion in the work area reducing efficiency. Some tasks are best performed by one person.

Shortcuts to constructing hauling systems are based on teamwork. By dividing the system into several manageable component parts, the team leader can assign team members to complete these tasks in a way that provides the most efficiency and the least effort in building the system.

Figure 12.15 Hauling with the 5:1 Piggyback

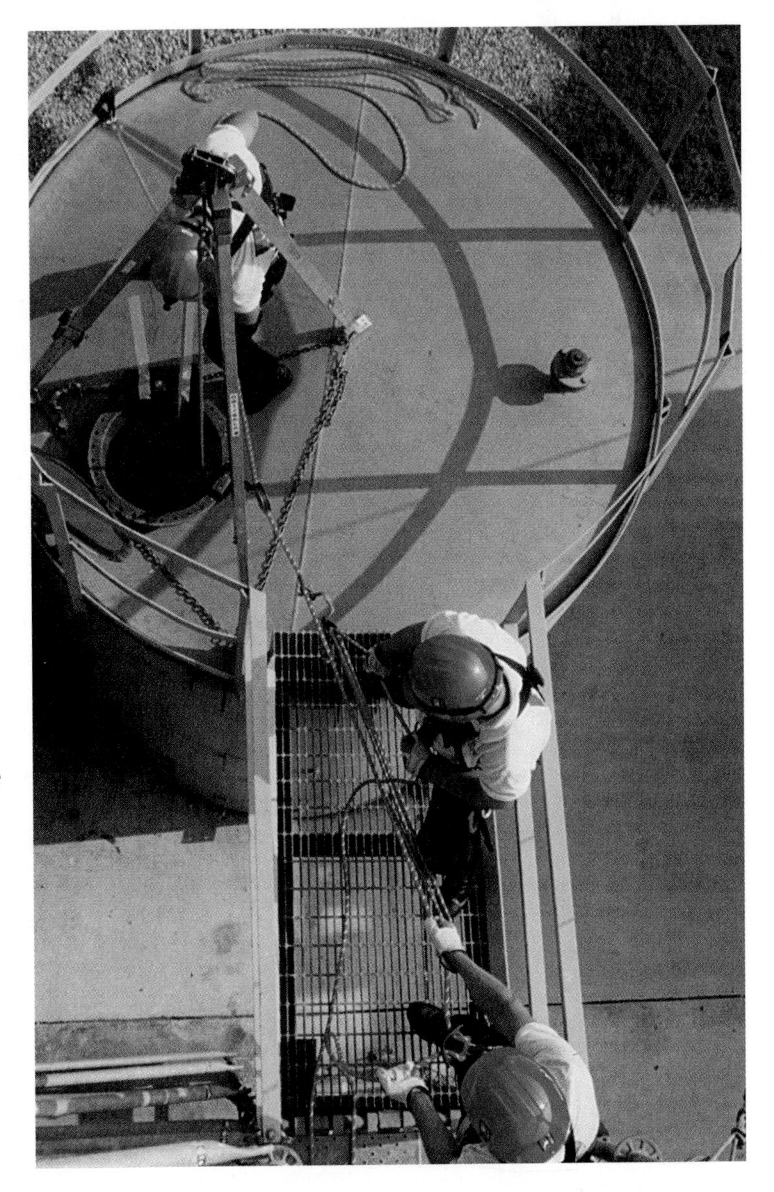

Shortcut for Building the Z-Rig

The following steps are not necessarily in the order that they should occur (see Figure 12.14). Many can occur simultaneously. The last two steps, however, are always the last two steps.

Here are the detailed steps:

1. Lay the main line out straight with the knotted end toward the load. You can bag the remaining line.
2. Attach two mechanical rope grabs to the main line, one behind the other, with their arrows pointing toward the load.
3. Attach a carabiner to the cam of the front rope grab.
4. Attach two pulleys to the main line, one behind the other.
5. Attach the rear pulley to the carabiner on the front rope grab. This rope grab becomes the haul cam. The pulley becomes the front traveling pulley.
6. Pull the front pulley and rear rope grab back toward the anchor. You must open the rope grab's cam to slide it along the rope. These two items become the rear directional pulley and ratchet cam.

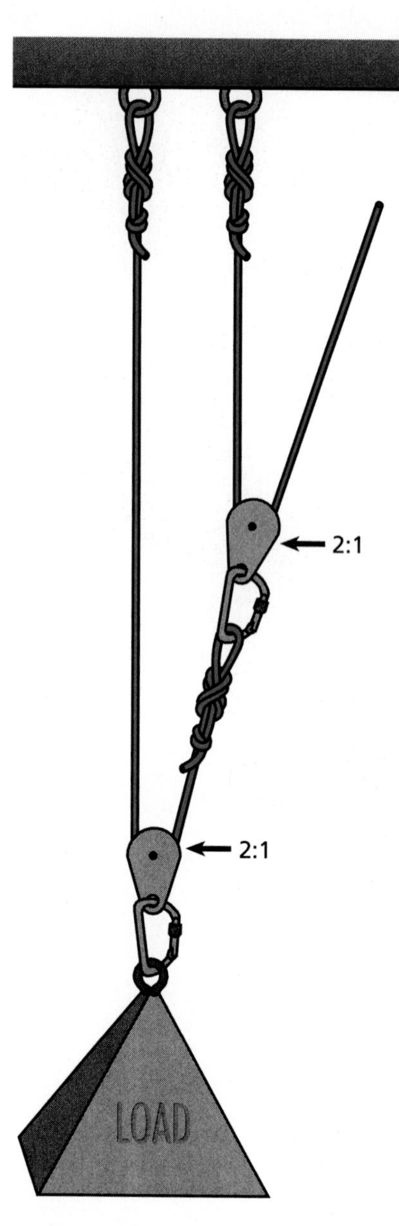

Figure 12.16 Progression of compound mechanical advantage—4:1 Compound System

7. Attach the rear directional pulley to its anchor.
8. Attach the ratchet cam to its anchor.
9. Rig a safety line belay system to back up the primary rescue system.
10. **Finally, secure the victim to the loose end.**
11. **Prepare to haul.**

This method can be remembered easily by learning the following two mnemonics:

1. **Cam, cam, pulley, pulley**—This is the order of attachment of the cams and pulleys along a single length of rope, starting from the knotted end (nearest the victim) and working back (toward the anchor). These components should be attached side by side, separated by only a few inches.
2. **Back to front**—This refers to the movement and attachment of the last component (the rear pulley) in the line of equipment to the first component (the front cam).

These two phrases can help a team to remember this shortcut in times of crisis.

Procedure and Communication

1. Remove all slack in the main line and extend the system as far forward as possible. This maximizes the length of the haul before resetting is necessary.
2. Confirm that the safety and main lines are attached to the load.
3. If possible, position the haul captain with a field of view of both the load or the load watch and the haul team.
4. Position the haul team members with the rope in their hands ready to haul.
5. The haul captain gives the verbal commands. Unlike the simple vertical system, the Z-rig can be reset, so the command, "slack" is appropriate.
   "Haul"—The haul team begins hauling while the ratchetman prevents the ratchet cam from jamming into the rear directional pulley.
   "Set"—The haul team stops hauling but keeps tension on the haul line. This command is repeated by the ratchetman when the ratchet cam has been moved as far as possible toward the load (forward). This removes all slack in the system and prevents the load from moving back down into the shaft during resetting.
   "Slack"—The haul team eases tension onto the ratchet cam and the lead haul member resets the haul cam. This can be performed most easily by grasping the carabiner to which the haul cam is attached and pulling it forward to expand the system to maximum extension.
   "Stop"—This command stops the operation and is for emergencies only. It can be given by any member of the team who sees that it is necessary.

Figure 12.17 4:1 Piggyback system

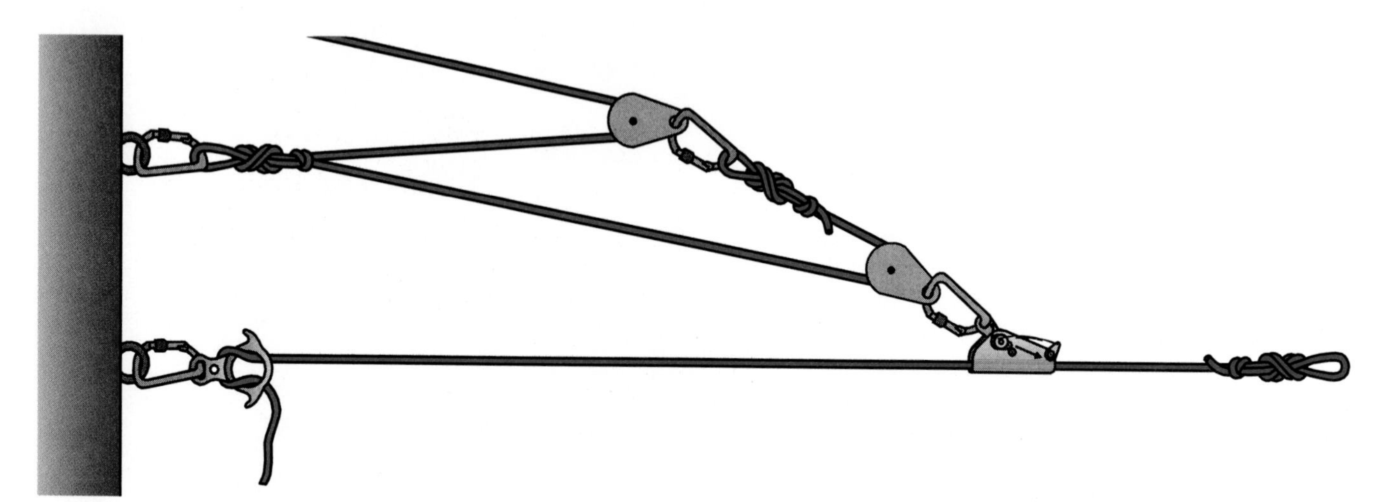

The haul team should never anticipate the haul captain's command for "slack." This can cause shocking of the ratchet cam, which may damage the rope.

Compound Mechanical Advantage Systems

The second type of mechanical advantage system used in hauling operations is the compound or "stacked" M/A. Compound systems are created by stacking two or more M/A systems onto the haul line of the other hauling system(s).

For example (see Figure 12.16):

1. A 2:1 system can be attached to the haul line of another 2:1 system. When this happens with a 100-pound load, the 100 pounds is reduced to 50 pounds by the first 2:1.
2. The second 2:1 is then attached to a 50-pound load, which reduces the force required to lift 25 pounds. Since the force required to lift the 100-pound load is only 25 pounds or $\frac{1}{4}$ of the load, the M/A is 4:1.

There is a much easier way to determine the M/A of a compound system: Identify the individual M/A systems in the stack and multiply them by each other. In this manner, a 2:1 stacked on a 1:1 would be a 2:1 ($2 \times 1 = 2$), a 2:1 on a 3:1 would be 6:1 ($2 \times 3 = 6$), and a 2:1 on a 2:1 on a 2:1 would be 8:1 ($2 \times 2 \times 2 = 8$). Virtually any system can be stacked onto the haul line of any other to create a compound M/A.

Compound M/A systems can be used for a variety of reasons. Primarily, they are used when a greater M/A is needed either due to a heavy load or fewer haulers. Improperly used, these systems can develop enough force to exceed the rated capacity of their component parts. Always limit the number of haulers appropriately and establish a load watch.

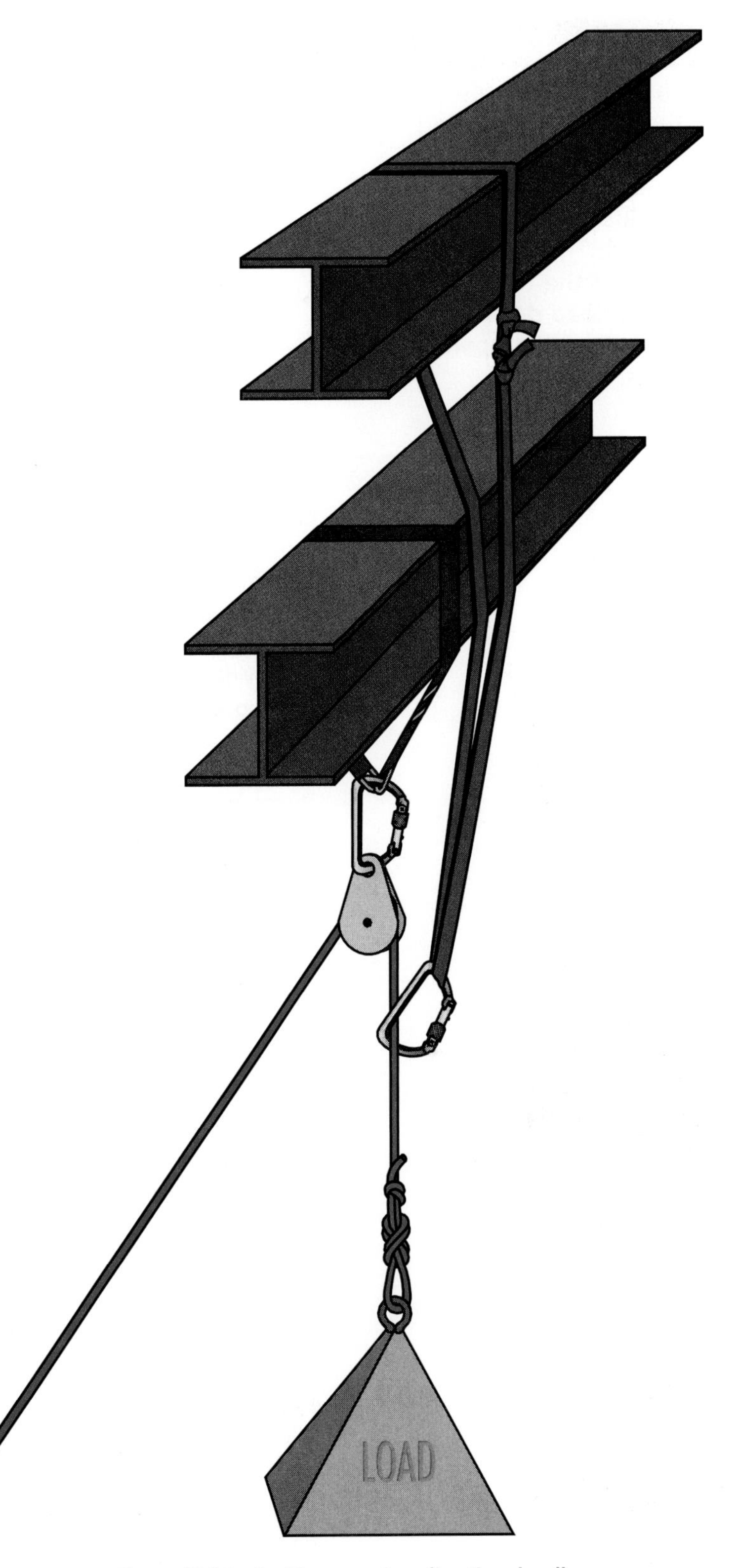

Figure 12.20 Backing up a top directional pulley

Piggyback Systems

In some situations, a vertical block-and-tackle system cannot be used because of the amount of rope needed to reach the bottom of a deep shaft. In these cases, rescuers can build a relatively short simple block-and-tackle M/A system. This system can be attached or "piggybacked" to a 1:1 system being used to lower a rescuer into a shaft or some other depth. In this manner, he or she could be lowered on a rope attached to a descent control device such as a rappel rack or figure-8 plate, and could be retrieved immediately in case of a problem with the "piggybacked" simple system. This piggybacked system is actually a compound M/A because a simple system (for example, a 3:1) has been stacked onto a simple 1:1 system to create a 3:1 M/A ($3 \times 1 = 3$). The greatest advantage of these type systems is that they can be used for both hauling and lowering. Also, they reduce the amount of rope needed because they are capable of being reset.

WARNING

The main line used with the Piggyback hauling system must meet the strength requirements for the load being supported. This rope will support the full weight of the load during lowering or hauling operations.

Any system can be used to create a piggyback for any properly built single-line rope lowering system. Some features are common to all piggyback systems (see Figure 12.17).

- The system is usually formed with two ropes: a main line and the haul line.
- The main line is attached to the patient and anchored to a descent control device such as a rappel rack or figure-8 descender. A figure-8 descender is recommended with piggyback systems as a ratchet device because it is easier to take up rope slack through it during hauling operations.
- The second rope is the haul line. This line is used to build the M/A system, which is then attached to the main line with a haul cam.
  - Both the M/A system and the main line should be anchored in line with each other. As with the Z-rig, the rigging plate works well in piggyback systems to keep components in line with each other while allowing enough separation between them to relieve congestion for easier operation.

Configuring a Piggyback System As mentioned previously, any system can be piggybacked. The most common systems for a piggyback are a 3:1 (see Figure 12.15), a 4:1 simple block-and-tackle system, and a 4:1 compound system.

A 3:1 simple system can be constructed easily or prerigged with a short section of rope (40 to 60 feet). It can be operated in either a 3:1 configuration or turned around to provide a 4:1 configuration and greater M/A. This depends on the haul team's working space.

The disadvantage of piggybacking simple block-and-tackle systems is that, depending on the number and size of the pulleys in the system, they can be difficult to reset. Therefore a 3:1 or 4:1 is recommended, rather than a higher M/A. The size of the pulley sheave has a significant influence on the drag created in the system. Use of pulleys with a sheave diameter at least four times the diameter of the rope allow easier hauling and resetting. However, these large pulleys (usually 3 or 4 inches) can also increase the weight and size of a system, creating more problems. There is another way to increase the efficiency of piggyback systems while keeping them compact and without compromising strength. Rescuers can use a smaller diameter rope (most $\frac{3}{8}$-inch rescue-grade ropes are at least 5,000 pounds minimum breaking strength) in conjunction with smaller pulleys (2-inch pulleys for instance) for construction of the piggyback hauling system. By using the smaller rope, the smaller sheave pulleys still meet the four-to-one rule and the system remains efficient. Because the system is distributing the load among several ropes (each approximately 5,000 pounds strong), the combined strength of the ropes in the system is sufficient for two-person loads (over a 15:1 safety factor). Since these piggyback systems incorporate a different type of ratchet mechanism in the form of a descent control device, a single small-diameter rope will not be subjected to the entire load at any time.

A 4:1 compound M/A system is another alternative to a piggyback system (see Figure 12.17). The advantages are that it requires at least 50% less rope and fewer pulleys (two traveling pulleys) than a simple 4:1 block-and-tackle. This makes it very efficient for hauling and resetting. The disadvantages are that most teams find it difficult to build. In addition, the system may be hauled only to half of its total extended length before resetting is required, making it difficult to operate in a confined work area. This is in contrast to a simple 3:1 or 4:1 piggyback which may be collapsed completely before resetting is required.

Equipment for the Piggyback

- One haul line rope
- Two pulleys (single-sheave)
- One rope grab device (haul cam)
- Steel locking carabiners and anchor rigging
- A separate safety line belay system

Personnel Requirements for the Piggyback This operation has a team consisting of the haul team, ratchetman, haul captain, safety person and load watch. The team

Building the Compound 4:1 Piggyback

1. Tie a very compact knot in the end of the haul line that will be used for the piggyback system.
2. Fold the rope in half.
3. Place the bight formed by doubling the rope near the rear anchor.
4. The knotted and loose ends of the rope should be placed toward the load.
5. Offset the rope slightly by making the loose end approximately 4 feet longer than the knotted end.
6. Tie an anchor knot such as a double-loop figure-8 in the loop.
7. Attach the anchor knot to the same anchor system as the descent control device or to one that is closely in line with the descent control device. Again, the rigging plate serves this purpose well.
8. Make a small bight (enough to accommodate a pulley) in the knotted end of the rope.
9. Reeve a traveling pulley into this loop.
10. Attach this pulley to the main line with a rope grab device and a carabiner. The haul cam should point toward the load. This step is the same regardless of the piggyback hauling system.
11. Make another bight in the loose end of the haul line. This bight should be very near the knotted end of the rope.
12. Reeve a traveling pulley into this loop as well.
13. With a carabiner, attach this traveling pulley to the knotted end of the rope.
14. Rig a separate safety line belay system to the load.
15. Recheck all connection points to make sure the load is attached to the main line properly. Prepare to haul.

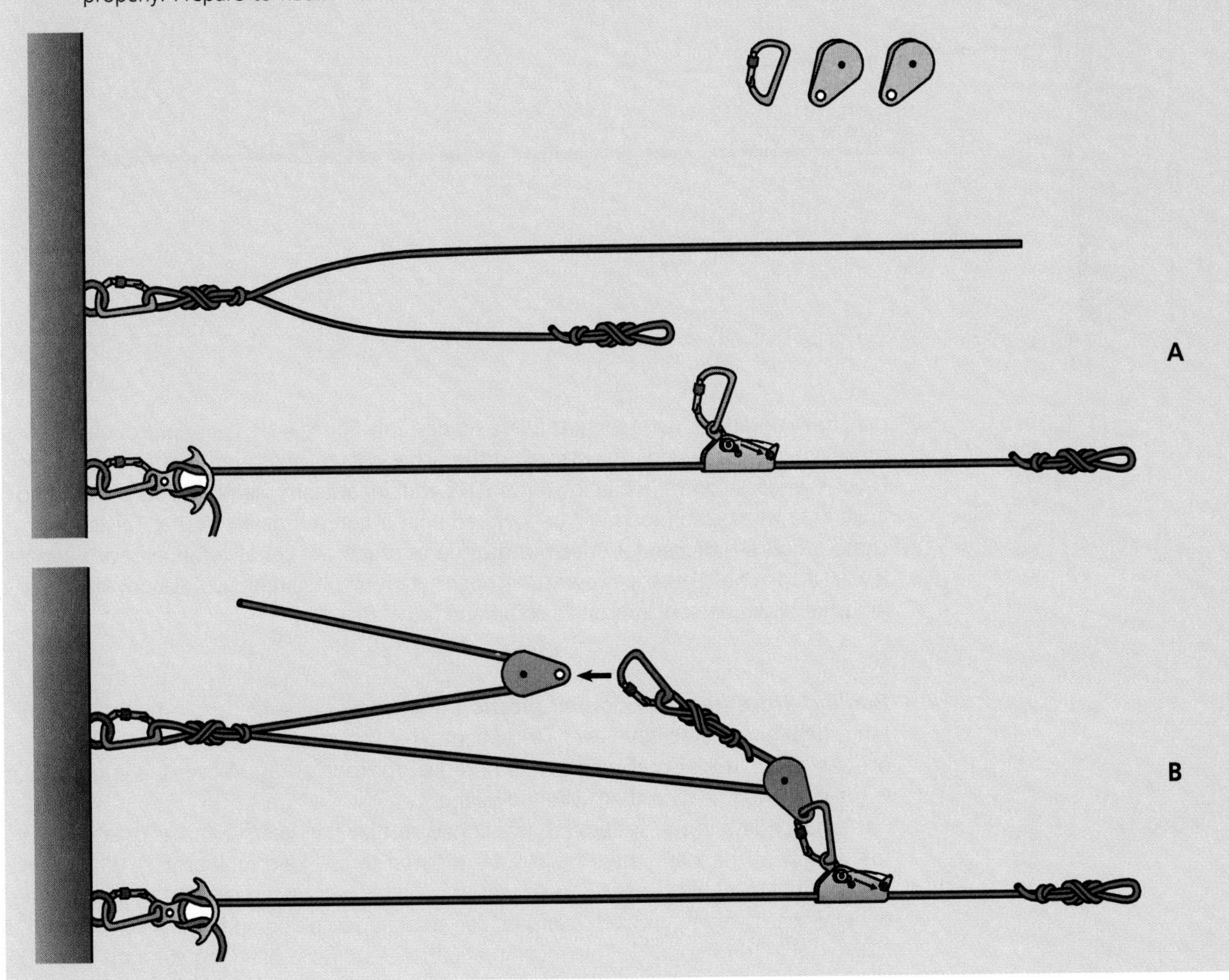

Shortcut for the Piggyback

The same principles for the Z-rig shortcut apply to the piggyback shortcut. However, the mnemonics are different:

1. Biner, pulley, biner, pulley—This is the order of attachment of components to the line being used to create the piggyback hauling system. The order starts at the knotted end of the haul line and progresses toward the loose end. The first carabiner is actually attached to the knot.
2. Front to back—This refers to the movement and attachment of the first component (the carabiner in the knotted end of the haul rope) in the line up with the last component (the rear traveling pulley).

To build a shortcut for the piggyback:

1. Lay out the main line in a straight line with the knotted end toward the load.
2. Attach the other end of the rope to the ratchet/brake device. You can bag the remaining line.
3. Lay out the haul line in a straight line with the knotted end toward the load. This line should be parallel to the main line.

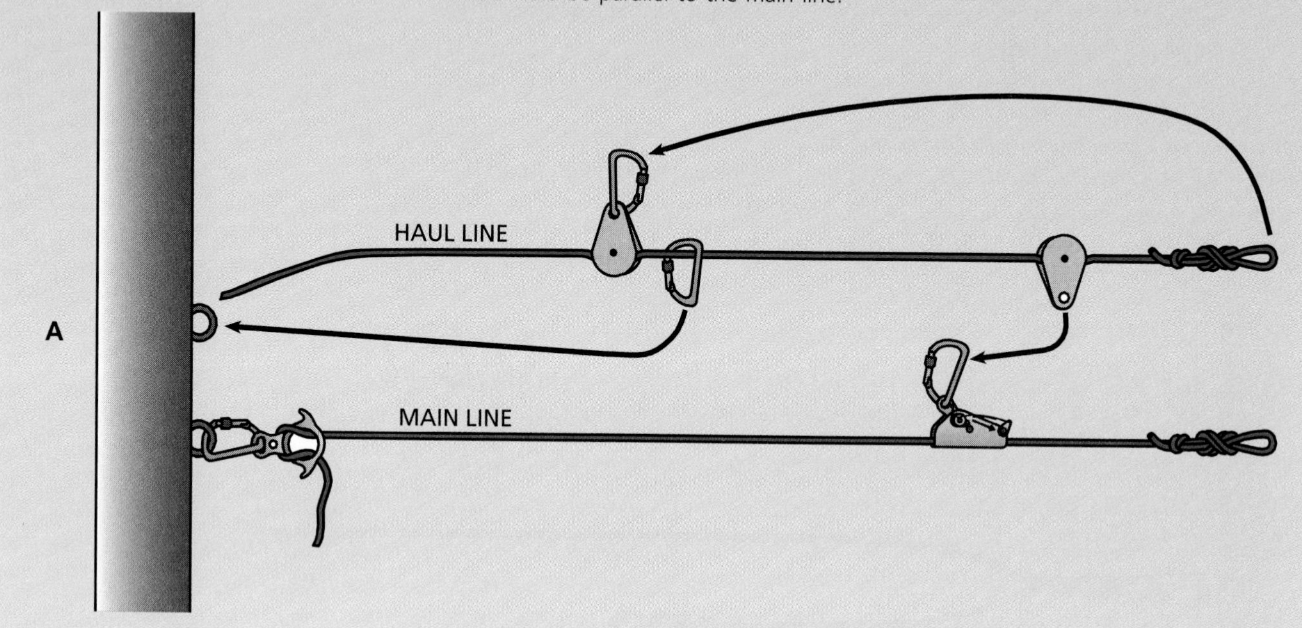

may have an additional member, a line tender, if a figure-8 descent control device is used alone for lowering. This backs up the brake person operating the figure-8 in case he or she loses control while lowering. This additional team member is recommended anytime a two-person load will be lowered with a figure-8 device alone. This is because a figure-8 descender does not provide as much control as a rappel rack during a lower. If the line tender is present, he or she performs a variation of a body belay behind the brake person to provide some additional friction.

Hauling Procedure and Communication Whenever possible, use a pulley to establish a high-point directional over the patient. This facilitates retrieval from a space or over an edge. This also eliminates the potential for rope abrasion over the edge, which is greater when hauling than when lowering.

Some pulleys in the system are positioned so that they receive forces greater than the weight of the load. These pulleys are referred to as "load multipliers." When these load-multiplying pulleys exist in a system, it is highly recommended that they meet the general-use (two-person load) standard for auxiliary rescue equipment as presented in NFPA 1983 (1995 edition). This recommendation requires a breaking strength of 8,000 force pounds. If a pulley used in this manner (such as a single high-point directional

4. Attach one mechanical rope grab to the main line with its arrow pointing toward the load.
5. Attach a carabiner to the cam of this rope grab.
6. Attach a carabiner to the knotted end of the haul line, followed by a pulley, another carabiner, and another pulley.
7. Attach the carabiner at the knotted end of the haul line to the rear pulley. This pulley will become the rear traveling pulley.
8. Attach the front pulley on the haul line to the carabiner attached to the rope grab on the main line. These two items become the front traveling pulley and the haul cam.
9. Pull the carabiner attached to the haul line between the two pulleys to the rear, forming a bight in the rope.
10. Tie an anchor knot in this bight and attach it to its anchor system.
11. Rig a separate safety line belay system to the load.
12. Recheck all connection points and prepare to haul.

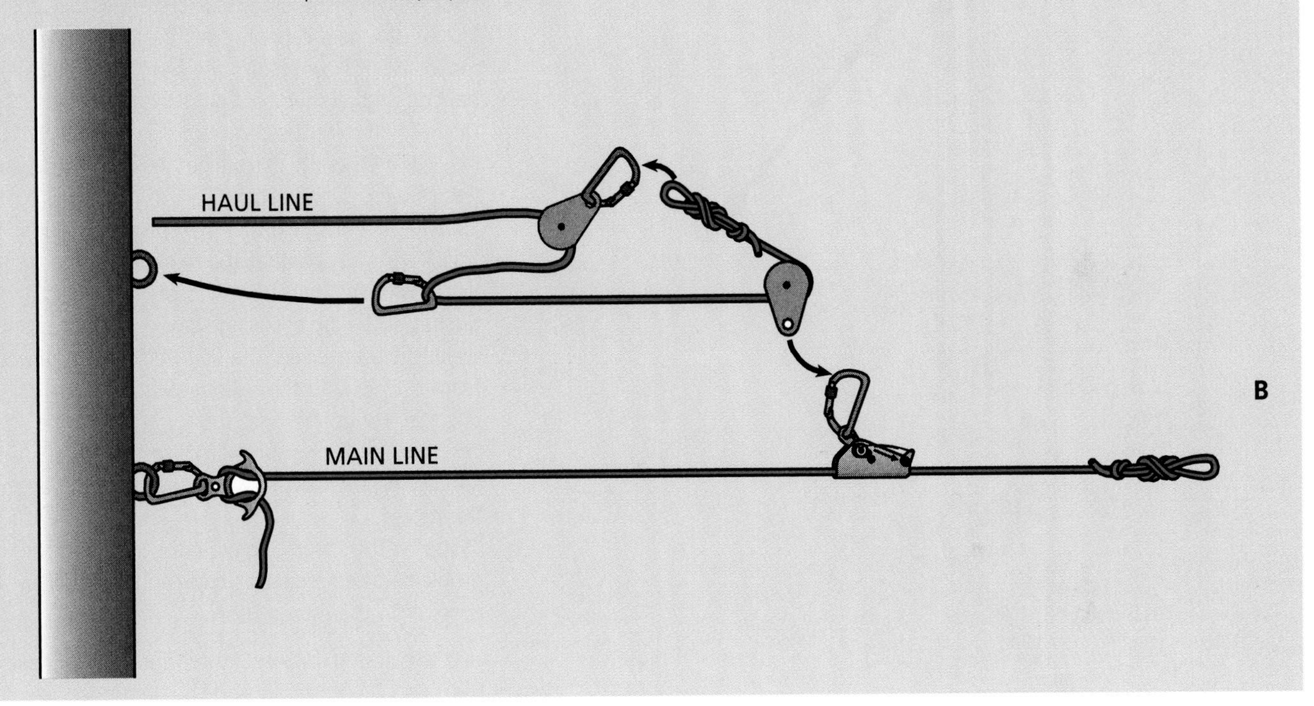

pulley) does not meet this standard, it should be reconfigured or backed up with equipment that does (see Figure 12.20). One way to accomplish this backup is by anchoring a separate piece of rigging (such as webbing, anchor straps, or rope) to an anchor point above the pulley. This rigging should meet strength requirements for two-person loads. Attach the other end of the rigging with a carabiner to the rope issuing from either side of the pulley. This carabiner should hang loosely below the level of the pulley (but not so far that it would cause significant shock loading). Of course, it is best to use the right piece of equipment for the job rather than to rig a backup. Whenever possible, replace substandard pulleys with pulleys that meet general-use strength standards.

Anchor the short (it may be long depending on available space) simple system to the same anchor as the lowering device or another anchor in line with the lowering line (see Figure 12.20). Moving out and away from the main line will cause the system to haul off center. This will cause the patient to settle back down a bit during resetting of the system.

Attach the other end (load end) of the system to the main line (1:1 system) using a mechanical rope grab. The rope grab acts as an extension of the load. When the piggybacked system is hauled, the rope grab grabs the main line, lifting the load. Used in this fashion, the rope grab is called a "haul cam."

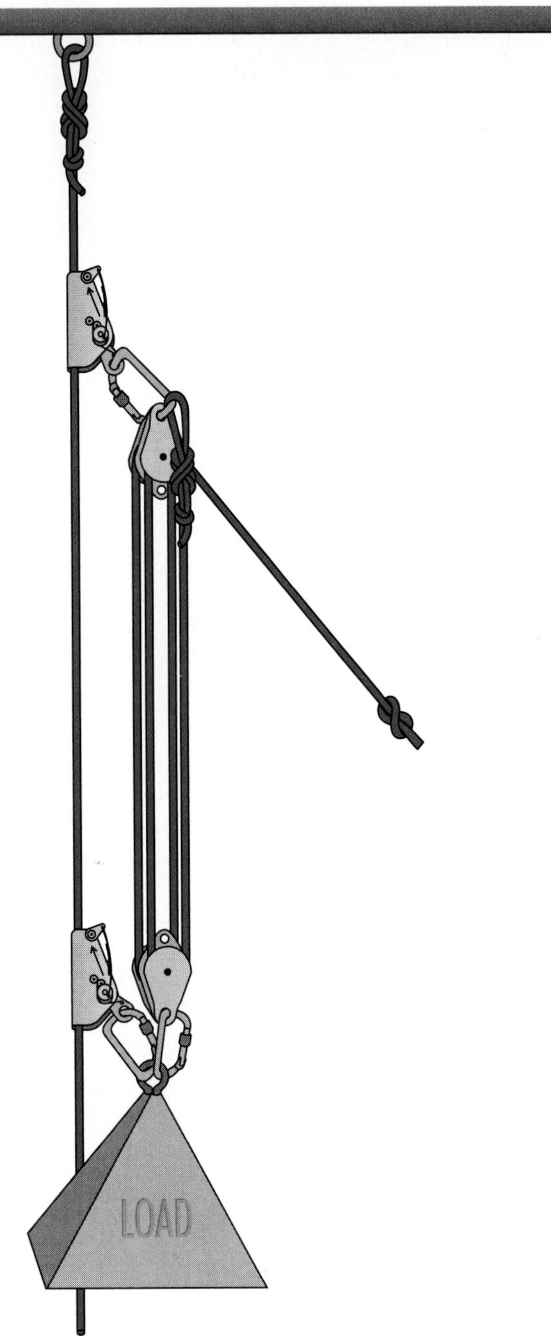

Figure 12.21 Inchworm Confined Space 4:1 Mechanical Advantage System

Remove the slack in the main line, making sure that both the safety line and the main line are attached to the patient. Then continue the haul. The haul captain gives the verbal commands:

- **"Haul"**—When the haul captain gives the "haul" command, the haul team begins to operate the system. As the piggyback system is hauled, the ratchetman (previously operating the descent control device) uses the descent control device as a ratchet, taking up slack as it accumulates in the main line. A figure-8 descent control device is recommended in this type of system because it makes taking up slack easier than other devices such as the rappel rack.
- **"Set"**—When the piggyback system is fully collapsed, the haul captain gives the "set" command. At this command, the haul team stops hauling and all members hold their positions. The ratchetman takes up remaining slack, after which he or she locks off the ratchet device and signals "set!" back to the captain.
- **"Slack**—The haul captain then gives the signal "slack" to indicate that the haul team is to gently transfer the load from its system to the ratchet device by releasing slowly. As soon as the weight is transferred, the first person on the haul team is to extend the system as far forward as possible. He or she does this by grasping the carabiner attaching the system to the haul cam and sliding the cam forward (toward the load) on the rope.
- **"Stop"**—The "stop" command is reserved for problems or emergencies and can be issued by anyone on the rescue team.

Once the system is reset, the haul captain reissues the "haul" command and the sequence repeats until the patient is retrieved.

Lowering Procedure Lowering with this system is the same as lowering with any single-line lowering system. The only significant difference is that the haul cam must be held open or removed from the main line to lower unencumbered.

WARNING

The inchworm is labor intensive and can quickly fatigue the rescuers operating the system. To prevent exhaustion, provide frequent relief for rescue personnel.

The Inchworm Confined Space System

The inchworm confined space system is a short 4:1 simple M/A system (see Figure 12.21) attached to and traveling along an anchored main line via a rope grab device. It is designed for use when rescue must take place through and around many objects that would hamper common hauling systems with added friction produced by the rope running across them. The practical application of this system is extremely limited, but it is an important tool. Though rare, situations arise in which its use is ideal. Some principles and considerations to be aware of when using the inchworm include:

- This system works best for horizontal hauls, but it will also function in short vertical hauls.
- This is the system of choice to perform rescue in industrial vertical vessels that contain horizontal trays or to operate through a series of horizontal ducts or pipes.
- The system is used to actually "inch" your way around the obstacles by using a short

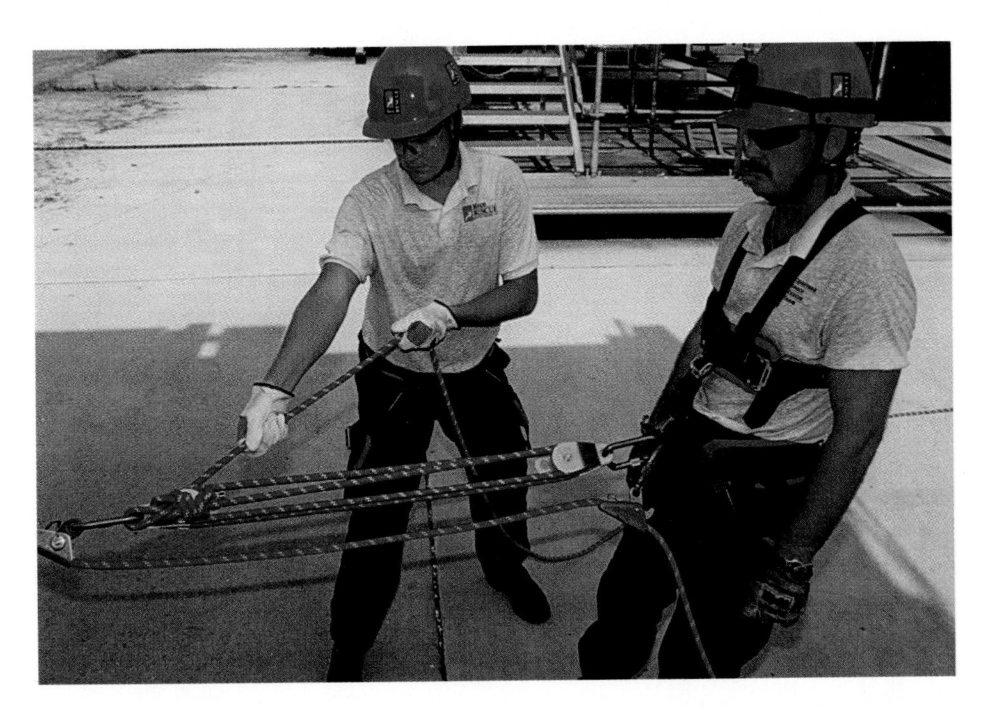

Figure 12.23 Hauling with the Inchworm System

hauling system attached to a fixed line.

- Do not attempt to enter a confined space without taking the necessary monitoring, safety, and personal protective precautions (See Chapters 13 and 14 for further information on confined space rescue).

Configuring the Inchworm This system uses a main line, anchored outside of the space, as an extended anchor for a short simple block-and-tackle M/A system. On one end, the system is attached to this main line via a rope grab device. The load is attached to the other end of the M/A system. As the system is hauled, the rope grab grips the anchored line, allowing the load to be pulled along the path of the main line until the system is completely collapsed. In horizontal applications, the system is then reset by grasping the carabiner attached to the rope grab device and pulling it toward the anchored end of the main line. In vertical applications, a second rope grab is necessary to temporarily transfer the weight of the load from the inchworm so it can be reset for continued hauling. In either case, the system is continually collapsed and reset as it moves along the path of the main line. This gives the system the appearance of an inchworm, which is where it gets its name.

Equipment for the Inchworm The equipment required for the inchworm system is:

- one short (18 to 20 feet) section of $\frac{3}{8}$- to $\frac{1}{2}$-inch-static kernmantle rescue rope

Building the Inchworm System

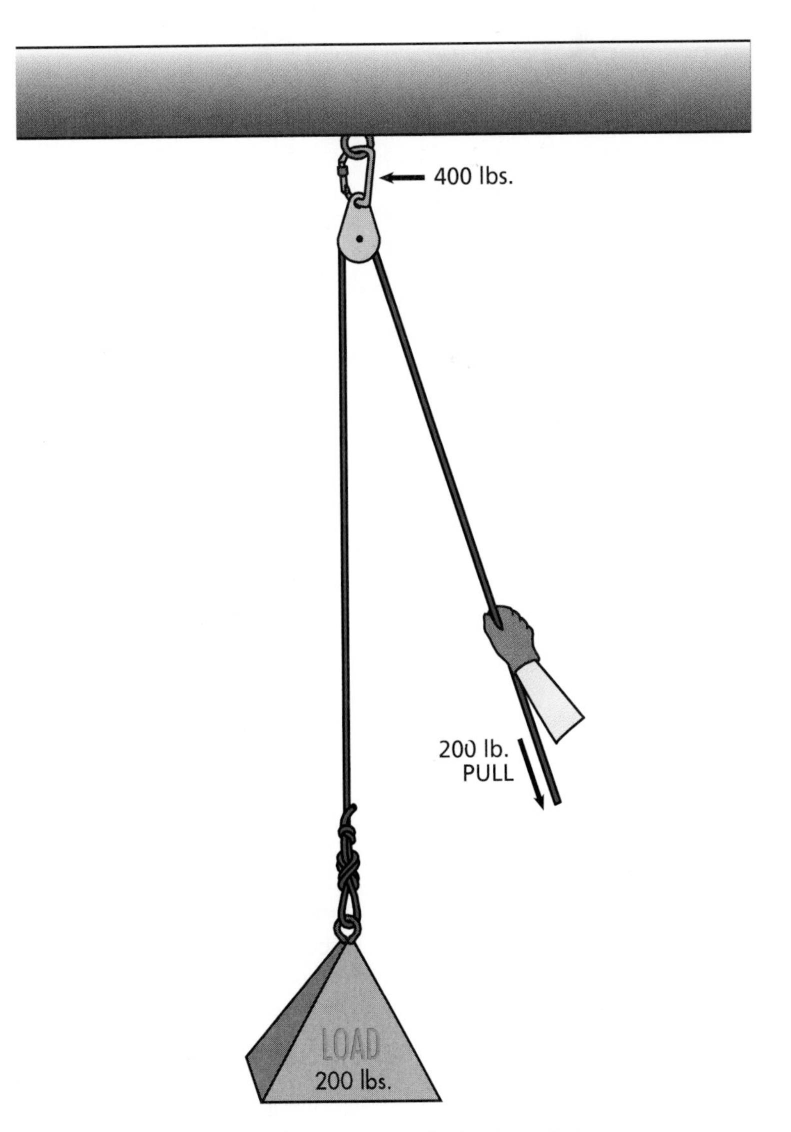

Figure 12.24 Example of a load multiplier

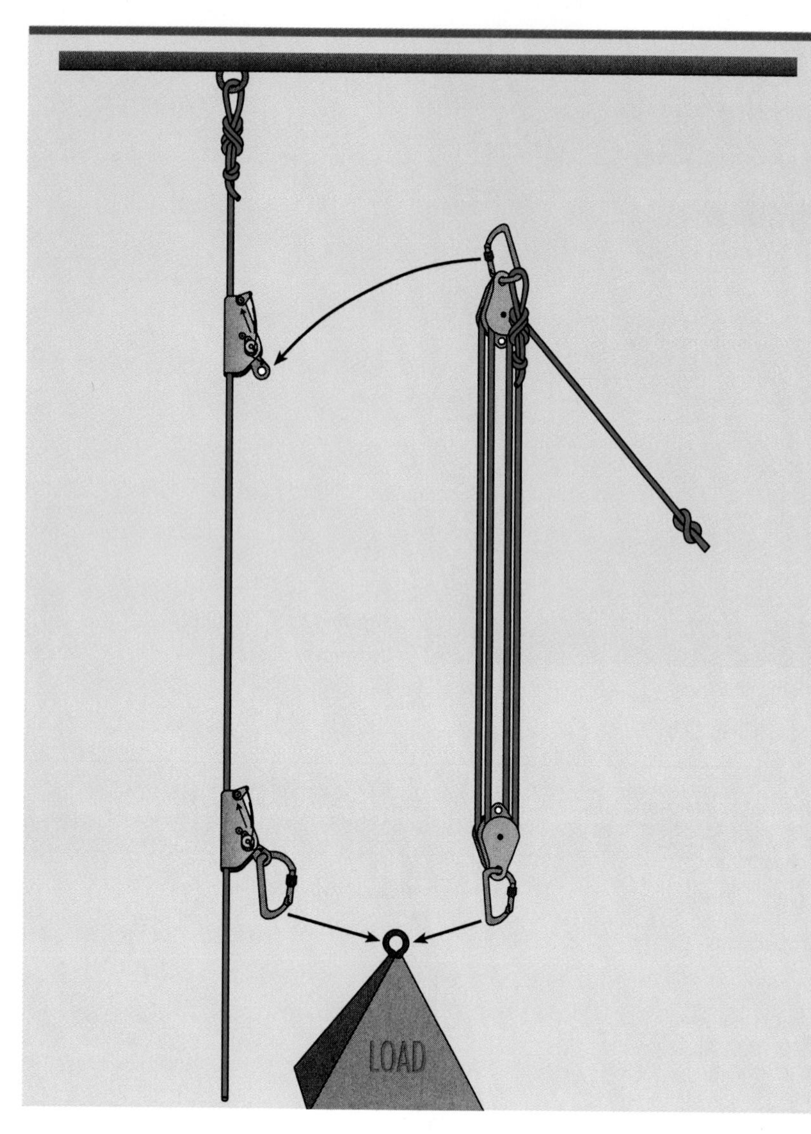

1. Anchor the main line outside of the space or entry area. Build a simple 4:1 M/A system as previously described. Do not attach the cams.
2. Tie a figure-8 stopper knot in the end of the rope to prevent the loose end from slipping through the top pulley.
3. Attach a rope grab device to the main line, arrow pointing away from the patient and toward the egress.
4. Attach the top carabiner of the inchworm to the rope grab.
5. Attach the bottom carabiner of the system to the patient's harness or litter bridle.
6. For short vertical hauls, attach another rope grab device to the main line below the inchworm attachment rope grab.
7. Connect the second rope grab directly to the patient's harness or litter bridle with one steel carabiner. This will allow the load to be held in place while the inchworm is reset in the vertical environment.
8. Always use a safety line belay system when hauling in a vertical application.
9. Recheck all attachment points and prepare to haul the patient.

- one main line ($\frac{1}{2}$-inch rope)
- two double-sheave pulleys (one traveling and one directional)
- two cams (Both are used to anchor the system to the main line. Only one is required for horizontal applications.)
- three carabiners (Only two are required for horizontal applications.)
- a separate safety line belay system when using the inchworm in a vertical application

Incorporating the Rope Grab Cams

The inchworm is the only hauling system presented in this chapter in which the arrow on the rope grab device points AWAY from the load. The bottom cam is designed to hold the load in place vertically while resetting the system. Therefore, the inchworm system can be used without the bottom cam in horizontal applications but should always be used WITH the bottom cam in vertical applications.

Personnel Requirements The inchworm system is designed to be operated by one rescuer in confined spaces. However, if it is possible to use other personnel to help manipulate the load, it reduces the fatigue associated with operation of this system. This is particularly significant when the inchworm is used in a vertical application.

Hauling Procedure

1. If the system (see Figure 12.23) will be used vertically, confirm that the safety line is attached to the patient and the safety person is ready.

2. Haul as far as possible.
3. Set the bottom cam (in vertical applications only) and release the load onto it.
4. Extend the inchworm by pulling the upper cam (nearest the rescuer) as far as possible along the static line toward the egress.
5. Repeat the haul procedure to "inch" the patient up or across to the desired destination.

The inchworm can be constructed quickly or prebuilt for rapid deployment. Although it has been shown as a 4:1 M/A system, it might be advantageous in some cases to turn the inchworm around to create a 5:1 M/A with a haul in the opposite direction.

The P Method

The P method is a theoretical means of determining the forces applied to, and the mechanical advantage of, various hauling systems. The *P* stands for "pull" in the system. While the P method provides theoretical information on mechanical advantage, it does not account for actual loss of efficiency due to friction produced by a system's components. The P method assumes that the rope legs issuing from the pulleys are parallel and at an approximately zero degree angle. It also assumes a pulley sheave diameter at least four times the diameter of the rope for maximum efficiency.

Load Multipliers

When you pull on a rope, you exert force in a straight line transmitted along the length of the rope. If a rope is attached to a suspended load weighing 200 pounds, then you must pull with a force of at least 200 pounds to move the object (see Figure 12.24).

If you pass the rope through a high-point directional pulley and attach it to a suspended 200-pound load, you still have to pull at least 200 pounds on the haul line to lift the load. However, this time there is 200 pounds of pull on each side of the pulley. There is 200 pounds of pull created by the load on one side of the pulley and approximately 200 pounds of pull created by the haul team on the other side of the pulley.

As long as the angle between these two rope legs is near zero degrees, the force exerted on the high-point directional pulley is about twice the load. This type of directional pulley is often called a "load multiplier." The forces are multiplied in the same manner on any pulley in a hauling system as long as the angle between the rope legs is near zero degrees.

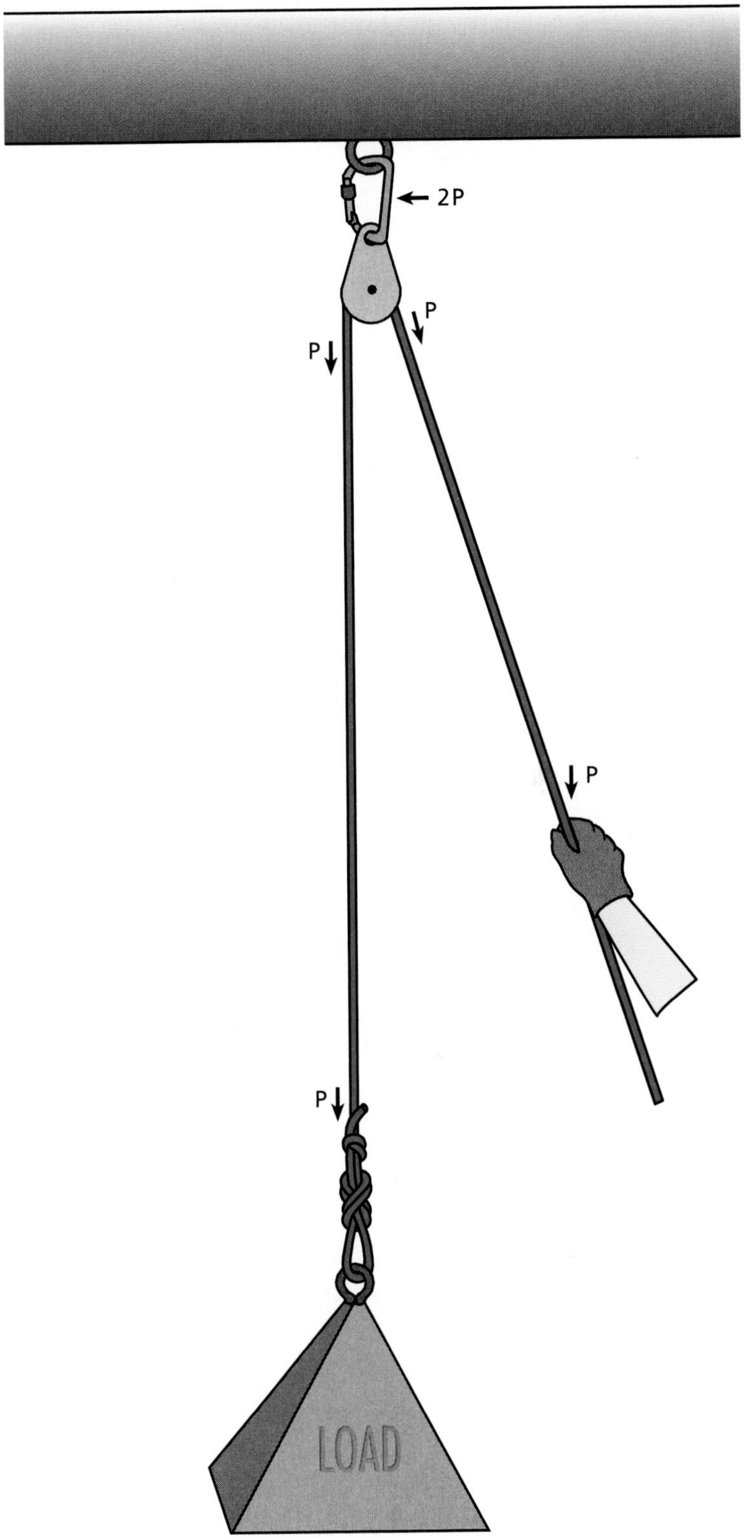

Figure 12.25 **Determining "P" for simple 1:1 vertical system**

Determining P for a Simple 1:1 Vertical System

Remember, the variable P represents the amount of "pull" on the haul line of a system.

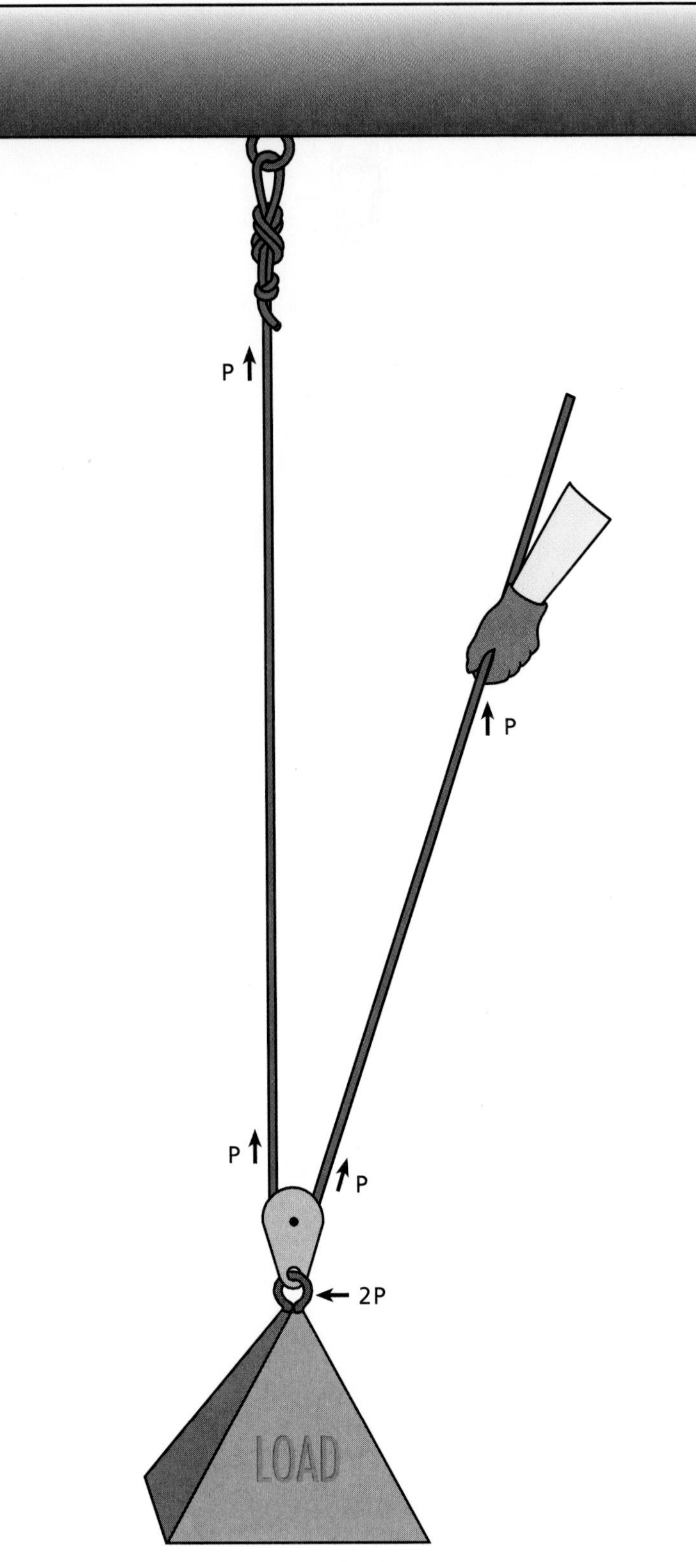

Figure 12.26 Determining "P" for simple 2:1 vertical system

- When using the P method, always start calculations at the haul line and work toward the load.
- The force (input force) being applied to the haul line is always P (which means 1 × P).

In the illustrated 1:1 mechanical advantage (M/A) system (see Figure 12.25), the force (P) exerted on the haul line is transmitted along the entire length of the rope and terminates at the load. The force is the same on both sides of the pulley. Since this is a load multiplier, the force applied to the pulley and its anchor is approximately twice the load or 2 P (2 × P). Since P is transmitted along the entire length of the rope, terminating at the load, the load is being pulled with 1 P (1 × P) amount of force.

If the force at the load is P, and the force at the haul line is also P, then the ratio is 1 P of load to the amount of force (1 P) required to lift the load. Comparing the number of P's at the load to the number of P's at the haul line, indicates that the mechanical advantage of this system is 1:1.

Determining P for a Simple 2:1 Vertical System

In the illustrated 2:1 M/A system, we start with P at the haul line (see Figure 12.26).

- The force travels along the entire length of the rope and ends at the anchor.
- The force exerted on each side of the pulley is 1 P. Since this is a load multiplier, the total force exerted on the pulley (and the load) is 2 P.

If the force at the load is 2 P, and the force at the haul line is 1 P, then the ratio is 2 P of load to the amount of force (1 P) required to lift the load. Comparing the number of P's at the load to the number of P's at the haul line determines that the mechanical advantage of this system is 2:1.

Determining the Forces on System Components

The P method also allows you to learn the forces applied to almost any part of the hauling system. In the previous example, the force exerted on the anchor point is 1 P or approximately $\frac{1}{2}$ the weight of the load (2 P). If the load is 200 pounds (or 2 P), then the force on the anchor is 100 pounds (or 1 P). The force on the anchor will never exceed 100 pounds as long as the load is allowed to move freely. If, however, the load were to catch on an object, the forces on the entire system would quickly increase based on whatever force the haul team can exert.

For example, seven strong haulers are hauling a 200-pound patient on a 2:1 system. During the haul, the patient's head catches under a steel I-beam. Now the haulers are pulling against a load that is not moving. As they pull harder in an attempt to move the load, the forces on the haul line and the system increase.

If the haul team pulls 1,000 pounds of force (P) on the haul line, then 1,000 pounds will be exerted on the rope and anchor rigging. Using the P method, if P is equal to 1,000 pounds, then twice that amount (2 P, or 2,000 pounds) will be exerted on the traveling pulley. Even worse, the rescuers are exerting 2,000 pounds of force on the patient's head.

The number of haulers is limited on a M/A system to avoid exerting too much pressure on the patient. This way, the haul team will be able to feel resistance if the load catches. Consequently, they can react quickly to prevent damage to the patient and/or system components. Therefore, there should be a load watch provided when any M/A system is operating. If a patient gets caught on something, it can be detected immediately.

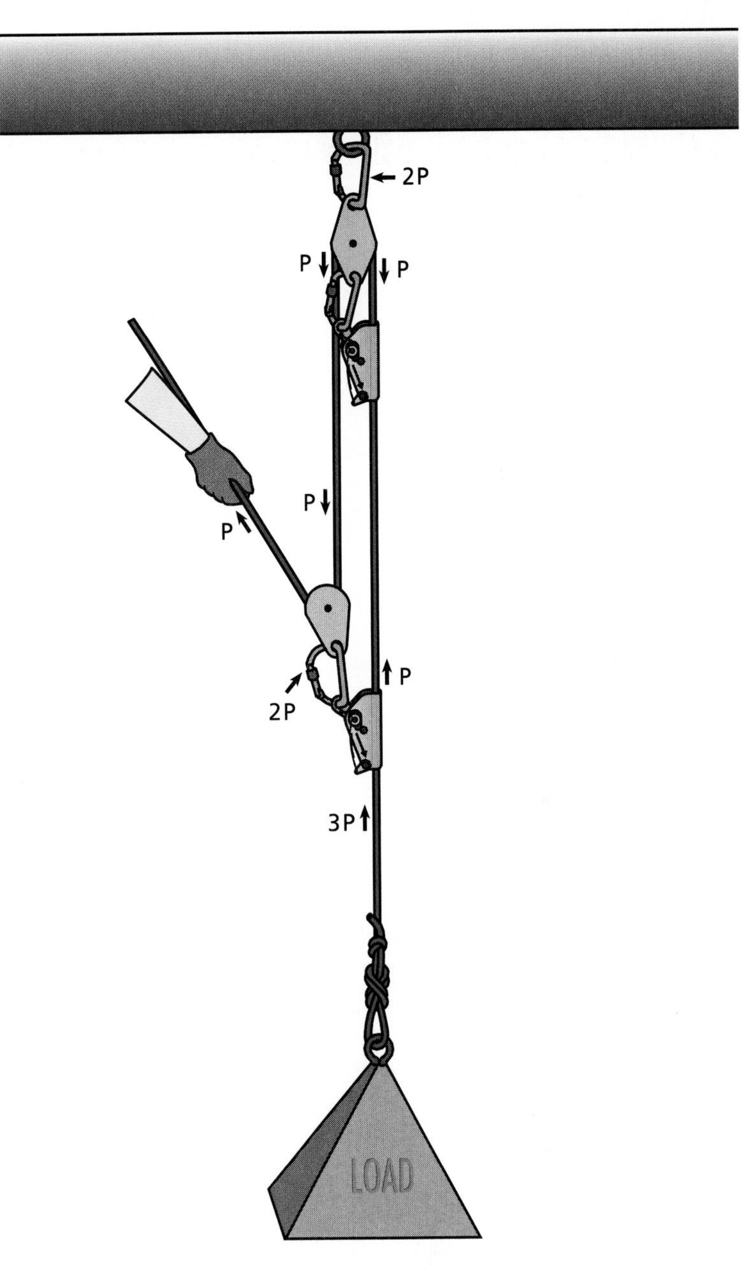

Figure 12.27 Determining "P" for 3:1 Z-Rig system

Determining P for a Simple 3:1 Horizontal System

To determine P for M/A systems such as the Z-rig and piggyback, use the formula given for calculating P for a simple 2:1 vertical system with one addition. That is, any time a rope grab device is used in the system, the forces exerted on the rope grab from various parts of the system must be added together. Whatever the total force produced on the rope grab, it will be transmitted along the rope (toward the load) from that point.

For example, the Z-rig system in Figure 12.27 shows:

- A force of 2 P is exerted on the traveling pulley.
- The traveling pulley is attached to a cam-type mechanical rope grab.
- The rope running through the rope grab has 1 P of force.
- The P coming into the rope grab must be added to the 2 P already exerted by the attached traveling pulley.
- The total force produced by the haul cam is 3 P.
  This force will continue to be transmitted along the rope, terminating at the load.

Therefore, the mechanical advantage of this system is 3 P to 1 P, or 3:1.

Summary

Hauling systems are one of the most useful tools in technical rescue. Systems that double for hauling and lowering are extremely versatile for confined space rescues. Mechanical advantage is the basis from which you will build the systems required for the job at hand. The information provided here is no substitute for training and hands-on application under supervision of a competent instructor.

CHAPTER 13

Confined Space Communications

The information in this chapter is provided as a basis for continued trainiing. Each rescuer should consult with his or her own team leader for the correct SOGs for the team. Topics covered in this chapter include:

- Introduction
- Overview
- Regulations and Equipment
- Communications Equipment
- Assignment of Duties

Introduction

Communications systems and their operations are often the last thing considered during a confined space emergency (see Figure 13.1). Nevertheless, they provide one of the most important elements of rescue practices. As in any rescue, communications are crucial to an effective team effort. During confined space rescue, the ability to communicate from outside the space to inside it is not only important, it is required by OSHA.

Much recent research has focused on equipment and methods for communications during confined space rescue. This section explores the practical applications, regulatory compliance, and intrinsic safety requirements for confined space communications equipment. It also offers suggestions for selection, deployment, and operating guidelines during a confined space emergency.

Overview

Before safe and reliable voice communication systems were available, rescue teams relied on shouting, tapping, and rope tugging to send messages back and forth. Deciphering how many tugs from the end of a 100-foot rope that goes around a corner or two is almost impossible. Yet for many teams this is the primary method of communication for "regulatory compliance." Although the "OATH" (OATH is a rope-tugging method of communication) method meets requirements for compliance, it should be used only in the context for which it was intended, "when you cannot speak and be understood," not as a primary method of communication.

The technology and the equipment for safe and reliable confined space voice communication is commercially available, so it is a needless risk to send someone into a space without the ability to simply ask for help.

*Most of the information in this chapter is derived from a report that has been compiled based on input from several nationally recognized rescue entities, both private agencies and municipal fire service organizations. This research and subsequent report were generated by Andrew Ibbetson of CONSPACE Communications Incorporated. This company, based in Canada, is a recognized leader in the field of confined space communications systems worldwide.

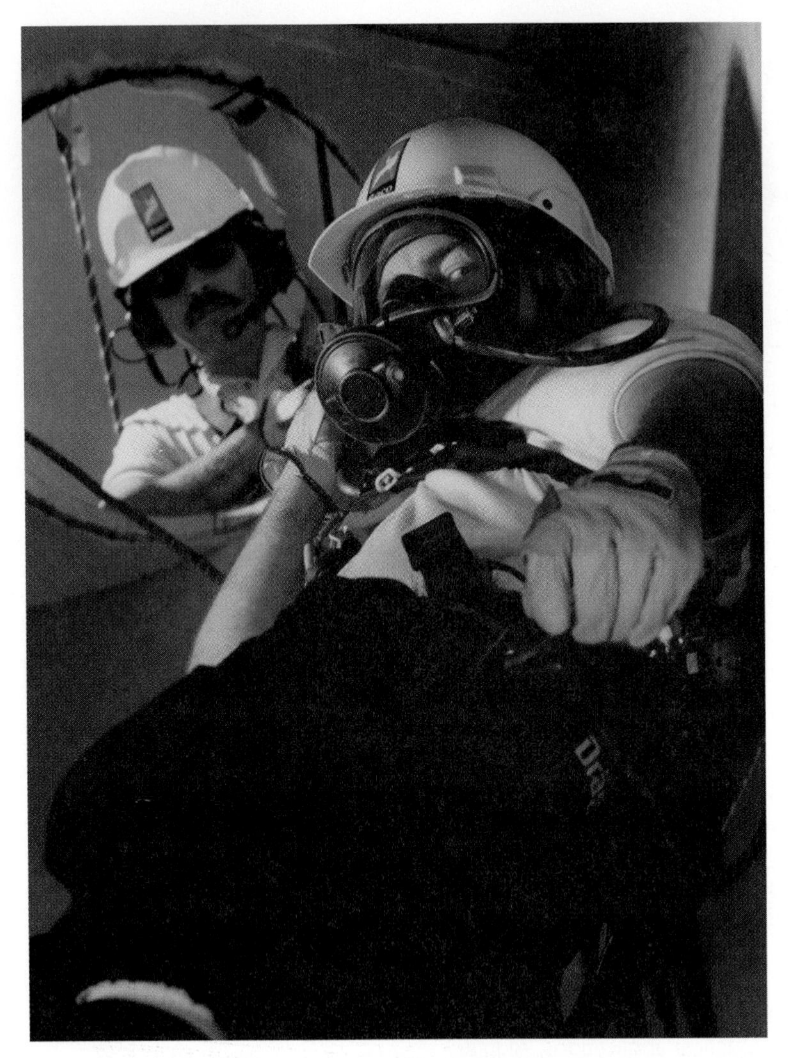

Figure 13.1 Con Space Communications

A correctly selected and used method of continuous voice communication can save a considerable amount of time during a confined space rescue operation. Instantaneous communication among the rescuers and rescue personnel who are outside a confined space can dramatically improve the entire operation. Rescuers inside a space can immediately call for equipment to extricate a patient or for additional support. They can also relay medical information or direct line hauling operations. Reliable communication among the attendant and rescue entrants has a calming effect on rescuers and reduces the likelihood of accidents caused by misunderstandings, confusion, or panic.

Communication among team members is primarily for the safety of the rescuers. However, other advantages to a correctly deployed communication system include:

- higher levels of perceived safety
- better training
- reduction of the stress experienced by rescuers due to claustrophobia or panic
- more efficient use of personnel
- faster rescues

Another characteristic of voice communication is the ability of rescuers to assess a victim's condition before the rescuers actually enter the space.

This chapter describes the major benefits of a properly selected and deployed hardline communication system for confined space rescue. Also included are considerations and points for discussion regarding the selection, deployment, and integration.

Experienced confined space rescuers know the drawbacks, pitfalls, and danger of not having reliable voice communication during a confined space rescue. Rescue teams must develop procedures and practices for its integration and recognize hardline communication equipment as a valuable rescue tool that will increase safety, save time, and save lives.

Practical Applications

Communication equipment is often the last piece of confined space equipment to be considered—after PPE, breathing apparatus, and gas detection, retrieval and ventilation equipment. It is the equipment, however, that ties together the whole rescue operation and allows a rescue team to work as a cohesive unit.

Communication and Retrieval Equipment

The developments in the area of retrieval equipment over the last few years have been remarkable. The advances in the types, styles, designs, and inner workings of this equipment have exploded since the Confined Space and Fall Protection Regulations were enacted by OSHA and federal law.

Tripods, hoists, and winches have become very popular. Of course, the best retrieval device in the world is useless unless the attendant recognizes a need for it. Communication equipment can save valuable time and mean the difference between retrieving a worker or recovering a body from a confined space.

In confined space rescue, manual haul systems are the preferred method of retrieval. The most common problems in rope rescue involve line tending and hauling.

The ability of entrants to communicate their needs regarding the paying out, taking up, or stopping of the rope is a great advantage. It makes a rescue operation proceed more smoothly.

Communication and Gas Detection

Gas detection equipment should be used in all confined space operations. Recent advances have increased reliability and decreased the size of many gas detection devices. Confined space entries are now routinely conducted with small gas monitors. Entrants can carry them and sample gases in the area in which the entrant is working. This type of gas monitoring complements monitoring at the point of entry. For this type of program to work properly and keep permit documentation current, the attendant should get periodic readings from the entrant monitor and note them on the permit. If an entrant monitor sounds an alarm, entrant(s) must immediately notify the attendant of the change in atmosphere.

If gas monitoring is done only at the entrance to a space, the need for communication becomes even greater. If an atmospheric alarm sounds while the entrant is working in high noise and/or out of sight, the attendant must have a way to inform the entrant of the hazard and tell him or her to evacuate the space immediately.

Communication and Breathing Apparatus

Breathing apparatus is common to confined space work and confined space rescue. The trend in apparatus for use in confined spaces is toward the supplied air respirators (SAR). This equipment is able to provide rescuers with a virtually unlimited supply of air, and also has physical and weight advantages (i.e., no air tank to carry).

Communication is a valuable link where SAR is concerned. If there is a problem with the supplied air system and an alarm sounds, the attendant can notify the entrant(s) immediately so they can switch to their emergency air supplies. If the problem is only momentary, communication can be used to coordinate between the use of emergency air and the normal air supply.

Communication and Ventilation Equipment

Ventilation equipment is used widely for confined space work. If there is a problem with the air flow or if an airborne hazard (e.g., carbon monoxide from vehicle exhaust) is introduced into a space, the attendant must inform the entrant(s) without delay.

Human Factors

Entering a confined space can subject personnel to claustrophobia or panic. The space they enter is harsh and unfriendly and was designed by engineers for an industrial process, not for human occupancy. Therefore, rescuers cannot rely on the surroundings for their psychological well-being (sense of security, being in control) and must depend on what they can take into the space with them.

The well-being of rescue entrants determines how well they function at any given moment. The study of ergonomics tells us that the better people feel, the better they perform their jobs. In an actual rescue, adrenaline and emotions can create a very stressful atmosphere. Personnel working outside their comfort zone are considerably prone to errors through poor decision making and bad judgment due to stress. Rescuers, no matter how experienced, are still human beings. Although an error due to stress outside a space might be corrected easily, the same error made inside a space could be someone's last.

The human voice has been proved to have a calming effect on people in isolation. Therefore, reliable, continuous voice communication can help to provide confined space entrants with the level of comfort needed to relieve the fears of entry, maintain an acceptable comfort zone for the duration of the rescue operation, and keep claustrophobia and panic in check. Industrial workers who routinely use a voice communication system for confined space work confirm this. They report feeling safer, more at ease, and less stressful. They also say that, as a result, they work better, are more efficient, and are much happier in their work. As an added benefit, safety attendants also react favorably to being able to communicate with entrants. It makes their job less boring and they feel more useful by being able to monitor entrants at all times. Close team work among entrants and safety attendants is possible with little or no effort.

Regulations and Communication Equipment

The industry regulation for confined space is governed by OSHA 29CFR 19210.146, Confined Space Standard for General Industry. All discussions regarding confined space rescue are intended to fully comply with this standard. Although the regulation does not specifically require a powered communication system, it is virtually impossible to fully comply without one. The regulations address the duties of those involved in any confined space operation in the context of an actual confined space environment.

The "duties of the authorized entrants" include alerting the attendant, giving updates on status, and listening for evacuation orders. This may not seem difficult, but when the entrant is 100 feet inside a pipe that has horizontal and vertical changes in direction and high ambient noise, the ability to communicate is very difficult. If the entrant is wearing breathing apparatus and hearing protection, the communication becomes even more challenging.

The "duties of attendants" include communicating evacuation alerts, monitoring entrant status, monitoring activities both inside and outside the space, and monitoring the entrants for behavioral effects of gases, vapors, and chemicals. The attendant must also watch for any situations outside the space that could endanger the entrants.

The most interesting communication requirement in the regulation is that the attendant monitor the entrant(s) for symptoms or behavioral effects of exposure to hazards. To do this requires a communication system capable of continuous communication (like a party line) and hands-free operation. This allows the attendant to monitor the entrant(s) continuously for slurring of speech, out-of-character responses, or irregular breathing.

Regulation Excerpts

The following are excerpts from OSHA 29CFR 1910.146 dealing with communication in confined Space:

(d) Permit-Required Confined Space Program
Under the permit-required confined space program required by paragraph (c)(4) of this section, the employer shall:

(4) Provide the following equipment (specified in paragraphs (d)(4)(i) through (d)(4)(ix) of this section) at no cost to employees, maintain that equipment properly, and ensure that employees use that equipment properly;

(iii) Communications equipment necessary for compliance with paragraphs (h)(3) and (i)(5) of this section.

(H) Duties Of Authorized Entrants

(3) Communicate with the attendant as necessary to enable the attendant to monitor entrant status and to enable the attendant to alert entrants of the need to evacuate the space as required by paragraph (iX6) of this section;

(4) Alert the attendant whenever: The entrant recognizes any warning sign or symptom of exposure to a dangerous situation or The entrant detects a prohibited condition.

(i) Duties Of Attendants

(2) Is aware of possible behavioral effects of hazard exposures in authorized entrants.

(5) Communicates with authorized entrants as necessary to monitor entrant status and to alert entrants of the need to evacuate the space under paragraph (i)(6) of this section;

(6) Monitors activities inside and outside the space to determine if it is safe for entrants to remain in the space and orders the authorized entrants to evacuate the permit space immediately under any of the following conditions:

- If the attendant detects the behavioral effects of hazard exposure in an authorized entrant;
- If the attendant detects a situation outside the space that could endanger the authorized entrants.

Communication Equipment and Intrinsic Safe Approvals

Intrinsic safe approval levels are covered in greater detail later in this chapter. The level of intrinsic safe approval is very important when choosing electrically powered equipment for confined space rescue. An intrinsically safe circuit is a circuit in which any spark or thermal effect is incapable of causing ignition of flammable or combustible material in air under prescribed conditions. Rescuers never know what environment they will be called upon to enter next. For safety, OSHA compliance, and liability concerns, equipment must be certified by a nationally recognized test laboratory (NRTL). For rescue use, electrical equipment should be approved at the highest level possible so that it can be used safely in the widest variety of rescue locations, environments, and conditions.

Rescuers should not enter a space unless the atmosphere is at or below 10% of the flammable materials' lower explosive limit (LEL). However, atmospheres in confined spaces are subject to rapid changes. Teams must prepare for the worst case and have reliable equipment.

Approval levels are often misunderstood. It is common for people to assume that equipment rated Class I, Division I, or simply "intrinsically safe" can be used anywhere. This is not correct. For example, you should never use equipment approved for a Class I (flammable vapors) environment in either a Class II (combustible dust) or Class III (ignitable fibers) environment. Doing so could be the last mistake you ever make.

All intrinsically safe approved equipment carries label(s) that list the name of a nationally recognized test laboratory and the class, division, and group levels of approval. If the label carries only the name of the test laboratory and a file approval number, contact a NRTL for a copy of the approval or the levels of approval for your equipment. Division marking is optional for all equipment except that in Division II, in which case the division marking is required.

The following is a condensed version of the National Electrical Code (NEC) classifications for hazardous locations. Also provided is a cross reference between the level of approval and possible rescue sites. The following classifications apply to ALL electrically powered equipment used in or around confined spaces or potentially explosive environments. This includes communication, equipment, lights, gas monitors, PASS devices, pagers, pumps, blowers, and so on.

WARNING

The term "intrinsically safe" is becoming a generic term. Some organizations advertise their equipment as "designed to intrinsic standards" or "meets intrinsic safe requirements" or simply "intrinsically safe." Using nonapproved equipment or equipment not approved for a specific hazardous environment could cause an explosion or accident, injuring or killing workers or rescuers. Check equipment approvals so that you are aware of the areas in which you can and cannot deploy your equipment.

National Electrical Code (NEC) Classifications for Hazardous Locations

- **Class I**—Locations in which flammable gases or vapors are present or may be present in the air in quantities sufficient to produce explosive or ignitable mixtures.
- **Class II**—Locations that are hazardous because of the presence of combustible dust.
- **Class III**—Locations that have the presence of easily ignitable fibers or filings.

Classes are also broken down into divisions:

- **Division I**—Locations with particularly hazardous materials in potentially flammable concentrations in the air continuously, frequently, or intermittently under normal operating conditions.
- **Division II**—Locations that might become hazardous in the event of mechanical breakdown, accidental failure, or abnormal operation or equipment.

The classes are further broken down into groups:

- Class I
  - Group A — Acetylene
  - Group B — Butadiene, hydrogen, ethylene oxide, propylene oxide
  - Group C — Acetaldehyde, ethylene, cyclopropane, ether vapors, unsymmetrical
  - Group D — Acetone, ammonia, benzene, butane, butyl alcohol, butyl acetate, ethane, eythl acetate, ethylene dichloride, gasoline, heptane, hexanes, isoprene, methane, methanol, ketones, propanol, petroleum, octanes,

pentanes, propane, ethanol propylene, styrene, toluene, vinyl acetate, vinyl chloride, xylanes

- Class II
  - Group E —Metal dust includes aluminum, commercial alloys, and magnesium
  - Group F — Carbon black, coal, charcoal, coke dust
  - Group G — Flour, starch, grain dust
- Class III
  - No groups

Examples of Classifications and Corresponding Rescue Sites

- **Class I, Division I and Division II**—Petroleum refineries, dry cleaning plants, petrochemical plants, hospitals, utilities, aircraft hangers, paint manufacturers, dip tanks containing flammable or combustible liquids, spray finishing areas
- **Class II, Division II**—Grain elevators, some coal-handling or preparation plants, flour and feed mills, confectionery plants, fireworks manufacturing and storage areas, grain ships, areas that package and handle pulverized sugar and cocoa, manufacturing and storage areas for magnesium, spice-grinding mills
- **Class III, Division I and Division II**—Wood-working plants, textile mills, cotton gins, cotton seed mills, flax-producing plants, knitting mills, weaving mills

__NOTE:__ Individual group classifications also apply to these sites and were omitted here for brevity. These lists are a guideline only. If you have specific sites you wish to categorize, please refer to the National Electrical Code or contact your local OSHA compliance officer.

Equipment certified intrinsically safe by test laboratories in Europe and other parts of the world are not accepted for use in the United States unless they carry a separate U.S. approval. The exception to this is equipment approved by the Canadian Standards Association (CSA). The approved equipment must actually have "NRTL" on the printed label (below the CSA logo). This denotes that the equipment has been tested following Underwriters Lab (UL) and ANSI test methods and is recognized by OSHA as safe for use in the United States.

Selecting Communication Equipment

Selection criteria for rescue equipment can be divided into two categories:

- Reliability—Technology here refers to the ability of the equipment to function reliably in the confined space environment. Electrically powered communication equipment is one of two basic types: wireless and hardline.
- Durability—The ability of the equipment to withstand the rigors of the job and to survive rough handling, exposure to chemicals, immersion in water, and so forth.

Confined space equipment must be designed and built to survive the environment in which it will be used regularly. Rescue teams must feel confident that their equipment will work in the worst conditions. The following are questions for rescuers to ask regarding communications equipment:

- Is the equipment subject to dead spots or interference? How is it shielded?
- Is it a private communication system? Can communication be interrupted by outsiders?
- Is voice communication continuous?
- What is the level of Intrinsic Safety?
- Is the equipment built to a standard of quality? Which standard?
- What type of warranty does it carry?
- What materials are used to construct the equipment?
- What is the chemical resistance of the equipment?
- Is the equipment waterproof? Immersion proof?
- What is the power source? batteries (type)? other?

- What is the battery life? Is there a low battery warning signal?
- Can it be used while wearing breathing apparatus?
- Are system components and accessories interchangeable?
- How quickly can the equipment be deployed?
- How easy is it to use? How much training is required?
- How many people can use the communication system simultaneously?
- Can the equipment establish communication with the victim prior to entry?
- What kind of accessories are available for the equipment?

Equipment Classification

Several types of communications systems are available to rescuers. Each has distinct advantages and disadvantages depending on the rescue situation.

Wireless Communication Systems

The advantages of a wireless system are that it has no hard lines, accommodates an unlimited number of users, allows freedom of movement, and uses existing radio equipment. The disadvantages of a wireless radio system for confined space rescue include:

- It is subject to dead spots and intermittent communication.
- It is not hands-free, requires push to talk.
- VOX accessories require fine adjustment and can lock the system open in high noise areas.
- Radio frequency interference can affect the readings of other safety equipment such as gas detectors.
- Continuous monitoring of entrants by the attendant is practically impossible.
- It is subject to electrical interference and static in the transmission due to equipment such as generators, welders, and power lines.
- Messages can be garbled and require repeating, particularly by people wearing face masks.
- Nonprivate network communications can be monitored and interrupted by outside sources.
- It is open to lockout by users on the same frequency.
- Portable radios used inside confined spaces are subject to considerable damage and high repair costs.
- Intrinsic safe radios typically have a limited level of approval.

Hardline Communication Systems

The disadvantage to any wired communication system is the physical restrictions of the hard line. Most emergency services personnel are comfortable with wireless (radio) communications. Wireless units may be preferable to hardline communications when users need to roam free, particularly over large areas and outside confined spaces.

However, the reverse is true in confined space operations. Hardline systems can provide rescuers with the high level of reliability they need to carry out a rescue operation safely and quickly. The advantages of hardline communication systems confined spaces include:

- clarity of communication
- hands-free operation
- continuous communication and entrant monitoring
- communication unaffected by electrical interference if hard line is properly shielded
- dedicated and private communication system for the entry team
- outsiders cannot monitor or interfere with team communication
- the hard line can be joined to an air line to create a single umbilical
- low maintenance and repair costs
- availability of high level intrinsic approved equipment

Communication Rope

Communication equipment designed for dive or high-angle rescue is sometimes used for confined space applications. This equipment uses communication wires embedded in a kernmantle rope. Considerations regarding this type of equipment include:

- The life of a rope is limited and replacement costs are ongoing.
- Life safety rope that has been shockloaded should be removed from service immediately. This can mean loss of communication.
- Interior wires cannot be inspected for wear or damage.
- Rope is very difficult to clean.
- Communications gear for diving usually does not carry Intrinsic Safe Approval.

Rescue teams considering this equipment should ask the manufacturer for a certificate of compliance with National Fire Protection Association (NFPA) Rope Standard.

Deployment of Communication Equipment

The deployment of a communication system varies from one rescue team to another. It depends on the number of people, operational procedures, policies, and the rescue strategies. Communication strategies for industrial confined space rescue usually combine two communication technologies:

1. hardline equipment used inside the space and
2. radio equipment used outside the space.

Positions and Tasks of Communications

To discuss the use of hardline communication systems for confined space rescue, it is important to have common terms for the structure of a confined space rescue team and for the tasks assigned to team members. Team positions listed are simplified for brevity. In many cases, the tasks are combined. For example, it is possible for a team leader to carry out additional tasks listed for the safety attendant and line tender.

Team Leader

The leader coordinates the entire rescue, is the focal point of communication, instructions, and information. He or she responds to requests for equipment and relays medical information.

Safety Attendant

This attendant is responsible for ensuring the safety of the entrants while they are in the confined space. He or she monitors for symptoms of exposure to hazards and ensures that there are no threats to the entrants in or around the entrance to the space. The safety attendant also manages lines and coordinates equipment to be sent into the space to assist in the rescue.

Primary Entrant

The first one into the space, this entrant is responsible for initial contact, assessment, and safe removal of the victim from the confined space. He or she must be able to communicate easily with other team members from inside the confined space to relay instructions and information. A minimum of one entrant on a two-person entry team should have voice communication.

Secondary Entrant(s)

This team member is a stand-by rescuer(s) and must be able to carry out the tasks of the primary entrants. He or she should be able to monitor communications of the primary entry team during stand-by mode. If called upon to enter the space, the secondary team should be able to communicate and be monitored by the attendant. A minimum of one secondary entrant on a two-person entry team should have voice communication.

Line Tender or Hauler
This member manages lines and ropes and equipment going into the confined space and assists with the rescue operation. On a communication system the line tender monitors the entry team and relays instructions as they relate to paying out or taking up rope, the air hose, and similar items.

Air Supply Officer
This person communicates issues regarding the fresh air supply (if applicable) for the entrants. More often this information is relayed through the team leader or safety attendant.

Deployment Configurations

As with any piece of rescue equipment, the application of a voice communications system varies according to the situation. Communication equipment selected for confined space rescue must be flexible and easily adapted to a variety of operational requirements.

Actual deployment of a communication system can be configured to include some or all of the above team members (or more, if required). The following three configurations present the most common hardline communication system deployments for confined space rescue operations:

- One attendant outside the space, a primary rescue entrant inside the space, and a secondary (back-up) rescue entrant outside the space
- One attendant outside the space, a rescue team leader directing operations outside the space, a primary rescue entrant inside the space, and a secondary (back-up) rescue entrant outside the space
- One attendant outside the space, two primary rescue entrants inside the space, and two secondary (back-up) rescue entrants outside the space

Integration of a Communication System

When a confined space rescue team introduces a voice communication system, members must design and integrate their own communication policies and protocols to complement their existing rescue methods. As with any equipment, team members must familiarize themselves with it and include it in simulations and training programs.

There are a variety of rescue training scenarios and rescue team deployments. There are no hard and fast procedures for the introduction of a communication system by rescue teams. The job description for a communications officer illustrates some key elements in successfully integrating a communication system into a rescue team's operation.

Communications Officer

The communications officer is the rescue team member responsible for integrating communications equipment into the team's procedures and protocols. He or she is responsible for maintaining safety, efficiency, and teamwork. This officer is also responsible for the care, maintenance, and deployment of rescue communication equipment.

The suggested roles and responsibilities of a communications officer are:

- Arranges with suppliers to provide equipment training and/or rescue training materials.
- Reviews product literature and becomes familiar with all of the accessories and possible configurations of a communications system.
- Monitors the testing and general upkeep of the equipment, including changing batteries and replacement/repair of lost and damaged equipment.
- Packs the systems to ensure quick deployment.

- Trains all team members in proper deployment and operation of the communications system. This includes but is not limited to:
  - Initiating and maintaining contact with the victim (if possible) upon arrival at the scene and communicating pertinent information, medical or other, to the team leader.
  - Assessing the rescue situation and determining the most efficient equipment configuration for the rescue at hand.
  - Outfitting the entrant(s) with the proper communication accessories and ensuring they wear it correctly for safe and optimum performance.
  - Performing final functional test before the entrant(s) are approved for entry.
  - Monitoring the entrant(s) while the rescue is in progress and communicating their needs to the team leader (if not already on the system).
  - Determining rules of conduct and developing suggested operating guidelines to be employed by the rescue team as it relates to communication.
  - Implementing an alternative method of communication, agreed to and understood by all team members, to be used in case of a failure.
  - Staying updated with the latest application methods and procedures developed during ongoing training programs.

Summary

The importance of communications systems for use in confined space rescue is obvious. Without reliable communications, regulations cannot be met and safe operations cannot be maintained. This vital element of the rescue equipment cache should be a first priority in promoting safe and efficient practices on the scence of any confined space rescue.

CHAPTER 14

Confined Space Rescue: Monitoring, Hazard Reduction, & Ventilation

The information in this chapter is provided as a basis for continued training. Each rescuer should consult with his or her own team leader for the correct SOGs for the team. Topics covered in this chapter include:

- Atmosphere Testing Procedures
- Monitoring and Retesting
- Hazard Reduction
- Rescuer Safety
- Forced Ventilation

Introduction

Atmospheric monitoring should take place continuously or at frequent intervals during a rescue in a confined space. All equipment for atmospheric monitoring should meet OSHA requirements. Equipment should also be maintained and calibrated according to manufacturer's recommendations.

Atmospheric Testing Procedures

The following testing procedures are recommended. The first set of tests should be performed by remote probe before anyone enters the space. Test all levels of the space because vapors have various densities (the weight of a vapor compared to air). All areas of the space to be occupied should be tested before entering (see Figure 14.1).

1. **Test to be sure there is an acceptable level of oxygen.** According to OSHA, air containing less than 19.5% or more than 23.5% of oxygen is unacceptable. An atmosphere that contains less than 19.5% of oxygen is oxygen deficient and may not meet normal breathing requirements of the worker inside the confined space. An atmosphere containing more than 23.5% of oxygen is oxygen enriched and enhances the flammability of combustibles.
2. **Check the atmosphere's flammability (measured in the percentage of the lower explosive limit [LEL] or lower flammable limit [LFL]).** The LEL is the lowest concentration of a product that will explode or burn when it contacts a source of ignition of sufficient temperature. According to OSHA, a confined space is hazardous if it contains more than 10% of the LEL. A flammable gas must reach 100% of its LEL to ignite and burn. Monitors are usually calibrated with a flammable gas such as methane, heptane, or pentane. Methane has an LEL of approximately 5% in air. Different gases have different LELs. A monitor calibrated to methane will give an inaccurate reading for a gas with a different LEL. A monitor

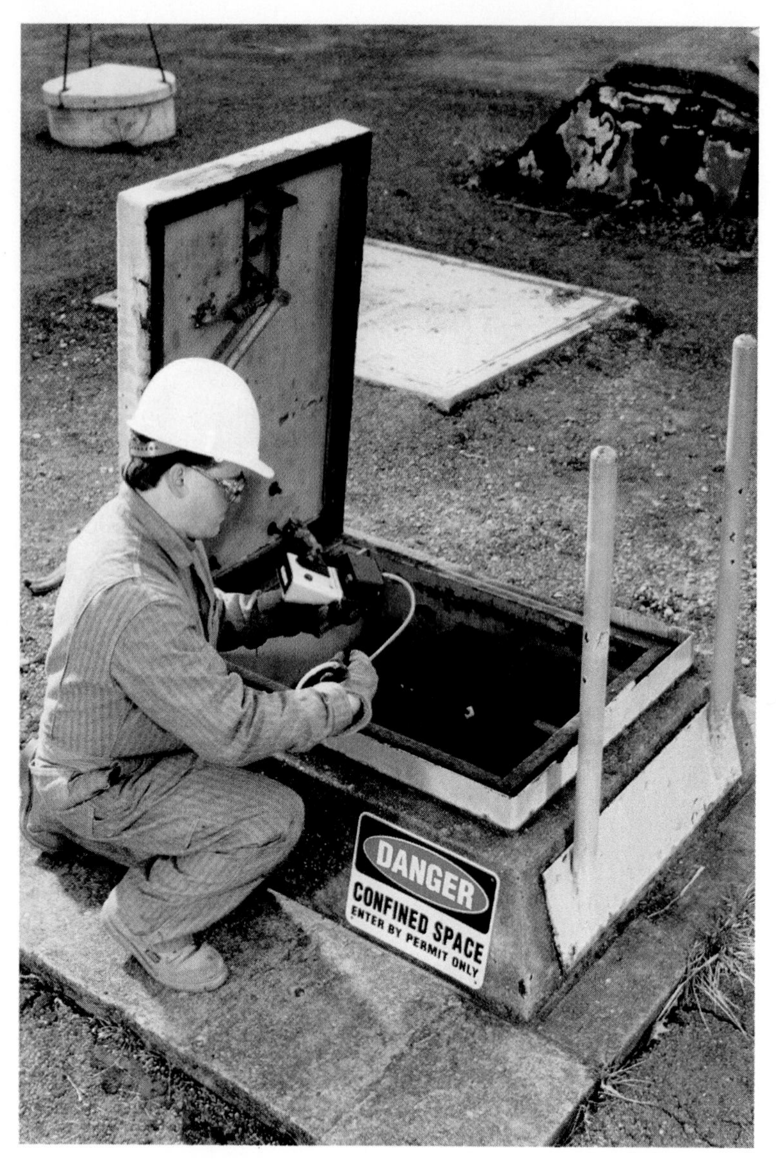

Figure 14.1 Atmospheric monitoring is a must

reading of 10% or less of the LEL should ensure that an atmosphere is below the LEL of most gases. The manufacturers of most atmospheric monitors can supply conversion charts to figure the percentage of LEL for gases by comparing them to the test gas for which a monitor is calibrated.

Note: *An oxygen-deficient or oxygen-enriched atmosphere can give a false reading because most flammability monitors are accurate only within a specified range of oxygen content.*

3. **Test for toxicity.** If the material in the space is known, use monitors specific to that chemical to test for these products. If the material in the space is not known, it is necessary to use meters that take readings and narrow the spectrum of chemicals until it identifies existing chemicals. At least two companies manufacturer tube systems designed to perform this type of broad-spectrum analysis. Toxicity may be measured in terms of the permissible exposure limit (PEL). The PEL is the concentration of a toxin that most people could safely be exposed to for 8 hour. Any toxin in a confined space greater than its PEL is hazardous.

If any of these hazards exists in a confined space, the hazard must be controlled before entry. Often, this is done through ventilation of the space. After the ventilation system is turned on, retest the air.

Monitoring Frequency

If a space is vacated for any length of time, retest the atmosphere before reentry. During rescue efforts, the atmosphere should be retested frequently or monitored continuously.

If conditions within the space cannot be compensated for with the use of personal protective equipment (such as fresh-air breathing apparatus), the rescuers should evacuate the space and discontinue the rescue until the problem can be corrected.

A wet-bulb globe thermometer measures the heat and humidity of a space. It should be used to test areas with the potential for heat stress. This device is not usually practical for rescue. However, it can help determine relief schedules for personnel working in the space to prevent exhaustion.

Note: *Monitors can read inaccurately due to the cross-sensitivity of certain chemicals. Address concerns about a monitor's cross-sensitivity to its manufacturer.*

Hazard Reduction

Reducing or abating the hazards of a confined space emergency is essential before entry is safe. In addition to the protective equipment to mitigate certain hazardous environments (fresh-air breathing apparatus), other things can and should be done externally to prevent dangerous conditions from developing inside the space. Without consideration of these procedures, injury or death can occur.

Secure and Isolate Energy Sources

Many forms of energy may be present as normal processes occur inside an operating

DANGER
DO NOT OPERATE
NAME
EMPLOYEE NUMBER
DATE
USE THIS TAG AND NO OTHER FOR LOCKOUT. DO NOT USE FOR ANY OTHER PURPOSE.
LOCKOUT TAG
TAGS & SIGNS UNLTD N.O. LA 1-800-274-0028 #LO1
DANGER
DO NOT REMOVE THIS TAG.
DESCRIBE EQUIPMENT AND REASON FOR LOCKOUT
OBSERVE PLANT LOCKOUT PROCEDURE
LOCKOUT TAG
SEE OTHER SIDE

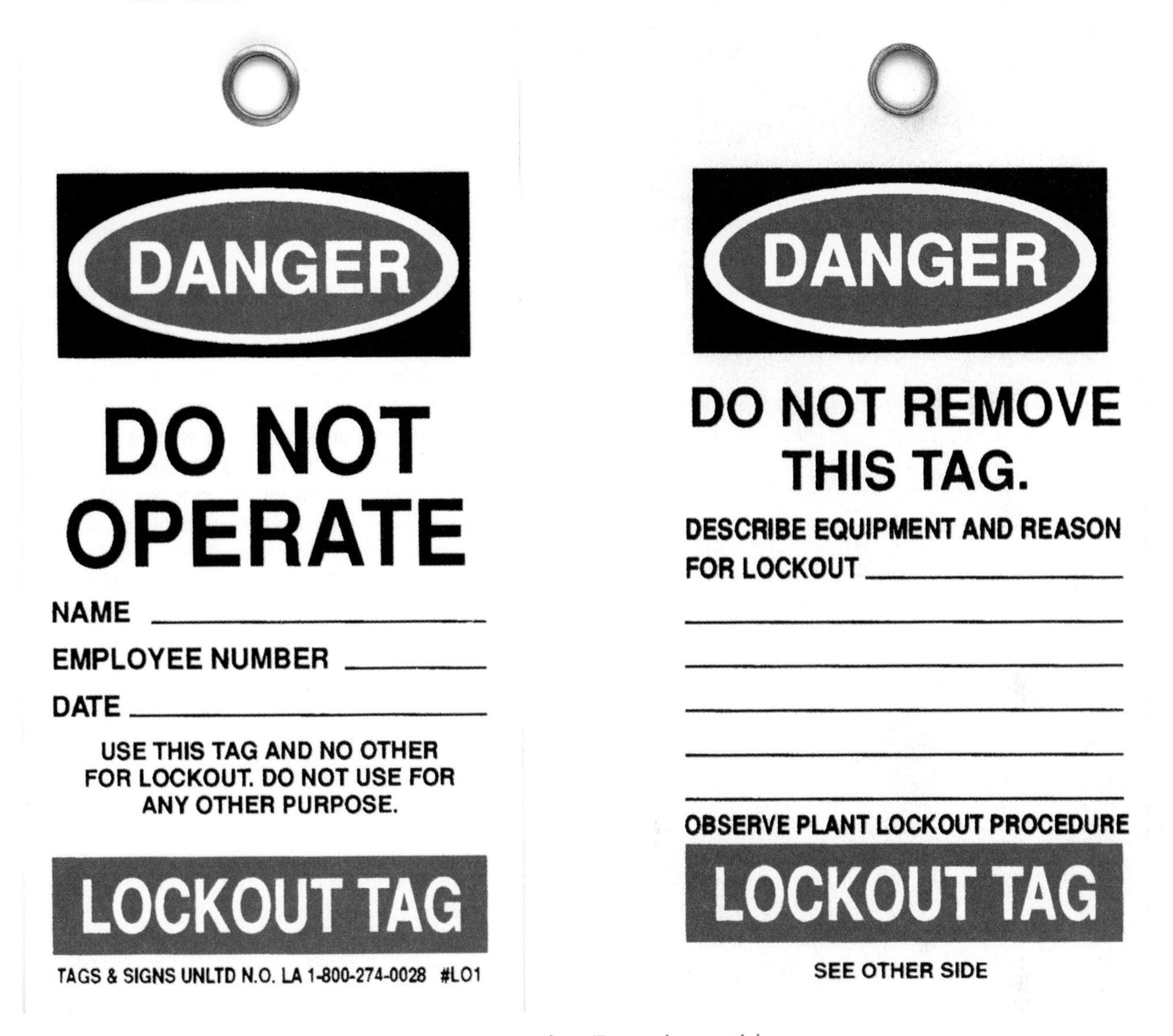

Figure 14.2 Lockout/Tagout is essential

unit or vessel. While the confined space is closed (buttoned up) and in operation, the processes inside do not normally present a threat to people working around the outside of it. Recognizing the need to isolate these dangerous forms of energy, OSHA requires that measures be taken before permit spaces are entered. When an emergency occurs in these spaces, the rescue team is obligated to ensure that proper precautions have been taken and that nothing has been missed. The emergency may have been caused by a failure to isolate dangerous forms of energy.

Several forms of energy must be secured prior to rescue entry:

Electrical

If sources of electricity are not completely isolated, electrocution of rescuers is likely. Electricity is dangerous enough in wide open areas. The restricted nature of confined spaces exacerbates the hazards. Electricity is usually isolated by a combination of (1) turning it off at the source and securing it with a lock device (lockout) and (2) placing a warning of some type (usually a label or tag) on the switch to deter someone from trying to turn it back on (tag-out) (see Figure 14.2). Most industrial facilities have policies concerning lockout/tag-out procedures. They may vary slightly, but all involve positively securing energy at the source and visual warning to keep it that way.

Hydraulic

In this text, "hydraulic energy" includes energy in liquids and finely divided solids that, if not secured, may cause chemical exposure or engulfment. These materials are usually introduced into a process by way of piping or other conduit. These pipes must be definitively isolated, by whatever method, to prevent the chance of even minor leakage of materials. The best means of accomplishing this is through physical separation of the lines at some point leading into the space. Segments of pipe or valves can be removed entirely and/or caps (blind flanges) placed on the exposed pipe end. This is the most secure method, but it may not be the most practical. Consideration of the vessel design, number of isolation points, the materials present, and work to be done all play a part in deciding on the method of isolation. Most industrial facilities use a combination of shutting off valves (blocking) and placing separators at pipe connections (blinds or blanks). Isolation by simply shutting off a single valve (blocking) is inadequate. If valves alone are used for isolation, they should be shut off in two locations on the same line. Then the isolated line must be completely emptied via a bleed valve between the two isolation valves that can eliminate residual vapors or liquids. This is sometimes referred to as "double block and bleed." Blinding or blanking a line provides a positive means of separating the product from the vessel to be entered. These devices are placed at a flanged pipe joint by eliminating the pressure on the pipe, removing some or all of the flange bolts, separating the pipes enough to slip in the blind, and resecuring the bolts after insertion. These blinds usually provide a visual indicator of their presence. Some blinds have a handle that resembles a skillet (skillet blind) that can be seen after the blind is inserted. Some have two disks joined side by side that resemble a pair of spectacles, one lens open and one solid. These spectacle blinds allow quick visual assessment of whether the pipe is isolated (open spectacle visible) or not (solid spectacle visible). All industrial facilities have policies governing procedures to isolate hydraulic energy prior to allowing a permit to be issued.

Mechanical

This includes energy from augers, blades, conveyer belts, gears, flywheels, and anything mechanical. They may move inside the space due to outside influences, weight distribution, or gravity. These forms of energy must be secured to prevent injury. The means of securement varies, but should include a tagout as well as ways to prevent people from accidentally returning the object to working order.

Other hazards

There may be other hazards either in a space or introduced into the space that must be mitigated. Falling debris from buildup of scale can be significant and capable of causing injury. Dropped equipment can also be a hazard. Tools and equipment should be secured. Helmets and other appropriate gear can be worn to protect the rescuer from falling objects.

WARNING

Most rope rescue hardware cannot be classified as nonsparking. It can be a source of ignition for flammable materials. Check with manufacturers of rope rescue hardware to determine construction features and methods of use least likely to generate sparks.

Rescuer Safety

Rescuers should never enter flammable atmospheres. However, an atmosphere that is initially clear may reach its LEL within a short time if flammables are introduced. When flammability hazards exist, rescuers consider intrinsically safe tools and equipment. It is a good idea to maintain the highest intrinsic level available any time a team must enter a permit space that previously contained a product that might be reintroduced.

Forced Ventilation

Forced ventilation is one of the most definitive methods to reduce or eliminate hazardous atmospheres in a space. Rescuers consider several things when using ventilation to "clear" a space.

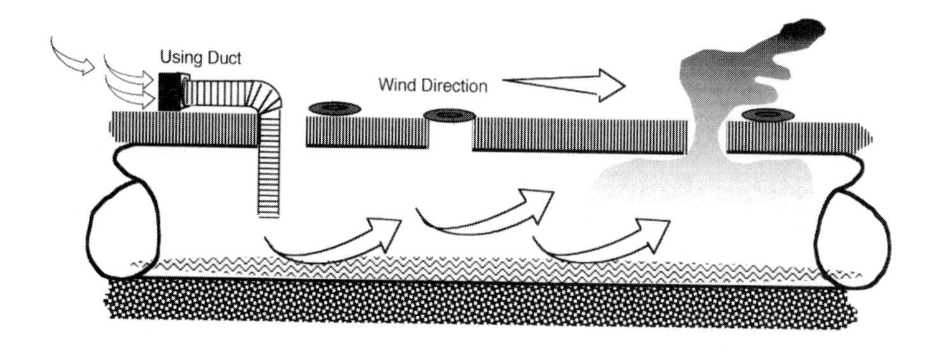

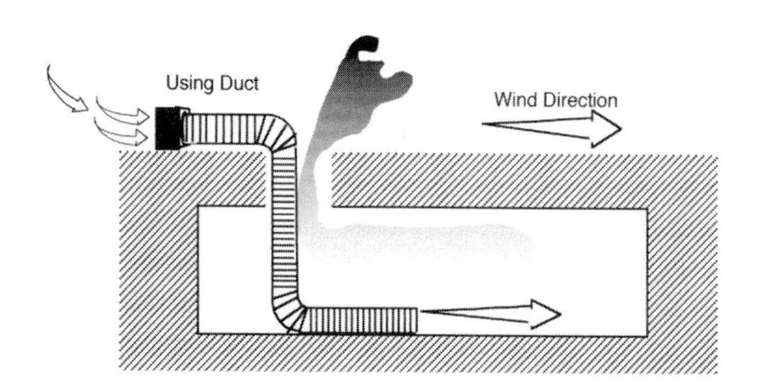

Figure 14.3 **Ventilating the air in a confined space**

Conditions/Risks

Many hazardous atmospheres in confined spaces have been introduced from outside sources. This is often due to chemical or vapor release elsewhere in the facility that literally flows into the open space. The same problem can be caused by improper attention to ventilation methods. Air introduced through positive pressure ventilation (pushing ambient air into the space) can be tainted by harmful vapors existing in ambient air outside of the space. Setting up this type of ventilation too near machinery,

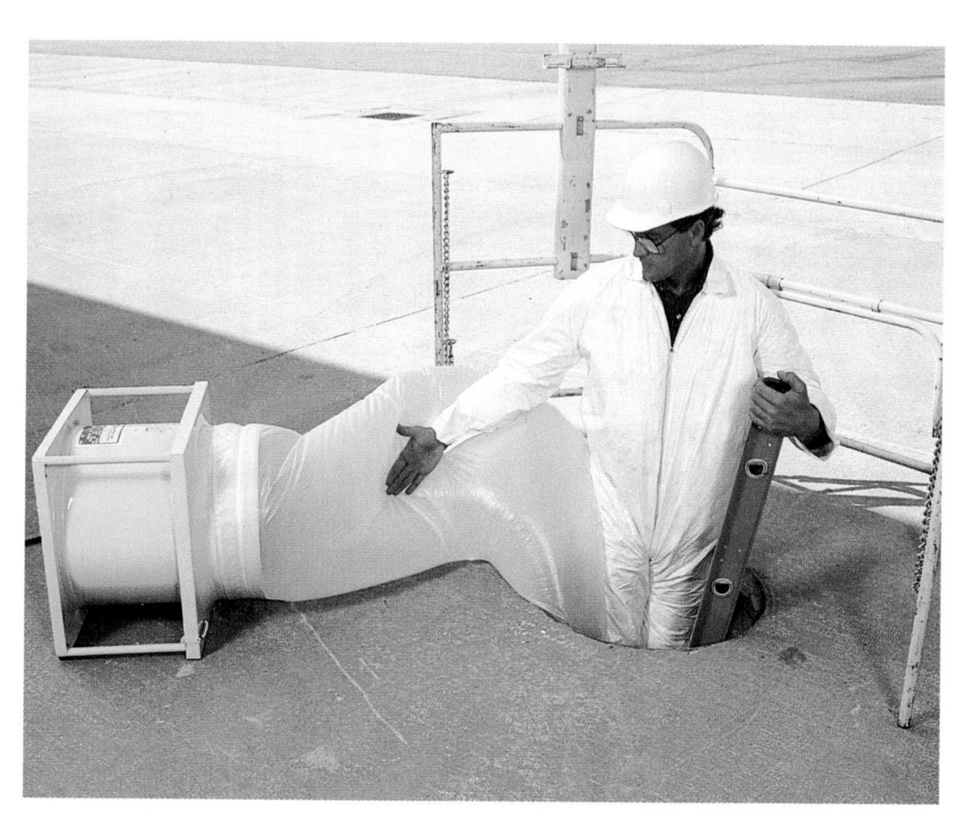

Figure 14.4 **Plastic duct in manway is flexible so that a rescuer can pass easily**

equipment, or work processes that produce harmful vapors can be extremely injurious to rescuers and to victims in a space.

Proper Ventilating Procedure

Another concern is the adequacy of backup power for electrically operated ventilators. If ventilation is keeping the atmosphere clear and it is lost as a result of a power failure, conditions inside the space can become unacceptable in a hurry to the unprotected patient. Rescuers must have appropriate back-up power.

However ventilation is set up, it should move air throughout the space (see Figure 14.3). Depending on the shape of the space, it may have pockets of dead air. There are many methods to ensure proper air flow including the use of ventilation and "L" ducts.

Ducting allows placement of a large tube from the ventilator to a specific point of entry on a vessel's exterior. The duct directs the air to the specified area without much loss.

Placed in an entryway, "L" ducts reduce the amount of space taken by the ventilation equipment (see Figure 14.4). This plastic appliance sits on the inner surface of the manway opening and can be flattened to allow more room in the opening should entry be required.

Rescuers consider increased ventilation when temperatures are warm inside a vessel. Higher temperatures can rapidly fatigue personnel working inside it. When heat is a problem in the vessel, it is usually better to blow air into the bottom of the vessel while providing negative ventilation (drawing air out) from the top. This moves the hotter air (at the top because hot air rises) out of the vessel fast, and replaces it with the cool air introduced from the bottom.

Other ventilation strategies and considerations not mentioned in this text may be of value to the confined space rescue team. Again, the manufacturer of ventilation equipment can be a valuable source of information.

Summary

The environmental hazards that exist in any technical rescue can pose significant risks to the rescuers involved. Add confined spaces to these common hazards and the risks increase tremendously. There is no place to run when an explosion occurs or a toxic atmosphere overwhelms a rescuer inside a confined space. The importance of identifying and mitigating confined space hazards cannot be overemphasized. The proper use of specialized tools, such as atmospheric monitors and ventilation equipment, combined with procedures for the isolation of harmful energy sources can ensure the safety of confined space entrants. These measures aid both in the safe entry of rescuers, as well as in the removal of hazards affecting victims inside the space. The personal safety of the rescuer and victim must be the highest priority. Without isolating the hazards, rescue becomes recovery and rescuers become victims. Following proper procedures can help to prevent such tragedies.

CHAPTER 15

Respiratory Protection

The appropriate OSHA, NFPA, ANSI, NIOSH, MSHA regulations will be referred to throughout this chapter. With this information the rescuer will have a better understanding of the various aspects of breathing systems. This information is provided as a basis for continued training. Rescuers should consult with their team leader for the correct procedures for the team. In this chapter, topics discussed are:

- Types of Breathing Apparatus
- Pre-Use Check
- Donning and Doffing
- Post-Use Inspection
- Changing SCBA Cylinders
- Breathing Techniques
- Supplied Air Systems
- Respiratory Protection Standards

Introduction

Rescuers realize that they are called to the scene of a confined space emergency because something is wrong inside that space. Often, rescuers are not able to determine with complete certainty what happened to the entrant(s) and what is the present situation. The rescuers must take appropriate precautions to determine the hazards and protect themselves.

It is not wise for the rescuer to rely solely on atmospheric monitoring devices. The only guarantee of a good atmosphere is solid monitoring by a qualified person on a correctly calibrated device *along with* verbal contact with an awake and alert patient or co-worker. This is sometimes jokingly referred to as the "canary check." It is no joke, however. It has been reported that 25% of atmosphere-related fatalities occurred in spaces where the original monitoring showed the space to be safe to enter.

Types of Breathing Apparatus

Both OSHA CFR 1910.134(g)(2) and ANSI Z117.14.2 direct that, unless the cause of the emergency can be established as NOT atmosphere related, fresh-air breathing apparatus must be worn. For this reason, rescuers should choose to wear these apparatus anytime the cause of the incident is in doubt or potentially related to the atmosphere.

Because fresh air is often necessary, it is important to address appropriate respiratory protection. Of foremost concern to most industrial rescuers are OSHA Respiratory Protection Standards. Most persons who perform rescue in industrial settings are subject to them.

There are two types of fresh-air breathing apparatus:

1. **SCBA**—Self-contained breathing apparatus and
2. **SAR**—Supplied air respirator, also known as air line respirators (ALR).

Self-Contained Breathing Apparatus

In July of 1983, OSHA required that all SCBAs supply air by positive pressure rather than by demand (CFR 29, Part 1910, Section 156). Positive-pressure units supply air to

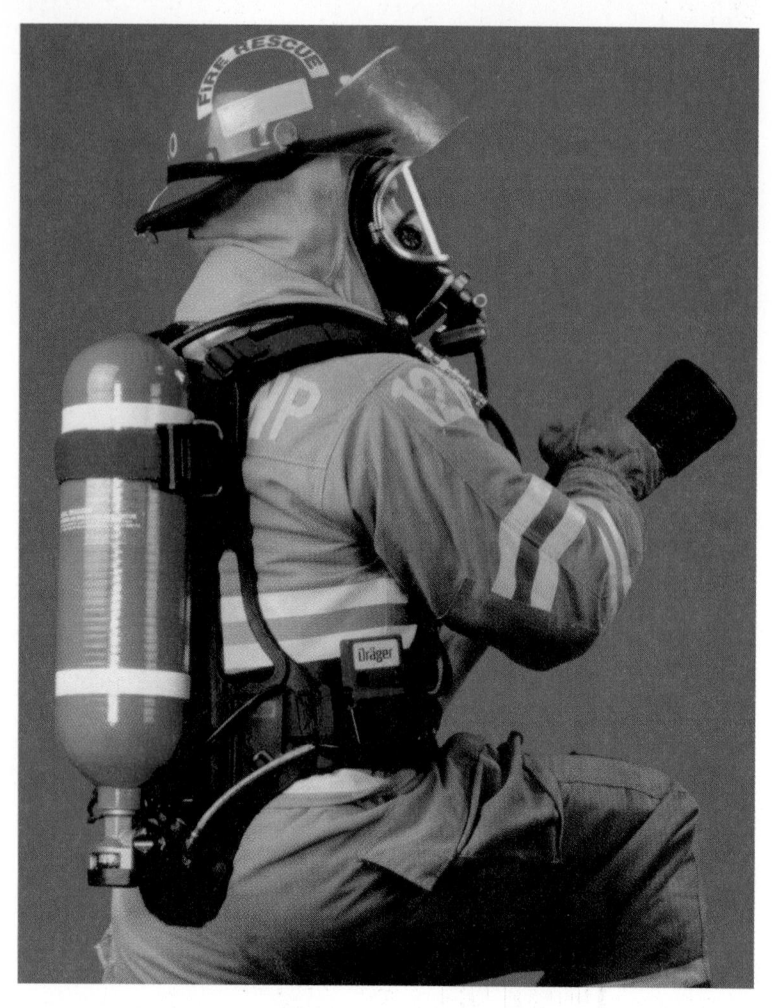

Figure 15.1 Open circuit SCBA

the face piece under a pressure greater than the surrounding atmosphere. Demand units supply air only when the wearer inhales and creates a negative pressure in the face piece.

It is also important to note that both the National Fire Protection Association (NFPA) and the American National Standards Institute (ANSI) require that only positive-pressure breathing apparatus be used in the fire service.

The advantage of positive-pressure apparatus is that it helps prevent contamination of the air inside the face piece if a leak occurs in the face piece's seal. It will not eliminate this possibility if the leak is significant.

Duration of Air Supply

Rescuers must know how much to expect from the air supply. But calculating this can be difficult because the wearer's personal characteristics affect the amount of air used in a given period of time. This is particularly true of open-circuit SCBA (open-circuit and closed-circuit SCBA are discussed below). References in regulations and by manufacturers often mention to the "rated" duration of air supply. The rated air supply generally does not correspond to the actual time air will be available. Even if the cylinder is full, the duration will vary according to an individual's breathing rate and the amount of physical activity. For example, a 30-minute rated unit may supply only 15 minutes with a moderate to heavy work load, and a 60-minute rated unit may supply only 45 minutes of air. The National Institute for Occupational Safety and Health (NIOSH) and the Mine Safety and Health Administration (MSHA) even require a manufacturer's statement to this effect:

> The user should not expect to obtain exactly 30-minute service life from this apparatus for each use. The work being performed may be more or less strenuous than that used in the MSHA-NIOSH test. Where work is more strenuous, the duration may be shorter, possibly as short as 15 minutes.

Although this statement implies a minimum duration of 15 minutes, the air supply can be depleted even sooner. It depends on the wearer and the degree of physical exertion. The rating of an open-circuit breathing apparatus should be considered the maximum amount of time available from the air supply. On the other hand, a one-hour closed-circuit unit is designed to provide a minimum of 60 minutes of protection, with less regard for the wearer's level of exertion. The most reliable means of determining how long an apparatus will supply air to individuals is through regular training and evaluation of their air consumption. Here is a rule of thumb for deciding safe working time in confined space rescue:

> $\frac{1}{2}$ the rated capacity of the cylinder − the amount of time from entry to patient contact = duration of air supply

Although not foolproof, this rule of thumb will help ensure enough time for egress when wearing SCBA. The goal is to egress BEFORE the low-pressure alarm is activated. When the alarm sounds in confined space operations, it may very well be too late to escape.

For this reason an accountability officer and documentation of times of entry and patient access are important. Without attention to this information, the rescuer's safety could be compromised.

Types of Self-Contained Breathing Apparatus

When using SCBA, the types of incidents to which rescuers respond dictate the type of apparatus.

1. **Open-circuit SCBA**—This type of breathing apparatus vents the wearer's exhalations to the surrounding atmosphere (see Figure 15.1). Open-circuit SCBA is currently the most used in industry and fire service. The air supply in these units is compressed air and can vary in pressure, volume, and weight according to the model and manufacturer. The quality of any fresh air supply should be at least grade "D."
2. **Closed-circuit SCBA**—This type of breathing apparatus recycles the wearer's exhalations after carbon dioxide and moisture are removed through a filtration process (see Figure 15.2). After "scrubbing," pure oxygen is added to the recycled air from a small cylinder before being returned to the wearer for breathing.
   - These units are usually of long duration, with air supplies of 30 minutes to several hours.
   - They usually weigh less and are lower profile than open-circuit units of similar rated capacity. This is because they use a smaller cylinder to introduce pure oxygen into the exhaled air of the wearer.
   - Closed-circuit units are now available as positive-pressure apparatus. The compressed oxygen in the system is supplied at a greater rate than that needed solely for breathing. This extra breathing air increases the pressure in the face piece during inhalation and exhalation.

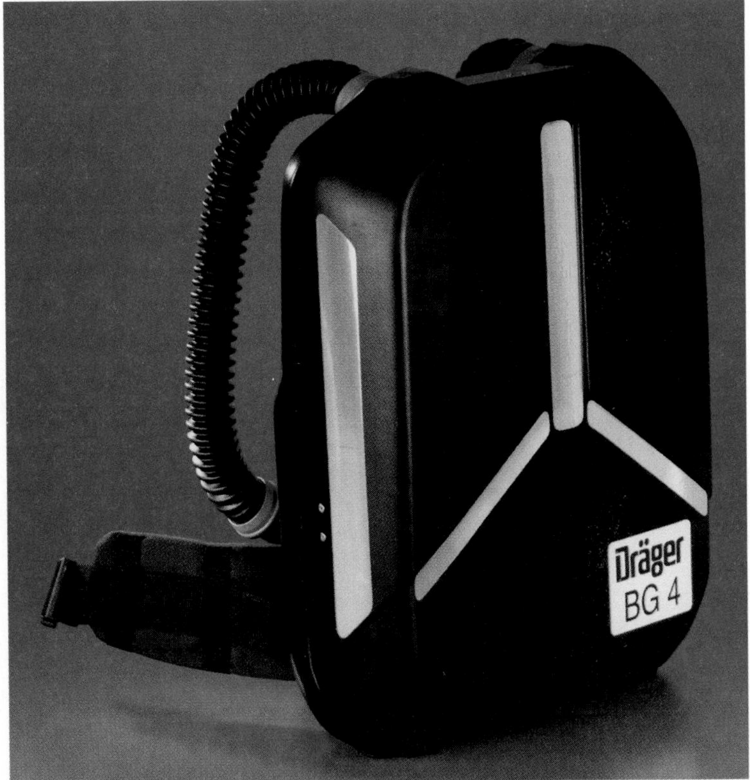

Figure 15.2 Closed circuit SCBA

While closed-circuit apparatus may seem like a solution to SCBA problems, there are disadvantages to their use:

- The increased supply (duration) may encourage the wearer to remain in the space, resulting in greater fatigue.
- These units, while of longer duration and lighter than open-circuit units, are generally more expensive to purchase and maintain. They also require more training and maintenance.
- The filtration process for most units creates heat as a by-product. This can be uncomfortable for the wearer. This problem is being addressed by some manufacturers.

Supplied-Air/Air-Line Respirators

In confined space rescue, an SCBA's size often makes it difficult to use. A SCBA should only be worn as directed by the manufacturer. Even if its use is possible, an SCBA small enough to pass through a narrow opening may limit the duration of its air supply to impractical levels. In these cases, a supplied air respirator (SAR) is a viable option.

An SAR consists of an open-circuit face piece, regulator, and egress cylinder attached via a low-pressure air line to a remote source of air supply (see Figure 15.3). By regulation, SARs are restricted to the maximum distance allowed by the manufacturer (usually no more than 300 feet) from the point of attachment. These points of attachment may be manifold-type units connected to larger diameter low-pressure air lines up to 300 feet long (see Figure 15.4). These lines may, in turn, be attached to regulated high-pressure manifolds engineered to span great distances from the original

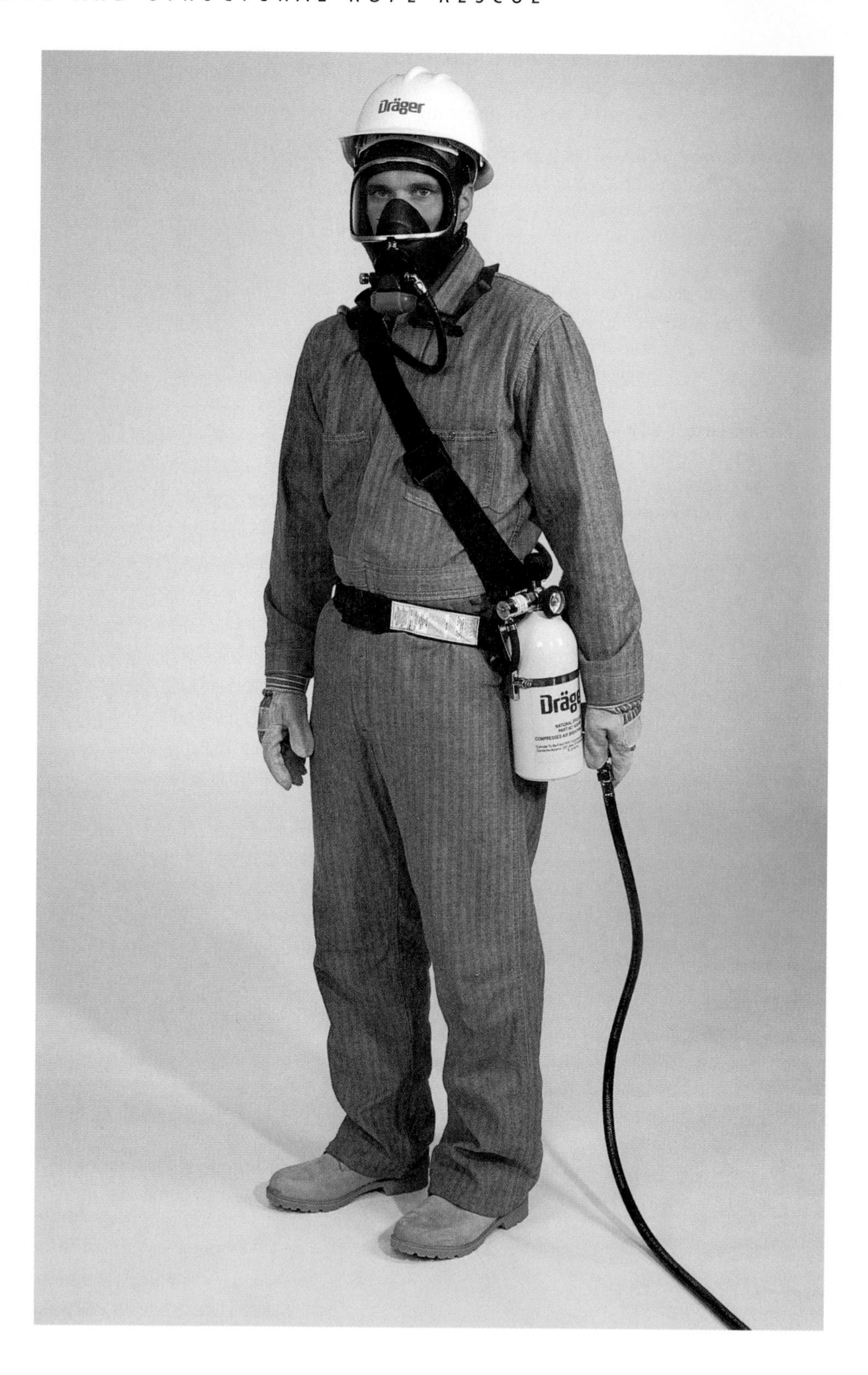

Figure 15.3 SAR

high-pressure source of air supply. This means that SAR units, while normally limited to 300 feet from point of attachment, can be ultimately supplied from distances much greater.

Never introduce any point of attachment into the hazardous atmosphere. They should remain in a controlled environment so they can be operated and monitored properly.

Because of their limitations, air line equipment is not feasible in confined spaces where distances greater than 300 feet from the entry point must be spanned or where severe entanglement hazards exist.

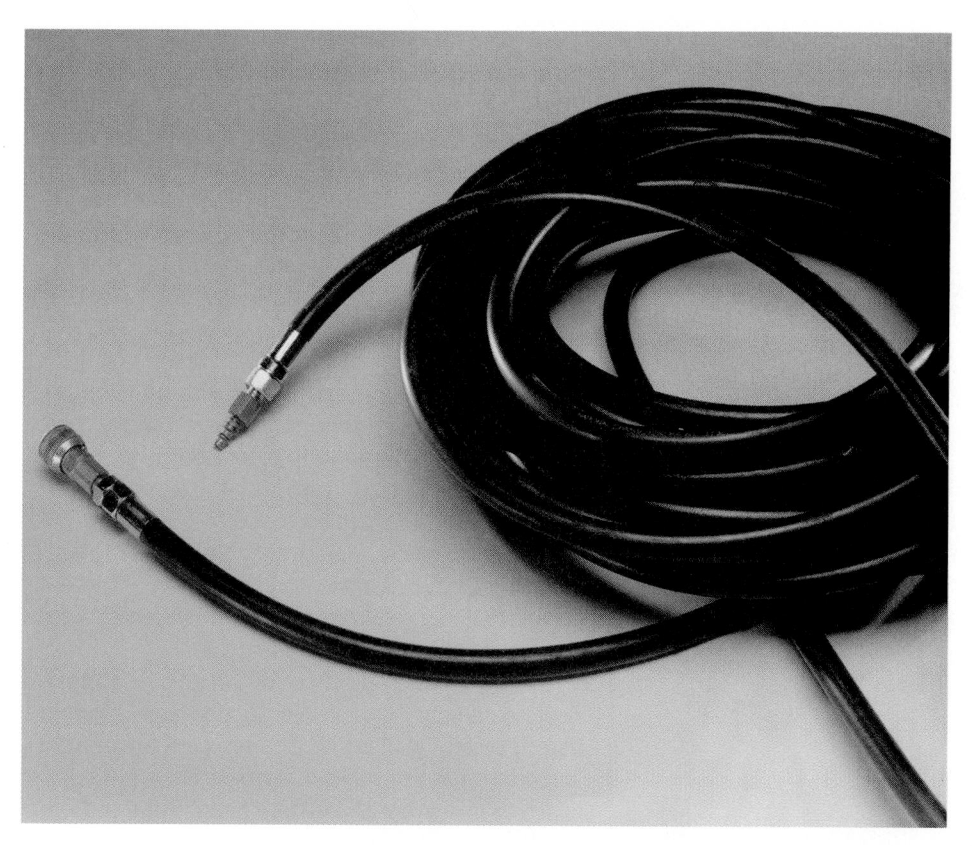

Figure 15.4 Low pressure airline

OSHA requires any SAR used in an atmosphere that is immediately dangerous to life and health (IDLH) have an additional supply. It must be capable of providing enough air for the wearer to escape the atmosphere in the event the primary supply is interrupted. This "escape" requirement is usually addressed by attaching very small breathing-air cylinders, usually rated for 5 minutes, to the SAR unit. The 5-minute cylinders are intended to provide enough air for escape, although they may be incapable of doing so. Several SAR units on the market now offer extended egress times of at least 10 minutes.

Although 5-minute egress may be possible from some spaces, rescuers should evaluate the suitability of the escape supply's duration based on their needs.

For rapid access to the patient, some rescue teams have developed a strategy of making entry on the egress unit's supply while waiting for the air line to be passed to them. This is not a wise policy. The egress supply is for escape only and should never be used alone for entry to a confined space. As will be discussed in detail, below, ANSI requires that to use the egress unit's air supply to perform entry, the self-contained breathing apparatus is required to have a rating of at least 15 minutes, and only 20% of that supply may be used for entry. It also must have low-pressure warning and other devices not included on SAR units. Some SCBA units meeting the requirements for entry have options for additional air line attachments. Depending on the circumstances, these units may make such a strategy feasible.

Safety and Use of Breathing Apparatus

Pre-Use Check

It is important to perform a pre-use safety check of all breathing apparatus. It is recommended that this test be performed daily or before each use if daily checks are not performed. The procedure should follow the specific recommendations of the manufacturer.

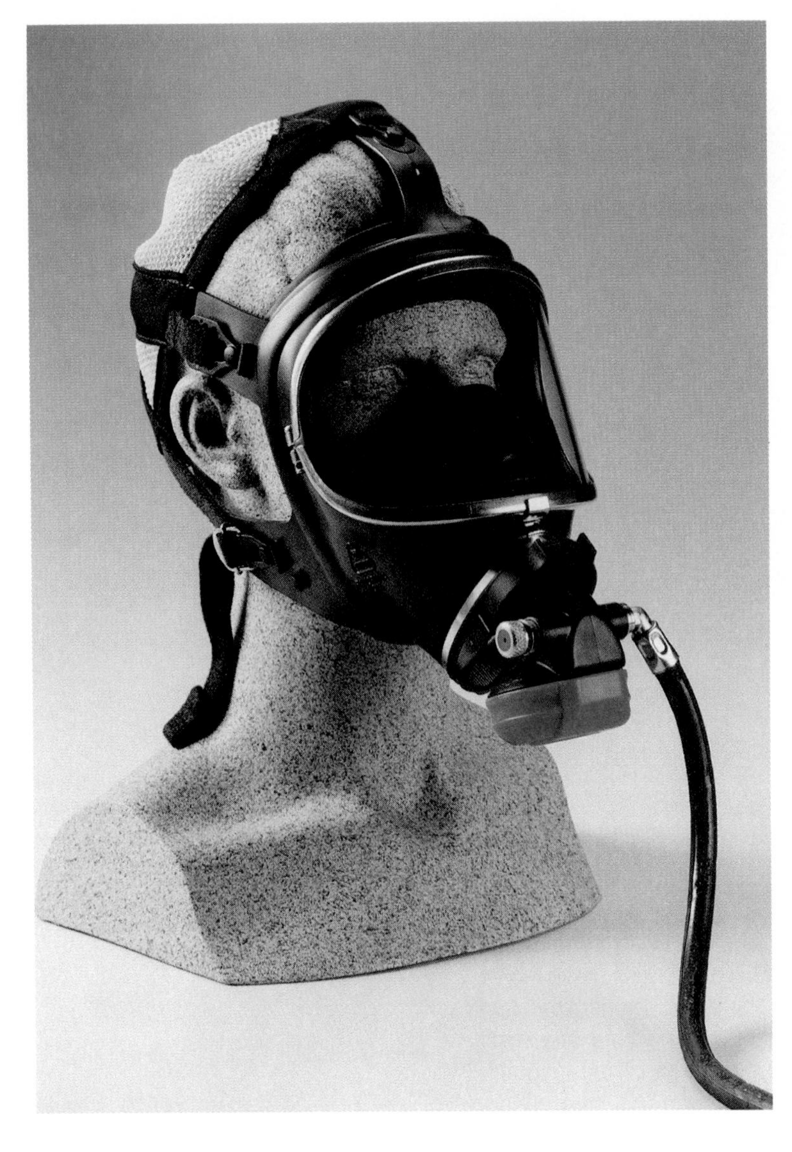

Figure 15.5 SCBA face-piece

Donning and Doffing the Breathing Apparatus

There are several methods for donning breathing apparatus. Donning (applying the apparatus) and doffing (removing the apparatus) procedures vary among units. As usual, rescuers should follow the manufacturer's recommendations, and perform the pre-use safety check if it has not already been done.

In certain extreme circumstances, a decision may be made to remove a breathing apparatus to traverse a narrow horizontal opening. If this is the case, it is extremely important to use a buddy system for controlling the unit to prevent it from dropping. Dropping could cause the rescuer's face piece to be pulled off, exposing him or her to a hazardous atmosphere. *Removal of the breathing apparatus cylinder harness or wearing it in any manner not intended by the manufacturer carries a serious liability and is not recommended.*

If the situation dictates such drastic measures (e.g., emergency escape due to a collapse), the buddy system may work. One rescuer removes the apparatus harness while leaving the face piece in place (see Figure 15.6). After checking the space he or she is about to enter, the rescuer then has the partner (buddy) secure the doffed unit while the rescuer backs through the horizontal opening. The rescuer's partner then hands the unit back to the rescuer for redonning. After the rescuer has donned the unit, the partner performs the same sequence with his or her apparatus, but negotiates the opening head first to move in the direction of the other rescuer.

When negotiating vertical openings where the rescuer's breathing apparatus must be removed, a buddy system will not be effective. In these cases, the rescuer must secure the unit to himself or herself or to the rope on which he or she will be lowered/hauled. The unit should be secured using rescue-grade equipment to prevent failure and dropping of the apparatus.

WARNING

When using SCBA, use caution when negotiating narrow openings, whether horizontal or vertical.

Post-Use Inspection

After each use, inspect all breathing apparatus and restore it to service. This should be done in addition to regularly scheduled inspection and maintenance. Inspection procedures should follow manufacturer's recommendations and will likely include at least the following:

1. Fully extend all harness and face-piece adjustment straps.
2. Replace expended air cylinders with full ones.
3. Turn on the system and check the unit for leaks. Perform all the other steps covered in the manufacturer's Pre-Use Safety Check.
4. Clean all parts, including face piece according to manufacturer's recommendations.
5. Document post-use inspection and restore the unit to service.

Changing SCBA Cylinders

Some agencies promote the changing of depleted SCBA cyclinders in hazardous environments. The authors DO NOT recommend the changing of SCBA cylinders while inside IDLH atmospheres. When changing the SCBA cylinders, the wearer should follow manufacturer's recommendations and should change the cylinders in a controlled area away from the hazard.

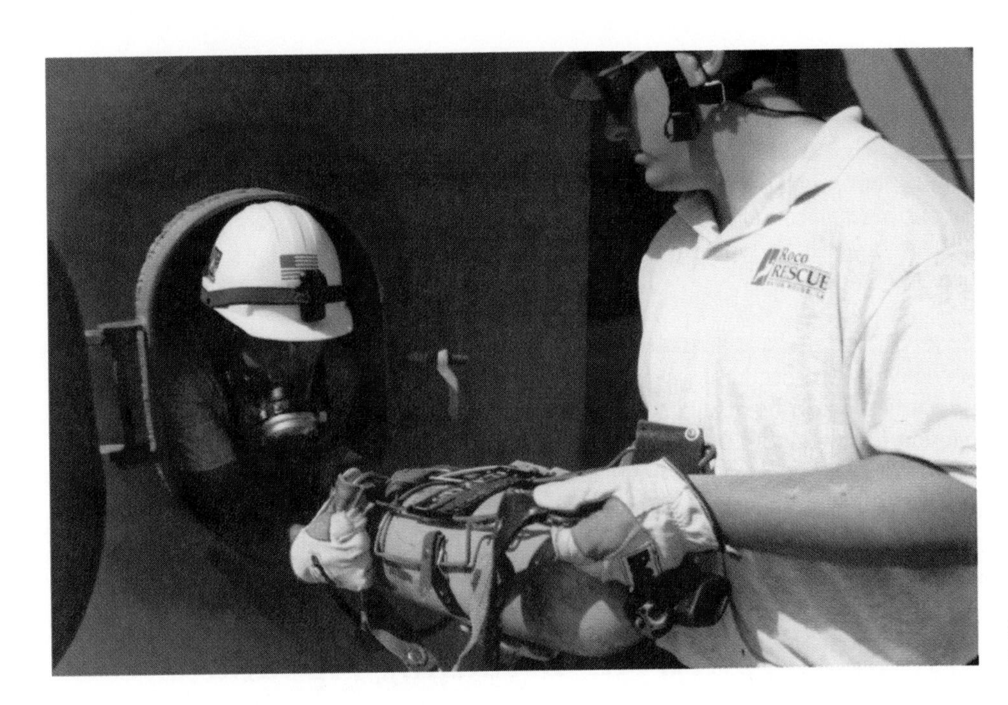

Figure 15.6 Using buddy system with the SCBA

Breathing Techniques

There are a several breathing methods to conserve the air supply of a breathing apparatus. Two of the methods are designed for use in emergencies only, and one is for normal work. To work properly, all methods require conscientious effort and concentration on technique.

Controlled Breathing Techniques

These techniques are used during normal work activity. Controlled breathing is based on the physiological reaction of the respiratory center in the brain to increased levels of carbon dioxide (CO_2) in the blood. In physiologically normal humans, when the brain senses an increase of CO_2, it causes the respiratory rate to increase in an effort to get rid of the waste product CO_2.

The face pieces of most breathing apparatus have exhalation valves near the base. If a person exhales in a random manner (such as panting), the exhaled CO_2 might be added to the ambient air in the face piece instead of exiting by way of the exhalation valve. The next breath taken (inhalation) might then contain increased amounts of CO_2. If this cycle continues, the increased levels of CO_2 in the blood cause rapid respiratory rates.

Controlled breathing dictates that the wearer inhale normally but exhale forcibly toward the exhalation valve. By pursing the lips and blowing the air forcefully toward the bottom of most face pieces, the wearer evacuates most of the exhaled breath from the face piece. This allows fresh air from the cylinder to enter the face piece and lungs on the next inhalation, avoiding increases in carbon dioxide. Nose cups also decrease the likelihood of CO_2 buildup in the face piece by reducing the area of the space from which must be evacuated.

Emergency Bypass Breathing

A sudden loss of air flow may occur because the regulator fails. A rescuer should immediately use the bypass, or purge, valve to allow air to bypass the regulator, and give him or her time to escape.

Bypass breathing is for emergencies only. If any mechanical failure of the breathing apparatus occurs during a rescue, the wearer must abandon the rescue and exit the space immediately.

Bypass valves are always red and, when activated, allow air to flow from the cylinder or first-stage regulator.

One procedure for bypass breathing is to stop, crack open the bypass valve several times, inhaling each time it is opened, then move several feet toward the exit. The process should continue in this manner (stop, breath, move) until egress is complete.

Bypass breathing will not remedy every type of mechanical failure of breathing apparatus, but it will handle most regulator failures. Other emergency procedures for various mechanical failures are considered advanced breathing apparatus techniques and are beyond the scope of this text. Consult the manufacturer for specific emergency procedures.

WARNING

Use of this technique in SCUBA diving can cause undesirable effects.

Emergency Skip Breathing

An emergency procedure designed to maximize the duration of the wearer's air supply is emergency skip breathing. Skip breathing simply invloves taking a normal breath, pausing for the length of time normally required to exhale the breath, then inhaling fully before slowly exhaling the breath. This is an emergency technique used only when the rescuer is stationary and must wait for help.

This breathing technique is designed for emergencies only. It is not intended for use below one atmosphere of pressure.

Use of Supplied-Air Breathing Apparatus

Regulations require the use of fresh-air breathing apparatus anytime the emergency may be related to an atmospheric hazard. Use of these apparatus should be promoted anytime the cause of the emergency is in doubt or potentially related to a hazardous atmosphere. Here are a few general tips for the use of fresh-air breathing apparatus in confined spaces:

Supplied air respirators are recommended for most confined space rescues because of the obvious time and weight limitations of SCBA. However, prior to using SAR for confined space rescue, rescuers should become familiar with OSHA compliance considerations for using SAR rather than SCBA.

Always use an additional "escape pack" when entering a confined space with an SAR. The escape pack consists of one or more small SCBAs worn on the rescuer's body. They contain enough air to allow him or her to make an emergency exit from the confined space if problems arise with the primary air supply.

Have an air supply officer to manage the fresh-air system and document information such as:

- The time of entry into the confined space.
- The amount of air at the time of entry (SCBA only).
- The time taken to reach the patient. Too long a time might indicate immediate egress by the rescuer because of physical exhaustion or limited air.

- Whatever the air supply, establish a maximum exposure time in confined spaces to prevent exhaustion.
- Monitoring devices such as a wet bulb globe thermometer can help decide the need for relief crews in confined spaces.
- Rescuers should use controlled breathing techniques with SCBA to maximize the duration of the air supply. It is a good idea when using any fresh air breathing apparatus, no matter the duration of the air supply.

When suspended on rope with fresh-air systems, fasten and snug all harness straps, with helmet in place over the face piece.

- When suspended in a seat harness, rescuers using SCBA should be aware that the weight of the unit might cause difficulty in maintaining an upright position while on line. If your full body harness does not have an upper front attachment point, you can fashion one by wrapping a utility belt or webbing loop around your upper body and attaching it with a carabiner to the load line. This will help you maintain an upright position.
- It is recommended that fresh air breathing apparatus be worn only as the manufacturer designed it.

Respiratory Protection Standards

The OSHA Standards

Federal regulations require that appropriate respiratory protective equipment be provided by the employer and be used in emergencies, or when feasible engineering or administrative controls are not effective in controlling toxic substances. Such equipment must be appropriate for the hazards of the materials involved and the extent and nature of work requirements and conditions.

The employer is also required to ensure that the user is trained in the proper use of the protective equipment. The respirators must be regularly cleaned and disinfected. If the respirator is used by more than one worker, it must be cleaned and disinfected after each use. No person is to be assigned tasks requiring the use of respirators unless it has been determined that he or she can physically perform the work and use the equipment. Breathing air must at least meet the requirements of the specifications for grade D breathing air.

If entries are made to a space where the entrant could be overcome by a toxic or oxygen-deficient atmosphere if the respirator were to fail, at least one additional person must be present. This additional person must be positioned such that he or she will not be affected by any likely incident, and must have the proper rescue equipment to assist the others in case of an emergency. Additionally, communications must be maintained among all individuals present.

Any time SCBA or SAR are used in IDLH atmospheres, safety harnesses and safety lines must be attached for lifting or removing persons from the hazardous atmosphere. The OSHA requirement also specifies that, in such a situation, "standby man *(sic)* or men *(sic)* with suitable *self-contained breathing apparatus* shall be at the nearest fresh air base for emergency use."

De Minimis Violations

De minimis violations occur when an employer violates a standard, but the hazard created by the violation is minimal or nonexistent. A *de minimis* violation has no penalty, does not need to be abated, and cannot be used as evidence of a history of violations for purposes of assessing penalties for later violations. In effect, classifying a violation as *de minimis* is like canceling the citation.

However, violation of the SCBA requirement will be classified as *de minimis* only if the following conditions are met:

1. An evaluation of the permit space to be entered has been done to determine which appropriate respiratory protection (SCBA or supplied air with SCBA) is best suited for the rescue, and the respiratory protection chosen is provided to rescuers.
2. The rescuer's respirators and air source meet the requirements of the 1910.134 standard.
3. The air source for the rescuer's respiratory protection is independent from that which is being used by authorized entrants.

The OSHA also recommends the following work practices for rescue services that choose to use SAR with escape SCBA:

1. Establish a policy requiring immediate withdrawal from the space whenever a respiratory protection problem develops;
2. Establish a policy for use and training on air line sharing "buddy breathing;"
3. Ensure that the rescuers wear full body harnesses and use life lines whenever practical;
4. Establish a policy requiring the minimum capacity of the air source to be twice the volume of the total needs of all rescuers connected to it for the anticipated duration of the rescuer's entry;
5. Establish a policy that mandates a minimum team of two rescuers for all permit space rescue entries.

NOTE: *This is an OSHA MINIMUM RECOMMENDATION for de minimis classification of breathing air violations. Neither OSHA nor the authors are suggesting that two rescuers are sufficient to constitute an entry rescue team.*

This particular provision has caused some concern in the rescue community. What happens if entry rescue is required through an opening too small for the rescuer to fit through while wearing the SCBA? Is the rescuer exposing himself or herself and the employer to OSHA penalties if he chooses to use SAR for rescue because SCBA will create difficulties with the rescue?

In a guidance document letter of interpretation, OSHA noted that the SCBA requirement is based on an out-of-date ANSI standard. The most recent version of the ANSI standard allows either a SCBA *or* a combination SAR with escape SCBA.

It is OSHA policy to accept compliance with a current national consensus standard that provides equivalent or greater protection from hazards, such as ANSI. A rescue service may use SARs in combination with SCBA (escape bottles) when performing rescue operations in a permit space whether or not it is an IDLH atmosphere. This would be considered a *de minimis* violation by OSHA.

In an attempt to correct this outdated standard, OSHA has proposed regulations for respiratory protection, which are pending approval. In the proposed standard, OSHA provides:

> 29 CFR 1910.134(g)(2)—The employer shall develop and implement specific procedures for the use of respirators in atmospheres where oxygen deficiency or the concentrations of hazardous chemicals are unknown and/or potentially immediately dangerous to the life or health (IDLH) of the employees.
>
> These procedures shall include the following provisions:
>
> 29 CFR 1910.134(g)(2)(I)—The employees shall wear positive-pressure self-contained breathing apparatus (SCBA) or combination full face piece pressure demand supplied air respirator with auxiliary self-contained air supply.

Rescuers and employers need to be aware of this pending standard and should keep abreast of its status. In addition to the changes regarding the use of SARs, other potential changes that affect rescuers include fit-testing requirements for respirators and medical requirements for rescuers.

The ANSI Standard

In addition to the OSHA requirements, rescuers should be aware of the ANSI standard for respiratory protection (ANSI Z88.2-1992). The ANSI standard provides accepted practices for respirator users and information and guidance on selection, use, and care of respirators. It also contains "requirements" for establishing and regulating respirator programs. The purpose of the standard is to protect employees against the inhalation of harmful contaminants and against oxygen-deficient atmospheres in the workplace.

It should be noted that although the standard speaks in terms of "requirements" and uses mandatory language such as "shall," ANSI is a *voluntary* standard. It does, however, provide useful information that can facilitate compliance with OSHA's regulations. As discussed above, it is OSHA's policy to accept compliance with a more stringent national consensus standard as fulfilling the requirements of an OSHA standard.

The respiratory standards are applicable to emergency and rescue teams as well as general employees. Additionally, ANSI specifically requires that the teams be trained properly in the use of respirators. ANSI requires that a suitable training program be established that includes emergency drills to ensure the proficiency and familiarity of team members with the respirators.

To comply with ANSI, the employer is responsible for providing "applicable and suitable" respiratory protection to protect the employee. The employer must also establish and maintain a respiratory protection program. The employer must also permit a respirator wearer to leave the hazardous area for any respirator-related cause.

The employee, for his or her part, is required to use the respiratory protection in accordance with instructions and training received. The employee must guard against damage to the respirator. If a respirator malfunctions, the employee is required to leave the contaminated area and report the malfunction to the person designated in the employer's written standard operating procedures. The employee must also report any change in his or her medical status that might affect the employee's ability to wear the respirator safely.

To meet the ANSI standard, respiratory training must include explanations and discussions of the following:

- The respiratory hazard and the effect on the wearer if the respirator is not used properly;
- The engineering and administrative controls being used and the need for respirators to provide protection;
- The reason for selecting a particular type of respirator;
- The function, capabilities, and limitations of the selected respirator;
- The method of donning the respirator and checking its fit and operation;
- The proper wearing of the respirator;
- Respirator inspection, maintenance, and storage;
- Recognizing and handling emergency situations;
- Applicable governmental regulations for specific substances.

Any person using a tight-fitting respirator must be fit tested, and the wearer must conduct an appropriate fit check of the respirator each time the respirator is donned and adjusted.

The respirator must be maintained according to the manufacturer's instructions and on a schedule to ensure that each wearer has a clean, sanitary, and properly operating respirator. Respirators must be stored in a convenient and sanitary location.

Respirator Selection

The very nature of confined space rescue and OSHA requirements makes the selection of respiratory protection very important. ANSI's requirements for respirator selection are particularly applicable to rescue. ANSI states that rescue teams must take into account worker activity, respirator use conditions, location of the hazardous area, and respirator characteristics, capabilities, and limitations.

Questions to be raised and answered when selecting respirators include the following:

- Is the worker in the hazardous area continuously or intermittently? Is the work light, medium, or heavy?
- How long must the respirator be worn?
- Is the respirator going to be used for routine, nonroutine, emergency, or rescue work?
- Where is the hazardous area with reference to the nearest safe area that has good air?
- What are the physical characteristics, functional capabilities, and performance limitations of various respiratory protection units?
- Is the service life of the respirator affected by the environmental conditions or level of effort required by the wearer? For example, extreme physical exertion can rapidly deplete the air supply in an SCBA.

Dangerous Atmospheres

Additionally, ANSI specifically addresses the selection of respirators for atmospheres immediately dangerous to life or health (IDLH), for use in confined spaces, or for use in reduced-pressure atmospheres. For purposes of the ANSI standard, an atmosphere is considered IDLH when:

- it is known or suspected to have concentrations above the IDLH level.
- it is a confined space that contains less that the normal 20.9% oxygen, unless the source of the oxygen reduction is understood and controlled.
- oxygen content is below 12.5% at sea-level atmospheric pressure.
- it contains total atmospheric pressure less than 450 mmHg (8.6 psi) equivalent to altitude of 14,000 feet or any combination of reduced percentage of oxygen or reduced pressure that leads to an oxygen partial pressure less than 95 mmHg.

If IDLH conditions are caused by toxic materials or a reduced percentage of oxygen, the required respiratory protection is a positive-pressure SCBA. Alternatively, a combination of a supplied-air respirator and SCBA can be used. This type of system combines the capabilities of SAR and SCBA into a single device. This system is divided into two groups: a combination-type supplied-air respirator with a SCBA having a rated service life of 15 minutes or more, and a combination-type SAR having a self-contained air supply rated less than 15 minutes. The combination unit rated at 15 minutes or more can be used to enter an IDLH atmosphere while the rescuer is breathing from the self-contained breathing supply IF not more than 20% of the rated self-contained air supply is used during entry. The combination with less than 15 minutes can be used to enter an IDLH atmosphere only if connected to the supplied air source, and the SCBA can be used only for egress.

Any time a respirator is worn under IDLH conditions, ANSI requires that there be at least one stand-by person in a safe area. The stand-by person must have the proper equipment to assist the person wearing the respirator if he or she encounters difficulty. Communications must be maintained between the stand-by person and the wearer. The respirator wearer must have a safety harness and retrieval lines. Other provisions for rescue can be used if they are at least equivalent to the safety harness/retrieval line requirement.

This is similar to the OSHA requirement that fresh air be used if it is unknown whether there is an oxygen deficiency or if the presence or level of toxicity is unknown (29 CFR 1910.134(g)(2). Given the time constraints of rescue, as well as OSHA's "timely response" requirement, this dictates in most cases, that fresh-air breathing apparatus be used for rescue. The rescue team cannot rely on atmosphere monitoring done prior to or upon its arrival because the emergency may be a result of improper monitoring or faulty monitoring equipment.

Summary

The respiratory system is vital to the function of the human body. Through respiration, the oxygen we depend on for life is introduced to our cells. However, many hazards associated with confined spaces can also be introduced through respiration, producing ill effects on rescue personnel. When a rescuer's respiratory system is inhibited or incapacitated, he or she becomes incapable of rescuing himself or herself, as well as others. The proper use of respiratory protective equipment helps to ensure that the rescuer will be isolated from hazards that would otherwise enter the body through inhalation. Each rescuer must possess the proper equipment and be trained in its use if he or she is expected to survive the rigors of confined space emergencies. Without continuous and extensive training with this equipment, the equipment is useless.

CHAPTER 16

Confined Space Rescue: Medical Considerations

The information in this chapter is provided as a basis for continuing training. Each rescuer should consult with his or her own team leader for the correct SOGs for the team: Topics covered in thic chapter include:

- Incident Size-up
- Medical Considerations
- Victim Assessment
- Trauma

Introduction

Industrial and structural rescues are usually required as a result of an injury caused by a preventable accident or by a serious illness. Rescues are usually caused by the following conditions alone or in combination:

- hazardous environments (e.g., hazardous atmospheres, extreme heat or cold)
- trauma (e.g., falls, falling objects, collapse)
- medical emergencies (e.g., heart attack, stroke)

By their very nature, confined spaces create potential for numerous kinds of injury. The word "confined" implies isolation from the outside and without normal means of ventilation. In the industrial situation this often means an overheated environment. Common problems include heat cramps, heat exhaustion, and heat stroke.

Without adequate ventilation, common industrial tools and machines quickly create dangerous atmospheres. Operating equipment such as small motors, welding equipment, and cutting torches create poisonous gases such as carbon monoxide that quickly reach dangerous levels in confined spaces. Small residues of chemicals or gases may remain in the space and can quickly become toxic or flammable. Gases such as nitrogen or carbon dioxide displace oxygen in confined spaces. The space may be so confined that there is not sufficient fresh air to supply a human's need for oxygen.

Incident Size-up

Before you attempt any rescue, you must

1. determine if the emergency was caused by a hazardous atmosphere,
2. identify the nature of the hazard, and
3. decide if you have the protective equipment, personnel, and training necessary to safely conduct the rescue in this environment.

If the answer to item 3 is "no," then do not consider the rescue until the environment can be cleared and entered safely or you can summon a specialized rescue team capable of dealing with that specific hazard.

4. If it appears certain that the patient could not have survived, do not risk human life to recover a body. Wait until the environment can be made safe for the recovery team.

Medical Considerations

When rescuing patients from hazardous atmospheres (toxic, flammable, or oxygen-deficient), time is crucial. Hazardous conditions may require you to immediately remove the patient to a controlled environment before you provide appropriate medical care. (See techniques for rapid patient access in Chapter 17.)

This principle is applied to rescuing patients found inside burning buildings, next to collapsing structures, or inside a burning car. Remove them immediately from the hazard, taking whatever precautions possible concerning the spine. In confined space emergencies, avoid resuscitative efforts for patients in IDLH atmospheres unless you can do so while effectively isolating them from the hazard and without wasting time.

WARNING

Do not administer oxygen where it may chemically react with a hazardous atmosphere.

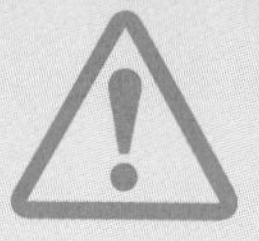

Airway and Breathing

In any case, if the patient can be isolated from the hazard (i.e., it is possible to put fresh air breathing apparatus on a breathing patient in an oxygen-deficient atmosphere), removal should not take priority over administration of appropriate care. Properly stabilize the patient prior to moving him or her.

Even in situations requiring immediate removal, always attempt to maintain spinal alignment. It may be impossible to perform proper spinal immobilization until patient and rescuers are in a safe and secure area. Spinal immobilization should be addressed simultaneously with the ABCs.

When rescuing patients from hazardous atmospheres, do not waste time on minor or stable injuries. Get the patient in the clear as soon as possible. You can then prioritize lesser injuries and treat them appropriately.

Another valuable treatment consideration involves administration of high-flow oxygen by nonrebreather mask to patients who are breathing but have been exposed to a respiratory hazard. This practice should be dictated by local protocol but is extremely useful in most situations of this type.

Spinal Immobilization

Consider possible head and spinal injury whenever you find a person lying unconscious due to an unknown cause. Immobilize the spine at the same time you open the airway (see Figure 16.1).

Decontamination

Review decontamination needs for both patient and rescuers as soon as you start your response. Organize decontamination procedures along with the rescue response. Have

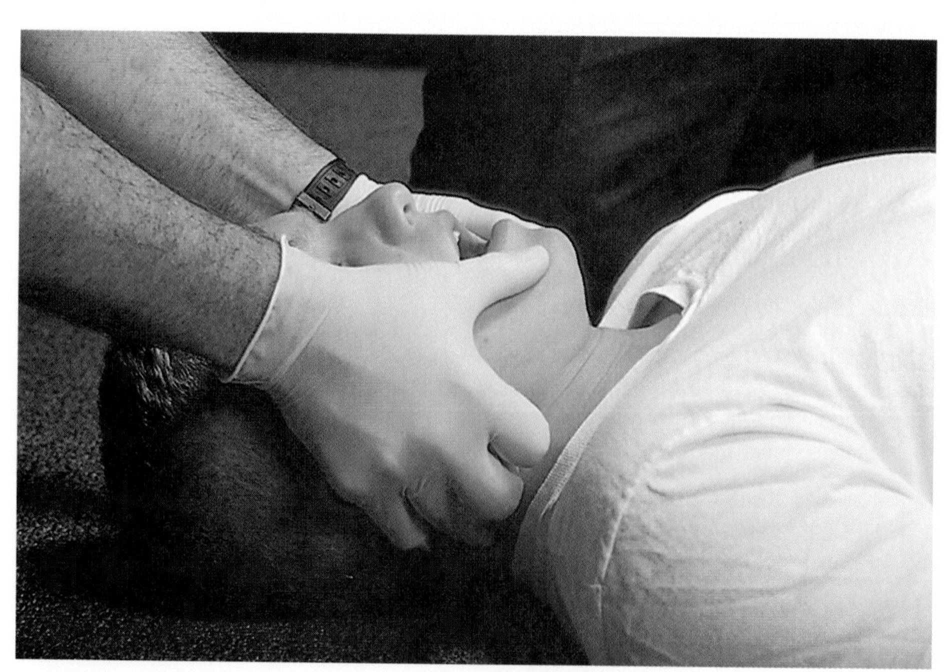

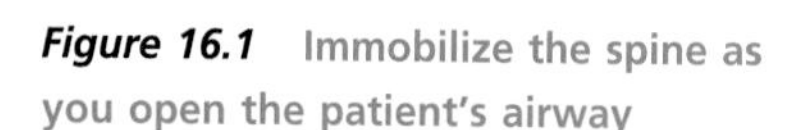

Figure 16.1 Immobilize the spine as you open the patient's airway

the decontamination procedures ready by the time the patient has been removed from the hazard and has been medically stabilized.

Patient Assessment—the ABCs

The first person on the scene of an accident or serious illness is the important first link in the chain of rescue and medical care. The first person on scene may also be the most important in saving the patient's life. This rescuer may have to start actions to remove life-threatening conditions or to protect the patient from problems that could cause permanent disability.

The primary survey relates to life-threatening conditions. For this reason, you must conclude the primary survey quickly. You should be able to complete the primary survey within 1 minute of making contact with the patient.

The Primary Survey

The most important first step in encountering the patient is the assessment—discovering what is wrong. The basic assessment must be done before a rescuer does anything else for or to the patient. The first part of the assessment is known as the "primary survey." The purpose of the primary survey is to quickly find any immediate threats to the patient's life or conditions that could cause disability. The primary survey is conducted in five steps in order of priority:

- **A** Airway and cervical spine management
- **B** Breathing
- **C** Circulation and bleeding
- **D** Disability
- **E** Exposure and protection from the environment

A—Airway and Cervical Spine Management

Make certain that the airway is clear. The airway can be obstructed by internal problems (such as the base of the tongue falling against the back of the throat) or external problems (such as food and vomit).

Consider the potential of cervical spine injury when opening the airway. Too much manipulation of the head and neck could cause neurological damage to the spine.

B—Breathing

After you are certain that the patient's airway is open, you must evaluate the quality and quantity of patient's ventilation. The main concern is "hypoxia," or inadequate oxygenation of the tissues of the patient's body.

C—Circulation

Even if the patient is breathing, the body must circulate blood to carry oxygen from the lungs to body tissues. Check for:

1. Pulse, including
   - Rate per minute
   - Regularity
   - Quality (strong or weak)
2. Capillary refill
3. Severe bleeding
   A significant loss of blood can lead to inadequate perfusion of the bodily tissue. You should take immediate measures to control severe bleeding.

D—Disability

Disability is a measurement of brain function by determining the patient's level of consciousness (LOC).

You can determine the patient's level of consciousness by assessing AVPU:

- **A—Alert.** The patient alert and at least somewhat oriented to events and surroundings.
- **V—Verbal.** The patient responds purposefully (with sound or movement) to your voice.

- **P—Pain.** The patient responds purposefully to pain induced by recognized safe methods (e.g., pushing neuro pressure points).
- **U—Unresponsive.** The patient does not respond to external stimulus.

E—Exposure and Protection from the Environment

Expose all parts of an injured patient's body to make certain there are no hidden injuries. Blood on clothing can be a distraction from identifying the most serious injuries. As a general rule, clothing is to be removed by the appropriate personnel at the appropriate location to thoroughly examine the patient's body. Whether prior to or after moving, the patient must be examined thoroughly as part of proper and complete assessment.

Once the patient has been examined completely, appropriate personnel replace clothing or use another cover to preserve body heat and to protect the patient from hazards. Once inside a protected (heated or air-conditioned, depending on outside temperature) examination area, such as the ambulance, the patient can be exposed as much as necessary.

Vital Signs

Take vital signs as soon as possible during assessment of the patient.

- **Pulse.** Check rate, strength, and regularity (e.g., the patient's pulse is 80, strong, and regular). Also check pulses below the site of an injury to an extremity. Poor or absent pulse, pale color, or coolness of the limb may all be indicators of circulatory damage or restricted blood flow.
- **Respiration.** Check the rate and volume of respirations (e.g., the patient's respirations are 32 and shallow).
- **Blood pressure.** Blood pressure can be measured with a sphygmomanometer, by auscultation, or by palpation. A quick rule of thumb can be used when equipment is not available. It is generally assumed that a palpable radial pulse indicates a systolic blood pressure of at least 80 mmHg. A palpable carotid pulse indicates a systolic pressure of at least 60 mmHg. Although limited, this information can be helpful when there is no other way to measure blood pressure.
- **Level of consciousness.** The LOC is part of a complete neurological examination that can be assessed with AVPU. We will discuss the neurological exam in greater detail later in this chapter.

If you are rescuing a trauma patient, continue to take these vital signs at regular intervals such as every 5 to 10 minutes. This will alert you of sudden and threatening changes in the patient's condition. Because this record can be very important later to medical personnel, have a copy available for ambulance or emergency room personnel.

The Secondary Survey

If during the primary survey you observe immediate life-threatening conditions that you cannot correct, transport the patient immediately to definitive medical care.

Once immediate life-threatening conditions are controlled, perform a "secondary survey." Start the secondary survey only after a complete primary survey.

The purpose of the secondary survey is to look for specific problems such as broken bones or bleeding sites. This is head-to-toe survey of the patient's body must be performed in a meticulous manner, so that you do not miss anything.

During the secondary survey, examine the body region by region. Begin at the head, progress to the neck, chest, abdomen, pelvis, and extremities. Finish with a detailed neurological exam of the patient.

At each region of the body, "look, listen, and feel."

- **Look** for unusual color, deformity, bleeding, or swelling.
- **Listen** for absence of or unusual sounds.
- **Feel** (palpate) each bone (see Figure 16.2).

Secondary Survey by Body Region

1. Head
   - Check scalp for:
     - Bleeding
     - Deformity
     - Swelling
   - Check eyes for:
     - Raccoon eyes
   - Check pupils for:
     - Size (pinpoint, dilated)
     - Symmetry (equal on both sides)
     - Responsiveness to light
   - Check ears for:
     - Discharge
     - Battle sign
     - Deformity
   - Check nose for:
     - Drainage
     - Singed nasal hairs
   - Check mouth for:
     - Bleeding
     - Foreign bodies
     - Singed lips
2. Neck
   - Check for:
     - Distended veins
     - Tracheal deviation
     - Subcutaneous emphysema
     - Deformity
     - Bleeding
3. Chest
   - Check for:
     - Deformity
     - Open wounds
     - Paradoxical movement
     - Flail segment
     - Equal symmetry (both sides rise and fall equally)
     - Pain
     - Unusual sounds
4. Abdomen
   - Check for:
     - Deformity
     - Swelling
     - Bleeding or discoloration
     - Pain on palpation
     - Rigidity
     - Guarding
     - Masses
5. Pelvis
   - Check for:
     - Deformity
     - Bleeding or discoloration
     - Pain on palpation
     - Open wounds
6. Extremities
   - Check for:
     - Distal pulses
     - Deformity or discoloration
     - Bleeding
     - Paralysis
     - Numbness and tingling
     - Capillary refill
     - Skin temperature and color (coolness and pallor)
     - Equal strength symmetrically

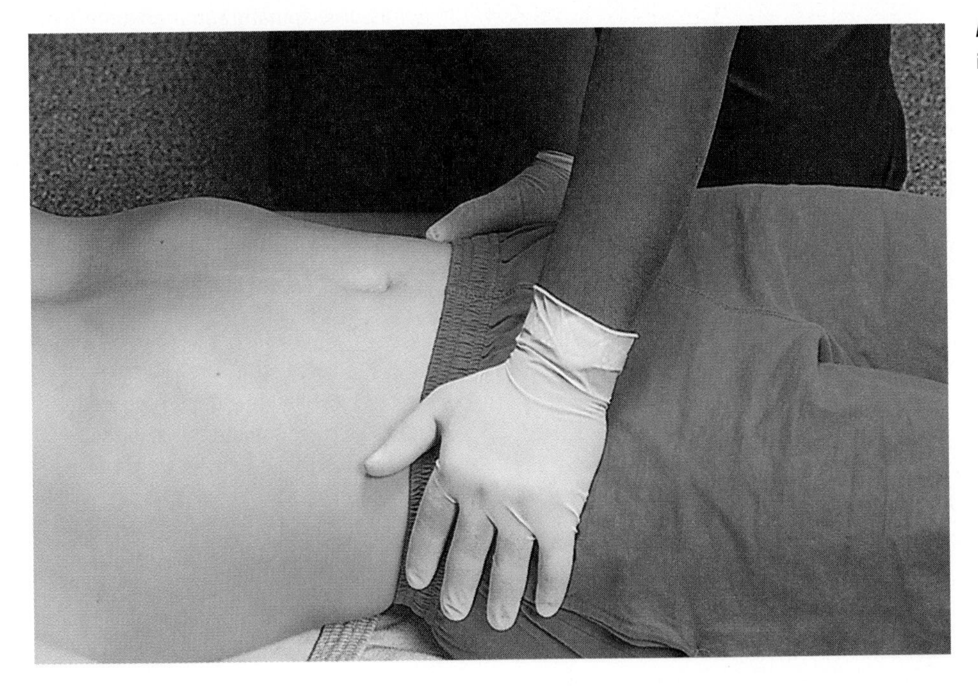

Figure 16.2 **Palpate each bone during the secondary survey**

Conclude the secondary survey with a neurological exam that includes

- assessment of the level of consciousness using a recognized coma scale (e.g., Glasgow Coma Score) or AVPU
- evaluation of motor and sensory function
- check of pupillary response

Trauma

Trauma is damage to the body caused by violent external means. Trauma includes injuries such as cuts, fractures, burns, crushing injuries, and amputations. Traumatic injury in confined space commonly results from a worker's falling or falling objects hitting a worker.

Secondary Injuries

Traumatic injuries are often secondary to some other problem. For example, a person may lose consciousness from hazardous atmosphere and fall, or might have a heart attack and fall. In these situations, the patient has a combination of problems, which the rescuer should recognize and treat properly.

Response to Trauma

1. Establish that the scene is safe and/or observe proper entry procedures.
2. Establish that safety precautions can be maintained during rescue.
3. Dispatch at least two (when possible) responders with medical training. This is particularly important if the patient is unconscious, needs spinal immobilization, or needs packaging for technical rescue.
4. If the patient is in a hazardous atmosphere, rapidly remove him or her to a safe area.
5. If the atmosphere is safe, perform ABCs (primary survey) simultaneously with cervical spine (c-spine) precautions. Do this by holding the patient's head in a neutral position while doing the primary survey (see Figure 16.3). Deal with life-threatening conditions encountered during the primary survey.
6. Place the patient on high-flow oxygen as appropriate and safe.
7. Decide if the patient needs spinal precautions. If the patient is unresponsive and the cause of unconsciousness is unknown, assume spinal trauma. If the patient is conscious, but has trauma to the head, neck, or back, assume spinal injury. Regardless of the patient's level of consciousness and presence or absence of pain, assume spinal trauma anytime the injury or mechanism of injury indicates it is possible.
8. While maintaining c-spine precautions, conduct the secondary survey.
9. Focus on and treat the serious, life- and limb-threatening injuries. Do not waste time examining and treating injuries such as minor fractures, cuts, and abrasions while life-threatening injuries need immediate attention. Address injuries in proper priority.
10. Package the patient for removal from the confined space or other location.
11. Monitor vital signs and level of consciousness frequently.

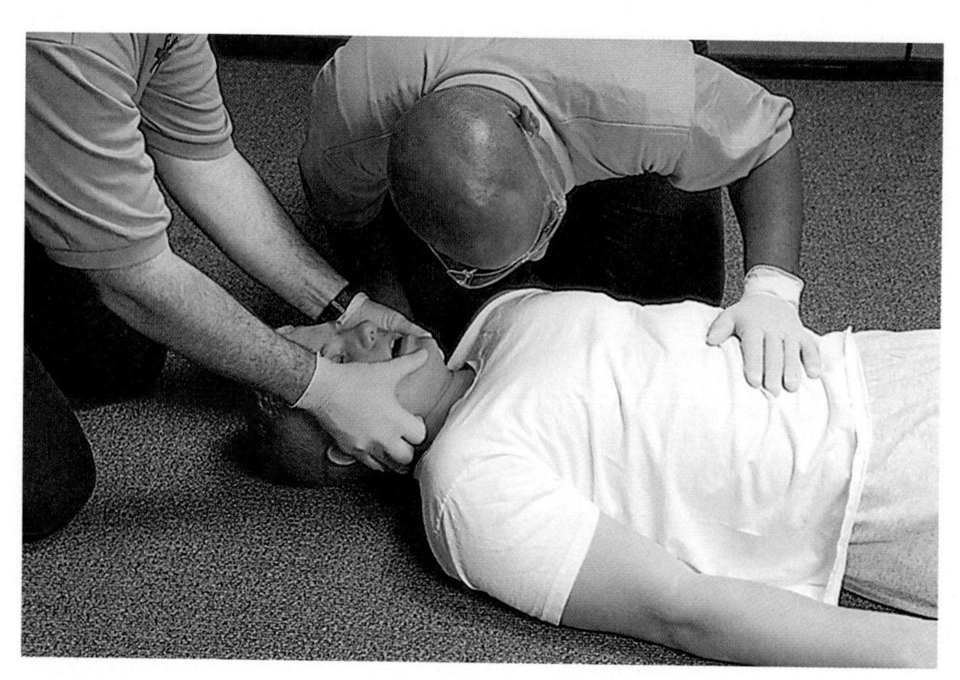

Figure 16.3 **Hold the patient's head in a neutral position during your assessment**

Spinal Immobilization in Confined Space

One of the most difficult challenges to rescuers is providing appropriate spinal care in confined space. The most important elements of patient care in a confined space are training and good judgment.

WARNING

Never attempt to perform a rescue in an unusual environment unless you have received the appropriate training.

Training and Judgment

Suitable medical training is the first step to providing proper care to any patient. Most standardized emergency medical training provides rescuers with the knowledge and skills to protect an injured person from further injury or harm. This awareness is particularly important when dealing with potential spinal injuries. Unfortunately, most basic training for emergency medical procedures only addresses care in nonhazardous environments.

Spinal Precautions

The following procedure assumes that you have completed the first seven steps listed under "Response to Trauma."

- For all trauma patients, maintain hands-on stability of the c-spine when you first reach the patient, during the primary and secondary exam, and until the rescuers immobilize the spine completely with immobilization devices or until rescuers can definitely prove there is no chance of spinal injury.)
- Maintain the head in a neutral position during examination and movement of the patient. This means that, if possible, one rescuer will be dedicated solely to maintaining c-spine precautions (although this is also a good position to monitor patient airway, breathing, and level of consciousness).
- Apply a rigid cervical collar on the patient (unless this is in conflict with your local medical protocol). Even with the collar in place, rescuers must maintain hands-on stability of the c-spine. The collar provides the following:
  - It helps stabilize the cervical spine.
  - It reminds a conscious patient to keep his or her head still.
  - It is a visual sign to all rescuers that they must practice c-spine precautions.
- Secure the patient in a spinal immobilization device. If possible, it is best to use a full backboard (see Figure 16.4). A full backboard serves two purposes:
  - It allows full immobilization of the entire body.
  - It requires fewer rescuers to move the patient as a unit.

If the space is too confined, then rescuers may use half body immobilizers. The half body immobilizers have built-in handholds. Do not use these handholds alone to perform vertical lifts of patients from vessels or other confined spaces. They may not provide the strength required for hauling vertically. Check with the manufacturer of the device for specific directions regarding its proper use.

You may place a full body rescue harness around both the patient and half body immobilizer in which he or she is secured. Again, this technique is subject to manufacturer's approval.

WARNING

Patients being evacuated in half body immobilizers require special precautions.

Shock

Most deaths in trauma cases are caused by shock. Hospital persons have several classifications for shock, but rescuers need to concern themselves only with the basic causes of shock and what rescuers should do for patients with possible shock.

Basic Causes of Shock

Three factors keep the healthy body from shock:

- functioning heart (good pump)
- sufficient fluid in the body (blood and plasma)
- adequate air exchange (for oxygen in the blood)
- intact vascular system (to deliver blood to tissues)

These three factors are needed to supply oxygen and nourishment to all body cells. If they do not receive this supply, body cells die and, eventually, the patient dies.

In trauma, two basic mechanisms disrupt circulatory system:

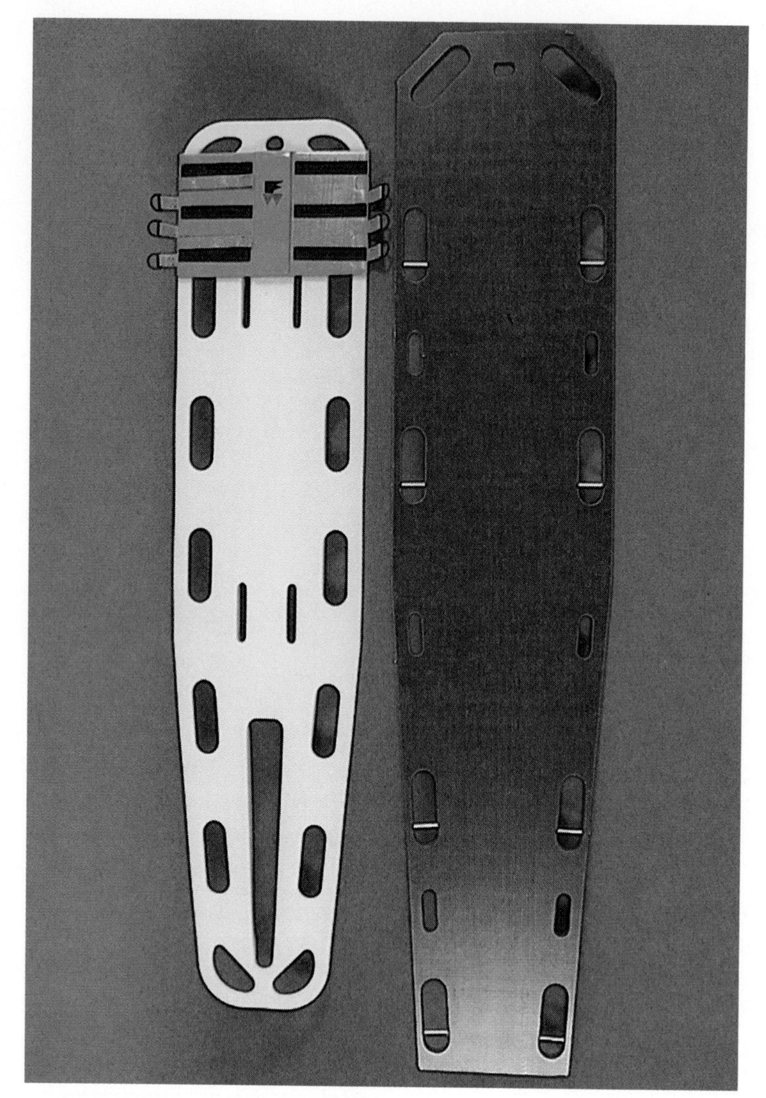

Figure 16.4 **Full backboards are best for spinal immobilization**

1. An injury causes the body to lose too much blood to the outside of the body or to have too much blood in the wrong places inside the body. There is insufficient blood in the circulating system to maintain volume and pressure to support life.
2. Some injuries cause the blood vessels to lose their tension or impair the pumping of the heart, which maintains healthy blood pressure. The result is the same: the body is unable to maintain volume and pressure to support life.

Treating Shock

Shock is a process of a body dying. The only certain way to reverse it is to get the patient to a hospital that has surgeons capable of repairing the damage that is causing shock. In general, there is very little that rescuers can do in the field to *reverse* shock. However, there are things rescuers should do that might *slow* the progress of shock. These things might also prevent permanent disability to the patient.

1. Avoid further damage to the patient during rescue. For example, some trauma can fracture bones that will damage organs and vessels. Further careless movement could cause greater damage.
2. Be aware of the ABCs when you first reach the patient *and throughout the rescue.* For example, a patient's airway may close or he or she might stop breathing without rescuers noticing. One rescuer should continue to monitor the ABCs.
3. If possible, maintain high-flow oxygen on trauma patients. Administered oxygen can help compensate for oxygen not being supplied naturally to the cells during shock. Shock robs vital organs of much needed oxygen. In the brain, oxygen-starved cells die quicker than anywhere else in the body, and can result in severe permanent disabilities. Although generally unrelated to shock, high-flow oxygen is particularly important in head injuries for the same reason.
4. Maintain c-spine precautions. Some spinal injuries can directly cause shock through damage to nerve pathways controlling the processes of blood vessel dilation and constriction. These vessels may dilate en masse, making it impossible for the body to supply enough blood to fill the void.
5. Move trauma patients to an ambulance or hospital as quickly as possible. This transfer should be done rapidly and safely while attending to immediately life-threatening problems.

Summary

It is obvious that the medical considerations associated with industrial rescues may differ from those in other emergencies. However, all emergencies require primary and secondary surveys, attention to spine and vital signs as presented here. It is not possible to attempt to address every aspect of this subject in a single chapter. It is the responsibility of every rescue team to ensure its adequate training in every major aspect of response including the often neglected but important area of emergency medical training. Technical rescue skills are of little use if the patient dies because of poor emergency medical care. Rescuers must be aware of the full scope of rescue operations and adequately prepare for all of them.

CHAPTER 17

Confined Space Rescue: Retrieval & Team Deployment

The information in this chapter is provided as a basis for continued training. Each rescuer should consult with his or her own team leader for the correct SOGs for the team. Topics covered in this chapter include:

- Standards and regulations
- Tripods and Winches
- Retrieval of Rescuers
- Team Deployment

Introduction

There are several options for retrieval of victims and rescuers from confined spaces during an emergency (some of them are discussed in Chapter 12, "Hauling Systems"). Team-constructed rope/pulley mechanical advantage systems offer the most versatility for rescue team personnel in confined space rescue. However, other manually operated mechanical devices are available that also may prove helpful.

Manufactured Portable Anchors and Winch Devices

Tripods (three-legged devices), quadpods (four-legged devices), and other manufactured portable anchors can be combined with winch devices. These systems are excellent for external retrieval when obstructions and configurations of interior vessels do not create entanglement hazards. Workers can set up these devices on the site of an entry and activate them immediately if a problem occurs inside the space. Rescuers should consider the patient's medical condition to ensure that a potential spinal or other injury is not aggravated by an external retrieval. Tripods are the most common portable anchors. There are guidelines to use of tripods and tripod/winch combinations.

Prefabricated tripods are manufactured by a variety of companies. The features of these tripods vary from model to model. Regardless of which tripod you choose, the following recommendations apply:

- Use only tripods designed and rated for human loads. Although not rated for such, several tripods on the market could be mistakenly used for human loads.
- Follow manufacturer's recommendations for assembly and use of the tripod. As with any equipment, a breach of the manufacturer's recommendations presents an issue of liability to the user.
- Although not required for efficient use, you may want to stabilize tripod legs with loose tag lines to prevent displacement of the legs while the load is being placed on or removed from the line. Do not pull these tag lines taut. This could cause uneven loading of the legs. Tripods are designed for use with a load evenly distributed on three legs.
- NEVER place more than one person's weight on a tripod unless it is approved by the manufacturer. Most tripods are only rated for a sustained load of 1,000 pounds.

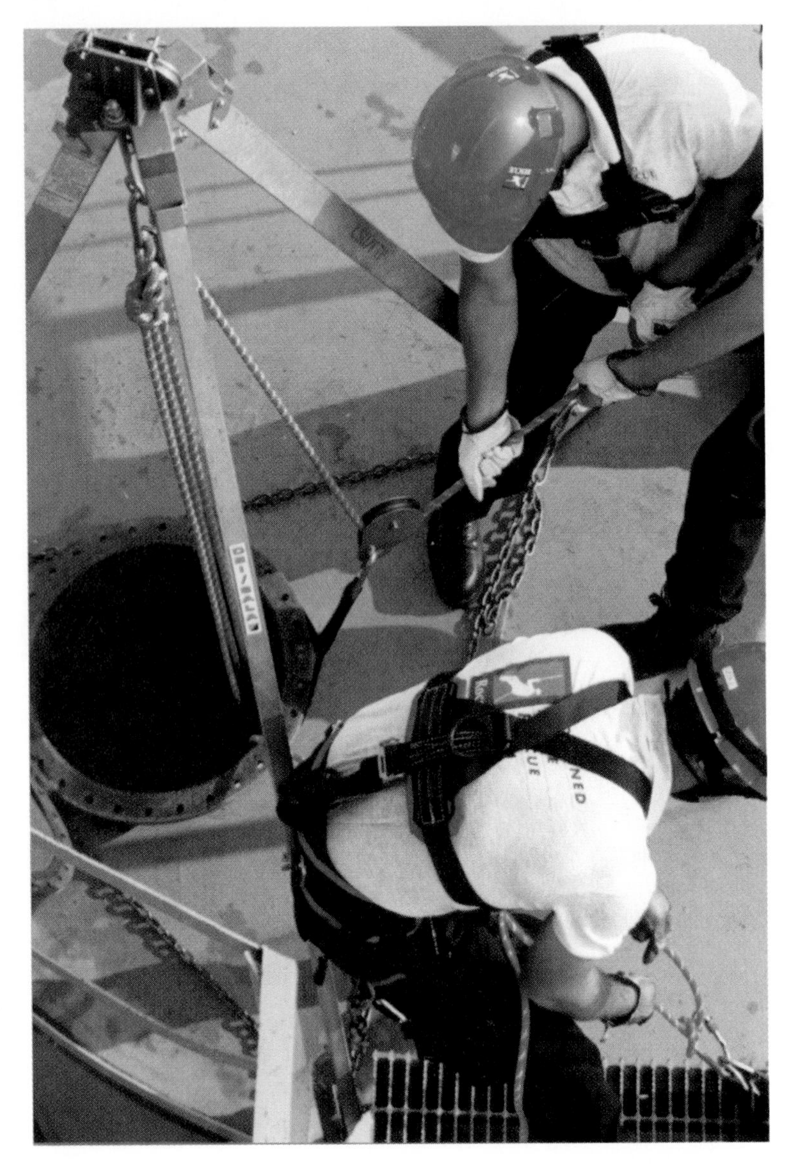

Figure 17.1 Tripod with bottom directional pulley and chains holding legs to a fixed radius

Investigate how the manufacturer rates the strength of its device. Strength ratings should be based on a sustained, even pull, not on the dynamic shock/impact capacity. Some tripods have been designed to handle the weight of two-person loads, usually with a 5:1 safety factor. Tripods are available that will not add significantly to the weight of the unit.

> Many tripods have height limits of 7 feet or even less; others extend much higher. The higher the tripod can extend, the more suitable it may be for complete extraction of packaged patients from a confined space. It may be advantageous to look for a tripod that has a maximum extension of 9 feet. Remember, though, the higher the tripod, the larger is the circumference of space necessary for the legs. In other words, as the height goes up, the legs go out.

- When using a rope hauling system, ALWAYS place a bottom directional pulley on the haul line. Place it as close as possible to the base of the tripod (see Figure 17.1). This helps prevent tipping of the tripod from a side pull.
- It is always a good idea to back up the rigging. If time permits in an actual rescue or certainly during training exercises, a backup can be rigged by wrapping the head of the tripod with a utility strap/belt or webbing and then clipping a carabiner to the hauling system in case the tripod's eyebolt anchor gives way.
- Mechanical winches must be designed for human loads and should be operated manually. Be sure the winch is capable of both lowering and hauling (known as "positioning"). Follow the manufacturer's recommendations for maintenance, use, and inspection. You should use a tripod/winch system that is also equipped with fall arrest apparatus. Do not use powered winches. They can injure the patient if entanglement occurs during retrieval.

> Mechanical winches are heavy and cumbersome. They are not suited for emergencies that call for the rescue team to go to the scene. They are ideal for situations where there is no internal congestion to cause entanglement. In those situations, the system should be set up and in place prior to initial entry.

These guidelines, although specifically for tripods and tripod/winch devices, can be applied generally to other manufactured portable anchors. Remember, follow manufacturer's recommendations.

Rescuer Retrieval

Tripod/winch systems can be employed in many cases to effect the retrieval of rescue entrants. However, rope/pulley mechanical advantage systems are generally more versatile for rescue applications that require multiple persons to enter the space. It is as important to provide a method to retrieve rescuers who enter the space as it is for workers who are injured in the space. It is likely to be a more important issue for rescue entrants, since one emergency has already occurred, which warranted the presence of the rescue team. This section concentrates on methods for retrieval of rescuers, although these systems are usually suited for workers as well as rescuers who must enter confined spaces.

Rope/Pulley Mechanical Advantage Systems

When using any retrieval device, the goal is to remove the entrant from the space without having to send personnel inside to do so (external rescue). Rope/pulley systems can be effectively employed to do this in most cases where the internal configuration of the space allows it. Even in situations where entanglement or ineffective retrieval may take place, it is a good idea to use a "locator line" to allow rescuers to find the fallen person quickly and with the least amount of effort.

The OSHA regulation CFR 1910.146 requires that all entrants to any type of permit required confined space wear a harness and retrieval line unless such rigging poses an entanglement hazard. OSHA further requires a mechanical retrieval system for workers who enter a vertical permit required confined space more than 5 feet deep. Rescuers should consider OSHA's criteria as the minimum. It is advisable to consider retrieval systems in conjunction with a prefabricated full-body harness for all rescue entrants, whether it is a horizontal or a vertical entry.

Consider a rescue taking place inside a steam drum or other long cylindrical vessel. The emergency external retrieval of this rescuer would be simplified through the use of a rope or rope/pulley system. Unless a condition (such as entanglement hazards) would prevent its use, a retrieval system should be used for all rescue entrants.

Selecting the Retrieval Device

Several considerations apply to the selection of the appropriate retrieval device. The depth of the space, the number of rescuers in the space to be retrieved, and the order in which they are to be retrieved are a few of these considerations.

Depth of Space

The depth of the space sometimes determines the type of rope/pulley system to use. For example, you might have a space 200 feet deep, but no ropes longer than 300 feet. In this situation, a smaller, resettable, hauling system piggybacked onto a single 300-foot main line might be better than a vertically configured 3:1 or 4:1 simple block-and-tackle system. The vertically configured system would require rope lengths greater than that available. Consider rope lengths of less than 200 feet to be generally inadequate for depths greater than 50 feet.

Number of Rescuers

If there is no need for spinal immobilization, one rescue entrant might enter the space and attach the victim to the hauling system being used for retrieval. This might be done without ever detaching the rescuer from the hauling system. For example, a rescuer enters the space by being lowered to a patient on a 4:1 vertically configured block-and-tackle hauling system. The rescuer reaches the patient, attaches the patient to the same hauling system via some type of suitable webbing link, then signals to the attendant to begin the extraction. Several considerations here include the need for greater mechanical advantage for a two-person load, the size of the opening the two persons must pass through, and anchorage suitable for two-person loads. Nevertheless, a single system can be used sometimes to provide both retrieval and extraction of two persons.

The authors recommend that at least two rescue entrants perform a confined space rescue—a first responder and an internal rigger. Multiple entrants in a situation requiring spinal immobilization must each remain attached to his or her method of retrieval at all times while working in the space (again, unless they encounter an entanglement hazard). The same single vertical system could be used to lower the first and second rescuer into the space, but would have to be detached to allow the second rescuer to be lowered into it. Unless both rescuers were attached to the same system and lowered into the space at the same time, the one system would not work as retrieval for both.

Even if one system were appropriate, which is likely not, there is the question of how to extract the victim. This would require another system to complete the rescue. The ultimate goal is to provide for retrieval of all persons in case they all go down at the same time. Although this is highly unlikely, it is the worst-case scenario and should be considered. The use of single-line systems that remain attached to each rescuer could provide retrieval for everyone if a catastrophe occurred. A mechanical advantage system could be piggybacked to any one of these single lines to retrieve the entrant if a problem arose. This emergency retrieval device need not be the same system used for extraction of the patient or even for routine lowering and hauling from the space. It is simply an emergency precaution in case everyone in the space became incapacitated.

For example, two rescuers are lowered into the space, one at a time, with the same 4:1 vertically configured block-and-tackle hauling system. Each time a rescuer reaches the bottom of the space, he or she detaches the system so it can be used by the next rescuer or victim for routine lowering or extraction. If each rescuer is attached to an additional single rope before being allowed to enter the space, this rope serves a dual purpose. It acts as the rescuer's safety line belay system during routine operations and it provides emergency retrieval should the need arise.

There may be several rescuers in a space, each attached to his or her own retrieval lines. Should an emergency occur, each rescuer could be retrieved individually through the use of an emergency hauling system piggybacked onto any one of the retrieval lines. If everyone went down inside the space, all rescue entrants could be retrieved, one at a time.

While this seems straightforward and simple enough, it is obvious that line management is necessary. Depending on the type of retrieval system, multiple lines can be present inside or outside the space. This increases the likelihood of entanglement, tripping, and confusion. Of course, each entrant is not constantly attached to a retrieval system. However, a single anchored retrieval system cable of being quickly attached to each entrant's line is acceptable to OSHA to meet its requirement for retrieval.

Poor housekeeping (improper line management) can quickly create problems on the emergency scene. Carefully set up lines so that they are out of the way and easily identified. Different colored ropes help avoid confusion as to which line belongs to whom. In cases where excess line is pooled in the space, slack should be removed or perhaps the rope coiled and secured with a small piece of electrical tape (so it will come apart easily if retrieval is necessary). These steps help ease the burden of the rescue team when it is providing retrieval systems. Because there may be communications lines and breathing air hoses in addition to rescue and retrieval lines going into one opening, line management is critical.

Order of Retrieval

Another important factor in rescues with multiple entrants is the order in which the rescuers must be retrieved. The question is, Does the first rescuer who enters the space need to be the first rescuer out? The key considerations are the patient's condition, rescuer fatigue, personnel requirements outside the space, and, if applicable, the type of fresh air breathing apparatus used in the rescue.

For example, two rescuers are entering a tank for an extended period. Conditions in the vessel are such (high ambient temperature) that extreme fatigue of the rescue entrants is expected within a short period of time. The first person in will probably need to be the first one out because he or she is likely to collapse from fatigue sooner.

The same point applies when rescuers use self-contained breathing apparatus or supplied air respirators. The SCBA air supply is limited. The first person in will likely be the first to run low on air and should be the first one out. The SAR has a virtually unlimited supply of air, so this would not be of great concern.

Some retrieval system configurations allow rescuers to make very efficient use of their lines. It is possible to place the first rescuer on the end of the retrieval line, lower him or her into the space, tie an in-line knot in the same line outside the space for the second rescuer, and lower him or her into the space on the same rope. This, in effect, allows both rescuers to have retrieval lines while it limits the number of actual ropes in the space. The problem with this system is that the first person in will be the last one to be retrieved in an emergency involving the collapse of all entrants. Although this system has some advantages, it might be inappropriate when severe rescuer fatigue is expected or when there is a limited air supply. In these cases, a retrieval system capable of individually recovering the rescue entrants in any order may be necessary. The order of retrieval is a factor in determining the configuration of the retrieval system.

Confined Space Retrieval System

A few rescue/retrieval systems allow for emergency retrieval of all rescuers should the worst case occur. These systems also allow for rescue of the victim. Note that some configurations use hauling systems for emergency retrieval that are different from systems used for routine lowering and hauling of entrants and victim. Some use the same hauling system for both. The following list shows advantages and disadvantages of a few configurations, referred to here as Confined Space Rescue (CSR) Systems 1 through 4. They do not work in all scenarios but may provide a solution for most.

CSR System 1

System type (see Figure 17.2)

- Piggyback hauling/figure-8 lowering system for normal use and emergency retrieval
- Shared safety and main line for all rescuers
- Ideal for situations with unlimited air supply and depth less than 50 feet with 200-foot rope.

Advantages

- The same hauling system works for both normal hauling and emergency retrieval operations.
- A safety line belay is always on the persons being retrieved.

Disadvantages

- The first person in is the last person out because of the knot attachments.
- There is a potential for rope entanglement inside the space.

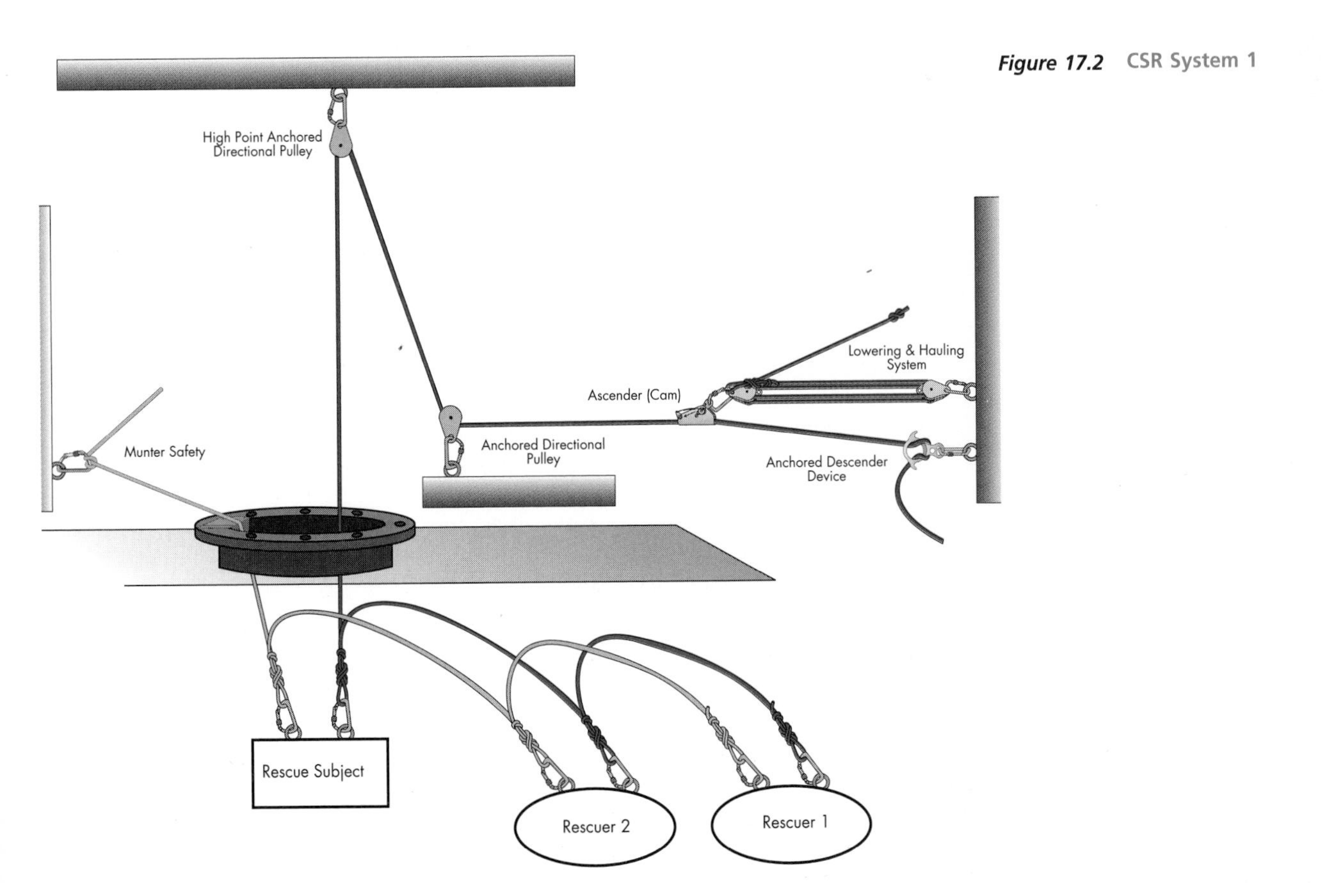

Figure 17.2 CSR System 1

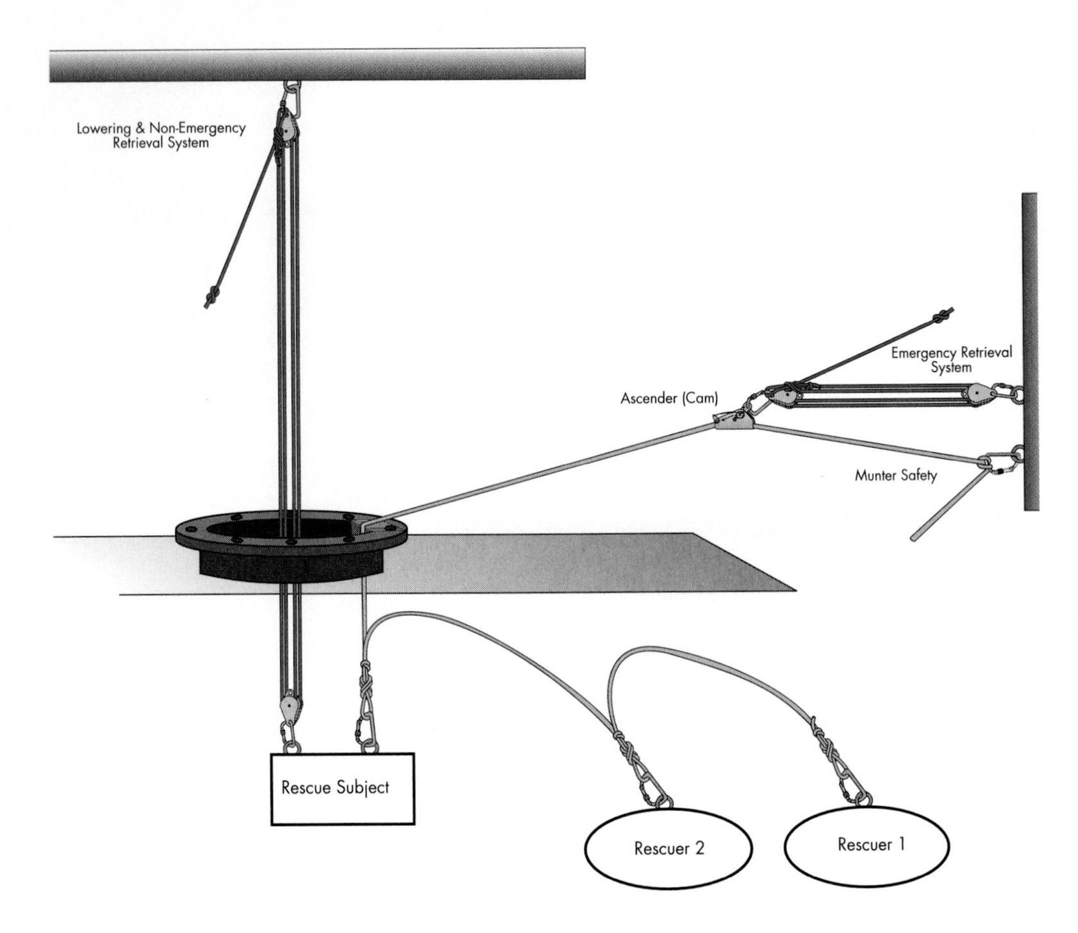

Figure 17.3 CSR System 2

CSR System 2

System type (see Figure 17.3)

- Vertical block and tackle simple system for normal lowering/hauling.
- Piggyback hauling system for emergency retrieval.
- Shared safety line for all rescuers.
- Also works in situations with unlimited air supply and depth less than 50 feet with 200-foot rope.

Advantages

- Fewer rope entanglement problems

Disadvantages

- Requires two separate hauling systems for normal hauling and emergency retrieval operations.
- The last person in is the last person out because of the knot attachments.
- There is no safety line belay system on the person being retrieved in a "worst case" emergency retrieval scenario.

CSR System 3

System type (see Figure 17.4)

- Vertical block-and-tackle simple system for normal lowering/hauling
- Piggyback hauling system for emergency retrieval
- Separate safety lines for all rescuers
- Idea for situations where SCBA is utilized and depth less than 50 feet with 200 foot rope.

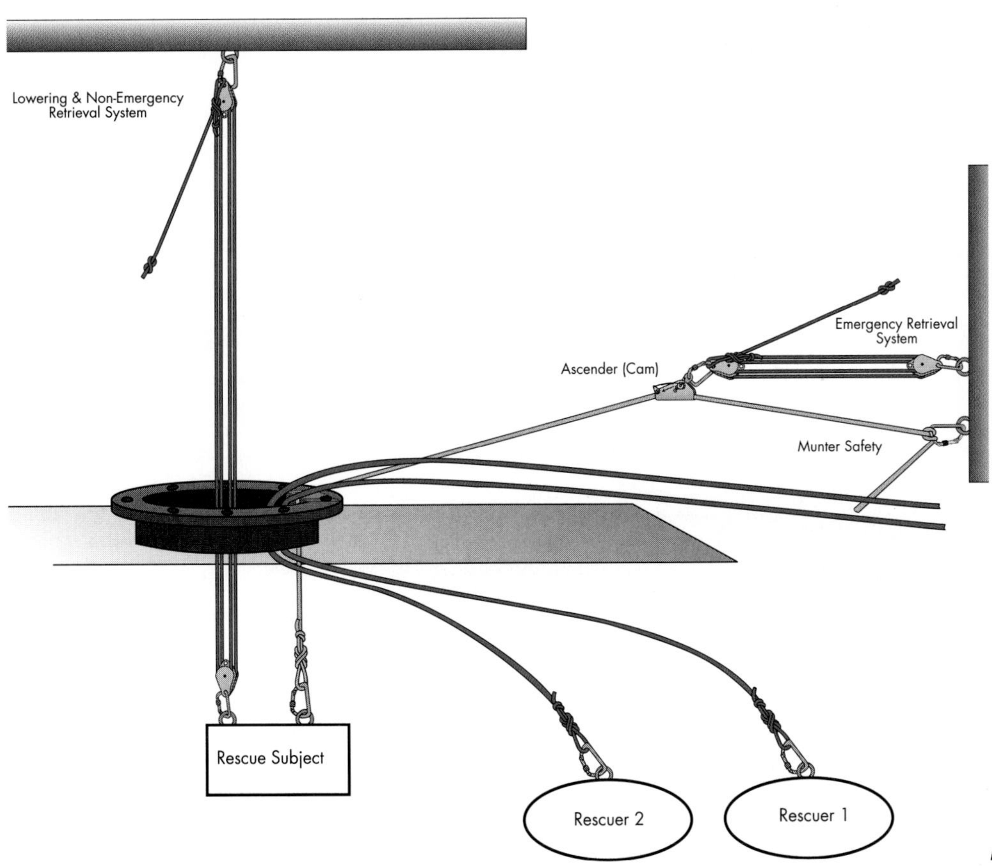

Figure 17.4 CSR System 3

Advantages

- ✚ Each person can be retrieved independently of the others. First in can be first out.

Disadvantages

- ✖ Requires two separate hauling systems for normal hauling and emergency retrieval operations.
- ✖ There is a potential for rope entanglement both inside and outside the space.
- ✖ There is no safety line belay system on the person being retrieved in a "worst case" emergency retrieval scenario.

CSR System 4

System type (see Figure 17.5)

- ➔ Piggyback hauling/figure-8 lowering system for normal use and emergency retrieval.
- ➔ Separate safety lines for all rescuers.
- ➔ Also works for situations where SCBA is utilized.

Advantages

- ✚ Each person can be retrieved independently of the others. First in can be first out.
- ✚ The same hauling system works for both routine hauling and emergency retrieval operations.

Disadvantages

- ✖ There is a potential for rope entanglement both inside and outside the space.
- ✖ There is no safety line belay system on the person being retrieved in a "worst case" emergency retrieval scenario.

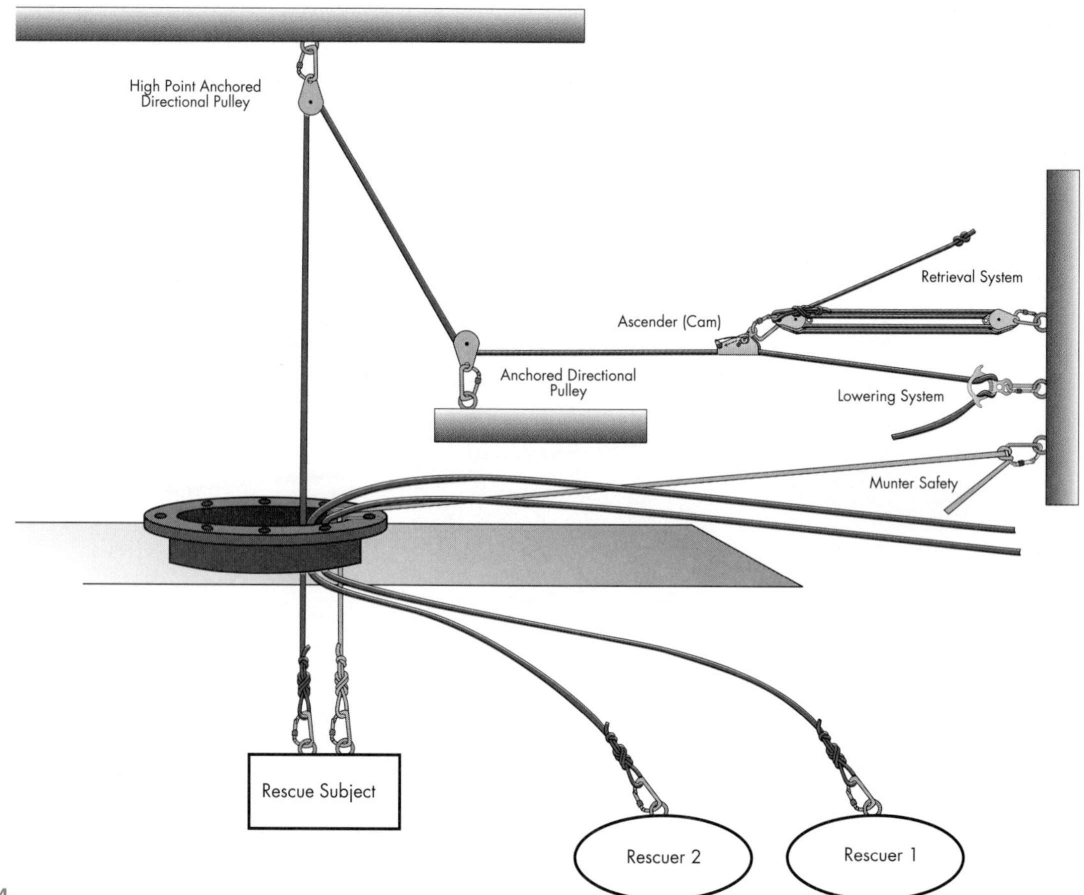

Figure 17.5 **CSR System 4**

Figure 17.6 **Using simple haul system to assist in horizontal drag**

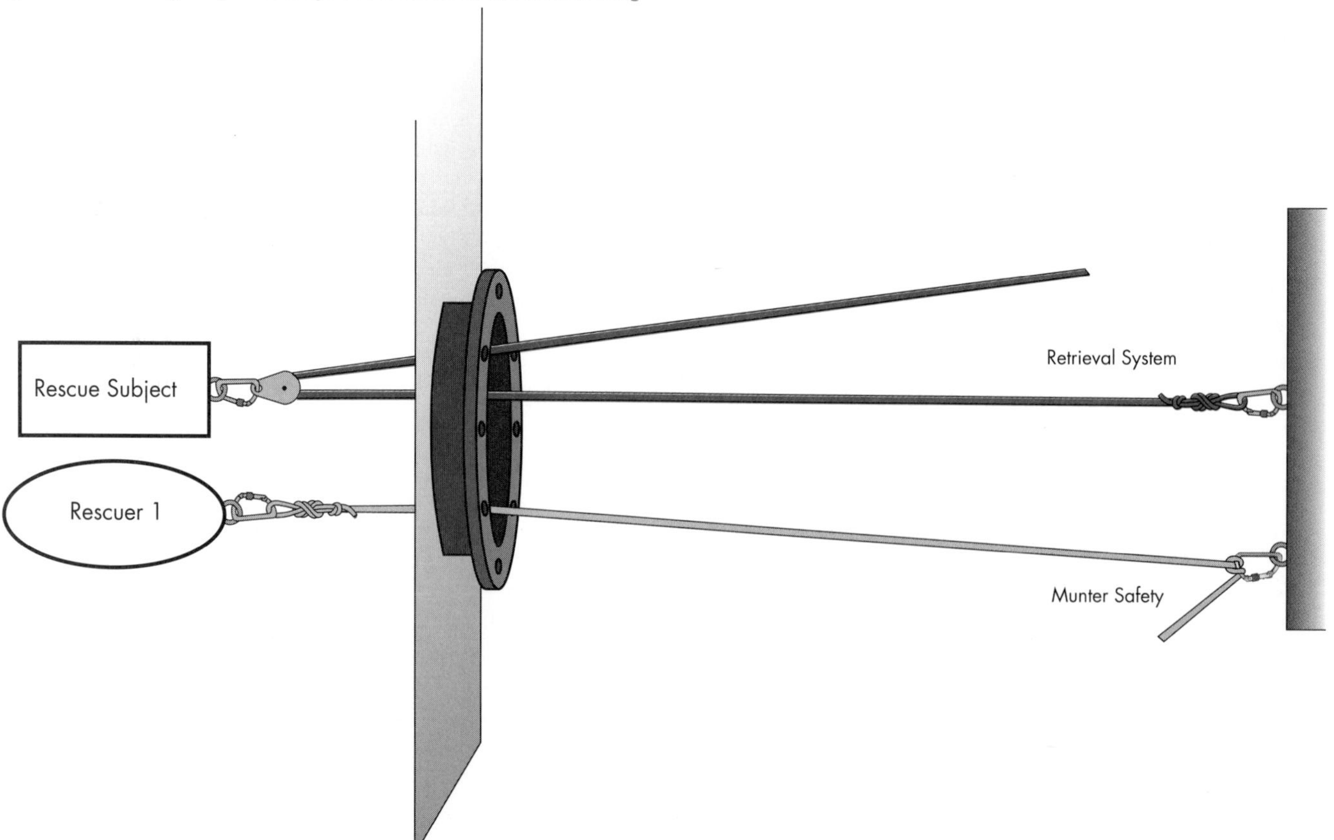

Line Management

The ropes in a rope/pulley retrieval system alone can be confusing. With air lines, atmospheric monitoring probes, and hardwire communications, the situation can seem impossible to manage. Here are a few things that might help you manage your lines properly:

- Use portable reels for air and communications lines. These reels, while expensive, provide an excellent means of managing excess lines.
- Marry air and communications lines. This can be done in a variety of ways. You can tape the lines together as they are fed into the space or you can prethread them into two-inch tubular webbing to create an "umbilical" that can be kept on a reel. If the type of retrieval system remains constant, you may even choose to include your rope in the marriage of lines. Be cautious! Various situations call for the use of communications without air line, air line without communications, rope without either, or any combination of the above. Be sure you can compensate for changing situations before you tie everything together.
- Color code ropes and air lines. This will help identify which entrant is connected to a particular line. The use of a different color of electrical tape at both ends of each line is one simple method of identification.
- Secure slack or unused lines both inside and outside the space. Place hoses in an area that eliminates trip hazards. Use electrical tape or some other means to secure excess rope slack in a coil. Creative use of plastic cable ties can be an effective means of securing unused coils of cable to handrails in the industrial setting. Use whatever means available to remove excess line from the work area (action perimeter).

Team Deployment Recommendations

CSR Considerations Prior to Entry

Several sources of information are available on the scene of a confined space emergency. Rescuers use all resources to develop a plan of action.

1. Locate the previous attendant for the entry. He or she can provide valuable information concerning the cause of the emergency.
2. Locate the unit supervisor or even an operator familiar with the usual processes in the space. These people can be extremely helpful in sizing up the internal configuration and eliminating hazards in the space.
3. Quickly assign a rescuer to attempt contact with the patient. By observing the patient, you can learn much about what you need for packaging and rescue. For example, if the patient is found unresponsive and lying in the bottom of the vessel, assume spinal injury. You will probably need a litter or similar device. A patient who can speak to you can let you know his or her level of consciousness. Get someone to the patient fast.
4. Observe the scene. As with any emergency, you can learn much from the surroundings. Placement of anchor points, overhead attachment points, and the mechanism of injury can be vital in determining the methods for rescue.
5. Brainstorm with the other rescuers. The axiom "Two heads are better than one" is particularly true in developing an action plan rapidly. Use the experience and advice of other rescue team members to determine your strategy. DO NOT rely on your expertise alone.

General Recommendations for Confined Space Rescue

Remember that regulations and standards represent *minimum* requirements to use as a guide for development of more rigid guidelines. Encourage your team to discuss and address procedures that need "beefing up." The following are only recommendations. Some may exceed or are not addressed by regulatory requirements.

- Always wear applicable personal protective equipment when working in confined space. Do not consider PPE an option that depends on personal convenience.

- Have at least one rescuer outside, ready and equipped for every one rescuer inside the confined space. These stand-by personnel are a valuable backup for rescue entrants. This function is particularly import when external retrieval is inappropriate due to entanglement hazards or an internal configuration that makes retrieval ineffective. In these cases, the only means of rescuing the rescuers is by entering the space.
- Proper PPE should be worn and required rescue gear should be immediately available to simplify rapid response. This is sometimes referred to as "warm stand by."
- Attempt to use at least a two-member rescue team for confined space entry. Although this is not a requirement nor, at times, even possible, it makes sense to use a "buddy system."
- Establish some method of back-up communications. This serves as a link to rescue entrants if the primary communications system fails. This is also a matter of recommendation and not regulation. However, when something goes wrong with such an important tool, lack of a back-up system can be devastating. Plan for the worst, hope for the best.
- Provide an attendant, known as a "hole watchs" for rescuers at all times. This is a requirement for any entrant. This person must devote attention to persons inside the space. If something goes wrong, this attendant calls the entrants out or notifies the proper personnel if rescue is needed. A trained rescue team member should provide this important service when rescue entry must be made. Because something has already gone wrong, a rescuer will be attuned to signs of additional trouble and can aid in the rescue.
- Never lower a rescuer into a confined space without an *immediate* means of retrieval. This retrieval system can be any safe manually operated mechanical system. It is strongly recommended that the guidelines for M/A systems in Chapter 12 be followed as they apply to retrieval systems. The only time retrieval systems are not required is when the use of such equipment will increase the overall risks of entry or will not contribute to the rescue. In such cases, its use can be waived. This should be considered the exception, not the rule. Most times, retrieval systems of some type can be used. Even if it does not provide an effective means of actual retrieval, a rope attachment can serve as a locator line in the event of trouble.
- Build vertical hauling systems on the ground before installing them at the site. This is more a matter of convenience. Some rope/pulley M/A systems are more easily handled if you build them in a controlled area before using them in the action perimeter.
- To prevent fatigue, do not allow the rescue entrants to rig the rescue systems. They may undergo tremendous work load once they have entered the space. This is conserve of energy. Although rescue entrant involvement is necessary in some cases for an effective rescue, avoid it if possible. Always allow the rescuer entrants to inspect the rigging prior to entry. They will be depending on its integrity.
- Make every attempt to reach the patient rapidly in a confined space emergency. Rapid deployment methods presented in this chapter can be effective for contacting the patient within 10 to 15 minutes of arrival on the scene. This average applies to most confined space emergencies with an atmospheric hazard that can be mitigated safely with ventilation and fresh air breathing apparatus. Of course, the time varies according to the complexity of the incident.
- Consider the rapid application of oxygen or fresh air to spontaneously breathing patients in the confined space. Remember, use of oxygen in the presence of hydrocarbons might not be advisable in a refining or chemical complex where there is potential reactivity.
- Consider the potential consequences of rescuing a dead victim. DO NOT risk a life to recover a body!

Checklist for Confined Space Rescue Entry

Although OSHA does not require a permit for rescue, the rescue team should be protected from hazards. One method of confirming all important safety issues prior to entry is to use a checklist. The checklist can remind the person in charge of necessary steps prior to allowing personnel into the space. It frees his or her mind to focus on the complex issues of performing the rescue. The following checklist is an example.

- ☐ Obtain information from resources (permit, MSDS, witness, etc.).
- ☐ Provide continuous atmospheric monitoring (O2, LEL, toxicity, wet bulb globe thermometer).
- ☐ Confirm lockout/tagout procedures and ventilate as needed.
- ☐ Wear fresh air breathing apparatus unless atmosphere is proven nonhazardous.
- ☐ Wear PPE (full-body harness, SAR, SCBA, clothing, etc.).
- ☐ Confirm primary and back-up communication.
- ☐ Assign an attendant.
- ☐ Provide a retrieval system unless inappropriate.
- ☐ Assign stand-by back-up personnel fully equipped as appropriate.
- ☐ Assign an air supply and/or accountability officer.
- ☐ Provide fresh air for patients who are breathing in bad atmospheres.
- ☐ Authorize each entrant prior to his or her entry.

Rapid Patient Access in Hazardous Atmospheres

When a patient is exposed to a respiratory hazard in a permit space and is still breathing, the most important thing is rapid access to give the patient fresh air or oxygen. This immediate life-threatening problem is one of the first elements in patient assessment (Airway, Breathing, Circulation). If the patient is not breathing, time is even more critical.

The goal is to get fresh air to the patient within 4 to 6 minutes; however, this is not realistic in most permit space emergencies that require entry for rescue. Rescuers can, however, expect to get to the patient within 8 to 12 minutes from time of arrival on the scene if they are deployed efficiently.

Once the tasks component of access have been identified, they can be assigned to individual team members. Although all situations differ slightly, a generic quick retrieval system may be suitable for rapid access to patients in most confined spaces. Although the system provides an effective first measure during rapid access, it can be cumbersome. Once you reach the patient and apply fresh air, you may have time to build a more appropriate and efficient system while packaging the patient. There are several tasks common to most confined space rescues:

1. Attendant/accountability officer immediately attempts indirect patient contact.
2. Monitor the space.
3. Conduct hazard abatement (lockout/tagout, etc.)
4. One or two rescuers, usually entrants, don air and communications equipment.
5. One or two back-up rescuers assist the entrants and don their own equipment.
6. One rescuer rigs a descent control device and rope for lowering the rescue entrant(s) into the space.
7. One rescuer sets up a block-and-tackle hauling system to be piggybacked onto the lowering line for emergency retrieval if needed.
8. One rescuer sets up and attends the breathing air supply system.
9. One rescuer rigs a safety line belay system, if required.
10. One rescuer sets up ventilation.
11. One team leader directs operations.

At this point, the focus is on the initial access and retrieval system for the rescuer only. Concern about the victim's egress system or high-point anchors comes at a later stage. A leader might group these tasks to provide an efficient assignment list like the following:

1. One rescuer to go immediately to the patient, establish communications, monitor the space, and act as the attendant/accountability officer.
2. One or two rescuers (entrants) don air and communications equipment.
3. One or two back-up rescuers assist the primary entrants and don their own equipment.

4. One rescuer rigs a descent control device and rope for lowering. The same rescuer hangs a prebuilt 3:1 or 4:1 block-and-tackle system (with a haul cam) to the same anchor point as figure-8.
5. One rescuer sets up and monitors the breathing air supply.
6. One rescuer rigs a safety line belay system.
7. One rescuer sets up ventilation.
8. One team leader directs operations and ensures hazard abatement.
9. After access/retrieval is in place, the available members of the team may meet for a brainstorming session to plan a more efficient method of patient/rescuer extraction.

Training for Rapid Access

The best way to get better at rapid access is through constant and appropriate training. Teams should first practice the elements of deployment without specialized equipment such as monitoring, air, communications, and ventilation. You can start by varying team member functions, then work with it and progress to achieving access in 4 to 6 minutes. Once you achieve this, use the following steps:

- Repeat the same session several times, each time adding another piece of specialized equipment such as monitor, communications, fresh air, and ventilation. This ties together all the equipment you might use in a real rescue and gives you time to become familiar with its proper use. The objective is to familiarize the team with the rapid setup of all equipment by incorporating it into a confined space rescue scenario that can be repeated many times. The team leader (rescue group or sector officer) should supervise this effort closely.
- Once the team becomes proficient in making rapid access to the patient at one practice site, move to new and unfamiliar locations. There, perform the same scenario a few more times with all equipment.
- This type of training should be repeated on a regular basis as scheduling allows. If you don't practice, you cannot maintain skills. Remember, USE IT OR LOSE IT.

Rapid access is possible in most situations. Training to do so will improve access times even in the face of unforseen circumstances. Without it, a rescue team is destined to fail.

Summary

Confined space rescue operations present one of the most formidable challenges for any technical rescue team. A thorough knowledge of the hazards and their safe mitigation is essential for success. Training and preplanning are the most significant tools in this race against the clock. A well-rounded program incorporates a serious study of the regulations governing entry and operations in and around permit spaces. Remember their primary purpose—to protect you, the rescuer.

CHAPTER 18

Confined Space Rescue: Regulatory Compliance

The appropriate OSHA, NFPA, and ANSI regulations will be referred to throughout the chapter. This information is provided as a basis for continued training. Rescuers should consult with their team leader for the correct procedures for the team. In this chapter, topics discussed are:

- Scope and Purpose of OSHA PRCS Regulations
- Issues of Compliance
- Training Requirements
- Evaluating and Equipping the Rescue Team
- Entry and Non-Entry Rescue
- ANSI Standards
- Civil Liability

Introduction

The industrial rescuer must be concerned not only with the outcome of a rescue, but also with OSHA's regulations. In other words, rescuers must know what will keep them prepared for confined space rescue as well as what will keep the employer in compliance with regulations. This text discusses the OSHA regulations that pertain to industrial rescue in permit required confined spaces. This chapter addresses the application of those regulations to confined space rescue and provides suggestions about documentation of compliance. It is important to remember that the law of each state must be considered. In "state plan" states, states that have authority to manage their own OSHA program in place of the federal OSHA program, the regulations are required to be at least as strict as federal law. In some cases, the law is more strict in the state plan states. For example, in California, which has authority to administer the federal program, the employer is required to "ensure that at least one standby person at the site is trained and immediately available to perform rescue."

Scope and Purpose of OSHA Permit Required Confined Space Regulations

As stated by the final rule effective on January 14, 1993, the scope and application of the Permit required Confined Space Regulations (PRCS) is to provide standards for the practices and procedures to protect employees in general industry from the hazards of entry into and rescue from permit required confined spaces. Agriculture, construction, and shipyard employment are exempt from these regulations. However, they are addressed in other regulations. To understand the scope and application of the general industry confined space regulations, determine how OSHA might apply and enforce these regulations, and develop a strategy for compliance, it is necessary to know what OSHA intended when it enacted the standard.

The published regulations require that the employer "ensure that the procedures and equipment necessary to rescue entrants from permit spaces are implemented and provided." Additionally, the proposed regulation allows the employer to have either an "in-plant rescue team or an arrangement under which an outside rescue team will respond to a request for service." The regulation requires that the employer ensure that the in-plant team be equipped and trained for rescue. It also requires simulated rescue operations in order to gain and maintain proficiency. However, the regulation does not explain the employer's duties as far as the capabilities of an outside service the employer might use. The law specifically requires only that the employer ensure that the rescuers be aware of the hazards at the facility "so that the outside rescue team can equip, train, and conduct itself appropriately."

OSHA notes that the term "employer" encompasses contractors. OSHA states that "a contractor whose employees enter permit spaces would be under the same obligation as any other employer to comply with this standard." To clarify that the regulations are applicable to arrangements for outside response, the final 1993 rule states that it applies to *all* employers who provide rescue services:

> "OSHA believes that it is important to protect employees who enter permit spaces to perform rescue duties regardless of who their employer is. The proposal did address the safety of rescue personnel in paragraph (h)(1); however, those requirements would have applied only to in-plant rescue teams. The proposal did not explicitly address the safety of rescuers of outside rescue providers. In the final rule, OSHA is applying provisions corresponding to proposed paragraph (h)(1)(final '1910.146(k)(1) to all employers providing rescue services). The Agency has determined that this action is necessary to provide protection for all employees of outside rescue services as well as those of in-plant rescue teams."

OSHA acknowledges that employers are not required to train or equip off-site rescuers. But that this does not mean that the employer who retains an off-site rescue service has no responsibility for the adequacy of the rescue services provided. OSHA specifically notes that the rule requires the employer "to take measures to enable the rescue of injured entrants." Although the employer is not required to train or equip the outside rescue service. However, the employer is responsible for any shortcomings in equipment or training.

On November 28, 1994, in response to a lawsuit challenging portions of the final regulation, OSHA issued another notice of proposed rule. OSHA proposed revising the standard so that it more clearly defined what an employer is required to do if it arranges to have persons other than its own employees provide permit space rescue and emergency services. Discussing the proposed provision relating to rescue services, OSHA stated:

> "[t]he proposed provision clearly indicates that host employers must evaluate a prospective rescue service's capabilities and verify that the needed capabilities are present before selecting that rescue service to perform permit space rescue."

Additionally, OSHA's current guidance for its investigators pertaining to permit required confined space regulations directs the investigators to determine how the employer evaluates proficiency in the duties required by the permit standard. It also instructs the investigators to examine how the employer determines if retraining is necessary. On August 2, 1995, OSHA further stated in a notice of informal public hearing that the proposed revision indicates that host employers must retain rescue services "that can respond adequately and in a timely fashion when summoned to perform rescues."

Although this proposed revision is not final as of the time of publication of this text, OSHA has clearly indicated how it interprets the existing regulations:

> "OSHA intended this rule making *simply to clarify the existing requirements* of '1910.146(k)(2). In particular, the Agency has attempted to indicate clearly that an employer who retains an off-site rescue and emergency service must ensure that the designated service has the equipment, training and overall ability to respond in a timely fashion when summoned to rescue a permit space entrant. OSHA does not thereby intend to require that host employers "guarantee" the performance of off-site services, to make compliance more burdensome for off-site services than for on-site services, or to prevent the use of off-site services. The Agency has consistently maintained that the purpose of [section] 1910.146(k) is to require that employers' provisions for rescue, by whatever means, are adequate. The proposed

amendment to [section] 1910.146(k)(2) (59FR60735) was intended solely to clarify the original intent of that paragraph."

Therefore, OSHA has clearly stated that this revision merely reflects its interpretation of the current regulation. It indicates the position OSHA is likely to take in enforcement proceedings, which should guide employers who are deciding how to comply with regulations.

Finally, OSHA directed that an employer who is using an off-site rescue service must verify the availability of the service *each time a permit space entry is scheduled or attempted.* OSHA further stated that if the off-site rescue service indicated that it would be unable to respond to a rescue summons for any reason, entry should not be authorized unless an adequate alternative rescue service is arranged.

Issues of Compliance

Several aspects of the permit required confined space regulations are not clear on how compliance should be accomplished. OSHA has given the regulated community a destination, but has not provided much of a road map to get there. This raises compliance issues that must be resolved by reading the regulations in conjunction with OSHA's stated intent.

The employer not only must provide rescue services. It must also ensure that the selected rescue service can respond to a rescue summons in a "timely" manner, that prospective rescuers are equipped and trained to perform confined space rescues at the host employer's facility, that the rescue service is aware of the hazards it may confront when called to perform rescue, and the rescue service has access to all permit spaces from which rescue might be necessary so that the service can develop appropriate rescue plans and practice rescue operations. According to OSHA, the intent of this regulation is to provide a level playing field for all rescue services, whether in-house or outside services.

Requiring "timely response" is sound logic, but there should be clearer guidance from OSHA, who offers no definition of "timely." Short of this guidance, the employer and rescuer must determine, by examining OSHA's intent in promulgating the standard, how OSHA might choose to apply and enforce the requirement for "timely response."

Although paragraph (k)(2) of the rule refers to employers who retain "off-site rescue emergency services," the agency has made it clear that paragraph (k)(1) applies to both outside rescue services and in-plant teams. According to OSHA, the intent of this regulation is to provide a level playing field for all rescue services.

> "The criteria . . . are designed to protect [employees who enter permit spaces to perform rescue and emergency services] from permit space hazards and to maximize their ability to provide effective rescue and emergency services. Paragraph (k)(1) applies both to rescuers employed by employers who are conducting permit space operations and to rescuers employed by outside rescue services."

In other words, on-site as well as off-site rescuers must be adequately equipped and trained to respond effectively (read "timely") to a rescue summons. Because permit spaces vary in their capacity to kill or permanently injure employees, timely response varies. OSHA indicates that it will look at circumstances to determine what is "timely." One primary concern includes permit spaces in which there is potential for death or injury due to hypoxia, a condition in which the brain is deprived of oxygen. Hypoxia can be the result of a number of conditions in confined spaces, (e.g., low oxygen, engulfment, and asphyxiation) and can cause permanent brain damage in 4 to 6 minutes.

Defining Response Time

In the fall of 1995, OSHA sought comments from the public on the timely response issue via a public hearing in Washington, D.C. The public hearings on the confined space regulations emphasized that there is a general lack of understanding about what responding to a rescue summons entails. It is necessary to analyze the rescue process in order to address this issue adequately. Does the term "timely response" refer to the time it takes the rescue service to arrive at the site or the time to complete the evacuation? Does it start from the time a problem is recognized or from the time the rescue service is notified? From the viewpoint of the professional emergency responder, a rescue consists of several distinct time blocks:

1. **Reaction time** is the time between the entrant having a problem requiring rescue response and the safety attendant's recognition that the entrant has a problem.
2. **Contact time** is the time taken by the attendant to contact the rescue team.
3. **Response time** is the time taken by the rescuers to arrive at the scene of the rescue after contact.
4. **Assessment time** is the time taken by a rescue team to size up the problem and determine the strategy to perform a safe, efficient rescue.
5. **Preparation time** is the time taken by a rescue team to set up for the rescue.
6. **Rescue time** is the time taken for the team to reach, treat, package, and evacuate the victim from the confined space.

Clearly, response time is only a portion of the process. All of the time blocks must be considered by the rescuer and the entry supervisor when they evaluate the timeliness of rescue services. Employers must use caution when evaluating the response time of their rescue services. A desired response time that includes access to the entrant should be a GOAL ONLY! This also applies to rescuers when establishing team protocols or suggested operating guidelines. Rescuers should not be pressured by a mandated time limit to enter a hazardous confined space. As OSHA has pointed out, the majority of confined space fatalities in multiple-fatality incidents have been rescuers. One paradox in confined space rescue is that the most immediately life-threatening situations (caused by hazards such as atmospheric conditions) require the most time for assessment and preparation.

Untimely Rescue Response

Although it is challenging to define "timely," it is certainly easier to define what is not timely. OSHA has stated in the preamble of 1910.146 that the rescue team should have a goal of response to a CPR emergency of 4 minutes. Therefore, if an entrant loses fresh air supply in an oxygen-free confined space, reaching him in 7 minutes is not timely!

Many confined space incidents involve severe traumatic injury. Professional emergency responders are familiar with "the golden hour" principle, which encourages patient delivery to definitive care within an hour of the injury. Therefore, if an entrant falls off of a ladder and suffers severe head injuries, reaching him or her in 45 minutes is not timely. Finally, consider victims who have become sick or suffered minor injuries in a good atmosphere but are unable to self-rescue. The possibility of psychological shock or long-term emotional stress due to lying injured, frightened, and isolated in a confined space demands a timely rescue.

Rescue Response Time Goals

If a rescue team can establish what is not timely, the logic follows that the team can determine its outside time limits. Considering the six rescue response time blocks, it is almost impossible for even an on-site team to respond to a rescue summons and reach the victim within OSHA's goal of 4 minutes—unless the team is set up at the site prior to entry.

Additionally, it is an appropriate goal to initiate patient transport to the hospital within 30 to 40 minutes of the incident. Working backwards, allow the team 5 minutes to size up and prepare their rescue. The team would need to arrive at the scene within 10 minutes of the call. This evacuation goal would normally require the team to reach the patient within 15 to 20 minutes. The team then should strive to have the victim out of the confined space within *approximately* 30 minutes. The chart below illustrates possible average times that could be considered:

1. Permit required confined space incident occurs and rescue team is called: 0–3 minutes.
2. Rescue team arrives at the scene within 10 minutes: 3–13 minutes.
3. Rescue team sizes up and prepares to initiate rescue: 13–23 minutes.
4. Rescue team reaches and rescues patient: 23–38 minutes.
5. Patient is transported and arrives at the emergency room: 38–53 minutes.

It is critical to note the frequent use of the term "goal." There are numerous legitimate reasons that a rescue response could require more time than the goals specify. OSHA requires employers to evaluate and verify the rescue service's *adequacy.* OSHA requires rescue teams to train and drill in order to prove *competence.* These times are goals to use in training and help establish standards to evaluate the team.

Rescue Response Decision-Making Criteria

Regulations also require emergency action plans for hazardous work. It is therefore imperative that appropriate rescue response be determined before each entry. Simply put, by using the above guidelines a qualified person (entry supervisor), ideally must decide along with a rescue team representative, whether to require the rescue team to stand by the entry or just be available and ready should they be summoned.

Rescue Standby (RS) requires the team to be present and able to enter the space immediately and reach the patient in 2 to 4 minutes. Obviously, to respond this quickly, the team must be prepared prior to the entry by having assessed the hazards, decided a strategy, made team member assignments, and prerigged necessary equipment.

Rescue Available (RA) requires the team to be able to respond to the entry site in about 10 minutes and reach the patient approximately 5 minutes later. If correct procedures have been followed and rescue personnel are at the work site, on-site teams should be able to meet these goals. The average response time of off-site teams can be evaluated by reviewing their documented response times, found in records that emergency response agencies are usually required to keep. In either case, for an on-site team or an off-site team, a controlled drill is one effective means to determine response capabilities.

Rescue response mode is the decision of the entry supervisor. This decision for RS and RA mode should be based on the following considerations:

1. **The severity of the hazard.** Is the hazard immediately dangerous to life and health? Examples include atmospheric and engulfment hazards for which rescue RS is required. Non–life-threatening entrapment or trip hazards require RA.
2. **Personal protective equipment required.** Supplied breathing air is a key issue. If it is required for safe entry, then RS should be required. A problem with the air source would probably result in severe injury or death, if the entrant were not reached within 6 minutes.
3. **The entrant's ability to self-rescue.** Under normal circumstances, the entrant can be expected to self evacuate without assistance, thus calling for RA mode. If the entrant needs assistance to exit a space (e.g., to manage air hose and safety lines while climbing a ladder), the entry supervisor could take this as an indication for RS mode.

What actions can an employer take prior to the entry to ensure that the rescue service can respond in a timely manner? Although there are no guarantees, classifying each entry may be the most effective means to determine rescue response. Each work area should be evaluated to determine (1) if it meets criteria for a permit required confined space, and (2) the extent and/or severity of the hazard presented by the space. An effective means of accomplishing this is to place permit required confined spaces into one of two categories: rescue standby or rescue available.

Rescue Response Categories for Permit Required Spaces

The categorization of all PRCS can be done in advance based on the usual hazards associated with each space. Of course, the entry supervisor must review the assigned category and possibly recategorize the space according to existing entry conditions.

Category I—Rescue Available: This category consists of permit required confined spaces that

- do not require entrants to wear fresh air breathing equipment,
- do not expose the entrant to any obvious IDLH or potential IDLH hazard,
- do not warrant rescue personnel standing by during the entry, and
- do not require the entrant to have assistance to exit the space, under normal circumstances.

Category II—Rescue Standby: This category consists of permit required confined spaces that warrant stand-by rescue personnel at the entry site. Examples of rescue stand-by permit spaces include

- spaces in which entrants are required to use fresh air breathing equipment,
- spaces in which an obvious IDLH hazard exists or potentially exists, and/or
- spaces from which an entrant would be expected to have difficulty exiting without help.

It is important to point out that the entry supervisor is responsible for the safety of the entrants and must have the authority to determine rescue response needs. Based on experience, the supervisor may decide that RS is necessary even if the entry does not technically fall in Category II. The supervisor should document why RS is necessary, but it should be the supervisor's decision. For example, the supervisor may decide RA is adequate even though the entry is an air because the entrants are utilizing supplied air as a precaution only, that is, when monitoring shows no apparent atmospheric hazards.

Although Categories I and II only encompass PRCS covered by 29 CFR 1910.146, all work spaces should be categorized in order to document that proper evaluation has occurred. During an OSHA inspection, documentation as to why a space was determined *not* to be a PRCS might be necessary; an OSHA inspector may think otherwise. This site-specific documentation can provide valuable insight that could persuade OSHA that the categorization was correct.

Importance of Categorizing Work Spaces

Once the spaces are categorized, an informed decision can be made as to what may be required to comply with the requirement of "timely response." Most PRCS's fall into Category I, in which the rescue service need only be available to respond in the event of an incident. Any serious incident that occurred in a Category I space would not be the result of a hazard presented by the space itself, but rather of unforseen medical emergencies (illness or injury) such as a heart attack or fall. If the space is properly categorized and the decision is documented, the task of justifying an "other-than-immediate response" to an incident has been made easier.

The rescue response *preparation* considered timely for an incident in a Category I space may not be considered timely for an incident in a Category II space. This is because the hazards associated with a Category II space should be recognized *prior to* entry. When the decision is made to expose an entrant to the hazards of a Category II space, RS is more appropriate than RA. Because the response should be immediate with RS, the requirement for a timely response would be satisfied. This categorization system balances the impracticality and expense of providing rescue standby for every entry and the necessity of rescue standby when entrants are occasionally exposed to obvious extreme hazards and might require immediate rescue response.

Although OSHA's stated intent in promulgating standards does not always prevail in administrative and judicial proceedings, the agency's interpretation is given great deference. Therefore, in attempting to comply with OSHA's permit required confined space standard, it is wise to consider OSHA's pronouncements of intent. In the instance of timely response, although OSHA has recognized the need for quick response, it has also recognized that it is not feasible to require that rescue teams be outfitted and standing by for every PRCS entry. Categorizing spaces to determine whether they are rescue standby or rescue availability is a common-sense approach.

Training Requirements

Employers want to protect employees who work in confined spaces, and they want to protect rescuers who respond to confined space incidents. They must comply with federal regulations, but must also consider plant production and personnel. How do they make sure employees are properly trained? Can rescues from confined spaces be performed at their sites in the safe, timely, and effective manner specified by OSHA?

There are numerous training considerations in complying with the rescue requirements of 29 CFR 1910.146. Employees must be trained in the proper use of PPE and rescue equipment. Each rescue team member must be trained to perform all assigned rescue duties safely. Each member must be trained as an authorized entrant and should be trained in attendant duties as well. Team members must be trained at least in basic first aid and CPR.

The primary question remains, How much actual hands-on rescue training is required? One common misconception is that a rescue team is required to train only once a year. Although section (k)(iii) requires annual training, that is not the complete picture. Section (k)(iii) requires that rescuers practice permit space rescues from actual permit spaces or spaces that simulate the types of permit spaces from which rescue is to be performed. Can each representative type of confined space be covered at each site during one training session per year? And, will the rescue service (whether using an on-site or off-site service) be able to competently effect a permit space rescue in a safe and timely manner? Section (k)(iii) of 1910.146 states:

> "Each member of the rescue service shall practice making permit space rescues at least once every 12 months, by means of simulated rescue operations in which they remove dummies, mannequins or actual persons from actual permit spaces. Representative permit spaces shall, with respect to opening size, configuration, and accessibility, simulate the types of permit spaces from which rescue is to be performed."

Examine these statements point by point. First, take special note that *each* member shall practice, not some or whoever is on shift, but *each* member shall receive hands-on practice using dummies, mannequins, or actual persons as simulated victims. Also note that practice "at least" once every 12 months is the *minimum* requirement. Depending on site specifics, once every 12 months certainly may not be enough to meet the performance requirements of the standard. OSHA points out in the preamble to the regulation that "periodic demonstrations . . . will provide the necessary feedback regarding the adequacy of the rescue equipment, the rescue procedures and the training." The key issue is whether the practice is sufficient to ensure the capability of the rescue team. Even if the team practices ten times in a year, it has not met OSHA's requirements if it is not capable of performing the rescue.

Then comes the phrase "by means of simulated rescue operations." The rescue trainer should provide realistic problem-solving scenarios to simulate confined space rescue operations.

Problem-Solving Scenarios

The use of realistic problem-solving scenarios highlights deficiencies or problems, which must be noted and corrected, in such areas as

- equipment and manpower,
- ability to operate from written preplans and suggested operating guidelines,
- shortcomings in the preplans and/or standard operating guidelines, and
- the competency, efficiency, and timeliness of the rescue service.

This section of the regulation further emphasizes that rescuers not only must receive hands-on practice, but that this practice must include the types of spaces they may face in an actual emergency. Realistic practice and rescue experience must be provided for rescue personnel by the use of similar representative spaces with respect to opening size, configuration, and accessibility. Obviously, it would be ideal for rescuers to practice in each actual permit space. However, in most instances, this simply is not possible. OSHA specifically states in the final rule that it is not always appropriate for employers to make the actual permit spaces available for entry simply to allow the rescue service to practice. Despite this, rescuers must develop and maintain familiarity with the types of permit spaces from which rescue might be required. A supervisor must carefully consider the factors in determining whether a space is representative of another according to the guidelines offered by OSHA as well as basic common sense.

To determine whether a space is representative for rescue purposes requires a working knowledge of rescue operations. The person making such an assessment must be familiar with rescue techniques, as well as equipment and personnel requirements. The assessment requires a comprehensive overview, taking into consideration the various obstacles that the confined space might present to rescuers during an emergency.

Although a facility may have hundreds of permit spaces, there may be only a few types of spaces once they are inventoried, assessed, and classified. Once the representative types have been determined, a training schedule can be developed to ensure that each rescuer receives the appropriate practice for each type of space on that site. This provides a practical approach to assessing rescue needs regarding training, equipment, and personnel as well as critical documentation for OSHA. The following describes one procedure for typing confined spaces. Modifications may be required for a particular site.

Typing Confined Spaces

Size of Opening

Based on OSHA guidelines, first consider the "opening size." The rule anticipates variations among opening sizes in permit spaces, so practice sessions are not required for every size of opening. A general consensus of experienced rescuers establishes 24 inches as a line of demarcation. If a portal (opening) is 24 inches or larger, a rescuer should be able to enter the space wearing SCBA and protective clothing. It also allows the rescuer to extricate an average-sized person in standard spinal immobilization packaging. An opening smaller than 24 inches presents a greater challenge to a successful entry and rescue. Therefore, spaces fall into two distinct classifications: (1) openings 24 inches or bigger and (2) openings smaller than 24 inches. Measurement should be made at the smallest point of the opening.

Configuration of Opening

The configuration, or shape, of the opening must also be considered when determining space types. Is the opening round (including ovals) or is it angular (rectangle or square)? Although the shape of the opening usually does not affect the rescue system (e.g., hauling or lowering), it does matter as far as rescuer entry and patient extrication. For example, a patient packaged in a rigid litter may not fit through a 20-inch round opening but might fit through a 20-inch square opening.

Accessibility

The OSHA regulations also consider accessibility, which has two meanings. The first is the passage into the space and the second is the approach to the space. Passage into the space refers to the angle of entry, which is either vertical (up or down) or horizontal (sideways). Approach to the space refers to the opening's height. Is the opening elevated or not elevated? This obviously affects the way the rescue is conducted. Will a hauling or lowering system be required for access to or egress from the opening? A rescue in which a victim is inside a space at ground level with a ground-level portal is much different from a rescue of a victim through an elevated portal. Extrication via the elevated portal obviously would be more difficult because the patient must be hauled to the opening and then would likely have to be lowered to the ground. Therefore, practice for an elevated extrication should constitute practice for extrication from a similar nonelevated opening. The converse is not true, however, for typing purposes. Consider diagonal portals as vertical access because the same type of rescue system can be used.

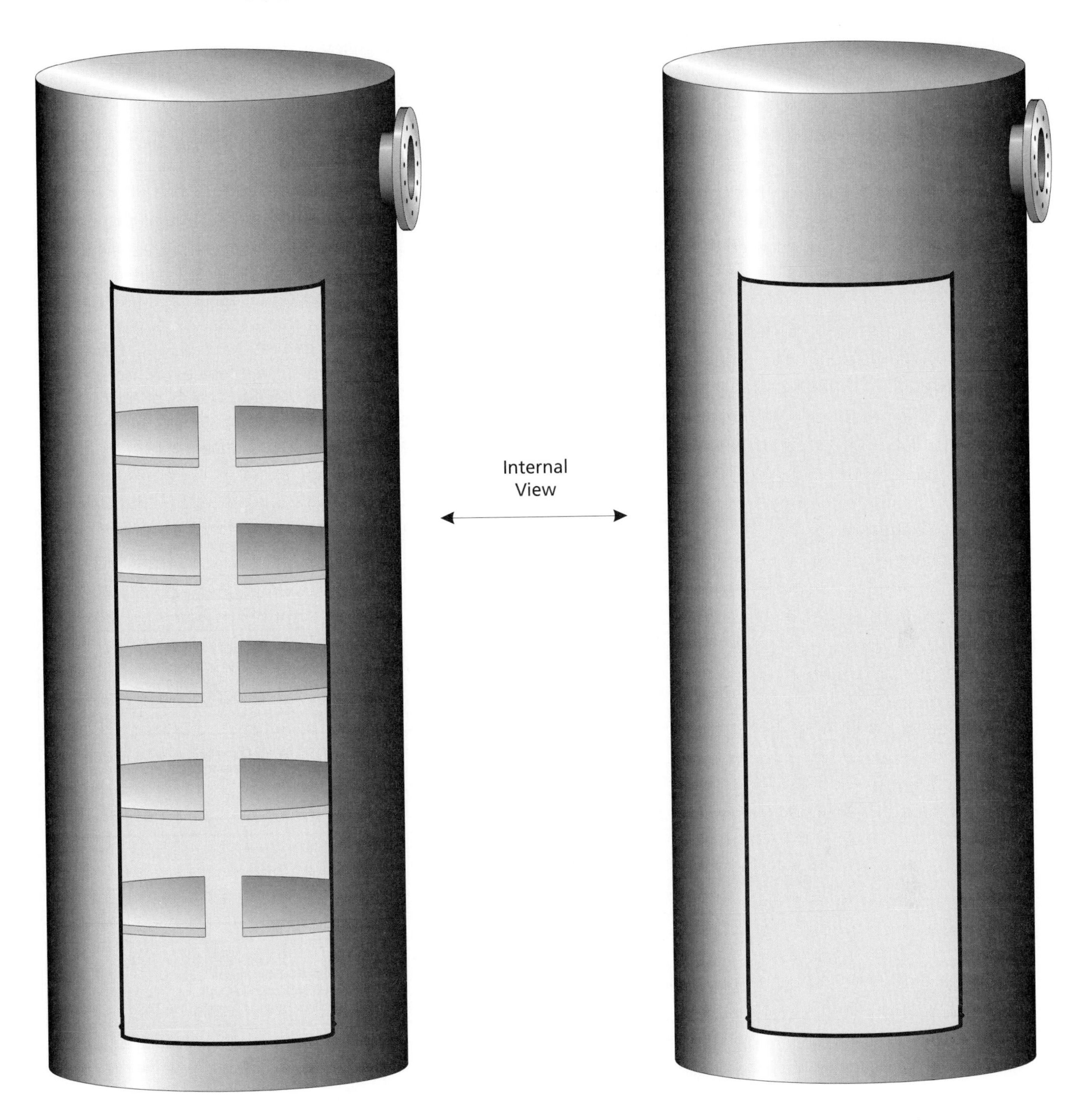

Figure 18.1 Two vessels that look alike on the outside may have very different internal configurations

Internal Configuration

The internal configuration of a permit space must be considered. Is it congested or noncongested? Two vessels that appear identical from the outside may require very different rescue plans due to internal configurations (Figure 18.1). Although one may be relatively noncongested, the other may contain a maze of internal obstacles. Internal congestion is usually the determining factor when considering external rescue (retrieval) versus entry rescue. OSHA points out that internal configurations that could entrap entrants are definite safety risks.

In confined space rescue, entanglement hazards are the norm and have a major effect on how a rescue is conducted. A vessel filled with internal trays and baffles can become an obstacle course for rescuers. It is critical that internal configurations be evaluated when considering rescue provisions, and that rescue personnel be trained and prepared to navigate various obstacles and scenarios. Proven capabilities in congested spaces should certainly suffice for capabilities in noncongested spaces. Additionally, many vessels that will be typed as horizontal entries according to accessibility will require vertical rescue systems internally. Reactor towers with side entries are a common example.

The following are examples of confined space types (see Figure 18.2). There are 12 routine types of permit spaces, and each type has a "sister" type if it is elevated. A trench would be classified as a vertically accessible rectangular type. Establishing such a system provides a method for evaluating and typing permit spaces in a facility.

The following table contains predefined types of confined spaces normally found in an industrial setting. Classifying spaces by types can be used to prepare a rescue training plan to include representative permit spaces for simulated rescue practice as specified by OSHA. These types focus mainly on the OSHA-specified criteria of opening size, configuration, and accessibility. Another important factor is the internal configuration (congested or noncongested) of the permit required confined space.

CS TYPE 1 / 1E elevated
Portal Size: Less than 24 inches
Configuration: Round / Oval
Accessibility: Horizontal Entry (vertical portal)

CS TYPE 2 / 2E elevated
Portal Size: 24 inches or larger
Configuration: Round / Oval
Accessibility: Horizontal Entry (vertical portal)

CS TYPE 3 / 3E elevated
Portal Size: Less than 24 inches
Configuration: Square / Rectangle
Accessibility: Horizontal Entry (vertical portal)

CS TYPE 4 / 4E elevated
Portal Size: 24 inches or larger
Configuration: Square / Rectangle
Accessibility: Horizontal Entry (vertical portal)

***CS TYPE 5 / 5E** elevated
Portal Size: Less than 24 inches
Configuration: Round / Oval
Accessibility: Vertical Top Entry (horizontal portal)

***CS TYPE 6 / 6E** elevated
Portal Size: 24 inches or larger
Configuration: Round / Oval
Accessibility: Vertical Top Entry (horizontal portal)

***CS TYPE 7 / 7E** elevated
Portal Size: Less than 24 inches
Configuration: Square / Rectangle
Accessibility: Vertical Top Entry (horizontal portal)

***CS TYPE 8 / 8E** elevated
Portal Size: 24 inches or larger
Configuration: Square / Rectangle
Accessibility: Vertical Top Entry (horizontal portal)

CS TYPE 9 / 9E elevated
Portal Size: Less than 24 inches
Configuration: Round / Oval
Accessibility: Vertical Bottom Entry (horizontal portal)

CS TYPE 10 / 10E elevated
Portal Size: 24 inches or larger
Configuration: Round / Oval
Accessibility: Vertical Bottom Entry (horizontal portal)

CS TYPE 11 / 11E elevated
Portal Size: Less than 24 inches
Configuration: Square / Rectangle
Accessibility: Vertical Bottom Entry (horizontal portal)

CS TYPE 12 / 12E elevated
Portal Size: 24 inches or larger
Configuration: Square / Rectangle
Accessibility: Vertical Bottom Entry (horizontal portal)

**Could include open sumps, pits, tanks, trenches, and so on.*

DEFINITIONS

(1) Diagonal Portal - Plane of manway or portal is at an angle (between perpendicular and parallel to the ground). To be considered a vertical entry/horizontal portal.
(2) Elevated Portal - Bottom of passageway is 4 feet or higher from ground level.
(3) Horizontal Entry - Access passageway is entered traveling parallel to ground level through a vertical portal.
(4) Manway or Portal - An internal or external opening large enough for a person to pass through.
(5) Rectangular/Square Portal - A four-sided opening with four right angles. Opening size is determined by measuring the shortest side of the opening.
(6) Round/Oval Portal - A circular or elliptical opening; also any polygon not having exactly four sides. Opening size is determined by measuring the smallest inside diameter.
(7) Vertical Entry - Access passageway is entered traveling perpendicular to ground level through a horizontal portal.

Importance of Typing and Establishing Training Plans

As mentioned previously, after all permit required spaces are typed, the training coordinator can design a matrix of training scenarios to ensure each team member receives the training required for compliance. Failure to implement a systematic approach to training in representative spaces can only result in a haphazard attempt to meet OSHA's training requirement. The time to evaluate and type the spaces is *before* an incident occurs, and *before* OSHA asks how the training is planned and conducted.

> "OSHA's measurement of a host employer's compliance with proposed paragraphs (k)(2)(i) and (k)(2)(ii) will not be based solely upon a rescue service's actual performance during any single instance, but instead upon the host employer's total effort prior to arranging for an outside rescue service to ensure that the prospective rescue service is indeed capable, in terms of overall timeliness, training, and equipment, of performing an effective rescue at the host employer's workplace."

Although this quote refers to an outside rescue service, OSHA's desire for a "level playing field" for rescue services should alert employers to the agency's intent. It is important to remember that OSHA is clarifying that what is already clearly applicable to in-house rescue services is equally applicable to outside services.

The training coordinator must decide how to best meet OSHA's requirement that *each* team member practice in *each* type of space by simulated rescues. If there are numerous permit spaces of a particular type, the logical choice is to look at worst-case scenarios. "If I can rescue here, I can rescue anywhere!" is a good theme for the trainer. The point is to prove rescue capabilities to the team itself, to plant management, and potentially to an OSHA inspector.

Practice of rescues from nonelevated spaces will *not* satisfy the practice requirements for rescues from elevated permit spaces. Elevated rescue scenarios afford increased difficulty and require special rescue techniques. Likewise, practice in noncongested spaces will not satisfy practice requirements for congested spaces. Therefore, practicing the more difficult scenarios would make the most efficient use of resources and training time, while satisfying requirements for compliance and preparedness.

By training each rescue team member in each type of space using the worst-case scenario (congested, elevated, etc.), the first of the two goals (compliance and preparedness) is *almost* achieved. Full compliance entails "proof of competency" in addition to proof of practice. Competence comes from confidence, which is derived from practicing in those worst-case scenarios. This does not mean simply practicing in the smallest, most difficult permit space on site will cover every imaginable space in the facility? It is possible to take the worst-case scenario theory too far. There are techniques and procedures that a rescuer might use in the worst-case scenario that, under normal circumstances, the rescuer would avoid. An extremely small opening may force the rescuer to "bend" standard medical protocol. Tight portals that dictate the use of wristlets (to decrease the patient's profile) may not allow the rescuer to use the ideal spinal immobilization procedures. Practicing in such spaces would not adequately prepare rescuers for extricating patients from larger openings in which spinal immobilization procedures and equipment can (and should) be fully utilized. These procedures must be practiced and proper equipment and techniques should be applied when circumstances allow. Although worst-case scenario is an effective method for practice, it should be used for each type of space.

Additionally, by establishing types of confined spaces, the rescue service can establish generic rescue plans for each type of space according to specific safety and efficiency needs. These generic plans will serve as rescue guidelines for that type of permit space. These plans can be further refined or customized for a specific permit space within that particular type. For example, the rescue service can develop confined space rescue systems (see Chapter 17, Retrieval and Team Deployment). When establishing the generic preplan, the rescue team can designate a particular CSR system to use for that particular space, and need only provide further details on such things as anchor points for that particular space.

Importance of Typing in Training Effectiveness

Once the training plan has been established for meeting OSHA requirements in the various types of spaces, the employer must ensure that the training provided is adequate and effective. Rescue training must produce results: It must provide rescuers the capability to perform rescues in a safe and timely manner from the spaces for which they are responsible. OSHA has stated its intent in the proposed clarification of the permit required confined space regulation:

> "An employer who retains an off-site rescue service and emergency service must ensure that the designated service has the equipment, training, and overall ability to respond in a timely fashion when summoned to rescue a permit space entrant . . . the purpose of 1910.146(k) is to require that employers' provisions for rescue, by whatever means, are adequate."

As mentioned, this quote refers to off-site rescue services, but OSHA has made it clear that it is equally applicable to on-site teams.

The required training must provide rescuers the necessary skills to perform their duties safely. What good is training that is inadequate for a specific site? And, what good is training that cannot be proved effective? Even though the most capable of rescue services can botch a rescue (and OSHA recognizes this), such an incident will certainly result in a closer examination of the service's capabilities. Documentation should be on file that written and performance-based evaluations have been conducted for each rescue team member. A program of organized and effective training, along with regular practice drills, prevents most errors from occurring during a confined space rescue. Should such an incident occur, however, a good training program should assist a positive close inspection by OSHA.

In its pending clarification of 1910.146, OSHA has proposed a *verifiable evaluation* of rescue team capabilities. OSHA currently requires that the employer "certify that the training required has been accomplished." This training must provide the trainee with "the understanding, knowledge, and skills necessary for the safe performance of the duties assigned." Further, OSHA's compliance directive looks at "how" the employer evaluates employee proficiency in the duties required by the permit space regulation, which necessarily includes rescue duties. An effective, and arguably the best, way to accomplish this is to conduct yearly performance evaluations of the rescue service. If an employer does not have the expertise to conduct these evaluations or if an independent evaluation is desired, a contracted evaluator can be hired to do the job. An employer should specify that complete, written documentation is required from the evaluator.

Although not specifically addressed by OSHA in training requirements, the training coordinator must also consider the use of breathing equipment during rescue training and practice drills. If a permit space requires breathing equipment, training without it would obviously not prepare rescuers for an actual emergency. They must be trained and experienced in performing rescue operations using full breathing equipment as required by conditions in the permit space. Other very important training considerations in preparing for realistic rescue scenarios include the provision for "air watch" personnel, rigging and performing rescues "on air," rescuer claustrophobia, working with air lines or SCBA, entanglement hazards for air lines, and communications. These are key components when preparing for actual rescue emergencies in permit spaces.

Meeting OSHA requirements can be a daunting task. Inefficient use of resources can lead to an improperly prepared rescue team. A coordinated, systematic approach saves time, money and, quite possibly, lives.

Evaluation of the Rescue Team

One of the challenges of arranging for rescue services is that the host employer is required to ensure that the rescue service is capable. Objective criteria should be used in evaluating a rescue team's capabilities. Such objective criteria will aid employers in deter-

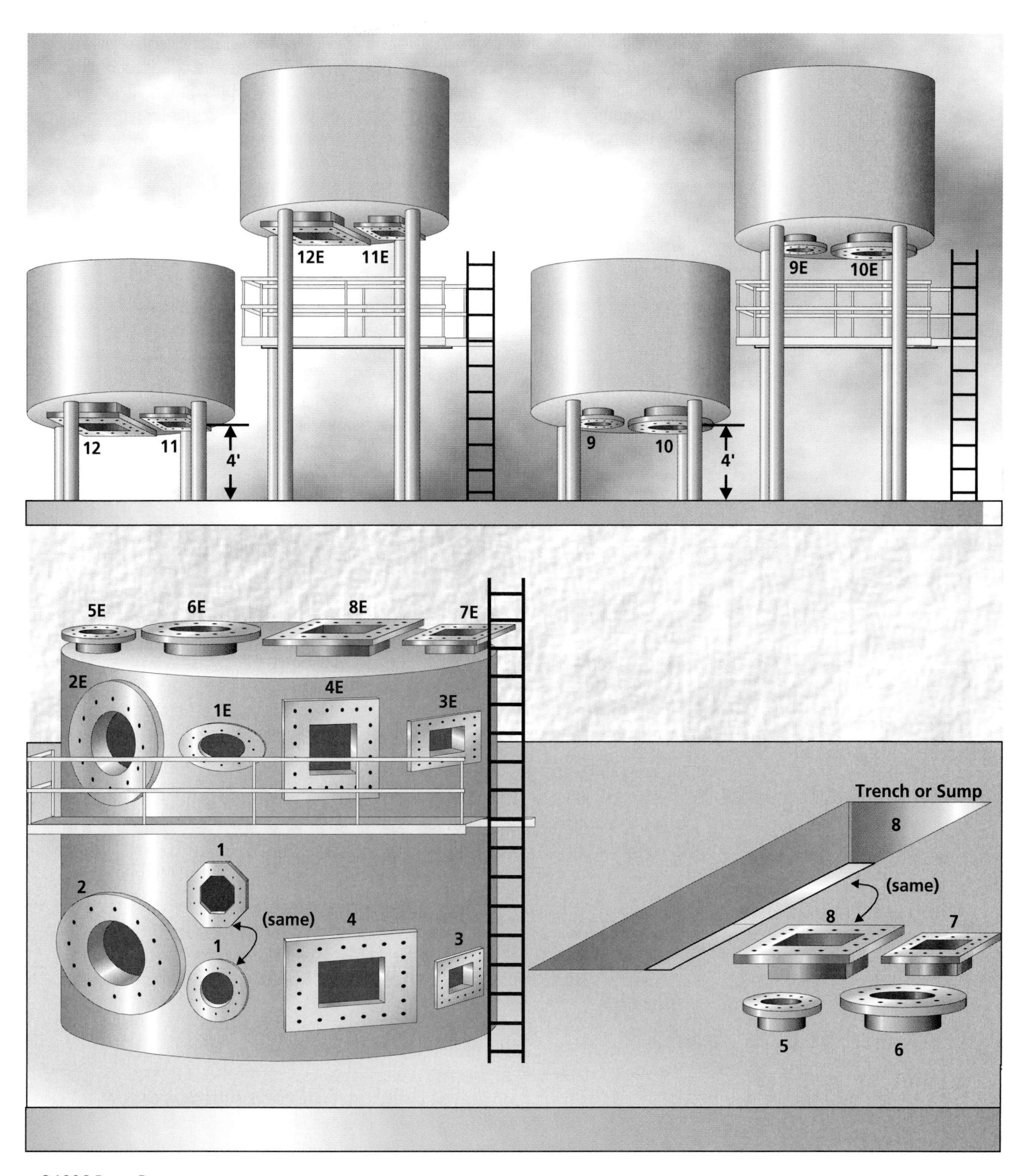

Figure 18.2 Illustrations of confined space types based on OSHA criteria

mining both whether their in-house service is adequate, and whether outside rescue services being considered are adequate. As discussed earlier, the same criteria and requirements applicable to in-house rescue services are applicable to outside rescue services.

The language of OSHA's proposed revision only requires that the employer ensure the *capability* of the outside service to perform confined space rescue, not that the employer ensure that every rescue is successful. As long as an employer properly determines the capability of the rescue service and the rescue service is indeed *capable,* the proposed regulation would not penalize the employer if the otherwise capable rescue service commits an error during a rescue. However, in the event of an error, OSHA will more than likely scrutinize the determination of the capability of the rescue service. Although the mere commission of an error does not mean the rescue service is incapable, this further underscores the necessity for some objective criteria documenting the determination of its capability made by the employer.

Under the proposed regulation, the employer will, as with other OSHA programs, be required to obtain sufficient expertise to determine the capabilities of its in-house or outside teams. Again, objective criteria for evaluating rescue service capabilities would facilitate this task. Given the typical employer's lack of expertise in confined space rescue and the immediacy of the issue, many employers hire an outside evaluator to assess the capabilities of outside rescue services. The employer should consider establishing guidelines to choose an evaluator and to document the criteria of the selection.

Most rescue experts agree that the most expeditious manner to accomplish verifiable evaluation of rescue capabilities, as proposed by OSHA, is to conduct an annual documented performance evaluation of the service. An evaluator can conduct and document the evaluation. It is recommended that this evaluation consist of, at a minimum, three simulated problem scenarios of the type the service is likely to encounter at the employer's site. Additionally, the evaluator should administer a written test designed to evaluate the team members' general rescue knowledge. This evaluation can be conducted in one day (8 hours). If successfully completed, it would document that the team has practiced in the spaces in which the simulations were conducted.

Suggested Evaluator Criteria

The qualified evaluator should, at a minimum, have received training meeting OSHA's criteria for confined space supervisor, entrant, attendant, and rescuer. The evaluator should also have received training in respiratory protection, hazard communications, HAZWOPER Awareness Level, personal protective equipment, and fall protection. Additionally, the evaluator should have documented, at a minimum:

1. 80 hours of formal training in confined space and structural rescue;
2. 1 year of experience as an emergency rescue responder; and
3. Successful completion of an 8-hour confined space evaluator workshop that consisted of
    - an overview of the pertinent regulations,
    - a written test of the prospective evaluator's knowledge of the regulations,
    - training on how to establish rescue scenarios,
    - training on grading (written evaluation form) a service's performance, and
    - how to use appropriate forms and disseminate compliance information.

Keep in mind that videos are training aids and should be used as just that—as an overview, as a demonstration, and as reinforcement of the hands-on training—not as a substitute for this training.

Equipping the Rescue Team

Regulation 29 CFR 1910.146(d)(4)(viii) requires that the employer provide

> "rescue and emergency equipment needed to comply with paragraph (d)(9) of this section, except to the extent that the equipment is provided by the rescue services."

Paragraph (d)(9) provides that the employer must

> "develop and implement procedures for summoning rescue and emergency services, for rescuing entrants from permit spaces, for providing necessary emergency services to rescued employees, and for preventing unauthorized personnel from attempting a rescue."

Simply stated, the employer must ensure that the rescue service, whether in-house or outside, is properly equipped. However, equipping the rescue team is not a simple matter, and there is no single checklist that can be used to purchase equipment that will work for every facility. The needs of the facility must be assessed in order to make this determination. Also, when purchasing equipment consideration must be given to the most difficult rescue operation that the facility might present.

The employer is only relieved of the responsibility to provide rescue equipment to the extent that the rescue service provides its own. If an outside service responds and is not properly equipped to perform the rescue presented, the employer is responsible. Therefore, it is critical that the employer analyze both a rescue service's capabilities, and the status of its equipment and the suitability of that equipment for rescue in that particular facility. A rescue service may be capable of performing a rescue in Facility A with the equipment it has, but not in Facility B. In such a case, the employer at Facility B has not met the regulatory burden if it retains this rescue service without requiring an equipment upgrade or providing the proper equipment for the team. A qualified outside evaluator can make this determination if the employer lacks the expertise. For this reason, however, if the employer is using the outside evaluator to assess the capability of the team, the evaluator must first assess the needs of the facility.

An employer should not only rely on assertions made by a rescue service that it is properly equipped. At the least, the employer should verify that the service has done a thorough assessment of the facility and the rescue requirements presented by the facility. Likewise, employers should be wary of relying on the assurances of other facilities that a team is capable. Again, the team may be equipped to handle a rescue in Facility A but not in Facility B. A reliable rescue service will insist on assessing the facility so that it can determine if it is properly equipped and to make the necessary adjustments to its equipment inventory.

Many new rescue teams prefer to purchase equipment for initial training. These equipment needs and much of the equipment required for subsequent training and rescue operations can be determined by the person performing the training. For that reason, equipment should be purchased *after* selecting a trainer. However, once training is completed, the rescue team should set about to determine additional equipment needs. This should be done even if an outside evaluator or trainer is consulted prior to making the initial purchase of equipment. For obvious reasons, the future rescuer is not capable of selecting the proper equipment until after he or she has received rescue training. Further, as the rescuers begin practicing in different permit spaces and with varying scenarios, they may discover that additional or more suitable equipment is needed. Also, as new permit spaces are constructed or installed, equipment needs may change. Therefore, assessment of rescue needs, including equipment, should be ongoing.

Entry and Non-Entry Rescue

In the permit required confined space standard, OSHA refers to both "rescue" and "non-entry rescue." "Non-entry rescue" is somewhat of a misnomer that has created some confusion. In practical terms non-entry rescue is "retrieval," and does not fall under the portions of the standard applicable to rescue. "Rescue" refers to entry rescue.

Whenever possible, OSHA urges the use of non-entry rescue. As stated by OSHA, non-entry rescue involves the least danger for rescuers and . . . a retrieval system (body harness attached to a lifeline extending outside the permit space) will generally be the appropriate form of non-entry rescue." However, OSHA further notes that there will be instances where non-entry rescue is not feasible. Accordingly, sections (k)(1) and (k)(2) of the final rule were included to pertain to rescuers entering permit spaces to perform rescues, and "to ensure that designated rescuers were adequately trained and equipped to safely (for both authorized entrants and the rescuers themselves) perform effective rescues."

The OSHA regulations define "rescue service" but not "rescue,"—entry or non-entry. Because of the failure to provide a definition for "rescue," there has been some confusion over the applicability of the requirements of sections (k)(1) and (k)(2). "Rescue service" is defined as "the personnel designated to rescue employees from permit spaces." In delineating the duties of attendants, OSHA requires in 29 CFR 1910.146(i)(8) that the employer ensure that each attendant "performs non-entry rescues as specified by the employer's rescue procedure." Does this mean that the attendant is "personnel designated to rescue employees from permit spaces" and is therefore subject to the requirements applicable to rescue services? At first glance it may seem so, but such is not the case. "Non-entry rescue" does not fall under the definition of "rescue" for purposes of the standard demonstrated by 29 CFR 1910.146(i)(4), which prohibits the attendant from performing "rescue" while still functioning as an attendant. This section requires the employer to ensure that the attendant remains outside the permit space during entry operations until relieved by another attendant.

When the employer's permit entry program allows attendant entry for rescue, attendants may enter a permit space to attempt a rescue if they have been trained and equipped for rescue operations as required by paragraph (k)(1) of this section and if they have been relieved as required by paragraph (i)(4) of this section.

Section (k)(1) specifically states that the section applies to "employers who have employees *enter permit spaces to perform rescue*." Section (k)(3) pertains to non-entry rescue, and in no way purports to make the remainder of section (k) applicable to non-entry rescue. The confusion between non-entry rescue, or retrieval, and entry rescue has caused some employers to mistakenly believe that every authorized attendant is subject to the requirements applicable to rescue services. Such is not the case unless the attendant is also specifically assigned to the rescue service. In any case, once he or she is relieved to perform an entry rescue, he or she is no longer the authorized attendant. The mere fact that an attendant performs non-entry rescue, or retrieval, from the permit space does not make the attendant a rescue service for purposes of the standard.

ANSI Standards for Confined Space Rescue

The American National Standards Institute has released its own standard for confined spaces, including rescue standards. Standards set by ANSI are based on a consensus of parties substantially concerned with the scope and provisions of the particular standard. Compliance with standards provided by ANSI are voluntary. ANSI standard Z117.1-1989 establishes minimum safety requirements for confined spaces.

Safety standards released by ANSI do not impose mandatory requirements on employers. However, they are important because they represent a consensus opinion on minimum performance requirements necessary in developing and implementing comprehensive programs, such as a confined space program, for the safety and health of personnel. Violation of these standards will not subject the employer to any sort of administrative penalty, such as those imposed for violations of OSHA standards. However, use of a consensus standard can establish reasonable care in a civil proceeding. (The issue of civil liability is discussed briefly in the next section.)

The ANSI confined space standard is intended to provide the minimum safety requirements for entering, exiting, and working in confined spaces at normal atmospheric pressure. It does not apply to underground mining, tunneling, caisson work, or similar tasks that have established national consensus standards. It is not intended to replace any existing specific standards and procedures, but rather to support existing standards and procedures that meet the confined space standard's performance objectives. In developing its confined space standard, OSHA considered and rejected the wholesale adoption of the ANSI standard. This was primarily due to the fact that

OSHA did not believe ANSI sufficiently addressed non-atmospheric hazards. The ANSI standard contains a wealth of information regarding other aspects of confined space rescue and is a valuable compliance tool, so long as consideration is given to the fact that it does not address non-atmospheric hazards.

Emergency Response Plan

The ANSI standard requires that the employer have a written emergency response plan with provisions to conduct a timely rescue if a confined space emergency arises. This emergency response plan shall include

1. a determination of what methods of rescue must be implemented to retrieve entrants,
2. designation of rescue personnel that are immediately available where permit required confined space entries are conducted,
3. the type and availability of equipment needed to rescue individuals,
4. an effective means to summon rescuers in a timely manner, and
5. training and drill of the attendant and rescue personnel in preplanning, rescue, and emergency procedures as outlined in the standard.

According to ANSI, this entails a review of the different types of confined spaces at the facility and the steps and equipment are required to rescue an entrant. ANSI does not provide a method to determine the types of spaces, however the method of typing spaces outlined earlier should suffice to satisfy this requirement. Like OSHA, ANSI states that the size and configuration of the confined space must be considered. ANSI likewise permits the use of off-site rescue personnel, provided they are capable of performing the rescue, are familiar with the facility, and can respond in a timely manner. ANSI further states that the off-site provider should be involved in the development of rescue procedures and drills. Additionally, ANSI suggests that consideration be given to the type of lighting in the confined space, communications devices, and any other special equipment that might be used for rescue.

Developing a Preplan

One method of complying with this standard is to develop a written preplan for rescue in the confined space, which addresses all of these requirements, plus any site-specific issues that will facilitate rescue at the facility. This type of preplan is space-specific, and is completed prior to entry of the particular space. This preplan should be used in conjunction with a general emergency response plan that addresses standard operating procedures to be followed in the event of an emergency.

Training Requirements and Evaluation

The ANSI standard also provides general training requirements for personnel responsible for supervising, planning, entering, or participating in confined space entry and rescue. This training should at a minimum include

1. an explanation of the general hazards associated with confined spaces,
2. a discussion of specific confined space hazards associated with the facility,
3. instruction on the use of personal protective equipment and other required safety equipment, including the reason for the PPE and/or equipment, the proper use of the PPE and/or equipment, and the limitations of the PPE and equipment,
4. an explanation of the permit system and other procedural requirements for confined space entries,
5. how to respond to emergencies,
6. individual duties and responsibilities, and
7. a description of how to recognize probable air contaminant overexposure systems and method(s) for alerting attendants.

Additionally, there are training requirements for emergency response personnel. ANSI states that this training shall include, at a minimum

- the rescue plan and procedures developed for each type of confined space rescuers are anticipated to encounter

- the use of emergency rescue equipment, CPR and first aid
- location of the work and configuration of the confined spaces in order to minimize response time.

In conjunction with these requirements, the rescue personnel should simulate actual rescue conditions by conducting practice drills. ANSI suggests addressing typical rescue problems in these drills such as egress restriction, ability to lift without injury, problems with rescue equipment, and fall hazards. The training in the use of rescue equipment should include any medical equipment rescuers would expect to operate during the rescue.

Compliance with the ANSI standard requires periodic assessment of the effectiveness of this training by a qualified person. ANSI defines a "qualified person" as a "person who by reason of training, education, and experience is knowledgeable in the operation to be performed and is competent to judge the hazards involved." The evaluation should consist of written as well as practical testing. ANSI recommends that personnel

1. be questioned or asked to demonstrate practical knowledge of confined space hazards in their work areas,
2. identify locations of confined spaces,
3. explain their roles in exercising proper permit procedures,
4. demonstrate and explain the use and donning of PPE such as respirators, and
5. explain their roles in response to emergency situations.

These training sessions must be repeated as often as necessary to maintain competence. ANSI explains that personnel who routinely enter the same confined space on a daily basis require less refresher training than those who only occasionally enter confined spaces. The periodic assessment will aid in determining the frequency of refresher training required.

The ANSI training requirements include training people who will monitor atmosphere. Practically speaking, this includes rescuers. Rescuers typically perform their own testing of the atmospheric conditions prior to entering a space, particularly in a situation where an entrant is unresponsive, possibly as a result of atmospheric conditions in the confined space. This training in the proper use of atmosphere-monitoring equipment includes field calibration, basic knowledge of the work being performed, the anticipated hazardous contaminants, and anything that could alter the original internal or external conditions of the confined space.

Where a contractor is involved, ANSI requires that the employer and the contractor establish who will serve as the rescue responder in an emergency and the means of notification of the rescue responder. If, for instance, the contractor plans to depend on the host employer's rescue services, this should be agreed upon before the entry. However, it should be noted that such an agreement in no way affects either party's responsibility under OSHA regulations.

Although the ANSI standard is not mandatory, it can help demonstrate compliance with OSHA standards, as well as contribute to a defense in civil actions. ANSI provides specifics in some instances where OSHA provides none. The ANSI standard is a good starting point for documentation of actions regarding worker safety in permit required confined spaces.

Civil Liability

Although there are too many issues involved with civil liability to provide a detailed analysis in this text, a brief note is warranted. This chapter discusses the regulatory issues relating to permit required confined space rescue. Although compliance with OSHA's standards will help the employer avoid administrative civil and/or criminal penalties, compliance with those standards will not necessarily provide a successful defense against civil liability in a personal injury lawsuit. OSHA requires a minimum standard for compliance, which may not satisfy the standard of reasonable care required to succeed in civil litigation. Therefore, the rescuer must be concerned with not only compliance, but also civil liability.

The OSHA regulations are very broad and are short on specifics. In a civil court, however, the specifics are important. The employer and rescuer will be called upon to explain not only what was done, but why. Why was rescue service A chosen over rescue service B? Why was equipment X not available? Was the employer or rescuer concerned simply with compliance at the cheapest cost rather than with providing a competent and well-equipped rescue team? Although compliance is important, civil actions are more concerned with action taken (or not) to protect the victim than with whether minimum government safety requirements were met. Therefore, when forming, equipping, or contracting for a rescue service, one should ask more than, What is required for compliance?

Finally, the interplay between contractors and host employers needs to be considered. Agreements between those parties can allocate civil liability, because in most states parties are generally free to enter into indemnity agreements with little restriction. However, a host employer must recognize that it may be held liable for an injury or death in a confined space even if it has a contractor perform the entry. Although the *responsibility* for the permit required confined space entry may be transferred by the host employer to the contractor, the *liability* does not necessarily follow. Because such legal actions fall under state jurisdiction, the particular laws for each state should be consulted to determine the extent of the host employer's liability.

Confined Space Rescue Compliance Guidelines*

Complying with OSHA's 1910.146 Permit-Required Confined Space Regulation poses quite a challenge for U.S. industries. Because it is a performance-based standard, it is difficult to understand exactly what is required for compliance. This, unfortunately, has led to a number of confined space fatalities for trapped workers and their improperly trained and equipped rescuers.

For the safety of your workforce as well as emergency response personnel, adequate preparation of confined space rescue is crucial . . . not to mention the probability of OSHA penalties and possibly even criminal prosecution. With this in mind, let's address some of the most commonly asked questions concerning compliance with OSHA's 1910.146.

1. **To whom does the standard apply?**
   In general, the requirements apply to any general industry employer that has employees enter confined spaces. It applies to host employers and contractors alike. It is important to note that the courts have upheld OSHA's assessment of fines and penalties against host employers for deaths in the workplace even when an independent contractor controls the work being performed. In one case, for example, the host employer and the independent contractor were *both* held liable for a worker's death because the court held that both were responsible for insuring the safety of their employees.
   Source: 29 CFR 1910.146(a)
2. **Are there any other standards that are applicable to confined space rescue?**
   Yes. Two consensus standards, the 1979 NIOSH Criteria Document and ANSI Z117.1-1989, address confined space rescue and are both cited by OSHA in the preamble to the regulation. The ANSI standard contains more detailed rescue provisions than the OSHA rule. Therefore, it is a good guideline for many rescue issues including the

* The information in this section is derived from "Confined Space Rescue Compliance Handbook", The Roco Corporation, 1997, and is protected by copyright. The compliance handbook was generated as a result of Roco's participation with OSHA in developing explanatory material to assist employers with compliance questions. Roco personnel are contracted by OSHA's solicitor as experts in confined space rescue compliance issues.

need for written response plans and team evaluation criteria. Additionally, NFPA's Technical Rescue Committees are formulating national operational and professional qualification consensus standards.
Source: 58 Federal Register 4467

3. **What is a "rescue service"?**
OSHA defines "rescue service" as "the personnel designated to rescue employees from permit spaces" and points out that an employer must prohibit "unauthorized personnel" from entering a space to attempt a rescue. Employers must clearly designate the individuals that are on the rescue team.
Source: 29 CFR 1910.146(b)

4. **Does this mean that an attendant who is required to provide non-entry rescue (referred to as retrieval) is a part of the rescue service?**
No. OSHA specifically states that the attendant *may* be a designated rescue service member, but may not perform entry rescue as part of the rescue service unless relieved by another qualified attendant. Purchasing retrieval equipment such as a tripod-winch combination and practicing non-entry rescues is *not* full compliance with the rescue requirements if entry rescue is potentially required.
Source: 58 Federal Register 4518

5. **How does OSHA address "non-entry" rescue?**
First, OSHA *requires* that whenever a permitted entry occurs, the entrant must wear a body or wrist harness with a retrieval line attached, unless either would endanger the entrant or not assist in a rescue. Also if a vertical entry occurs in a vessel more than 5 feet deep and non-entry rescue is planned, a "mechanical device" for retrieval must be available. The space should be evaluated to determine if non-entry retrieval is possible, and if so, how it will be accomplished.
Source: 29 CFR 1910.146(k)(3)(ii)

6. **What is a "mechanical device" for retrieval?**
OSHA does not define "mechanical device." It defines a "retrieval system" as "the equipment used for non-entry rescue of persons from permit spaces." This includes a retrieval line, chest or full-body harness, wristlets, if appropriate, and a lifting device or anchor. From a rescue standpoint, this can consist of a tripod with a hand winch, or block and tackle, or other rescue systems consisting of ropes, pulleys, and belay or cam devices that create a mechanical advantage.
Source: 29 CFR 1910.146(b)

7. **What does the standard generally require of the employer as far as rescue is concerned?**
Section (d)(9) of the standard requires that the employer develop and implement procedures for:
   1. Summoning rescue and emergency services,
   2. Rescuing entrants from permit spaces,
   3. Providing emergency services for rescued employees; and,
   4. Preventing unauthorized personnel from performing rescue.

   Source: 29 CFR 1910.146(d)(9)

8. **Is an employer required to have an in-house rescue team?**
OSHA allows in-plant teams, outside rescue services, or a combination of the two. OSHA's concern is the response and performance of the team, not the source.
Source: 58 Federal Register 4527; 29 CFR 1910.146(k)

9. **What does OSHA look for when evaluating a rescue service?**
OSHA's compliance directive keys its inspectors to several items to look for when evaluating the employer's rescue capabilities. If the employer chooses to provide an in-house rescue service made up of its own employees, OSHA will:
   (a) identify those individuals,
   (b) verify their training,
   (c) determine current first aid and CPR certification,
   (d) compare rescue procedures to the written program, and
   (e) note work shifts of rescuers and compare them to the entry permit times.

   Additionally, OSHA's new clarification requires the employer to evaluate and verify that an outside rescue service is capable in terms of timely response, training, and

equipment. One can assume that an in-house team would be judged by the same criteria. The best method to evaluate a rescue team's capabilities is to perform an annual scenario-based, graded performance evaluation.
Source: OSHA Compliance Directive, "Application of the Permit-Required Confined Spaces (PRCS) Standard, 29 CFR 1910.146," Document No. CPL2.100, April 15, 1995 (hereinafter "OSHA Compliance Directive")

10. **What about an outside rescue service? Can't I just list "911" for emergency response?**
No. If an outside rescue service is used, OSHA will address several questions to determine whether the arrangement meets compliance requirements, such as:
    1. Who will provide the off-site services and where is that service located?
    2. How is the arrangement documented? Is it by contract, letter, verbal agreement?
    3. How does the employer determine, in relation to the hazard, whether the off-site rescue service's response time, experience, and training are adequate?
    4. Has the rescue service met the training requirements found in paragraph (k)(1)?
    5. What method is used to summon the rescue service?
    6. Is the rescue service on-site or on-call when the permit space entry is taking place?
    7. What is the response time for the rescue service?
    8. How does the employer verify that the rescue service will be available during the time of the employee entry?

Source: Compliance Directive

11. **Because the entry supervisor is required to verify that the rescue service is available, what should be the procedure when using an outside service such as a fire department?**
The employer's representative, the entry supervisor, must contact the fire department prior to the entry. If he finds out the rescue unit is on an extended call or is otherwise out of service, no entry can take place unless an adequate alternative service is available. Taken a step further, there should be a notification procedure in the event that the rescue service responds to another rescue call or otherwise goes out of service after the entry has begun. In this case, the entry should be suspended until the rescue service is again available.
Source: OSHA Compliance Directive

12. **What about an outside rescue service consisting of public employees, a municipal fire department, for example—are they required to follow OSHA regulations?**
Municipal employers are subject to OSHA only in those "state-plan" states that specifically include public employees. There are 25 states that have authority to administer approved OSHA state plans. The PRCS regulations in these states are at least as stringent as the federal regulations, and in some cases, are more stringent. Municipal employees in states not having authority to administer approved state plans are not protected by OSHA. However, a private employer in those states is still responsible for OSHA compliance, even if the service relied on is a municipal service. The private employer must ensure that the service is capable and that the service's members are trained to the same standard as the on-site team. Additionally, the fire chief who chooses to send his firefighters into permit-required confined spaces without the appropriate training or equipment certainly exposes himself to greater civil liability because the existing OSHA and ANSI national standards provide guidelines that protect his employees.

13. **What about a combination team?**
If there is a combined response consisting of an in-house and outside rescue service, OSHA will want to see a copy of the rescue plan describing the role of each party. OSHA will assess the arrangement to determine if the combined service enables the employer to comply with the rule.
Source: OSHA Compliance Directive

14. **Is an employer required to provide rescue equipment to the rescue service?**
Only to the extent that the rescue service does not supply the needed equipment. From a practical standpoint, this would require the employer to verify that the rescue

service has all of the equipment necessary to perform rescue from the particular spaces for which it is responsible. The employer can then make available any additional equipment needed by the service.
Source: 29 CFR 1910.146(d)(4)(vii); 58 Federal Register 4526-27, 4529.

15. What equipment is required for rescue?
OSHA provides no specific equipment requirements, only that the employer ensures that the rescue service has the equipment necessary for making rescues from permit spaces. Additionally, OSHA requires that the necessary rescue equipment be listed on the entry permit. Rescue equipment is "that equipment which has been designated by the manufacturer as rated for rescue."
Source: 29 CFR 1910.146(d)(4)(viii); 29 CFR 1910.146 (f)(11)

16. How can employers verify that the outside rescue service has the necessary equipment for rescue from permit spaces?
This is tough for the employer who has no one on-staff with the expertise to verify rescue equipment requirements. However, the employer should require that the rescue service prepare written rescue plans for all spaces. Because the plans should list the necessary rescue equipment for each space, the employer can verify that the equipment is available. This will also alert the rescue service to any equipment that is lacking. By attaching the plan to the entry permit, the employer will fulfill OSHA's requirement that the rescue equipment be listed on the permit.

17. Are the general training requirements in the standard pertinent to the rescue team?
Yes. Rescuers must be trained so that they:
(a) have a clear understanding of their job responsibilities and its risks;
(b) obtain *sufficient* formal education to perform a possible technical rescue; and,
(c), can repeat learned rescue skills during a critical incident.
These three requirements can only be met with quality training and structured practice sessions.
Source: 29 CFR 1910.146(g)(1)

18. How much training will satisfy this requirement?
The training must establish proficiency. Proof of proficiency can be demonstrated by a performance evaluation conducted by a qualified person. A specific amount of initial training is recommended, as well as refresher training, to achieve the dual goals of compliance and preparedness.
Source: 29 CFR 1910.146(g)(3), ANSI Z117.1-1989 15.5.1 Verification of Training-Periodic assessment of the effectiveness of employee training shall be conducted by a qualified person. Note: Training effectiveness may be evaluated by several techniques. Written, as well as practical testing is recommended . . .

19. Does the employer have to certify that the training has been done?
Yes. OSHA requires that the employer certify that the training has been accomplished. The employer must also document the training by providing records containing the employee's name, the signature or initials of the trainer, and the dates of the training.
Source: 29 CFR 1910.146(g)(4)

20. What are the training requirements specific to rescue?
Sections (k)(1) paragraphs one through four contain training requirements specific to rescue.

- Paragraph One requires the employer to ensure that each member of the rescue service is provided with and is trained to use the necessary PPE and rescue equipment for making rescues from permit spaces.
- Paragraph Two states that each member of the rescue service must be trained to perform the assigned rescue duties and must have received authorized entrant training.
- Paragraph Three specifies the minimum required hands-on training.
- Paragraph Four specifies that each person on the rescue service must have had first-aid and CPR training, with at least one person being currently certified.

Source: 29 CFR 1910.146

21. **Is attendant training required for members of the rescue team?**
No. In fact, the standard prohibits an attendant from entering the space to perform rescue. However, it is recommended that all team members be trained as authorized attendants. If possible, team member should act as an attendant during a rescue entry to expedite communication with the rescue entrant.
Source: 29 CFR 1910.146(l)(9); 58 Federal Register 4518

22. **How much actual "hands-on" rescue training is required by OSHA?**
Each member of the rescue service is required to practice rescue operations at least once every 12 months from the actual spaces they may encounter, or from representative spaces that closely simulate the types of spaces they are responsible for. Because practicing from the actual spaces is not feasible in most cases, the rescue team needs to determine the various types of spaces they may encounter. The training officer can then design a training matrix that will allow each member of the rescue service to practice rescue operations for each type of space.
Source: 58 Federal Register 4528; 29 CFR 1910.146(k)(1)(iii)

23. **So, the standard requires more than one "hands-on" training session every 12 months?**
Absolutely! Don't forget that this is a performance-based standard. The key is that the employer must ensure the team is proficient or competent. Even if there is only one type of confined space in the facility, OSHA's minimum training requirement for "hands-on" training once every 12 months may not be sufficient to ensure proficiency. Remember, ***each team member*** (not just those who showed up for a particular drill) must practice simulated rescue operations (not just setting up equipment or tying knots) for ***each type of space*** (not just the same training prop or location repeatedly).
Source: 29 CFR 1910.146(g)(3) & (k)(1)(iii)

24. **How does the rescue team determine how many different types of confined spaces it has responsibility for?**
The rescue team can design a typing system using OSHA's criteria of a representative space . . . simulating the actual space with respect to portal opening size, configuration, and accessibility. Or, the team can use a typing method which has been reviewed by OSHA and found acceptable such as the one included in this text. This method of classification identifies 12 types of confined spaces (see page 312). It is important to note that although the in-house team need only practice in the particular types of spaces found at its facility, the off-site team responding to various facilities should document practice in all 12 types of spaces.
Source: 29 CFR 1910.146(k)(1)(iii)

25. **Explain how this method is used to "type" confined spaces.**
This method uses OSHA's three criteria for a representative space. These criteria are considered in relation to rescue techniques and strategies. For example, a rescue from a small, round opening would be performed differently than a rescue from a large, square opening. This method takes both OSHA's criteria and practical rescue experience into consideration.

26. **A portal opening can be any imaginable size. There could be hundreds of different sizes. How is this addressed?**
It is not necessary to practice from every different size opening in the facility. A general consensus of experienced rescuers establishes 24 inches as a line of demarcation. Why 24 inches? If a portal is 24 inches or larger, a rescuer should be able to enter the space wearing breathing equipment and protective clothing. It also allows a rescuer to extricate an average-size person using standard spinal immobilization procedures. An opening smaller than 24 inches presents a greater challenge to rescuers in making a successful entry and rescue. Therefore, spaces can be classified as those with openings 24 inches or larger, and those less than 24 inches.

27. **What is meant by "configuration of the opening," and how is this factor addressed?**
Configuration refers to the shape of the opening. Is the opening round or oval, or is it square or rectangular? The shape of the opening affects rescuer entry and patient

extraction. For example, a patient packaged in a rigid litter or on a spine-board usually will not fit through a 20-inch round opening. But the same patient usually will fit through a 20-inch square opening.

28. What does "accessibility" mean?

Accessibility actually has two definitions:

- passage (through the portal), and
- approach (to the portal).

Passage through the portal refers to the angle of entry into the space. There are vertical entries, meaning that the rescuer must enter either up or down through a horizontal portal; and, horizontal entries, meaning the rescuer must enter sideways through a vertical portal.

Approach to the space refers to the portal's elevation. Is the opening elevated or non-elevated? This will obviously affect the way in which the rescue is conducted. Will a hauling or lowering system be required for "access to" or "egress from" the opening? A rescue in which a victim is located inside a space at ground level with a ground level portal is much different than extracting the same victim from an elevated portal.

29. What if I have two spaces that are the same type, but one is elevated while the other is not?

Practice should only be necessary from the elevated space, if it is identical to the non-elevated, except for the elevated portion of the rescue. Therefore, practice from the elevated space, which is more difficult, should preclude practice from the non-elevated space. However, the converse would not be true. While there may be hundreds of actual PRCS at one facility, the typing chart identifies only 12 types of spaces. If any one of those types have multiple locations, both ground level as well as elevated, practice should only be required in the worst case scenario—the elevated space.

30. What about the inside of the space?

One of the factors OSHA considers in determining if a confined space is "permit-required" is if it has an internal configuration that could trap or engulf the entrant. The internal configuration of the space can be congested or non-congested, which could refer to converging walls, trays, pipe racks, or any other imaginable obstacle. But, as with the elevation issue, this does not create another OSHA "type." Because a rescue from a space that is internally congested is more difficult than a rescue from a non-congested space, practice from the congested space will constitute practice from the same type non-congested space. In fact, many times non-entry rescue, or retrieval, can be performed from non-congested vessels.

31. How does typing the spaces aid with training?

Remember, OSHA requires "hands on" training for each type of space by each team member at least once every 12 months. Once the spaces are typed, the training coordinator can determine how many practices are necessary to meet the minimum requirements for "hands on" training. Also, this will aid the training coordinator in determining how many additional practices may be necessary to meet the proficiency standard. Finally, it provides documentation to aid in demonstrating to OSHA that the rescue service's training covers all types of spaces in the facility.

32. Couldn't the rescue service simply practice on the most difficult space in the facility once every 12 months ... "worst-case scenario" approach?

The "worst-case scenario" approach is fine *within space types*. However, for example, practicing to vertically extricate a patient from a 16-inch round portal utilizing a "half-board" for spinal immobilization does not prepare the rescue service for extracting an entrant from a 24-inch square portal on full-board immobilization. That is why the spaces must be typed in the first place ... to assure that the proper techniques for the particular space and circumstances are practiced.

33. Are there any other benefits to typing spaces?

Typing spaces allows the rescue service to predetermine rescue techniques required for a particular type of space. Those techniques can then be incorporated into the customized preplan for a particular space.

34. **OSHA's new clarification ruling for confined space rescue emphasizes timely response. Will the agency have expectations of a timely rescue response?**
Yes. OSHA expects that the rescue response will be "timely." Recall that OSHA instructs its inspectors in the compliance directive to identify how the employer determines that the rescue service's response time is adequate. While OSHA does not define what is timely, the agency has indicated that it will look at the circumstances involved to determine adequate response.
35. **What does OSHA mean by "circumstances?"**
An example would be that the inability to breathe would require a quicker response than, for instance, a simple bone fracture.
36. **If CPR should be initiated in 4 to 6 minutes, does this mean that my rescue team must be capable of a 4-minute response time?**
No. OSHA has stated that it isn't reasonable to require a 4-minute response for all situations. However, OSHA has said that because permit spaces vary in their capacity to kill or injure employees, what constitutes "timely" will vary accordingly.
Source: 58 Federal Register 4526
37. **So, how can I anticipate the need for a 4-minute response?**
Look at the hazards presented by the entry or the work to be performed. If existing or potential hazards are immediately life threatening, response should be immediate. An example would be hazardous atmospheres. If you purposefully send someone into a "bad" atmosphere on supplied breathing air, you should anticipate that there could be a problem with the air supply and that an immediate response would be needed to save that person.
38. **Is there any way to respond within 4 minutes?**
Yes. If the rescue team is standing-by at the entry site, rigged and ready for rescue.
39. **I understand that in certain cases the rescue service should have a team of two or more rescuers standing by before the entry is made. What about the rest of the time?**
A plan can be formulated that considers the circumstances affecting what is timely, and that a successful rescue in an IDLH environment might be possible only if accomplished immediately. Entries can be categorized as "Rescue Standby," in which the rescue team is standing by at the site; or, "Rescue Available," in which the rescue service is on-call and available to respond should the need arise (see figure 18.3).

RESCUE RESPONSE
DECISION-MAKING CRITERIA

***Rescue Stand-by* (RS)** requires the team to be staged at the entry site during entry in order to be able to enter the space *immediately* and reach the patient within two-to-four minutes. Obviously, to effect a rescue in a timely manner, the team must be prepared *prior* to the entry by assessing the hazards, deciding a strategy, making team member assignments, and pre-rigging necessary equipment.

***Rescue Available* (RA)** suggests the team to be able to respond to the entry site in about ten minutes and reach the patient approximately five minutes later. If correct procedures have been followed and rescue personnel are at the work site, on-site teams should be able to meet these goals. The response time of off-site teams can be determined by their documented Average Response Times—records that emergency response agencies are usually required to keep. In either case, for an on-site team or an off-site team, a controlled drill is one effective means to determine response capabilities.

Figure 18.3 Rescue Response Decision Making

Figure 18.4 Determining Rescue Response

DETERMINING RESCUE RESPONSE . . .
RESCUE STAND-BY VS RESCUE AVAILABLE

The entry supervisor must decide which of the two response modes is appropriate by answering three simple questions . . .

(1) Is the hazard or potential hazard immediately dangerous to life or health?
(2) Is breathing air required for entry?
(3) Would the entrant have difficulty exiting the space unassisted?

If the answer to any of these questions is yes, then stand-by rescuers would be required. If the answer to all three questions is no, then the appropriate response mode would be on-call or available.

40. How can this be done?
The response criteria should be based on the ***severity of the hazard*** or potential hazard, the PPE required (especially SCBA or SAR), and the ability to self-rescue. Refer to Figure 18.4 for determining the appropriate rescue response.

41. Should each space be classified as Rescue Available or Rescue Stand-by?
No. Each ***entry*** into the space should be classified with the rescue response category required. The classification would take into account the circumstances surrounding each entry. For example, a clean space that is being entered by an inspector to examine a weld does not pose the same hazards as does an entry when the welding is being performed.

42. Who is responsible for determining the rescue response mode required for each entry?
The entry supervisor is ultimately responsible for a safe entry. The supervisor is required to determine if the rescue service is available and that there is operable means to summon the service. The supervisor should categorize the entry as "Rescue Stand-by" or "Rescue Available" based on personal knowledge of the entry. The supervisor should have the authority to categorize an entry as "Rescue Stand-by" even if he or she answered "no" to the three questions used to determined response mode. The supervisor's instinct or experience may indicate there could be a serious problem with a rescue from that particular space.

43. What should the response time be for Rescue Stand-by as opposed to Rescue Available?
There should be a goal in "Rescue Stand-by" to reach the patient within 2-to-4 minutes. This is possible because the team is rigged and ready for entry. The goal in "Rescue Available" is to arrive on the scene within approximately 10 minutes and to access the victim about 5 minutes later.

44. Why are these times a goal, rather than a definite time limitation?
Goals are needed to measure proficiency in training and to help determine adequacy. A prospective outside rescue service with a documented response time of 20-30 minutes to a particular facility is not adequate. On the other hand, mandated timely response could result in inadequate assessment of the situation prior to entry of the rescuers. We certainly want to afford rescuers the opportunity to "look before they leap." Remember, the objectives of the rescue provisions in the regulation is to avoid rescuer injuries and fatalities. Therefore, it is unreasonable to pressure the rescuer into entering the space before he or she is fully prepared.

45. Is a specific amount of rescue training recommended?
The amount of training recommended is directly proportional to the types of spaces and the category of entries for which a team may be responsible.

The following chart (Chart 18-2) shows the amount of initial formal training required for those facilities that would never utilize Rescue Stand-by. In other words, all entries are classified as Category I-Rescue Available.

Chart 18-2 - Initial Rescue Training Recommendation

Category 1 - "Rescue Available"

Number of Confined Space *Types*	Initial Training Hours for *Team Members*	Initial Training Hours for *Team Leaders*
1 - 2	24 Hours	80 Hours*
3 - 6	40 Hours	80 Hours*.
7 - 12	80 Hours	120 Hours*

** Training for Team Leaders may be extended to two years, if necessary.*

Chart 18-3 - Initial Rescue Training Recommendation

Category 2 - "Rescue Stand-By"

Number of Confined Space *Types*	Initial Training Hours for *Team Members*	Initial Training Hours for *Team Leaders*
1 - 2	40 Hours	120 Hours*
3 - 6	80 Hours	120 Hours*.
7 - 12	80 Hours *(on-site)*	120 Hours* *(on-site)*

** Training for Team Leaders may be extended to two years, if necessary.*

A team that is responsible for only one or two types of spaces could probably prepare themselves with only 24 hours of formal initial training. However, the team leaders should receive at least 80 hours of training to have the experience and knowledge necessary to run team drills. Most medium-sized facilities with three to six types of spaces could probably prepare themselves with 40 hours of formal initial training. Again, team leaders need additional training hours. Larger facilities with seven or more types of spaces would need at least 80 hours of formal training to prepare themselves for the large number and different types of spaces.

The second chart (Chart 18-3) indicates the amount of initial formal training recommended for those facilities with Category II-Rescue Stand-by entries, during maintenance shut-downs, for example. Even if Rescue Stand-by is only required periodically, the rescue team must be prepared and capable. Because of the dangers and complexities of Category II entries, team leaders should be more knowledgable in order to plan and coordinate team practice sessions. Note that formal *on-site* training is recommended in certain cases, so that the training can be more customized for the particular spaces being entered.

These charts, designed for the newly created rescue team, refer to initial training requirements. Existing teams should work with a competent rescue professional to determine on-going training needs. Management must be committed to the rescue team's training, as well as follow-up practices, to ensure that the team is capable.

46. How much follow-up practice is necessary to meet compliance requirements?

The recommendation for the number of follow-up practice days of training per year must meet two important goals: Compliance and Preparedness.

Hands-on rescue practice must be documented for each team member in each type of representative space. In calculating the number of practice days needed, let's look at a couple of assumptions:

Assumption 1 - A minimum of 2-to-3 practice exercises for each type of space will be needed.

Assumption 2 - A rescue team will be able to stage and practice a minimum of two confined space types (consisting of 2-to-3 exercises per type) in an 8-hour training day.

Assumption 3 - The rescue team will practice in one group.

Figure 18.5 Formula for Determining Practice Days

FORMULA:

[for compliance with 1910.146(k)(1)(iii)]

$$\frac{\text{Number of CS types}}{\text{2 types practiced per day}} = \begin{array}{l}\text{Total Number of CS Practice Days Annually} \\ \textit{(required for each team member)}\end{array}$$

These assumptions can be compiled to create a formula for calculation of practice days (see Figure 18.5).

Two-to-three practice exercises should be conducted for each *type* of confined space. Repetition of an exercise helps to ensure that mistakes are corrected and that proficiency is achieved. It also gives the team an opportunity to determine the most efficient technique, while allowing team members to practice different assignments within the chosen rescue technique.

NOTE: If your team practices in two or more groups, you would need to multiply the above calculated total number of practice days times the number of team groups to get an *overall* total number of practice days per year.

In addition to *Confined Space practices,* specialized training is required for rescue personnel. Rescue team members must practice with and be trained to use PPE, monitoring, ventilation, communications, and fall protection equipment. All CS practices must include elevated rescue techniques.

Additionally, OSHA's clarification and ANSI's standard both require verified evaluations of the rescue team's capabilities. Team members should be individually evaluated by a formal skills test, while the team is put through a graded, scenario-based performance evaluation. These evaluations should be conducted annually by a qualified person. Depending on the size of the team, allow two days to complete Individual Performance Evaluations (or IPEs) and one day to complete the Team Performance Evaluation (or TPE). It is necessary to add three evaluation days to the number of practice days to arrive at a facility's ANNUAL COMPLIANCE MAINTENANCE requirements.

Now, let's apply all of this information to an example ....

A 16-person rescue team is responsible for 8 confined space types. In order to meet work schedule requirements, the team practices in two groups. So, 8 confined space types divided by 2 types covered per day would equal 4 practice days annually per team member. *(*2-to-3 practice exercises per type)*

Then multiply the 4 practice days times the 2 team groups for a total of 8 practice days annually. We now must add the 3 days for individual and team performance evaluations to arrive at 11 total days necessary for ANNUAL COMPLIANCE MAINTENANCE.

CHAPTER 19

Rescue Involving Hazardous Materials

Various OSHA regulations and NFPA standards will be referred to throughout the chapter. This information is provided as a basis for continued training. Rescuers should consult with their team leader for the correct procedures for the team. In this chapter, topics discussed are:

- Ludwig Benner's General Hazardous Materials Behavior Model
- OSHA Levels of Training
- Chemical Protective Clothing
- NFPA Standards for Chemical Protective Clothing
- Factors Affecting both CPC and the Rescuer
- Respiratory Protection
- Decontamination

Introduction

For this chapter, a "hazardous substance" is any substance that, when not properly contained, poses an unreasonable risk to life, the environment, or property. Hazardous substances are considered hazardous materials if there is a future use for them. They are considered hazardous wastes when there is no additional use for them.

"HazMat rescue" is a phrase that is not often heard. Many organizations in the industrial and municipal emergency response arena have invested considerable amounts of time and money to prepare for product control whenever toxic chemicals are released. Unfortunately, they disregard the concept of rescue. Because of misunderstanding and awe of chemicals, many incident commanders assume that everyone exposed to hazardous materials will instantaneously die upon exposure.

In fact, a chemical release primarily presents a rescue situation. That rescue challenge continues throughout the event, and includes dealing with three types of victims. A percentage of the workforce will be untouched (physically) by the event. A second group will be exposed or contaminated but ambulatory (the walking wounded). A third group will be unaccounted for, or missing in action (MIA).

Most of the "walking wounded" need no help leaving the area but need to be directed to decontamination, medical treatment, and debriefing. The ambulatory victims need some small assistance in exiting the area of highest contamination. They need to be directed or escorted to a decontamination corridor and then to a triage and treatment facility.

The MIA group elicits the greatest resistance to thinking in a positive rescue mode. Many factors affect the incident commander's assessment and selection of a search-and-rescue mode. Unfortunately, one common defense of the "don't bother rescuing" program hinges on protective clothing. The thinking is, "If I have to wear a Level XYZ suit to reach them, they are already dead."

If that thought is applied to the fire ground, it quickly falls apart. Imagine telling the fire chief at the scene of a multiple-alarm apartment fire, "Hey, if I need to wear all this structural firefighting gear and SCBA to reach them, they are already dead." Experience shows that there are survivors of fires where there has been significant exposure to fire, toxic gases, and heat. Not all personnel in the area at the time of the fire are lost. Whether a rescue is attempted on the fire ground depends on many factors. Many of the same factors influence decisions about rescue mode at the scene of an emergency that involves hazardous materials.

Ludwig Benner's General Hazardous Materials Behavior Model

What rescue teams do in an emergency depends on the event's time table. Since the early 1970s many people have been using Ludwig Benner's General Hazardous Materials Behavior Model. It still works. The model is valuable when determining the following:

1. What would happen if I did nothing?
2. Can this emergency be mitigated safely by using a strictly defensive strategy?
3. Is it safe enough to perform offensive operations? Would these operations greatly affect the outcome of the incident?

The behavior model asks several questions:

1. Where is the hazardous material or container likely to go when released (in this location)?
2. How will the hazardous material or container get there?
3. When will the hazardous material or container get there?
4. What harm will occur when it does get there?

Hazardous Materials Behavior

Hazardous materials are dynamic. Consider what has happened, what is happening now, and what may happen as the incident progresses. Four factors affect the behavior of hazardous materials during an event:

1. the inherent properties and quantity of the hazardous material(s) involved in the incident
2. characteristics of the container
3. natural laws of physics and chemistry
4. the environmental conditions including the terrain and the weather conditions.

Sequence of Events

When a hazardous material is released, it usually indicates the following general sequence of events:

1. **Stress.** The hazardous materials container is stressed.
2. **Breach.** If the container is stressed beyond its capability, it opens.
3. **Release.** When the container is breached, the contents can escape. This may involve the release of the product, container, energy, or all three.
4. **Dispersion.** As the product, container, or energy travels away from the point of release, the natural laws of physics and chemistry govern the pattern it will follow.
5. **Exposure.** As the product, container, or energy moves away from the point of release, it may contact exposed persons, the environment, or property.
6. **Harm.** Hazardous materials, the container, or energy may injure the things they contact.

Size-up the Incident

When the concentrations of the released material are known, the following steps are used to decide the extent of danger to health and safety in the area of a hazardous materials incident.

1. **Collect data.** Remember to properly protect your personnel when collecting data and to survey the scene in a 360-degree pattern. Also, use the buddy system for all survey personnel.

2. **Record and plot the data.** Always put the data on a site map. A clear overlay can help. Documenting the time of the survey and the weather conditions is also important.
3. **Compare the data to established exposure levels for health and safety implications.** Three possible resource guides for comparison are the NFPA flash point index (flammable range data), the American Conference of Governmental Industrial Hygienists (threshold limit values), and the NIOSH *Pocket Guide to Chemical Hazards.* Material safety data sheets (MSDS) also serve as an excellent resource for the hazardous properties of a specific material.
4. **Estimate the impact of exposure to personnel in the endangered area.** Remember to factor in the use of shielding, engineering controls, or PPE. It is always important to consider the impact of the weather (temperature and wind) and to review the released material's physical properties (vapor density, volatility, specific gravity). Do not overlook the duration of the exposure to personnel.

OSHA Levels of Training

The HAZWOPER regulation (OSHA) says that training shall be based on the duties and functions to be performed by each responder of an emergency response organization. Consequently, it is possible to identify the operational expectations at each level.

The emergency response to hazardous substance releases is addressed in section (q) of 29 CFR 1910.120. The five training levels all require an annual refresher course or demonstration of competency.

Awareness Level

The OSHA First Responder Awareness specifies no minimum number of training hours. First responders at the awareness level are individuals likely to witness or discover the release of a hazardous substance. These individuals have been trained to initiate an emergency response sequence by notifying the proper authorities of the release. They would take no action beyond notifying the authorities.

Operations Level

The OSHA First Responder Operations requires a minimum of 8 hours of training. First responders at the operations level respond to releases or potential releases of hazardous substances as part of the initial response to the site. Their responsibility is to protect nearby persons, property, and the environment from the effects of the release. They are trained to respond in a defensive fashion, not to actually try and stop the release. Their function is to contain the release from a safe distance, keep it from spreading, and prevent exposures.

Technician Level

The OSHA Hazardous Materials Technician has a minimum training requirement of 24 hours. Hazardous material technicians respond to releases or potential releases to stop them. They assume a more aggressive role than a first responder at the operations level. They approach the point of the release to plug, patch, or otherwise stop the release of a hazardous substance.

Specialist Level

The OSHA Hazardous Materials Specialist requires a minimum of 24 hours of training. Hazardous materials specialists respond with and provide support to hazardous materials technicians. Their duties parallel those of the hazardous materials technician, but they require a more directed or specific knowledge of the various substances they may be called upon to contain. The hazardous materials specialist also acts as site liaison with federal, state, local, and other governmental authorities concerning site activities.

Incident Commander

The OSHA On-Scene Incident Commander also has a minimum training requirement of 24 hours. On-scene incident commanders assume control of the incident scene beyond the first responder awareness level. This level requires at least operations level training, as well as training specific to a hazardous materials incident commander as outlined in the law.

Chemical Personal Protective Clothing

The purpose of chemical protective clothing (CPC) is to protect the wearer against the effect of toxic or corrosive/caustic products that could enter the body (inhalation, skin absorption) or damage tissue upon contact with the skin. These harmful products could be in vapor, liquid, or solid form. One type of material is not compatible with every type of chemical. Although it may provide excellent resistance against one chemical, the same material may provide very poor or no protection against another chemical.

Selection of the proper chemical protective clothing for a specific action must take into account the following factors:

- the identity of the released material
- the physical state of the material (solid, liquid, gas)
- the presence of flammable vapors
- the temperature of the released material
- the likelihood of direct contact with the material
- the atmospheric concentrations of vapors (below TLV/TWA, above TLV/TWA, below IDLH, above IDLH)
- the presence of ionizing radiation
- the material's route of entry to the body
- the likelihood of cuts, tears, and abrasion of the protective clothing
- the entry to confined or crowded spaces
- the potential for explosion, blast, pressure wave, or fragmentation hazards

The four levels of personal protective clothing are Level A, Level B, Level C, and Level D.

Levels

Level A personal protective clothing consists of a full-body, gas-tight, vapor-protective garment. The garment is constructed of protective clothing material to isolate the body from direct contact with dangerous gaseous or liquid chemicals. There is also a positive-pressure fresh air breathing apparatus. Level A clothing provides the highest level of respiratory and skin protection. Level A clothing is appropriate when the hazard is identified and requires the highest level of protection for skin, eyes, and the respiratory system. Level A is also used where there is a high concentration of gases and vapors and when there is a high potential for splash, immersion, or exposure to unexpected gases/vapors/particulates that are harmful to the skin, or can be absorbed through the skin.

Level B personal protective clothing includes a full-body splash-protective (not gas-tight) garment and a positive-pressure fresh air breathing apparatus. This clothing provides the highest respiratory protection, but a lesser level of skin protection. Level B protection is used when the type and atmospheric concentration of the substance has been identified. It requires a high degree of respiratory protection but less skin protection. Level B is also appropriate when the atmosphere contains less than 19.5% oxygen and unidentified gases/vapors are not suspected of containing high levels of chemicals that are harmful to or can be absorbed through the skin.

Level C protective clothing is made of a full-body splash-protective (not gas-tight) garment and an air purifying respirator. This clothing provides a lesser level of respiratory protection and a lesser level of skin protection. It is worn when the concentration(s) and type(s) of airborne substance(s) are known, and the criteria for using air purifying respirators is met (the atmosphere is not oxygen deficient). Level C protection is appropriate when the atmospheric contaminants, liquid splashes, or direct contact will not adversely affect or be absorbed through any exposed skin. This level of protective clothing is required when air contaminants have been identified and measured, and can be removed by an air purifying respirator or when the use of air purifying respirators has been authorized by the incident commander.

Level D protective clothing consists of a work uniform that includes coveralls, a hard hat, eye protection, and safety shoes. This provides minimal protection, and is used only for nuisance contamination. This level of protection also includes structural firefighting clothing with a fresh air breathing apparatus (minimal skin protection against chemical attack) and chemical protective clothing without respiratory protection. Level D protection is appropriate when the atmosphere contains no known hazard or when work functions preclude splashes, immersion, or the potential for unexpected inhalation of or contact with hazardous levels of any chemical.

Types

Three types (designs) of Level A and Level B chemical protective clothing are available. Each has specific advantages and disadvantages.

Type I Suits

An advantage of the Type I suit (with the respiratory protection on the inside) is that it protects the self-contained breathing apparatus from contamination or chemical damage. Type I garments are easy to decontaminate because there are few places for contaminants to be trapped. A disadvantage of Type I garments is their tendency to be bulky (to be large enough to cover both the wearer and self-contained breathing apparatus). They also have limited visibility because of the location and design of the face shield. In addition, they weigh more than garments of other designs because they require greater amounts of fabric.

Type II Suits

The advantage of the Type II suit (with the respiratory protection on the outside) is the good visibility it provides because the face shield is separate. Mobility is also good because the suit is compressed by the straps on the self-contained breathing apparatus. Exposing the SCBA to damage and contamination is one disadvantage of Type II garments. Decontamination is difficult due to the trapping of contamination under the breathing apparatus.

Type III Suits

The advantage of the Type III suit featuring a supplied airline (with the respiratory protection located inside or outside the suit) is longer operating time due to uninterrupted air supply. The disadvantages include limited mobility due to the air line, and a limited entry distance because of the air supply hose (300 ft. from point of attachment). In addition, the incompatibility of the air hose material and the hazardous material(s) could result in air line failure.

Composition

- butyl—97% isobutylene, 3% isoprene copolymer
- chlorobutyl—butyl rubber with chlorine atoms substituted randomly for hydrogens
- chlorinated polyethylene—polyethylene with 36 to 45% by weight chlorine atoms substituted randomly for hydrogens
- EVA/PE—blend of 14% ethylene/vinyl acetate copolymer, 86% polyethylene
- EVOH—ethylene/vinyl alcohol copolymer
- fluorine/chloroprene—viton chloroprene laminate
- fluorinated ethylene propylene resin (FEP)—hexafluoropropylene/tetrafluoroethylene copolymer
- FEP/TFE—FEP/tetrafluoroethylene blend
- natural rubber—isoprene
- NBR, nitrile—random or alternating acrylonitrile/butadiene copolymer
- neoprene—chloroprene

- neoprene/SBR—chloroprene/styrene-butadiene blend
- neoprene/natural—chlororprene/isoprene blend
- polyethylene—ethylene
- PVA—vinyl alcohol
- PVC—vinyl chloride
- PVC/nitrile—blended vinyl chloride and random or alternating acrylonitrile/butadiene copolymer
- saran—85% vinylidene chloride, 15% vinyl chloride copolymer
- saranex—laminate of polyethylene and saran
- SBR—25% styrene, 75% butadiene random copolymer
- silver shield, 4 H—laminates of polyethylene and EVOH
- viton—hexafluoropropylene/vinylidene fluoride random copolymer
- viritle—Viton/nitrile blend
- urethane—condensation product of a polyisocyanate and a polyol

Guidelines for Procedures

Although OSHA does not apply these requirements specifically to confined space rescue, they provide excellent guidelines for these operations.

Safety Procedures

1. Participate in a medical surveillance program.
2. Conduct routine exercises and training in donning, using, and doffing PPE.
3. Arrange a program on preventing heat stress that includes proper physical conditioning.
4. Incorporate reliable communications equipment into a system that has two back-up systems (radio, evacuation alarm, public address).
5. Aggressively inspect and maintain PPE.
6. Use the buddy system for all entries.
7. Assign back-up personnel to stand by to rescue personnel in the hot zone.
8. Establish a decontamination corridor prior to entry into the hot zone.
9. Have emergency medical personnel (advanced first aid or higher training) standing by with transportation.
10. Maintain tight site security to prevent surprises (train movement, investigative reporters, environmental action groups).
11. Monitor the atmosphere continuously.
12. Medically assess personnel on scene before, during, and after entry.
13. Put in place a rehabilitation program to replenish fluids and allow for rest and recovery.

Emergency Procedures

1. Evacuate the exposed personnel.
2. Conduct rapid decontamination.
3. Search for missing personnel.
4. Remove and isolate all protective clothing for further decontamination and study.
5. Medically assess all personnel.
6. Transport all exposed personnel for evaluation.

NFPA Standards for CPC

Personal protective equipment must prevent entry of hazardous materials into the body. There are four primary ways chemicals enter the blood stream:

1. **Inhalation** through the respiratory tract. Respiratory hazards include high heat resulting from combustion, oxygen deficiency, and toxic materials.
2. **Absorption** through the skin or mucous membranes.
3. **Ingestion** by eating, drinking, or smoking in a contaminated area.
4. **Injection** through a puncture or laceration in the skin. Some hazardous materials harm the skin on contact.

Vapor Protective Suits for Hazardous Chemical Emergencies, NFPA 1991

This standard specifies minimum documentation, design criteria, performance criteria, and testing methods for vapor suits designed to protect emergency response personnel from exposure to specific chemicals in vapor and liquid splash environments during hazardous chemical emergencies.

Liquid Splash Protective Suits for Hazardous Chemical Emergencies, NFPA 1992

This standard specifies minimum documentation, design criteria, performance criteria, and testing methods for liquid splash suits designed to protect emergency response personnel from exposure to specific chemicals in liquid splash environments during hazardous chemical emergencies.

Support Function Protective Garments for Hazardous Chemical Operations, NFPA 1993

This standard specifies minimum documentation, design criteria, performance criteria, and testing methods for garments worn by personnel in support functions during hazardous chemical operations. The standard applies to use outside the hot zone in support functions.

Factors Affecting CPC

Compromising Protective Fabric

There are three ways that a barrier (protective) fabric can be compromised.

1. **Penetration.** This is the movement of a material through a suit's closures, which include zippers, buttonholes, seams, flaps, and other design features. Hazardous materials can also penetrate CPC through cracks or tears in the suit's fabric. Protection against penetration is vital. A regular and routine inspection program can uncover conditions that could allow penetration. The CPC must be properly stored and regularly maintained and tested to ensure that it can still provide the proper level of protection.
2. **Permeation.** Permeation is the movement of a chemical through fabric on a molecular level. The three phases of permeation are adsorption, diffusion or absorption, and desorption or chemical breakthrough. The breakthrough time and permeation rate vary according to the barrier fabric selection. The breakthrough time is measured as the time elapsed between chemical exposure and detection of the substance on the other side of the barrier. The permeation rate is the average constant flow of chemical after breakthrough. Permeation rate and breakthrough times are important factors in selection of PPE including CPC. The fabric of choice has the greatest resistance to breakthrough and lowest permeation rate of hazardous substances to which a rescue team is likely to be exposed.

   Different fabrics have different resistance levels to chemical permeation, and all will absorb chemicals over time. NFPA Standards 1991, 1992, and 1993 provide guidelines for manufacturers' permeation testing and certification. Before buying CPC, make sure that it meets, and has been certified as meeting, the appropriate standard. When choosing CPC for use at an incident, the HazMat technician must be sure that the garment protects wearers from the type of hazardous materials to which it is going to be exposed. In any event, the wearer is advised to use extreme caution. Available data does not cover every situation the responder may encounter.
3. **Degradation.** Degradation is the physical and visibe change in a piece of barrier fabric that diminishes its level of protection. Degradation of CPC can be either chemical or physical. Degradation means an increased likelihood that a hazardous material will permeate and penetrate the garments, thus endangering the health of the responder. Chemical degradation can be minimized by avoiding unnecessary

contact with chemicals and by effective decontamination procedures. It is important that the garments a responder wears are chosen according to their ability to protect him or her from the chemicals involved in an incident. In addition, CPC must have breakthrough times consistent with its expected use. CPC wearers should recognize the physical limitations of their garments and make every effort to avoid circumstances that could damage the material.

There are seven indications of degradation of chemical protective clothing: swelling, shrinking, blistering, discoloration, onset of brittleness, stickiness, and delamination.

Factors Affecting Rescuers Wearing CPC

Stress

Many physical and psychological stresses affect users of specialized protective clothing. Specialized protective clothing, particularly fully encapsulating garments, increases the stress of a responder to a hazardous materials incident. Persons wearing chemical protective clothing usually experience a loss of dexterity and mobility. The higher the level of protection, the greater this loss. Their visibility is restricted, and their communications are affected. In addition, wearing CPC increases the likelihood of heat stress and heat exhaustion. Reductions in dexterity, mobility, visibility, and communication, in turn, create additional physical and mental stresses.

It is important that the hazardous materials technician be aware of these stressors and receive adequate rest and rehabilitation to compensate for them. It has been found that drinking fluids such as water before one dons CPC reduces some effects of excess heat. Although, while this reduces heat stress, it might also increase urinary frequency. The time a person must remain inside the CPC without relief should be a consideration.

Temperature

Wearing air-cooled jackets, water-cooled jackets, and ice vests may help cool personnel in CPC. The air-cooled jacket allows the body's usual cooling mechanism to function normally. The body releases perspiration to the surface of the skin so it can evaporate and carry away heat from the blood vessels along the surface of the body. Most air-cooling systems require an air line and large quantities of breathable air. The air line adds weight to the wearer and increases resistance to movement. An air-cooled system demands a large air source fed into a vortex cold tube. The tube spirals the air and reduces the temperature of the air as it enters a network of tubes that bathe the wearer in cool breezes.

One very popular method of cooling emergency responders is with a water-cooled jacket. A reservoir of cold water or ice and water is carried on either the chest or hip of the wearer. A small battery-powered pump circulates cold water through a network of tiny tubes to create a conductive cooling effect. This technique is used in NASA space suits to maintain the body temperature of crew members working outside their space craft. The reservoir adds weight and bulk to the suit. A supply of cold water or ice and water is necessary to place the jacket into operation.

There are also vests that can hold frozen coolant packs. The vests are insulated on one side so that the cooling effect is not lost to the outside environment. A series of pockets hold frozen packets of ice close to the wearer's body. This requires a supply of the frozen coolant packs at the scene. The vests add weight to the wearer's burden.

Respiratory Protection

Due to OSHA's 29 CFR 1910.120 (q)(3)(iv) ruling, all emergency response efforts begin with the wearing of positive-pressure self-contained breathing apparatus.

"Employees engaged in emergency response and exposed to hazardous substances presenting an inhalation hazard or potential inhalation hazard shall wear positive-pressure self-contained breathing apparatus while engaged in emergency response. They shall continue to do so until the individual in charge of the incident management or command system (IMS or ICS) determines with air monitoring equipment that a decreased level of respiratory protection will not result in hazardous exposures to employees."

Selection

There are many factors to consider when selecting the proper form of respiratory protection. They include:

- identity of the contaminant
- oxygen level or deficiency
- concentration of contaminant
- confined space operation
- requirement to wear Level A or Level B protective clothing
- moisture content of ambient air
- toxicity of released substance
- limitations of personnel, such as training and environmental factors
- duration of work mission

Components of Air Purifying Respirators

Face Piece

The face piece provides a system to retain the equipment on the wearer's face in an air tight fashion. It also provides protected forward visibility.

Cartridge

The cartridge holds the appropriate material to absorb, chemically react and/or filter out selected airborne contaminants. The cartridge threads onto a special gasket-equipped face piece port. The face piece port is fitted with a one-way valve to allow air to flow into the mask only.

Exhalation Valve

This is a one-way valve that allows air to exhaust from the mask.

Components of Supplied Air Respirators

Face Piece

The face piece provides a system to retain the equipment on the wearer's face in an air tight fashion. It also provides protected forward visibility.

Breathing Tube

This tube brings air from the supply hose or regulator to the wearer's face.

Regulator

The regulator takes the high pressure of the remote air supply and reduces it for supply to the wearer. Some systems have two regulators. One is positioned close to the air supply. The second regulator is on the user's body to meet the individual's pressure demand.

Air Supply Hose

This line brings the air from the remote air supply to the wearer.

Remote Air Supply

The air supply may originate from an air compressor, a cascade system, or a tube truck filled with class D breathing air.

Exhalation Valve

This is a one-way valve that allows air to exhaust from the mask.

Advantages and Disadvantages of Air Purifying and Supplied Air Respirators

Air Purifying Respirators (APR)

- **Advantages.** Air purifying respirators weigh less than any other respiratory protective device. APRs are the least expensive type of respiratory protection.
- **Disadvantages.** APRs can become saturated with particles or contaminants, which create difficulty in breathing. APRs do not supply oxygen to the wearer. At least 19.5% oxygen must be present and the contaminant must be fully identified. Atmospheric monitoring must continue while personnel are wearing the APRs so that changes that require upgrading the respiratory protection can be identified rapidly. OSHA specifically prohibits use of APRs during emergency response efforts unless atmospheric monitoring documents its safe use. APRs cannot be used in IDLH concentrations.

Supplied Air Respirators

- **Advantages.** SARs and ALRs can be used for protection against all particles or gases. They can be used in oxygen-deficient atmospheres. Duration of the unit is limited only by the size of the air supply. Supplied air respirators keep the wearer cooler than air purifying respirators because the supply of cool air is continual.
- **Disadvantages.** Maximum allowable hose length is 300 feet from point of attachment to air source. The wearer must enter and exit the area along the same path. The air line hose can be attacked by some chemicals. In the event an IDLH atmosphere is to be entered, the rescuer must wear a bottle with enough air to escape if the primary air supply is interrupted.

Decontamination

Contamination can exist as a solid (particulate), liquid, or gas. There are four forms of contamination. The first form is fixed, in which contaminated particles adhere to a surface and are not easily removed. The second form is loose, surface contamination, in which contaminated particles adhere to a surface and are easily removed. Airborne is the third form, in which loose, surface material can be suspended in the air. The last form is waterborne (liquidborne) contamination, in which contaminated particles are suspended in water or other liquid.

Why Decontamination is Necessary

Decontamination is necessary because hazardous materials may have immediate short-term effects. For example, contact with a corrosive material or inhalation of a highly toxic material can both have immediate effects. In addition to the short-term effects, there may be long-term effects. For example, exposure and contamination to carcinogens can cause cancer, teratogens can damage a fetus, and mutagens can cause genetic damage.

Personnel must consider the impact of failure to decontaminate effectively. Accidental ingestion of hazardous materials while working on activities of long duration can affect one's ability to decontaminate. Tissue can be damaged by continued exposure to materials not removed from the skin. Another impact can be the contamination of other workers, equipment, and work places, as well as the contamination later of a responder's home and family.

Location and setup of the decontamination corridor should be in an area between the area of highest contamination (hot zone) and the areas that are contamination free (cold zone). The contamination-reduction corridor is in the warm zone where it meets the hot zone.

A large area (at least 50 ft. by 50 ft.) is necessary for decontamination and related support activities. Establishing the corridor on flat ground facilitates the retention of contaminated water and decontamination solutions. If a level area is not available, consider methods for runoff control. Water under pressure must be available at the decontamination corridor.

The configuration of the decontamination corridor is specific to the situation and product. The number of stations required to remove the contaminant safely and effectively is based on how hazardous the product is and/or the degree of difficulty in removing it from contaminated surfaces. Each of the decontamination stations in the corridor is separated to prevent cross-contamination. The stations in a decontamination corridor are set up in such a way that as a contaminated individual, vehicle, or equipment moves through the corridor, contamination is reduced and contained at each station. One side of the corridor is designated as "clean" and the other as "dirty." Contaminated protective equipment and disposable items are placed in containers on the "dirty side." There is one way in and one way out of the corridor, with entry and exit points clearly marked. The entry dressing station must be separated from the exit redressing station.

Methods of Decontamination

There are seven methods of decontamination. Each method has advantages and disadvantages.

Washing with a Surfactant

Surfactants such as detergents reduce the adhesion of the contaminant to the surface being cleaned. The advantage of surfactants is that water, detergent, and hoses are commonly available and washing is easy to perform. The disadvantage is that the properties of the material are not changed and this method requires the disposal of wash and rinse water.

Dilution

Dilution is the use of a solvent such as water to lessen the concentration of a contaminant. The advantage of dilution is that it is easy to perform and it is the best method to decontaminate skin. Dilution is the most common form of decontamination. A disadvantage of dilution is that some materials are not soluble in water. Use of this method expands the volume of material that will require treatment, storage, or disposal.

Neutralization

This method adjusts the pH level of the product closer to a neutral pH of 7. An advantage to neutralization is that the process renders harmless a challenge chemical. A disadvantage is that every product is completely specific and requires specialized knowledge and materials.

Degradation

This involves the use of one chemical to attack and alter the chemical properties of another. An advantage to this method is that the hazard is removed and rendered harmless. A disadvantage to the degradation process involves the use of additional hazardous materials, the generation of heat, and the likely production of harmful by-products.

Absorption

In this process, the product is mechanically pulled in or soaked up by the sorbent. The advantage to this method is that it is usually used for equipment and property on flat surfaces and not on responders or their protective equipment. Materials for this method can be natural or synthetic. A disadvantage to this method is that the absorbent material must not react with the product being absorbed. Generally this method does not change the hazardous properties of the chemical. For example, a flammable liquid that has been absorbed is now contained, however, it is still flammable. An exception to this rule is in the case of trying to absorb an acid spill with soda ash or limestone. This would both absorb the product and make it easier to move and neutralize the acid.

Dry Decontamination

This process uses a pressurized air chamber with filters or a vacuum system. The advantage to this method is that it works well for water-reactive chemicals, dusts, asbestos fibers, and radioactive particles. A disadvantage is that comprehensive dry decontamination requires special equipment intensive and can be costly.

Solidification

This process involves the use of a chemical agent to solidify the contaminant for removal. An advantage to this method is that, similar to absorbents, it eases the removal of a product. A disadvantage is similar to adsorbents and chemical degradation in that the reaction can produce heat or a more dangerous product. Costs of solidification agents can be prohibitive.

Testing Decontamination Effectiveness

The OSHA regulations require that the effectiveness of decontamination operations be checked. Decontamination methods vary in effectiveness for removing different substances. The effectiveness of decontamination methods should be assessed at the start of operations and on an ongoing basis. If decontamination is not effective, the method must be changed. Four methods for testing decontamination effectiveness include are:

1. **Visual observation** in natural or ultraviolet light can reveal visible stains or residue contaminants may leave. Some substances can be detected only in ultraviolet light.
2. **Wipe sampling** provides an after-the-fact analysis. Inner and outer surfaces of protective clothing are wiped with cloth or paper, which is then subjected to analysis.
3. **Cleaning solution analysis** analyses the decontamination solution at the last rinse to detect the remaining contaminants.
4. **Permeation testing** requires that a sample of the protective clothing be submitted for test. Some CPC has a tab of fabric on the exterior of the garment for this purpose.

Technical Decontamination and Emergency Decontamination

Technical decontamination involves the routine operations performed to remove contaminants from PPE and tools. When the primary problem is contamination, the efforts of decontamination personnel are focused on being very thorough. In contrast, emergency decontamination centers on removal of contaminants from persons who were contaminated and injured. In an emergency, the primary concern is to prevent further injury and loss of life.

Emergency Decontamination

If a victim has immediate life-threatening injuries such as cardiac and/or respiratory arrest, decontaminate the head and chest area. If the victim has major bleeding, complete decontamination can be delayed until after initial care. This does not mean that rescuers should not take whatever precautions are necessary to prevent injury and exposure to themselves. Contamination may be contained by wrapping the patient in a blanket or sheet. This will permit initial emergency medical care prior to complete decontamination.

If a victim has suffered a major trauma such as a fall from height or a crushing injury, decontaminate him or her with special concern movement of areas of injury. In the event of injury that does not present an immediate threat to life (e.g., broken bones, strains, sprains, etc.), decontamination should be performed using normal procedures.

Technical Decontamination

The following procedure for technical decontamination involves a six-station Level B decontamination corridor.

- **Station 1—Gross/Tool Drop.** The gross drop is a container for the temporary storage of contaminated tools and equipment. The crew drops in any tools that might be used again in the hot zone.
- **Station 2—Gross Shower.** The gross shower consists of a liquid retention pool and a simple shower for rinsing PPE. Gross contamination is washed off or diluted (if soluble) by a water spray.
- **Station 3—Wash/Rinse I.** Wash/Rinse I consists of a liquid-retention pool, a bucket containing decontamination solution, two brushes, and a nozzle and wand for rinsing PPE. Washing with a surfactant loosens nonsoluble contaminants or assists in the dilution of those that might be soluble in water.
- **Station 4—Wash/Rinse II.** Wash/Rinse II consists of a liquid-retention pool, a bucket containing decontamination solution, two brushes, and a nozzle and wand for rinsing PPE. Washing with a surfactant loosens nonsoluble contaminants and assists in the dilution of those that might be soluble in water.
- **Station 5—Undressing Area.** The undressing area to remove PPE and SCBA consists of chairs and containers for potentially contaminated items (disposable and reusable). Personal protective equipment is removed while preventing potentially contaminated surfaces from contacting unprotected areas of the body.
- **Station 6—Medical Monitoring.** An interview of the patient is the first step in the medical monitoring process. This should be performed immediately outside the undressing area and outside the decontamination corridor in the cold zone. Minimum medical monitoring includes pulse, blood pressure, body temperature, and cognitive assessment. If personnel have been exposed to a hazardous product or have been injured, further examination and medical surveillance is required.

Completing the Decontamination Process

Completion of the decontamination process requires that personnel perform the following:

1. Remove all clothing.
2. Shower thoroughly.
3. Don clean clothing.
4. Perform required recordkeeping such as completion of a work log.

If the personal shower is not completed at the incident site, it must be performed as soon as possible after personnel leave the site. If personal clothing has been contaminated (such as in the event of a suit breach), immediate removal of the clothing and a personal shower is essential.

Summary

Hazardous materials exist in almost every aspect of our daily lives. As long as these hazards are properly contained, the potential for danger to those around them is practically nonexistent. Unfortunately, hazardous materials accidents and their sometimes catastrophic consequences are all too familiar. Rescuers respond to these accidents to help the victims. However, the rescuer's priority during the rescue attempt must be to maintain his or her own personal safety. Without a thorough knowledge of diagnostic resources, safe operating guidelines, and personal protective measures, the rescuer may cause the victim to lose the most valuable resource available—the rescuer. Following the guidelines presented in this text can help to ensure the rescuer's safety.

CHAPTER 20

Managing the Rescue

Specific topics covered are:

- Safety Systems Approach to Rescue
- Incident Management System
- Crisis Decision Making
- The Response Evolution

Introduction

Management of the rescue is not much different from management of any emergency. The safety procedures, incident command (management) system, and the elements of response are similar. The greatest differences between a rescue and other emergencies are the tasks needed to accomplish the goal—to remove the person from the hazardous area to a safe area without doing additional harm. For instance, a structural fire may require such tasks as search and rescue, ventilation, attack (suppression), salvage, and overhaul before the incident is concluded. Although the need for human rescue certainly occurs in the framework of a fire or HazMat incident, the tasks of industrial rescue involve a different set of elements including location (of the patient), hazard abatement, access, stabilization, packaging, and egress. This chapter focuses on those elements of management specific to the rescue effort.

Safety Systems Approach to Rescue

Safety is as important in rescue as it is in any emergency. Safety must be pursued meticulously, both in preparation for and during the emergency. Rescue practices are inherently dangerous and must be treated as such. Even when rescuers take every precaution, things can happen that expose them to danger. If rescuers fail to recognize the danger, they are sure to be caught by it. Safety is an attitude, an observant, cautious attitude. There is no room for carelessness or apathy.

Assessing the Situation

Rescuers must evaluate their ability to conduct safe rescues from dangerous environments. There are situations for which a team is not prepared. It could be a scenario with no viable solution. In these cases, a difficult decision must be made: attempt rescue, or not? Some considerations in making that decision are the appropriateness of *personnel, equipment,* and *training.* If any of these three elements is found lacking, the only safe choice is to refuse to perform the rescue until capable resources can get to the scene.

Another factor is the consideration of the patient's viability. If, due to the situation, it is determined that the patient is not likely to survive, the risk to personnel must be compared to the expected benefit or outcome of the situation. It may be difficult to make rational decisions in these situations. In an industrial/structural rescue situation, the potential rescuer may know the victim. However, it is senseless to risk a human life for a dead body.

A decision not to rescue may be a conscious decision not to risk lives of more people. In these cases, the plan of aggressive attack changes to a more reserved posture. The best action may be to contain the incident and wait for someone qualified to do the recovery. Some cases require considerable time to abate existing hazards before recovery efforts can take place. In either case, this is now most likely a "body recovery" and rescuers must go into "recovery mode." This is an uncomfortable situation at best. The only way to prepare for it is to train for it.

Even more difficult sometimes are situations in which the rescue attempt has failed. Unsuccessful rescues have significant emotional and psychological impact on rescuers, particularly when the failed attempt is associated with injury or death of fellow rescuers. Safety is one of the greatest allies in the war against failure. Doing the right things in the right way can help avoid mistakes. By being prepared to respond properly to an adverse situation, you can save lives. Preparation is the key. Preparation means safety.

Safety in Planning

The planning phase of a rescue is extremely important. Safety relates to almost every phase of planning for a team's development and operation. It is the focal point from which our plans are derived. Some planning elements that require safety as a major consideration are team goals, membership criteria, and suggested operating guidelines. The section entitled "The Response Evolution," later in this chapter, reviews some of these elements. It provides a format for analyzing previous incidents to plan for safer operations in the future. This is one of the most important aspects of post-incident debriefing.

Safety in Training

A systems approach to safety can be instituted only through training. The way rescuers function during training often dictates how they act during an emergency. Humans are creatures of habit. Safe actions in training usually mean safer operation on the scene of an emergency. Most rescue organizations spend more of their time in training and preparation for incidents than in response to actual incidents.

Instructor Qualifications

Some significant characteristics of a safe instructor are dedication and attitude toward the job, good communication abilities, and thorough knowledge of the subject. Persons truly dedicated to their task will overcome many obstacles to reach their goal. The ability of an instructor is often in direct proportion to his or her dedication and enthusiasm. This is sometimes called "attitude." Attitude is not a measurable trait. It is, however, easily recognized. The proper dedication and attitude of an instructor toward training includes real concerns and zeal for the safety of his or her students and their practices.

An instructor must be well qualified through a combination of training and experience. Instructors should be students first and always, striving to learn more each day. A truly knowledgeable instructor knows enough to realize how much he or she still has to learn. This is a safe attitude. Overconfidence might be a first sign of danger. A person who feels he or she knows it all already, is obviously not experienced enough.

Still, there can be too much emphasis on experience. Experiences can be both bad and good. Performing an unsafe practice for many years is bad experience. Time on the job alone does not display competence. There are people who have been on the job for 20 years whose experience equals one year . . . repeated 20 times. An appetite for knowledge in combination with practical experience make the safest instructors. The organization responsible for instructor training should thoroughly investigate the potential instructor's background and experience.

In addition to qualifications and ability of an instructor, good communication is one of the best means of providing safety in training. Good communication among instructors and between instructors and students provides better organization and less confusion, thus, a safer working environment.

Steps to Promote Safe Training

A few of the things an organization can do to promote safety in training are:

- **Review established safety standards before every class.** Know the rules and apply them correctly and completely. Do not compromise on issues of safety. If there are no safety standards, create them! Suggested operating guidelines take much of the guesswork out of training. They are important to safe practices.

- **Control the number of students.** An instructor must not try to teach more students than he or she can safely and effectively supervise. This rule is called "span of control," which usually ranges from three to seven persons. Five students to one instructor is generally considered ideal although a 6:1 ratio is practical for most rescue training exercises.
- **Use back-up systems in training exercises.** Safety line belay systems can be used in field training exercises. When used properly, these systems can compensate for missed procedures that could cause disastrous results. They provide a separate and complete secondary system capable of catching the load in case a primary system fails. It is a good idea to use safety belay systems whenever a student is suspended on rope.

  Another form of belay called a "body belay" or a "bottom belay" can provide backup for a rappeller should he or she lose control or pass out during descent. The body belay does not back up the rope system itself but provides a back-up operator for the rappeller's descent control device.

  Other safety systems include the use of personnel to support the operation of descent control devices in lowering operations. These persons, sometimes called "line tenders," can back up the primary operator of the control device when only one is used in a rope rescue system. If the operator loses control of the device, the line tender helps rectify the situation. Line tenders are also useful in keeping ropes free of knots and tangles as they feed into the descent control device(s).
- **Maintain training equipment and keep thorough documentation.** This is one of the most important aspects of rescue training. It provides important data for establishing maintenance and determining when equipment is no longer safe and must be removed from service.
- **Establish emergency procedures for incidents that occur during training.** The time to figure out how to deal with an emergency is not after it happens. Set a procedure for "rescue mode." This mode should be activated whenever a student gets in trouble while performing practical rescue evolutions. *Be proactive, not reactive. Prepare for the worst, hope for the best.* Implement the rescue mode immediately anytime anyone recognizes a problem and alarms the rest of the group. To activate the rescue mode:
  - Designate verbal and/or hand signal to alert group members such as, "This is a real deal!"
  - Stop all other evolutions in the area if necessary so that other instructors can respond to assist.
  - Instructors may choose to use and direct other students to assist in the rescue.
  - Instructors must remain calm and relay that attitude to those around them.
  - Notify emergency services as necessary.

  When to prepare for rescue mode:
  - Incidents are most likely to occur when beginning-level students are in control of their own descent, such as with rappelling. Beginners often get clothing, hair, gloves, or other things caught in the descent control device. This can cause the student to be stuck on line, unable to free himself or herself and out of reach of other rescuers.

  How To prepare for rescue mode:
  - Preset the equipment necessary to perform the rescue based on problems most likely to occur.
  - Preassign the location of rescue equipment so it can be deployed easily to the appropriate areas for rescue.
  - Prerig the entire system if possible. If not, predetermine all anchor points and prerig as much as possible.
  - Preassign personnel to specific tasks.
  - If possible, practice deployment to ensure the effectiveness of the system.

Preestablish emergency communications for several reasons:

> To alert the group to a real emergency. The signal should be familiar to both instructors and students. Establish a signal for a problem (e.g., "real deal!").

> To check the condition of a live person playing the role of a patient. If a simulated victim is "playing dead" and has a real problem, it may go unnoticed and be perceived as part of the act.

> To ensure they are truly okay. Establish a code word that can be relayed between the instructor and the simulated patient to check and recheck the "patient's" condition. For example, The instructor can give the verbal signal "green!" The "patient" gives an identical response or moves head or hands. If there is no response, the simulated patient is assumed to have a real problem and rescue mode is implemented.

Safety in Response

Safety hazards multiply during response to any emergency. These issues should be addressed in suggested operating guidelines developed according to federal, state, and local regulations. Response is discussed in greater detail later in this chapter.

Safety on the Scene

On-scene safety is so important in emergency management that it has a specific staff function in the incident command (management) system. This person, the safety officer, is responsible for observing the scene for safety hazards. The job has such a high priority that, in matters of safety, the safety officer usually has authority over the person in charge of the incident. On an incident involving rescue, each rescuer should consider him- or herself equally responsible for the safety of their rescue systems. Team members should constantly back each other up by checking and double-checking the rigging and operation of rescue systems and their components. This is the "buddy system" in the truest sense. Humans can make mistakes easily under pressure. The rescue team cannot afford mistakes that can cost lives.

Post-Incident Safety

Just as most injuries in the fire service occur during the overhaul phase, many accidents occur on the scene of a rescue occur after the rescue. This "clean-up" phase finds rescuers excited and jovial or perhaps tired and frustrated. Either way, it is easy for them to forget the hazards that still exist even though the emergency is over. Dropped equipment is one of the leading causes of accidents during cleanup. Rescuers must be alert to this and take precautions to avoid this possibility.

Do not lay equipment near an edge or on industrial grating. It could find its way to the ground without being carried. Do not disassemble equipment while it is hanging over an edge. Pull it in onto the deck on which you are standing, before taking it apart. This reduces the chance of dropping the heavy items on someone several levels below. Do not remove your safety equipment during cleanup. The helmet that protects your head during the emergency might prevent injury during the cleanup.

Do not restrict consideration of postincident safety hazards to emergency incidents. One of the greatest risks of injury to the rescuer exists during the clean-up phase of a training exercise. People often are in a hurry to pack up and leave after a training evolution. Sometimes, safety is sacrificed for quick egress. Consider all phases of training serious enough to use safe practices.

In short, safety is a state of mind, an attitude. A rescue team member must set the example from the start.

Incident Management System

In some disciplines, such as urban fire, the incident command system (ICS) is known as the incident management system (IMS). Whatever its name, the system sets forth an organized means of directing the incident. Sometimes elaborate organizational flowcharts that depict an incident of major proportion can be intimidating. The important thing to remember about the IMS is that it is similar to a tool box. The entire system may seem huge and exhaustive but rescuers need only take the components that apply to the incident at hand. The IMS can be used on all incidents, large or small. The functions are still carried out relative only to the needs of the incident. For instance, in the overall incident management system, staff positions are assigned to the incident command (IC) to help handle the elements of scene safety (safety officer), distribution of information to the public (public information officer), and liaison with incoming resources from other agencies (liaison). These roles may each be assigned to a different person in a large incident, but the IC may handle all these functions at a small one.

There are many excellent texts and even national standards detailing the overall IMS. These volumes address the many aspects of managing the incident from the top to the bottom of the chart. This text is concerned with one element of the IMS, the rescue sector. Sectors represent geographical or functional areas of operation. Sectors in the IMS operations section show delegated and decentralized tasks that must be performed on the emergency scene. If the operations chief were directly responsible for each part of the organization below him or her in the structure, the ability to control would soon be taxed. The rescue sector is a functional area of operation and, like all sectors, is assigned specific personnel and equipment (the rescue team). A sector officer is assigned to each sector. In this case, the sector officer is the team leader.

Unity of Command

"Unity of command" describes the concept of having each person report to only one person, despite position in the command structure. Every person in an organization should have only one person to whom he or she reports at any one time. Without this very important principle, people or units could receive multiple and conflicting orders from higher levels in the command structure.

The team leader is usually the person designated as the rescue sector officer. This organizational relationship between team members and officer must be well established to issue and receive orders properly and to report progress to the officer. This principle is often applied within the rescue sector when two or three team members are sent to perform a given task. The sector officer may designate one member of this unit to be in charge. It now becomes evident that the other members of this unit report to the person placed in charge and this person reports directly to the sector officer. Each person knows to whom he or she must report.

Division of Labor

Tasks must be assigned to individuals or units in an organized manner to accomplish the desired result. These tasks must be well thought-out, each accomplishing a part of the overall plan of action. The more of these functions that can be assigned and completed simultaneously, the faster the plan will come together. Assignments must be based on the function to be performed and according to the qualifications and capabilities of team members. Some specific functions for the rescue sector include search and locate, hazard assessment and abatement, access, assessment and packaging of patient, and egress.

Span of Control

Span of control refers to the number of persons or units one can manage effectively. This number varies with the manager and with the difficulty of the tasks being performed, but it is most often from three to seven people, with the ideal being five. If a leader exceeds the effective span of control, things may be missed and accidents are more likely to occur due to poor management of the rescue effort. Due to the relatively small size of most rescue teams, tasks can usually be delegated to stay well within the officer's span of control.

Crisis Decision Making

Since every rescue is different, decisions must be made on the methods to use based on the situation at hand. Crisis decision making can be performed effectively with the help of all team members. As they respond to the scene, whether as a unit or individually, each member of the team begins to consider what needs to be done to perform the rescue. This is commonly referred to as "size-up." In most fire ground operations, size-up is performed by the officer. But most rescue operations dictate that every team member take an active part.

Standard operating procedures should dictate how to respond, where to respond, and who will be in charge when everyone arrives at the scene.

Two important events begin the decision making:

1. A team leader must be established (if this has not already been decided).
2. The team must come together.

Brainstorming

1. **"Huddle" the team** so the leader can give them all pertinent information relative to the incident. When he or she has distributed this information, the following should be done:

   If the patient's location is known, send someone immediately to contact him or her.

   Physical contact may not be possible initially. At a minimum, attempt to make verbal contact. This will give clues as to the level of the patient's consciousness, his or her injuries, and his or her level of apprehension (fear, pain, panic). Some communications devices allow remote assessment of a patient's condition without direct contact.

   Keep talking. The patient may be able to hear you, even if he or she appears unconscious. Explain what is happening at all times.

   Report findings to the team leader as soon as possible. This input is valuable to the team as it decides on the proper rescue methods.
2. **Begin brainstorming.** The team leader solicits the ideas of the team members, one at a time, to help formulate an action plan. Free-for-all conversation must be controlled. Ideas should be presented no matter how feasible or infeasible they appear. The team leader will sift through them to formulate an appropriate action plan.
3. **Form the action plan.** Once all members have presented their ideas, the team leader makes the final decision on what action to take.

   NOTE: *At this point, the leadership method turns more to autocratic than democratic. Nevertheless, although the leadership is not purely democratic, a good team leader readily accepts feedback from team members. Only a foolish person refuses information in the constantly changing rescue environment.*
4. **Make assignments.** Having decided on a plan, the team leader assigns personnel to the various task-level functions of the operation. Several things should be considered when making assignments:
   - Make instructions clear, short, and to the point. There is no better way to tell people what you want done than to show them what you want done. If possible, use drawings of various systems to illustrate the function to which you wish to assign them. A picture is worth a thousand words.
   - After each assignment, ask the team members if they understand. This indicates whether clarification of the assignment is necessary.
   - As a team member, do not hesitate to tell the team leader if you do not understand exactly what he or she means.
   - Do not allow individual members to drift away from the group after assignments have been given. Keep them together until the last assignment is made. This keeps all members informed of the overall plan.

This suggested planning phase in the operation of the rescue sector is not commonly used for most emergency operations. It is somewhat specific to rescue based on the diverse nature of rescue operations. At first glance, it may seem to take a considerable amount of time, as long as 3 or so minutes; however, this is a small price to pay to ensure the team's direction. Taking some time to plan can save precious minutes in the overall rescue operation. Teams that do not plan experience confusion and delays in their operations.

5. **Carry out the plan.**
   - Complete assignments.
   - The team leader disperses the team to complete its assignments.
   - As soon as they complete their assignments, team members must report completion to the team leader.
   - Do not allow rescuers to "freelance" after completion of their assignments. They should not attempt other tasks or join other teams without being assigned.
   - After each team member reports, the team leader either reassigns the team member to another task, or places them in a personnel pool (staging) for later assignment.

This entire process of crisis decision making seems very simple on the surface and contains many basic principles of the IMS. However, many teams have difficulty maintaining the structure necessary to fully take advantage of this approach. It takes a concerted effort and continued practice to make crisis decision making work. Rescue teams can try the technique in training sessions and explore variations that will work for them.

The Response Evolution

There are several distinct phases of "the response evolution" (see Figure 20.1). This system is a tool for planning, organization, and evaluating the rescue team's performance. Each phase represents a specific link in a chain of events that take place and come full circle in the response evolution. The following section presents a brief outline of organizational and operational elements encompassed by each phase.

Preplan

This preplanning phase involves development of every aspect of the initial and ongoing organizational structure. It includes development of team members, training, and SOGs.

1. **Develop the rescue team.** Develop equipment specifications based on the working environment and the type of anticipated use. Team member selection criteria must be established and qualified personnel chosen.
2. **Develop a training program.** Decide the type of training needed based on the environment in which it will be used (e.g., industrial, structural, or wilderness). Talk to several established teams and agencies for their recommendations.
3. **Develop team membership criteria.** The *attitudes* of prospective members are important. What is their motivation (desire, fun, money, or just to get out of work)? Are they enthusiastic? *Physical requirements* Technical methods do not require superb physical fitness; however, obesity can cause problems. An annual physical exam is recommended. Consider the *availability of the member* (administrator, operator, etc.). Will members be available in case of an emergency? The *right number* of members on the team should be based on plant size and work assignments, shifts, turnaround requirements, and so forth.

   Generally speaking, six members should be the minimum for adequate response and operation for simple rope rescues. Several more than this may be required for confined space rescue.
4. **Develop SOGs** which are extremely effective in reducing liability. Develop SOGs for
   - membership criteria
   - operational guidelines for various types of rescues
   - training and quality control

Figure 20.1

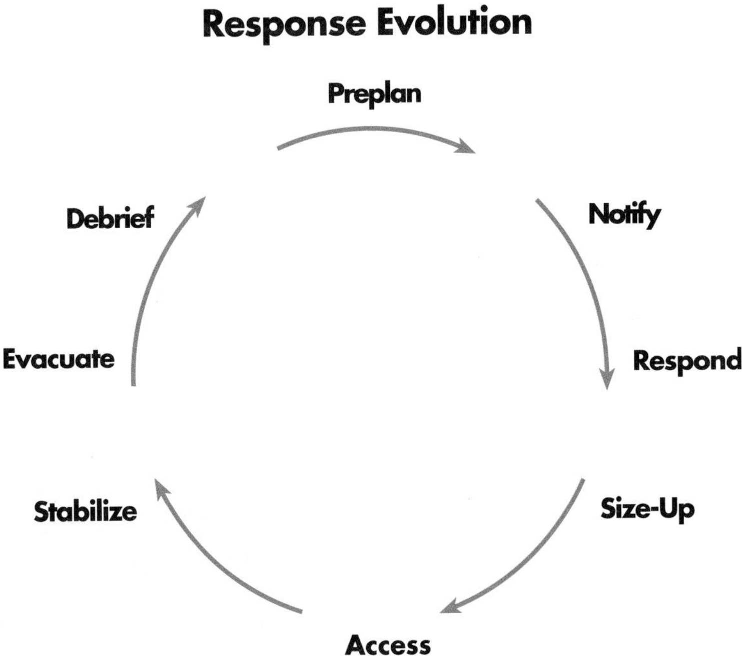

- rules and regulations (including a mission statement)
- command structure (including authority and responsibility for each position)

5. **Review past incidents to develop plans for the future.** Investigate and evaluate:
   - the types of rescues that have occurred.
   - Problems that have occurred during rescues. (See "Confined Space Rescue Preplan" form at the end of this chapter.)

Notify

The notification phase covers the actions and considerations in the notification process.

- Who notifies the team? SOGs should spell it out.
- Who is responsible? Authority and responsibility for this action must be assigned. The person responsible must know how and whom to call. Responsible persons must document all parts of the incident. They must also solicit and relay all information accurately.
- How are they notified (phones, pagers, radio, etc.)?
  - Are people on call to respond?
  - Give only necessary information when dispatching the team.
  - Keep the message short and to the point.

Respond

The response phase covers not only the guidelines for responding to emergencies but where the team members should go once they get to the scene. Staging is an important aspect of response, especially for many industrial facilities that maintain volunteer rescue teams who come from different parts of the plant at different times.

A *staging area* (a stand-by area for personnel and equipment ready for immediate use) must be established to maintain safety and organization. SOGs must establish who designates the staging area. The team leader is the best choice to make this decision, based on the dispatch information received during notification.

Authority for *type of response* (lights, sirens, etc.) must be established by SOGs. What can and cannot be done during response? SOGs must also designate a person to get rescue vehicles and equipment. This is especially important where the equipment does not have crew ready for response around the clock, for example, in volunteer response organizations.

Size-up

This evaluator phase actually begins long before the incident. There are many considerations in performing size-up for rescue.

- Size-up comes primarily from notification and takes into consideration the information received to start the formulation of an action plan. Information on items such as location, injuries, hazards, personnel, and equipment are all considerations in size-up.
- When sizing up for action, rescuers must remember that *things change in a crisis!* They must be able to adapt. The plan should account for changes due to
  - the human factor
  - injuries
  - the location
- EVERYBODY sizes up. Information is derived from
  - observations of the scene and the patient(s).
  - witnesses. (*Caution*: they may not be accurate.)
  - other team members.
  - the patient. (How did it happen? What hurts?)
  - the mechanisms of injury (the objects and processes that caused injury).
- Crisis decision making is necessary. Decisions should be based on the size-up of each team member and the subsequent brainstorming. The team leader makes the final decision on the plan of action. The team leader may have to make the hardest decision of all if the circumstances dictate: not to do the rescue! This is a difficult and awesome responsibility. The team leader must be capable of assuming this responsibility.

Access

The access phase involves getting to the patient. In most industrial rescue situations, knowing the location of the patient is not a problem. However, circumstances do arise that mean a search must take place to locate the patient. Although not included in the outline, location would take place here.

How do rescuers access the patient?

- The method of access need only get the rescuer to the patient. The method of egress may require the removal of a litter and an attendant.
- The method of reaching the patient is often different from the method of removing the patient.
- Rescuers must consider the potential for personal exhaustion when making access. Carrying heavy equipment or working in confined spaces can create serious problems. Consider the number of personnel available and establish regular relief for team members.

Stabilize

Assessment and subsequent stabilization of the patient must take place as quickly as possible. It will do no good to perform a technical rescue if the patient is killed by poor or inappropriate care.

- Consider immediate treatment of life-threatening injuries and quick, appropriate packaging for rapid removal of patients from hazardous areas.
- Consider the ABCs and stop severe bleeding.
- Consider spinal immobilization simultaneously with the ABCs.
- Do not waste time attempting to package insignificant injuries.
- Do not attempt to resuscitate pulseless, nonbreathing patients in a hazardous atmosphere. Package and remove them quickly to a safe area where more definitive and effective care can take place.

Evacuate

Most of the rope rescue techniques practiced are focused on evaluation. Removing the patient from the hazard is what rescue is all about. As previously mentioned, the egress route will most likely differ from the access route.

There are two important factors in choosing the evacuation method: safety and efficiency (Keep it simple—simplicity generally signifies safety.)

Proper rescue training generally focuses on evacuation techniques with an emphasis on care and packaging of the patient.

Team members should follow the team leader's orders, although they may not agree with them. This is an important team concept. The team leader should have a view of the overall situation, which the individual team members may not. The team members should always provide feedback to the team leader about changing circumstances. The team leader should review this feedback immediately and evaluate its importance. If there is time, the team leader should explain controversial actions to the team members to avoid argument.

Debrief

After any incident, it is appropriate to debrief, or critique. This phase outlines one method of debriefing which encompasses all of the other phases of the rescue evolution. These debriefings must be documented and the information analyzed to decide its applicability to future incidents. Without analysis and application, the debriefing has no value.

As usual, immediately following an incident, make the equipment ready for the next response. Be certain to document information about rope and equipment.

It is recommended that the debriefing not be performed immediately following the incident. Initially, rescuers are too emotional (happy, angry, etc.) to think clearly. Give them time to gather thoughts and write down the good and bad points for discussion.

Meet as a team, within 24 to 48 hours after the incident, to debrief. After 48 hours, recall of the details of the incident may not be accurate.

- Meet and debrief in a structured way. Cover both good points and bad points (good points first). Use the sequence of events in the response evolution to give structure to the debriefing. Discuss the effectiveness of the preplan, the notification process, the response, and so on.
- Consider calling in a rescue authority to provide an educated and objective review of the incident.
- Document the debriefing. Assign a secretary to record all the events of the discussion.
- Use the debriefing of the incident to further develop the team's safety and effectiveness. *Use the past to predict the future.* Apply this information to SOGs (preplan).

CSR On-Scene Prioritized Action Plan

1. **Priority One: Make the Scene Safe**
   - Assess Hazard–Approach the space and consider entrance into the space
   - Mitigate Hazard–Control or remove the hazard
2. **Priority Two: Victim Contact by Primary Responder**
   - Establish Victim Location
   - Perform Primary Survey (ABC's)
   - Determine Mechanism of Injury
   - Begin Psychological First Aid
3. **Priority Three: Size-Up**
   - Gather Information
     - Resource Identification
     - Primary Responder Report
   - Brainstorm Strategy–Risk/Reward (Go/No-Go)
   - ICS/IMS
     - Team Member Assignments
4. **Priority Four: Preparation**
   - Rescuer PPE
   - Anchoring & Rigging Rescue Equipment
   - Authorized Entrant Review
5. **Priority Five: Access Victim**
   - Designate Access Team Leader
     - Include All Rigging & Entrant Away Teams
   - Utilize Rescuer Retrieval (High-point)
   - Designate Back-up Personnel
6. **Priority Six: Stabilize & Package Victim**
   - Provide First Aid to Life-Threatening Injuries
   - Secure Packaging for Rescue Transport
7. **Priority Seven: Evacuate**
   - Move Victim to a Safe Location
   - Provide Medical Report to Emergency Medical Services
   - Remove Rescuers
     - Emergency Retrievals
8. **Priority Eight: Response Termination**
   - Pick-up and Inventory Gear
   - Decontaminate (if necessary)
   - Rebuild Gear Packages for the Next Call
   - Conduct Field Evaluation of Rescuer's Mental State

Critical Incident Stress Management

Historically, the combat zone has produced "shattered nerves" and "shell shock." Similar symptoms were noted in rescue workers throughout the Vietnam era of the 1960s and early 1970s. During the late 1970s and early 1980s, the Critical Incident Stress Debriefing (CISD) process was developed to address the physical, emotional, mental, and spiritual dilemmas proposed by the trauma of rescue work. This process or the management of critical incident stress does not provide definitive solutions for all rescuers. It does, however, offer a process that supports rescue workers in their quest for recovery and ability to cope with the consistent level of trauma to which they are exposed.

Three types of this stress are recognized: (1) acute—immediate reactions to the event, (2) chronic—immediate and lasting reactions, and (3) delayed—reactions that are not present until weeks or possibly months and years after an event or series of events.

The attention first given to this syndrome was in support of the social need to return to work. Presently, however, the health and well-being of the individual is becoming the focus of the recovery process. The concept of Critical Incident Stress Debriefing centers around the need for immediate and brief treatment approaches to immediate and sudden onsets of trauma. The stress model of CISD intervention views the onset of the crisis event as a precipitating event that surpasses the level of coping skills or abilities of the rescue worker. This untreated reaction to crisis might then evoke a pathological reaction in the rescue personnel.

The CISD model is a peer-led, peer-supported group to deal with the stress of the emergency service worker. As noted earlier, rescue workers respond better to peers than nonpeers in the venting process following a traumatic event. Two types of support group have volunteers to aid the rescue workers in the recovery process: (1) mental health workers, whose role is to assist in identifying the signs and symptoms that might lead to deeper emotional trauma and to assist in the development of the "group" process and (2) clergy, whose role is to address the spiritual issues that often arise or intensify when "bad things happen to innocent or good people."

It must be emphasized that peers lead and direct the debriefing process and are supported by the others. As supporters, mental health and religious professionals do not lead and direct the debriefing. Limitations on the effectiveness of treatment are noted when the process becomes a mental health "group therapy."

The CISD process is briefly defined in the following seven phases reprinted by permission of Jeffery T. Mitchell PhD.:

1. **Introduction phase:** Give names of participants, guidelines of the meeting, out of service; stress confidentiality.
2. **Fact phase:** Discuss facts that will not jeopardize an official investigation of. Speak of the facts and actions in which you participated. This is an attempt to recreate the event for all attendees.
3. **Thought phase:** Recall first thoughts during the event. Your personal thoughts are as important as the facts.
4. **Reaction or feeling phase:** Move from facts to feelings. What did each person feel during the event or in the hours immediately following?
5. **Symptom phase:** Peers describe cognitive, physical, emotional, and behavioral signs and symptoms—those occurring at the scene, hours later, or perhaps still being experienced.
6. **Teaching phase:** Relay information regarding stress reactions and what can be done to alleviate them. Normal reactive symptoms will subside with time. Specific instructions may be given here.
7. **Reentry phase:** Wrap up the debriefing. Review emotions or behaviors that have been covered. Encourage group interaction. Distribute hand-out material to take home and peruse later.

Summary

Some of the information touched upon in this chapter has been discussed in previous chapters because incident management is a consideration common to almost every aspect of rescue. Good management is important whether it relates to business or the emergency incident. The most significant difference between these two areas is the element of time. Rescuers must strive to make the most efficient use of time and effort on the scene. Proper incident management contributes significantly to this goal.

CONFINED SPACE RESCUE PREPLAN

DATE:

SPACE DESIGNATION: *(Unit/Vessel Name % ID #)*

SPACE LOCATION:

STAGING AREA:

SPACE CATEGORY:
☐ Category I - Rescue Available (RA)
☐ Category II - Rescue Stand-by (RS)

SPACE TYPE (1-12): ________
Elevated: Y N
Congested: Y N

MEANS TO SUMMONS RESCUE SERVICE:
❒ Phone ❒ Pager ❒ Radio ❒ Audible Signal ❒ Intercom ❒ Other:____________________

METHODS OF RESCUE ❒ *Confirm that attendant has been trained in emergency respone procedures.*

☐ External (Retrieval):	☐ Internal:________________ (Congested:________________)
☐ Hauling System Required	☐ Victim-Lowering System Required / Lowering Area:________________
☐ Anchorage: Overhead: ________	Pre-rigging Required? ❒ Yes ❒ No

Anchorage: ❒ Beam ❒ Stairwell ❒ Welded Steel Handrail ❒ Anchored Steel Pipe ❒ Support Strut ❒ Support Column ❒ Other:________________

SUGGESTED CSR PREPLANNED TECHNIQUE:
CSR#________ (1-5)

RESCUE EQUIPMENT REQUIREMENTS: *(Indicate Quantity Needed)*

	Hauling Systems		Carabiners		Pulleys
	Ascenders		Prusiks		Shock Absorbers
	Anchor Straps		Webbing		Rigging Bags

RESCUE ROPES NEEDED: *(Indicate Quantity Needed)*

	Main Line(s)		Hauling Systems		Lowering Line(s)
	Safety Line(s)		Line-Transfer System(s)		

MEDICAL & PACKAGING EQUIPMENT NEEDED: *(Indicate Quantity Needed)*

	Spinal Immobilization Device:		Stretcher Device:
	C-Collar:		Medical Kit:

ADDITIONAL PPE: *(See Permit / MSDS)*

DESIGNATION OF RESCUE PERSONNEL: *(Last Name, First Initial)*
- First Responder(s): ________________
- Team Leader: ________________
- Safety Line(s): ________________
- Back-up Rescuer: ________________
- Rigger: ________________
- Attendant: ________________
- Air Watch: ________________

SPACE DESCRIPTION:

SKETCH OR DIAGRAM OF SPACE: *(Use Back of Page if needed)*

ENTRY SUPERVISOR:	PHONE #	DATE:

REPORT COMPLETED BY:

CHAPTER 21

NFPA Standards for Rescue Operations and Professional Qualifications

Introduction

The National Fire Protection Association (NFPA) has had great impact on the operations of fire service and other emergency response agencies worldwide. As mentioned in earlier chapters, the NFPA is a consensus standard, one that does not carry the weight of law unless adopted as such by a governmental body. However, many safety professionals consider the NFPA a national benchmark for safety. In addition, this benchmark will likely be a factor, if not the prime reference, in litigation resulting from incidents involving rope and rope rescue related activities. Thus far, this text has only discussed NFPA equipment standards. The relation of these standards to manufacturing and quality assurance in the rope, harnesses, and other auxiliary equipment used by rescuers is very important and has been documented in earlier chapters. The NFPA realizes the need for standards that will influence both the components used to perform rescues and the actual operations involving and surrounding the use of these components.

This chapter examines some new standards proposed by the NFPA to provide a basis for Technical Rescue operations for a variety of disciplines at both the organizational and individual levels. At the time of this writing, two such standards are in varying degrees of completion. Since both standards are unfinished, the accuracy of the information contained within this chapter must occasionally be reexamined. However, both documents are due to be published by 1999 and are close enough to completion to allow an accurate overview of their content.

NFPA 1670 - Operations and Training for Technical Rescue Incidents

NFPA 1670, Standard on Operations and Training for Technical Rescue Incidents, is the first effort by the NFPA to develop a standard directed for organizations operating at various levels of capability in a variety of technical rescue disciplines. This standard helps an organization evaluate itself and determine if it can function at any of three levels (awareness, operations, and technician) in a given technical rescue discipline. It focuses on the actual operations required by an organization in a specific rescue specialty or discipline. In providing the organizational requirements for agencies wishing to perform a technical rescue discipline at a given level, the standard also creates guidance for training they must perform to comply.

There are seven different technical rescue disciplines covered by this standard. Many of these disciplines involve the use of high-angle rope techniques in their operations. In fact, so many technical rescue disciplines include rope rescue operations that "Technical Rope Rescue" was listed as one of the seven. This differs from other disciplines covered by the standard in that all others involve a particular environment in which the rescue is to be performed. Rope Rescue is not an environment, but a function. These technical rescue disciplines are currently covered by NFPA 1670:

- Structural Collapse
- Rope Rescue
- Confined Space
- Vehicle and Machinery
- Water
- Wilderness Search and Rescue
- Trench and Excavation

Each discipline sets forth requirements of the organizations wishing to operate as a rescue team within the specific environment. The organization may choose to meet standards for one or more disciplines and may decide to maintain different levels of capability within each discipline chosen. For example, a response agency might choose to become compliant with the NFPA 1670 Rope Rescue requirements at the highest level (technician). The same response agency may decide to maintain a confined space capability at only the awareness level. This agency would have a Technician level Rope Rescue capability and an Awareness level Confined Space capability. NFPA 1670 allows agencies to pick and choose in which disciplines and to what capability levels they will function.

As previously stated, NFPA 1670 is a technical rescue standard directed at the organization wishing to provide a rescue capability. What about individuals wishing to be qualified as rescuers within those disciplines? That is where NFPA 1006 steps in.

NFPA 1006 - Professional Qualifications for Rescue Technicians

Like NFPA 1670, NFPA 1006 deals with many different technical rescue disciplines. Unlike 1670, this standard deals with the job performance requirements for **individuals** (rather than organizations) wishing to be qualified for these disciplines. Another difference involves the lack of multiple levels of capability within NFPA 1006. At this time, the standard addresses only professional qualifications for rescuers at the Technician level. In other words, these are the minimum requirements to achieve the highest level of capability for an individual rescuer within a given discipline. In the future, the NFPA may consider creation of criteria for additional lower levels. For now, however, a rescuer may certify only as a Technician.

The disciplines listed in NFPA 1006 are similar to 1670:

- Rope Rescue
- Surface Water Rescue
- Vehicle and Machinery Rescues
- Confined Space Rescue
- Structural Collapse
- Trench Rescue

The list of disciplines in 1006 is not as exhaustive as those found in NFPA 1670, but future editions of the 1006 will probably expand.

Another important feature in the process of becoming a rescue technician for a particular discipline is the requirement for all technicians, whatever their discipline, to achieve an identical core of job performance requirements. This is sometimes referred to as "core plus one." The committee involved in development of this standard identified many common job performance requirements among rescuers of all disciplines. They then created a "core" of performance requirements within the document known simply as "Rescue Technician." These core requirements must be met first by any person wishing to become a technician in a specific discipline. For example, a person wishing to become a Rope Rescue technician must first complete the job performance requirements (JPRs) of Rescue Technician core and then complete those within the Rope Rescue Chapter. While the Rescue Technician core is common to all disciplines, it is important to note that it forms a prerequisite only, not a qualification in itself. There is no generic "Rescue Technician." There are only rescue technicians of a specific discipline or disciplines.

Questions and Answers from NFPA 1006

Since this text will be read mostly by individuals seeking to develop or improve upon their skills in various aspects of structural rope and confined space rescue, we will explore the NFPA 1006 document in greater detail than 1670. The authors have posed a series of questions concerning the standard that might accurately represent your questions. In answering these questions, we hope to provide a more thorough explanation of NFPA 1006 in its present form. Keep in mind that these explanations represent the opinions of the authors based on the information available and may not exactly match the thoughts of the NFPA committee. They should, however, accurately represent the general intent of the standard and therefore may be useful to you, the reader.

What is NFPA 1006?
NFPA 1006 establishes the minimum job performance requirements necessary for fire service and other emergency response personnel who perform technical rescue operations.

Is NFPA 1006 a team or individual standard?
NFPA 1006 is an individual standard. It specifies the minimum job performance requirements for service as a rescuer in an emergency response organization. NFPA 1670 addresses team requirements.

Does NFPA 1006 set a priority or order in which the requirements must be mastered?
No. The authority having jurisdiction is responsible for establishing the priority of instruction, along with the content of the training program, in preparing individuals to successfully meet the performance standards set by the standard.

Who is the "authority having jurisdiction" (AHJ)?
The "authority having jurisdiction" is defined as the organization, office, or individual responsible for approving equipment, an installation, or a procedure. The AHJ may be, for example, a fire chief or the management of an industrial plant.

Who evaluates the performance of the standard's requirements?
Performance of the requirements will be evaluated by individuals approved by the authority having jurisdiction.

The standard refers to the terms rules, regulations, procedures, supplies, apparatus, and equipment. What does this mean?
According to NFPA, these terms imply that it is the rules, regulations, procedures, supplies, apparatus, and equipment that are available to or used by the authority having jurisdiction. Therefore, they may vary from organization to organization.

Must an individual consider other NFPA standards or Occupational Safety and Health Association (OSHA) standards for the proper performance of each requirement?
To the extent such standards would otherwise be applicable, yes. For example, in a state where federal OSHA standards are not applicable to municipal departments, a municipal firefighter would not need to consider federal OSHA standards in the performance of the requirements.

Does NFPA supply its own definitions applicable to the standard, or do generally accepted definitions apply?

NFPA 1006 supplies its own definitions. These definitions contain some generally known terms, along with other definitions specific to the standard. Although the rescue terms are designed to meet the commonly accepted definitions, this does not rule out the possibility that definitions used in the standard might conflict with regionally accepted definitions of certain terms. Therefore, when preparing for evaluation, a candidate for testing should be familiar with the definitions found in the standard.

Do the performance requirements focus strictly on rescue techniques, such as building rope systems, or do they include ancillary skills, such as air monitoring or ventilation, which might be necessary in some situations?

NFPA 1006 assumes that such skills are necessary rescue skills rather than simply "ancillary" skills. Knowledge of such skills is necessary for the performance requirements.

What chapters of NFPA 1006 are applicable to confined space rescue?

Applicable chapters include Chapter 1 (Administration), Chapter 2 (Rescue Technician), Chapter 3 (Job Performance Requirements), Chapter 4 (Rope Rescue) and Chapter 7 (Confined Space Rescue). All of the knowledge and performance requirements found in these chapters must be mastered to attain the level of Confined Space Rescue Technician. Technically, only Chapter 3 (Job Performance Requirements) and Chapter 7 (Confined Space Rescue) need be completed for the confined space rescue portion. However, in reality, most of the skills found in Chapter 4 (Rope Rescue) should be mastered to perform rescues required for the Confined Space Rescue Specialty.

What requirements must be complied with before beginning training activities or performing rescues?

NFPA 1006 provides that a candidate must meet the following requirements:

- Age requirement established by the authority having jurisdiction.
- Medical requirements established by the authority having jurisdiction.
- Minimum physical fitness as required by the authority having jurisdiction.
- Emergency medical care performance capabilities for entry-level personnel as developed and validated by the authority having jurisdiction.
- Minimum educational requirements established by the authority having jurisdiction.

What are the minimum requirements for certification?

Minimally, the rescue technician must perform all of the job requirements from Chapter 3 (the core elements) and all job performance requirements in at least one of the specialty areas.

What areas do the core Job Performance Requirements cover?

The core job performance requirements assess the common knowledge and skills related to site operations, victim management, maintenance, and ropes/rigging.

What is included in "site operations?"

- Being able to identify the necessary resources for a rescue incident, including scene lighting, management of environmental concerns, personnel rehabilitation, and ensuring that the support operation helps the operational objectives of the rescue.
- Sizing up the rescue incident based on background information and reference materials to decide vital information such as the type of rescue, number of victims, and last known location of the victims.
- Managing the incident hazards. This involves reducing, isolating, or otherwise mitigating hazards inherent to the specialty being evaluated.
- Managing the resources that are being used in a rescue incident.

- Conducting a search of the incident scene to locate victims.
- Properly terminating the incident.

What is included in "victim management?"

- Assessing the victim.
- Basic life support stabilization of the victim.
- Triage of victims according to local protocol.
- Appropriate packaging of ill or injured victim(s) with basic equipment.
- Moving a victim in a low angle environment using transport equipment, litters, victim removal systems, or other specialized rescue equipment that are appropriate to the specific rescue environment.
- Transferring the victim to EMS according to local medical protocol. All pertinent information must be passed from the rescuer to the EMS provider.

What is included in the "maintenance" requirements?

- Inspecting and maintaining hazard-specific PPE clothing or equipment given for the protection of rescuers, including respiratory protection, cleaning and sanitation supplies, maintenance logs or records, tools and resources indicated by manufacturers for assembly or disassembly of components during repair or maintenance. Damage, defects and wear must be identified and reported or repaired as needed, equipment must function as designed, and preventive maintenance must be performed and documented consistent with manufacturers' recommendations.
- Inspecting and maintaining rescue equipment.

What is covered by the ropes/rigging portion of the Job Performance Requirements?

- Knot tying in rope and webbing. The knots must be properly dressed, recognizable, and safetied.
- Constructing a single point anchor system.
- Constructing a simple rope mechanical advantage system.
- Directing a team in the operation of a simple mechanical advantage system.
- Constructing a lowering system.
- Directing team in the operation of a lowering system.
- Constructing a safety line belay system.
- Operating a safety line belay system during a normal lowering or raising operation.
- Operating a safety line belay system to catch a falling load.
- Performing a system safety check as specified within the standard. This includes a visual, tactile, and verbal confirmation of all components in the system.

What is covered by the "Rope Rescue" specialty (discipline) area?

The Rope Rescue specialty area covers rope system skills necessary for performing rope rescue. Some of these skills involve rope rescue skills required for the "ropes/rigging" section of the Job Performance Requirements, while others are separate skills necessary for the specialty area.

What are the specific skill areas required for the "Rope Rescue" specialty?

- Constructing a multi-point anchor system.
- Constructing a compound rope mechanical advantage system.
- Constructing a fixed rope system, which is an anchored line that could be used for any number of purposes including rappelling.
- Directing the operation of a compound rope mechanical advantage system.
- Completing an assignment while suspended from a rope rescue system.
- Moving a victim in a high angle or vertical environment. This simply involves moving the victim from one place to another with the rope system.
- Directing a team in the construction of a high line system. High lines are rope systems designed to move victims or rescuers across expanses. There are sometimes necessary when negotiating wide open areas (such as ravines) or getting over obstacles present

on the ground. These systems may run between two points of equal height or between points of different heights (diagonally). Highlines are seldom required in the structural/industrial environments because these needs can generally be met with a combination of lowering systems and tag lines. For this reason, Highline methods are not described in this text.

- Directing a team in the operation of a high line system as a member of the team.
- Ascending a fixed rope. This may be as simple as using Prusik hitches to ascend an anchored rope for self-rescue or as complex as using mechanical ascent devices to climb out of a pit. NFPA does not require a certain ascent height or system but does set forth requirements that would prevent injury if the person were to lose control of the ascent. They simply require ascent of a fixed rope.
- Descending a fixed rope. Again, the distance or system used is not dictated, but safety requirements are.

What is covered by the "confined space rescue" specialty?

The confined space rescue specialty area covers skills and knowledge necessary for safely assessing confined spaces and performing rescue from confined spaces.

What are some items specifically addressed by the "confined space rescue" specialty?

- Completing a confined space rescue preplan in accordance with local, state, and federal guidelines and a preplan form.
- Assessing the incident given a preplan of the space and/or size-up information.
- Controlling hazards specific to the incident.
- Preparing for entry into a confined space.
- Entering into a confined space.
- Properly packaging the victim for removal from a confined space.
- Removing the victim and rescuers from confined spaces with internal entanglement hazards and converging walls.
- Controlling access to the confined space during the termination phase of the incident.
- Continued monitoring of the space as required.

The NFPA, A True Consensus

Perhaps the most interesting aspect of any consensus standard deals with its creation. They are developed through a "consensus" of input from people considered knowledgeable in the field for which the standard is being written. This means that the group of people agreed (for the most part) on the end result. NFPA committee members go through a rigorous application and screening process and are selected based on their proven knowledge and experience in a given area. The result is a compilation of efforts by those often considered leaders in their chosen fields of expertise. The product created by such a grouping of "experts" might be suitable for most recipients of the standards. However, NFPA takes this process a step further by encouraging input from the general public during various stages of the standard's development. This ensures a consensus both of the committee members chosen to develop the standard and of any person wishing to have input. This makes NFPA standards valuable tools for organizations seeking safe and effective methods for providing a rescue capability.

Summary

There are many other consensus standards that may be helpful to organizations and individuals wishing to develop or improve the quality of their rescue capability. Standards such as those produced by the American National Standards Institute (ANSI) and the American Society for Testing and Materials (ASTM) are as valuable as the NFPA and are often referenced within laws and even other consensus standards. The Society of Professional Rope Access Technicians (SPRAT) has completed a standard for those workers using ropes to position themselves for specialty work, such as window cleaning and bridge inspection. Consensus standards such as the NFPA, ASTM, SPRAT, and ANSI are dedicated to improving the quality of operations and the overall safety of rescuers and victims in situations that would otherwise prove extremely hazardous. It should be our goal as rescuers to seek out and use any guideline that can make our operations safer and more efficient.

APPENDIX A

Confined Space Rescue Regulations Information

The following are excerpts from ***OSHA's Compliance Directive*** *for Permit-Required Confined Spaces. This does not include the entire document. Readers are encouraged to review the document in its entirety.*

OSHA Instruction CPL 2.100 / Directorate of Compliance Programs
APPENDIX D: "PRCS Program Evaluation Considerations"

I. INITIAL INFORMATION

C. Evaluate the process by which the employer identified any permit spaces, as follows:

3. Analyze the evaluation method and equipment used.

a. Was the determination made based upon historical data? If so, how reliable is that data?

b. Were the substance's hazards appropriately identified and evaluated to comply with paragraph (d)(2) of the standard? All the hazards that can affect the safety and health of entrants must be determined; e.g., gasoline is flammable but also contains benzene, which can be a health hazard.

c. Were the sampling methods and / or testing equipment appropriate for each substance?

d. Are mechanical and other non-atmospheric hazards, for the space or for the work to be performed in the space, addressed in the employer's evaluation method?

4. If the employer has arranged to have some other party (consultant or insurance carrier) evaluate the workplace, request a copy of the report presented to the employer in order to assess the adequacy of the evaluation.

D. Are contractors performing permit space entries? If so, determine who they are and their work location.

1. Are these spaces multi-employer worksites?

2. Did the contractor develop the permit space program in use? If not, whose program is being used or followed by the contractor? If so, how was their program coordinated with the host employer's PRCS program?

3. What measures have the employers taken to facilitate coordination and safety for multi-employer worksites? Examples of these measures might be communications systems, postings, assignments of liaison personnel, or contractual agreements.

II. TRAINING

A. Employees:

1. What is the employer's policy with regard to employee entry referenced in paragraph (c)(2), and how are the employees informed of the policy?

2. How are the affected employees referenced in paragraph (g)(2) identified? Who are they?

3. How are the affected employees informed of the employer's policies on permit space entry?

4. How and when are new or reassigned employees informed of the existence and locations of permit spaces?

5. Is the employer's PRCS program used in employee training?

B. The trainer:

1. Who are the individuals conducting the training, and what training are they providing?

2. For the training being presented, is the trainer knowledgeable about the subject matter in general and with the particular permit space situations at the workplace?

C. The employer:
1. How does the employer verify that the training has been provided?
2. How does the employer evaluate employee proficiency in the duties required by the permit space program?
3. What criteria does the employer use to decide if re-training is necessary?

V. RESCUE

Review the employer's policy to determine which rescue procedures are being employed. If non-entry rescue has been ruled out, ascertain which of the entry rescue options has been implemented.

A. Non-entry rescue:
1. If non-entry rescue is being practiced, what equipment is used?
2. If non-entry rescue is not being practiced, what are the employer's reasons for not using it?
3. Does the employer review each space to be entered to determine whether to employ or not to employ non-entry rescue?

B. On-site rescue services: (A host employer's own employees)
1. Determine the number of employees assigned to perform rescue, verify training for each member of the rescue service, and find out which of them have a current first-aid and cardiopulmonary resuscitation (CPR) certification.
2. Review the rescue procedures as they compare with the written PRCS program, and with the requirements of paragraph (k)(1).
3. Note the work shifts of the rescuers and compare them to the permit entry times.

C. Non-host employer rescue employees (off-site):
1. Who provides the off-site rescue service and where is the service located?
2. How is the arrangement between the employer and the off-site rescue service documented (contract, letter of agreement, verbal agreement)?
3. How does the employer decide, given the identified permit-space hazards, that the off-site rescue service's response time, experience, and training are adequate?
4. Have the rescue service training requirements in paragraph (k)(1) been met?
5. What method is used to summon rescuers?
6. Are rescue services on-call or on-site when permit space entry is underway?
7. What is the response time for the rescue service?
8. How does the employer verify that the rescue service will be available during the time of employee entry?

D. Combinations:
1. If combination of on-site and off-site rescue services is employed:
   a. Obtain a copy of the rescue plan which describes the roles of each party, and
   b. Verify that the on-site and off-site rescue services employees have trained together as a team.
   c. Determine if the combined rescue services enable the employer to comply with the requirements for rescue services.

Excerpts from:
APPENDIX E: "Questions and Answers for PRCS Standard Clarification"

Section (a) - Scope and Application

7. **Must an employer covered by an industry-specific standard perform the initial workplace evaluation required by 1910.146 (c)(1)?**
   Yes. Employers with spaces covered by a specific industry standard must still determine if they have spaces which would qualify as a permit space not covered by the industry specific standard. Therefore, all employers must do an initial evaluation under 1910.146 (c)(1).

Section (b) - Definitions

1. **Under what circumstances will stairs or ladders constitute a limited or restricted means of egress under the standard?**
   Ladders, and temporary, movable, spiral, or articulated stairs will usually be considered a limited or restricted means of egress. Fixed industrial stairs that meet OSHA standards will be considered a limited or restricted means of egress when the conditions or physical characteristics of the space, in light of the hazards present in it, would interfere with the entrant's ability to exit or be rescued in a hazardous situation.
2. **Does the fact that a space has a door mean that the space does not have limited or restricted means of entry or exit and, therefore, is not a "confined space"?**
   A space has limited or restricted means of entry or exit if an entrant's ability to escape in an emergency would be hindered. The dimensions of a door and its location are factors in determining whether an entrant can easily escape; however, the presence of a door does not in and of itself mean that the space is not a confined space. For example, a space such as a bag house or crawl space that has a door leading into it, but also has pipes, conduits, ducts, or equipment or materials that an employee would be required to crawl over or under or squeeze around in order to escape, has limited or restricted means of exit. A piece of equipment with an access door, such as a conveyor feed, a drying oven, or a paint spray enclosure, will also be considered to have restricted means of entry or exit if an employee has to crawl to gain access to his or her intended work location. Similarly, an access door or portal which is too small to allow an employee to walk upright and unimpeded through it will be considered to restrict an employee's ability to escape. OSHA published a technical amendment to the preamble in Federal Register / Vol. 59, No. 213 / Friday, November 4, 1994, page 55208.
3. **Can the distance an employee must travel in a space such as a tunnel, to reach a point of safety be a determinant for classifying a space as a confined space?**
   Yes. The determination would most likely be a function of the time of travel to the point of safety.
4. **How will OSHA assess a space which is entirely open on one plane, such as a pit, in determining whether a space has limited or restricted means for entry or exit?**
   In determining whether a space has limited or restricted means for entry or exit, OSHA will evaluate its overall characteristics to determine if an entrant's ability to escape in an emergency would be hindered. Thus, a pit, shaft or tank that is entirely open on one plane can be considered a confined space if the means for entering the space (stairway, ladderway, etc.) are narrow or twisted, or otherwise configured in such a way as to hinder an entrant's ability to quickly escape (See question No. 1 of this section). Similarly, the pit, shaft, or tank itself may be confining because of the presence of pipes, ducts, baffles, equipment or other factors which would hinder an entrant's ability to escape.
6. **How will OSHA address a space that does satisfy the criteria for a confined space but that potentially contains a hazardous atmosphere?**
   Employers must comply with the permissible exposure limits and other requirements contained in standards addressing specific toxic substances and air contaminants, to the extent applicable, in all spaces in which employees may be present. In addition, the respiratory protection standard, 29CFR 1910.134, applies where an employee must enter a space in which a hazardous atmosphere may be present and no other specific standard applies. The respiratory protection standard contains special precautions for working in atmospheres that are oxygen deficient or immediately dangerous to life or health.
7. **Are the hazards posed by a confined space to be considered in determining whether a space meets the definition of a confined space?**

The determination whether a space has "limited or restricted means for entry or exit" within the meaning of the standard's definition of "confined space" should include consideration of whether, in light of the hazards posed by the particular space at issue, the configuration or other characteristics of the space would interfere with an entrant's ability to escape or be rescued in an emergency situation.

8. **Can a space that is initially designed for continuous human occupancy become a "confined space" because of changes in its use?**
   If the changes alter the character of the space or if new or more serious hazards are introduced, those changes require reevaluation of whether the space is fit for continuous employee occupancy. If the space is not fit for continuous employee occupancy and the other criteria of the confined space definition are met, the space should be reclassified as a confined space.
9. **Does the characteristic "contains or has a potential to contain a hazardous atmosphere" in the definition of "permit-required confined space" refer only to those atmospheres which pose an acute hazard?**
   Where employees are exposed to atmospheric or toxic hazards which do not present an immediate danger of death or disability that would render the employee unable to escape from the confined space, e.g., air contaminants which as arsenic or asbestos, OSHA's health standards for those hazards apply rather than 1910.146, and employees must be appropriately protected in accordance with those health standards. The PRCS standard is intended to protect entrants against short-term, acute hazards (not exposures at or below the permissible exposure limits); other standards address a broader range of health and safety concerns.
   As noted in the definition of "hazardous atmosphere" relating to atmospheric concentration of any substance for which a dose or permissible exposure limit is published in Subparts "G" and "Z", any substance that is not capable of causing death, incapacitation, impairment of ability to self-rescue, injury, or acute illness due to health effects is not covered by the PRCS standard.
10. **The definition of permit-required confined space contains the phrase "any other recognized serious safety and health hazard" as one of its hazard characteristics which would result in a confined space being classified as a permit space. The "Types of Hazards" listing in the Confined Space Hazards section of OSHA's Confined Space Entry Course No. 226 identifies hazards. Does the mere presence of a non-specified hazard such as physical hazards (e.g. grinding, agitators, steam, mulching, falling / tripping, other moving parts); corrosive chemical hazards; biological hazards; and other hazards (i.e. electrical, rodents, snakes, spiders, poor visibility, wind, weather, or insecure footing), which do not pose an immediate danger to life or health or impairment of an employee's ability to escape from the space, constitute a hazard which would involve this characteristic?**
    When a hazard in a confined space is immediately dangerous to life or health, the "permit space" classification is triggered. The list referenced above is only illustrative of the general range of confined space hazards which could, but not necessarily always, constitute a hazard which would present an immediate danger to life or health, such that "permit space" protection would be required. The determination of whether the resulting exposure to a hazard in a confined space will impair the employee's ability to perform self-rescue is the aspect that must be addressed by the employer.
    In order for "serious safety and health hazard" to be recognized as being an impairment to escape, its severity potential for resulting physical harm to an employee must be considered.

Section (c) - General Requirements

1. **Are employers covered by the PRCS standard in violation of paragraph (c)(1) of the standard if they have not evaluated their workplace to determine if any permit-required confined spaces?**

Yes. As of the effective date of the standard (April 15, 1993), employers were required to evaluate their workplace to determine if any spaces were permit-required confined spaces. Employers who have not performed the evaluation would be in violation of paragraph (c)(1) unless the workplace does not and could not contain **any** confined spaces.

13. **What are the employer's responsibilities in multi-employer permit space entries?**
Coordination between employers who have employees entering a particular permit space is required by 1910.146 (c)(8)(iv), (c)(9)(ii) and (d)(11). The host employer who arranges for a permit space entry by contractor employees has a duty to instruct the contractor on the hazards or potential hazards and other factors that make the space a permit space. The contractor who will have employees enter the permit space is responsible for obtaining that information prior to entry. All employers who will have employees in the permit space are responsible for developing and implementing procedures to coordinate entry operations (for example, determining operation control over the space, affected employee training, rescue, emergency services, and all other aspects of the standard requiring coordination). Any one of the employers having employees enter the permit space could have operational control over the permit space during dual entry. There should be absolutely no doubt, by any permit space entrant, attendant, and entry supervisor regarding who the controlling employer is and whose policy and permit space practices are to be followed.

Section (h) - Duties of Authorized Entrants

1. **Can an employee be both an Entry Supervisor and Authorized Entrant for an entry?**
The standard allows an employee to be both an entry supervisor and entrant as long as the employee has had the appropriate training and the duties of one activity do not conflict with the duties of the other.

Section (i) - Duties of Attendants

1. **When a single attendant is monitoring more than one permit space, is there a limit on how far the attendant can be from any of the spaces monitored?**
The bench mark for monitoring multiple spaces by a single attendant is his / her ability to perform **all** their (attendant) duties without compromising the safety of **any** entrants in **all** the permit spaces being monitored by the attendant. There is no minimum proximity requirement.

Section (j) - Duties of Entry Supervisor(s)

1. **Does an employer have to verify the availability of the off-site rescue service each time a permit space entry is scheduled or attempted?**
Yes, the employer has overall responsibility for employee safety. If the off-site rescue services indicates, for any reason, that it would be unable to respond to a rescue summons, entry shall not be authorized unless an adequate alternative rescue service is arranged.

Section (k) - Rescue Service

1. **Does an off-site rescue service have to have a permit space program?**
No, a complete program is not necessary. However, rescue plans and procedures are necessary. Rescue services (on-site and off-site) are required by paragraph (k) to have members who are trained, equipped, and practiced for safe entry into the particular permit spaces from which they will be expected to rescue entrants.
2. **What is OSHA policy on "horizontal" non-entry rescue?**
When practical, non-entry rescue is required by paragraph (k)(3) of the standard and is the preferred method of rescue, even for horizontal entries. OSHA recognizes that the danger of entanglement due to lifelines or lanyards snagging or

obstructions within a permit space may be greater for horizontal permit spaces than for vertical spaces.

3. **Would a rescuer entering an Immediately Dangerous to Life and Health (IDLH) atmosphere using a supplied-air respirator in combination with SCBA (escape bottle), be in violation of OSHA regulations?**

Yes, however, under the conditions addressed below, the violation can be considered as *de minimis*.

The PRCS standard, because of its performance nature, does not specify the personal protective or rescue equipment necessary for rescue. The OSHA standard for respiratory protection is 1910.134. Currently paragraph 1910.134(e)(3)(iii) requires, when an IDLH atmosphere exists, ... A stand-by man or men with suitable self-contained breathing apparatus shall be at the nearest fresh air base for emergency rescue.

The 1910.134 standard published in the June 27, 1974, issue of the Federal Register was derived from a now out-of-date voluntary standard (ANSI consensus standard Z88.2-1969). The most recent (1992) version of this same standard for respiratory protection for working in IDLH conditions has been changed. The new change specifies either a SCBA or a combination supplied-air respirator with SCBA for IDLH conditions.

It is OSHA policy to accept compliance with a provision in a current national consensus standard (ANSI) that provides an equivalent or greater level of protection from the hazards.

A rescue service can employ the use of supplied-air respirators in combination with self-contained breathing apparatus (SCBA) when conducting rescue operations. If a rescue service employer chooses to use combination supplied-air respirator with SCBA over the SCBA specified in the respiratory protection standard 1910.134(e)(3)(iii), for permit-required confined space rescue, the violation will be considered as *de minimis* as long as the following minimum conditions are also employed:

1. An evaluation of the permit space to be entered has been done to determine which appropriate respiratory protection (SCBA or Supplied-air with SCBA) is best suited for the rescue.
2. The rescuer's respirators and air source meet the requirements of the 1910.134 standard.
3. The air source for the rescuer's respiratory protection is independent from that which is being used by the authorized entrants.

We also would recommend the following policies and work practices for the rescue services which choose the supplied-air respirators with SCBA option:

a. Establish a policy requiring immediate withdrawal from the space whenever a respiratory protection problem develops.
b. Establish a policy for use and training on emergency air line sharing "buddy breathing."
c. Ensure that the rescuers wear full-body harness and use life lines whenever practical.
d. Establish a policy requiring a minimum capacity of the source air to be twice (2X) the volume of the total needs of all rescuers connected to it for the anticipated duration of the rescuer's entry.
e. Establish a policy which mandates a minimum team of two rescuers for all permit space rescue entries.

AN OVERVIEW OF ANSI Z117.1-1989 "American National Standard Safety Requirements for Confined Spaces"

The following is an overview of ANSI Z117.1-1989 and concentrates on rescue aspects of the standard only. Some portions have been paraphrased. It is recommended that the entire ANSI document be thoroughly examined.

AMERICAN NATIONAL STANDARD Z117.1-1989:

DEFINITIONS:

Attendant: A person who is assigned as standby to monitor a confined space process or operation and provide support or react as required.

Confined Space: An enclosed area that has the following characteristics:

(a) its primary function is something other than human occupancy.

(b) has restricted entry and exit.

(c) may contain potential or known hazards.

Examples of confined spaces include but are not limited to:

Tanks, Silos, Vessels, Pits, Sewers, Pipelines, Tank Cars, Boilers, Septic Tanks, and Utility Vaults.

Tanks and other structures under construction may not be considered confined spaces until completely closed.

Restricted entry and exit means physical impediment of the body, e.g., use of the hands or a contortion of the body to enter into or exit from the confined space.

Entry: Ingress by persons into a confined space which occurs upon breaking the plane of the confined space portal with his / her face; and all periods of time in which the confined space is occupied.

Permit Required Confined Space: A confined space which after evaluation has actual or potential hazards which have been determined to require written authorization for entry.

Qualified Person: A person who by reason of training, education and experience is knowledgeable in the operation to be performed and is competent to judge the hazards involved.

Shall: Denotes a mandatory requirement.

Should: A recommendation that is a sound safety and health practice; it does not denote a mandatory requirement.

IDENTIFICATION AND EVALUATION

3.1 Confined Space Survey. A survey shall be conducted of the premises, or operations, or both to identify confined spaces as defined in this standard. The survey shall be conducted by a qualified person.

NOTE: The purpose of the survey is to develop an inventory of those locations or equipment, or both, which meet the definition of a confined space so that personnel may be made aware of them and appropriate procedures developed for each prior to entry.

3.4 Confined Space Classification. Based on the evaluation of the hazards, a qualified person shall classify the confined space as either a permit-required confined space (PRCS) or non-permit confined space (NPCS).

5.0 Permit Required Confined Spaces (PRCS)

5.1 Entry Permits. A permit shall be established for all PRCS entries. This document shall include:

. . . 5.1.6 the type of equipment which will be necessary for a rescue and how aid will be summoned in the event of an emergency . . .

12.0 Safeguards

12.2 Retrieval Equipment. Appropriate retrieval equipment or methods shall be used whenever a person enters a PRCS. Exception: If the retrieval equipment increases the overall risks of entry or does not contribute to the rescue, its use may be waived.

NOTE: The type of retrieval equipment required is dependent on the specific circumstances. Consideration should be given to the size and location of the opening to the space, obstacles within the space, number of occupants, type of retrieval equipment, and whether or not the rescue would be vertical or horizontal.

12.2.1 A mechanical device shall be available to retrieve personnel from vertical type PRCS's greater than five feet in depth.

NOTE: In general, mechanical lifting devices should have a mechanical advantage adequate to safely rescue personnel.

14.0 Emergency Response

14.1 Emergency Response Plan. A plan of action shall be written with provisions to conduct a timely rescue for individuals in a confined space should an emergency arise.

NOTE: These rescue provisions will normally be present in the form of emergency response procedures.

Included in these provisions shall be:

14.1.1 determination of what methods of rescue must be implemented to retrieve individuals;

NOTE: A review should be conducted of all the different types of confined spaces which will be entered and what steps / equipment it will take to get someone out. Consideration should be given to the size and configuration of the confined space and the body size of entering personnel.

14.1.2 designation of rescue personnel that are immediately available where PRCS entries are conducted;

NOTE: Off-site emergency response personnel may be used provided they are capable of performing a rescue, are familiar with the premises, and can respond in a timely manner. Emergency treatment should generally begin within four minutes for a person with cardio 365 365

pulmonary arrest. If outside emergency organizations are to be used as rescuers, these organizations should be involved in rescue procedure development and drills.

14.1.3 type and availability of equipment needed to rescue individuals;

NOTE: Harnesses, lifelines, and mechanical lifting devices (for vertical entries) are normally required. Breathing equipment and medical aid equipment may also be necessary. Consideration should also be given to what type of lighting would be used in the confined space, communication devices, and any other special equipment which might be used for rescue.

14.1.4 an effective means to summon rescuers in a timely manner;

NOTE: Audible alarms, two-way radios, telephones, etc., are some of the possible means of summoning aid and rescue personnel. Consideration will be given to providing occupants a method of informing the attendant that there is an emergency.

14.1.5 training and drill of the attendant and rescue personnel in preplanning, rescue and emergency procedures according to section 15 of this standard.

14.2 Breathing Equipment. All rescue personnel must use self-contained breathing apparatus (SCBA) or Combination Type C Airline / SCBA breathing equipment, when entering the confined space to rescue victims.

If it is established that the cause of the emergency is not a hazardous atmosphere, rescue breathing equipment is not required.

NOTE: In some instances the entrance to the confined space may be such that an SCBA unit on the rescuer will not fit through the opening of the confined space. This should have been pre-determined in hazard identification and evaluation or drills. In this event, the rescuer may be required to use Combination Type C Airline / SCBA type breathing equipment.

14.3 Rescue Equipment Inspection. All rescue equipment shall be inspected periodically by a qualified person and prior to start of work to ensure that it is operable.

NOTE: Rescue equipment which is taken out of service should be replaced with similar equipment.

15.0 Training

15.1 General Requirements. Personnel responsible for supervising, planning, entering or participating in confined space entry and rescue shall be adequately trained in their functional duties prior to any confined space entry . . .

NOTE: Training, whether basic or advanced, formal or informal, should be commensurate with the complexity of the confined space entry requirements.

15.4 Training for Emergency Response Personnel. Training shall include:

15.4.1 the rescue plan and procedures developed for each type of confined space they are anticipated to encounter;

NOTE: Emergency response personnel should simulate actual rescue conditions by conducting practice drills. Rescuers should be timed to determine if adequate time was allotted for successful cardiopulmonary resuscitation (CPR) and first-aid techniques.

Typical potential rescue problems which should be addressed are egress restriction, ability to lift without injury, problems in using rescue equipment, and fall hazards.

15.4.2 use of emergency rescue equipment;

NOTE: Individuals involved in rescues should receive training in the use of rescue equipment including medical equipment they would be expected to use or operate during an emergency rescue.

15.4.3 first aid and cardiopulmonary resuscitation (CPR) techniques;

NOTE: Persons performing CPR or first aid or both, should possess current certification.

15.4.4 work location and confined space configuration to minimize response time.

NOTE: Rescuers should be able to effectively locate the emergency site without undue delay.

15.5 Verification of Training

15.5.1 Periodic assessment of the effectiveness of employee training shall be conducted by a qualified person.

NOTE: Training effectiveness may be evaluated by several techniques. Written, as well as practical testing, is recommended. Personnel should be questioned or asked to demonstrate their practical knowledge of confined space hazards that are in their work areas, to identify locations of confined spaces, their role in exercising proper permit procedures, use and donning of personal protective equipment, such as respirators, and their role in response to emergency situations.

15.5.2 Training sessions shall be repeated as often as necessary to maintain an acceptable level of personnel competence.

NOTE: Personnel who are routinely entering the same confined spaces on a daily basis will require less refresher training than employees who only occasionally enter a confined space. Periodic training verification will determine the frequency of refresher training.

NOTE: Documentation should be maintained in a central location and periodically reviewed to ensure proper follow-up for refresher training.

16.0 Medical Suitability. The physical and psychological suitability of persons to do confined space work shall be considered prior to working in confined spaces.

NOTE: Since confined space entry work may require the use of respiratory protection, possible exposure to various physical stresses such as thermal, humidity, noise, vibration, etc., and psychological stresses such as claustrophobia, and vertigo; these concerns need to be addressed by a physician or other licensed medical practitioner. Physical qualifications for respirator use are contained in ANSI Z88.6.

The physical and psychological capabilities of potential candidates for confined space work can be evaluated during training exercises for the confined space work.

17.0 Contractors

17.2 Identification of Rescue Responder. The employer and contractor shall establish who will serve as the rescue responder in an emergency and what system will be used to notify the responder that an emergency exists.

NOTE: Pre-planning should be conducted between the contractor and the employer to establish who will be responsible to perform rescue and provide medical services in the event of an emergency situation. If the contractor expects to use the employer's rescue capability, this should be agreed upon before the entry and the method of contacting the rescue responder established.

Glossary

Access The nature of the passage through, or the approach to, a specific confined space portal. 1. The passage (through the portal) refers to the angle of entry into the space, either vertical or horizontal. 2. The approach (to the portal) refers to the portal's elevation as it relates to grade.

Accessory Cord Small diameter rope, usually of kernmantle construction, used in a variety of techniques including self- rescue and in creating Prusik Loops.

Action Plan A written plan that describes basic mechanisms and structures a rescue response agency will use to mobilize resources and conduct activities in managing a specific anticipated rescue emergency.

Air Supply Officer The person within the Incident Management structure responsible for evaluating and coordinating fresh-air breathing apparatus supply resources on the scene of an emergency.

Anchor See Anchor Point

Anchor Point A single structural component used either alone or in combination with others to create an anchor system that can sustain the actual or potential load on the rope rescue system.

Anchor Strap A prefabricated rope system component of fixed or variable length designed to secure system components to each other or around anchor structures. It usually consists of webbing of varying lengths with ends sewn into loops, or to buckles or rings, that provide ease of attachment to other rope system components.

Anchor System One or more anchor points rigged in a way to provide a structurally significant connection point for rope rescue system components.

American National Standards Institute (ANSI) Serves as a clearinghouse for nationally coordinated voluntary safety, engineering, and industrial consensus standards developed by trade associations, industrial firms, technical societies, consumer organizations, and government agencies.

Ascender (ascent Device) An auxiliary equipment system component, a friction or mechanical device used alone or in combination to allow a person to ascend a fixed line.

Ascending (line) A means of traveling up a fixed line with the use of one or more ascent devices.

Assessment An appraisal of the circumstances or conditions concerning a specific matter.

American Society for Testing and Materials (ASTM) A consensus standards-making organization responsible for developing many currently used procedural documents including materials testing and safe operations. Many of these documents are cited as requirements within other laws and standards.

Atmospheric Monitoring The use of specialized equipment to assess the atmospheric conditions within a given area. The assessment may include (but not limited to) oxygen content, flammability, toxicity, and ambient temperature.

Attendant (Rescue Attendant) The U.S. federally regulated industrial workers who are qualified to be stationed outside one or more confined spaces, who monitor authorized entrants, and who perform all of the following duties: 1. remain outside the confined space during entry operations until relieved by another attendant, 2. summon rescue and other needed resources as soon as the attendant finds that authorized entrants might need assistance to escape from confined space hazards, and 3. perform non-entry rescues as specified by the rescue procedure listed on the permit (*See Entry Permit*). This term can also be used to designate rescue personnel assigned to perform the task of attendant during rescue operations involving entry-type rescue. In this case, the term "Rescue Attendant" is used.

Authorized Entrant A worker designated and authorized by the authority having jurisdiction to enter a specific confined space.

Awareness Level The National Fire Protection Association (1670—Standard on Operation and Training for Technical Rescue Incidents) term that describes the minimum operational capability by a response agency that, in the course of regular job duties, could be called upon to respond to, or could be the first on the scene, of a technical rescue incident. This level can involve search, rescue, and recovery operations. Members of a team at this level are generally not considered rescuers, but are trained to recognize hazards and contact additional needed resources.

Back-up Any component or system that provides a reserve safety mechanism in case of a malfunction of the primary component or system.

Basket Litter A transportation device designed for use with rope rescue systems, shaped as an oblong basket large enough to hold a sick or injured person.

Belay The method by which a potential fall distance is controlled to minimize damage to equipment and/or injury to a live load.

Bend A knot that joins two ropes or webbing pieces together.

Bight The open loop in a rope or piece of webbing formed when it is doubled back on itself.

Block and Tackle A form of simple mechanical advantage system constructed of a single rope reeved through a series of pulleys.

Bombproof A term used to refer to a single anchor point capable of sustaining the actual or potential forces exerted on the rope rescue system without possibility of failure.

Bottom Belay A maneuver in which a person at the bottom of a rope pulls down on the rope as someone is descending. This creates additional friction on the descent control device to slow or stop the person's descent.

Brake Bar Rack A type of descent control device that uses rope threaded through a series of metal bars to create friction capable of controlling the rate of descent.

Brakeman The person responsible for operation of a descent control device during a lowering operation with a rope rescue system.

Breathing Air System The system used to provide appropriate respiratory protection to personnel working within an area that contains an actual or potential respiratory hazard.

Bridle A harness, usually constructed of rope and/or webbing, used to connect certain rescue system components. The term usually refers to a bridle used for connection of a litter to a rope rescue system.

BTLS Acronym for Basic Trauma Life Support, a course of study specializing in assessment and management of traumatic injuries.

Buddy System The use of a partner to provide a safeguard when working within hazardous or potentially hazardous areas.

Cam An offset wheel mounted on a rotating shaft used to produce variable or reciprocating motion in another engaged or contacted part. Sometimes used to describe a rope grab device used in a rope rescue system such as a rope/pulley mechanical advantage system.

Carabiner An oval or D-shaped metal, load-bearing connector with a self-closing gate, used to join components of a rope system.

Closed-circuit SCBA A type of breathing apparatus that recycles the wearer's exhalations after carbon dioxide and moisture are removed through a filtration process.

Command Structure See Incident Command System

Communications Officer The person within the Incident Management structure responsible for evaluating and ensuring communications on the scene of an emergency such as a confined space rescue.

Complex M/A A rope mechanical advantage system created by incorporating a portion of one simple or compound rope/pulley mechanical advantage system within a portion of at least one other simple or compound system. This is different from the stacking effect characteristic of a compound rope/pulley mechanical advantage system.

Compliance The act of complying with a wish, request, or demand.

Compound M/A A rope/pulley mechanical advantage system created by stacking the load end of one rope mechanical advantage system onto the haul line of another, or others, to multiply the forces created by the individual system(s).

Confined Space By OSHA definition, a space that is large enough and so configured that a person can enter and perform assigned work, and has limited or restricted means for entry or exit (for example: tanks, vessels, silos, storage bins, hoppers, vaults, and pits), and is not designed for continuous human occupancy. See additional notes pertaining specifically to the National Fire Protection Association's definitions under Permit-required Confined Space.

Confined Space Rescue The removal of a live entrapped, sick, or injured person from a confined space or Permit-required confined space.

Confined Space Survey The OSHA general industry requirement of an employer to survey their facility to determine where Permit- spaces exist, identify them appropriately by physically marking them, and educate their employees of their location.

Controlled Breathing A breathing technique that creates efficient use of existing fresh-air supply when performing normal work functions and wearing fresh-air breathing apparatus.

Critical Incident Stress Management The management of psychological trauma resulting from a person's involvement in an emergency incident operation.

De mnimis A legal term commonly used to refer to violations of law considered small or trifling. The Occupational Safety and Health Administration defines de minimis violations as those that violate a standard not immediately or directly related to an employee's safety or health. OSHA further clarifies that a de minimis violation carries no penalty, need not be abated, and cannot be used as evidence of a history of violations for purposes of penalty assessments for future violations.

Debriefing A session held following an emergency incident to critically analyze all conditions and actions taken in the management of that emergency. The purpose is to determine effectiveness of operations and how to improve them when managing similar incidents in the future.

Decontamination To make safe by eliminating poisonous or otherwise harmful substances, such as noxious chemicals or radioactive material.

Descent Control See Descent Control Device

Descent Control Device A friction or mechanical device used with rope to control the descent of a load.

Directional Any method or component used to redirect the path of a rope or rope system (such as a directional pulley).

D-Ring A metal load-bearing connector shaped like a "D" used as an attachment point in rope rescue systems.

Dynamic Rope A rope designed to have significant elongation properties that provide a degree of shock absorption when used in rope systems where a likelihood of falls exist.

Elevated Rescue A rescue of a victim from heights where normal means of egress are not available.

Emergency By-pass Breathing An emergency technique for use with self-contained breathing apparatus, intended for situations where normal regulator function is impaired and the regulator must be by-passed in order to breathe from the unit.

Emergency Response Procedures See Action Plan.

Emergency Response Rescue Plan See Action Plan.

Emergency Skip Breathing An emergency breathing technique intended to create maximum conservation of existing fresh-air supply with self-contained breathing apparatus.

Entrant See Authorized Entrant

Entry Includes ensuing work activities in a space. It is considered to have occurred as soon as any part of the entrants body breaks the plane of an opening into the space.

Entry Permit A written or printed document, established by an employer in applicable U.S. Federally regulated industrial facilities for non-rescue entry into confined spaces, which authorizes specific employees to enter a confined space and contains specific information as required.

Evacuate To withdraw from a threatened area.

Fall Arrest Stopping a fall.

Fall Factor A calculation used to estimate the impact forces on a rope subjected to stopping a falling person. It is expressed as a ratio that indicates the relation between rope length and the distance the person falls.

Fall Protection Methods, equipment, and/or systems used to prevent (or render survivable) falls from heights.

Figure 8 Descender A descent control device shaped like an offset "8" that may be used for rappelling and lowering. A large ring on one end of the device is affixed to rope in a configuration to create friction. The small ring on the opposite end of the device may be used to attach to a harness or anchor system.

Figure-8 Weave A specific lashing configuration for securing a person to a long spine immobilizer.

Flexible Litter A transportation device made of flexible materials and designed to wrap around a person to create a secure litter. These devices usually gain rigidity once they have been applied in the manner intended by the manufacturer.

Full Body Harness An arrangement of materials secured around a person's waist, around thighs or under buttocks, and over shoulders. It is used to support them when performing work or rescue suspended from a rope, cable or other system.

General Use A National Fire Protection Association (NFPA) 1983 standard term meant to imply a particular equipment component or system is suitable to support two-person (600 lb.) loads.

Hard Link A term sometimes used to describe a potentially dangerous non-flexible attachment of components within a rope rescue system.

Haul Cam Term referring to a metal rope grab device used within a hauling system that grabs and moves a rope when the system is activated.

Haul/Lower Team Rescuers who lift or lower a victim.

Hauling Pulling or dragging forcibly; tugging.

Hazard Reduction The control or abatement of specific hazards within a given area.

Hazardous Material A substance (solid, liquid, or gas) that, when released, is capable of creating harm to people, environment and property.

HAZWOPER An acronym that refers to the OSHA Hazardous Waste Operations and Emergency Response standard (29CFR1910.120).

High Point Anchor A point of attachment for a rope rescue system or component elevated above the level of a given object or area.

Hitch A knot that attaches to or wraps around an object. When the object is removed, the knot will fall apart.

Inchworm Confined Space System A specific rope rescue system configuration designed to facilitate movement of persons around many obstructions. Repeated shortening and lengthening of the short rope/pulley mechanical advantage system within the rope rescue system creates an appearance similar to an inchworm. This system is ideal for drags along a horizontal plane, but will accommodate short vertical hauls with minor system modifications.

Incident Command System (Incident Management System) An organized system of roles, responsibilities, and standard operating procedures used to manage emergency operations.

Incident Commander A function within the incident command system used to designate the person (or persons depending on the type of command structure) responsible for directing the overall incident.

In-Plant Rescue Team A rescue team located on-site within the confines of a given facility such as a plant or mill.

Intrinsically Safe Equipment designed to be resistant to the possibility of generating a source of ignition when used in a specific potentially hazardous environment.

International Society of Fire Service Instructors (ISFSI) A membership organization dedicated to the advancement of fire service training and instructor development.

Kernmantle A type of rope construction consisting of an interior core (kern) which supports most of the load on the rope and a sheath (mantle) that is primarily designed to protect the core and support a minor portion of load bearing capability.

Kevlar Dupont trade name for a type of aramid fiber.

Laid Rope A type of rope construction consisting of fiber bundles twisted around one another.

Leg Wrap An emergency technique involving several wraps of rope around a person's leg to slow or stop an uncontrolled fixed line descent.

Line Tender The person designated to manage a specific loose rope within a system to prevent tangling or provide other additional safety mechanisms.

Line Transfer A technique for transferring a person suspended from a line or lanyard to a rope rescue system.

Litter Attendant A person attached, directly or indirectly, to a litter device within a rope rescue system for management of the litter around obstructions or projections and to provide patient care.

Load Limiter A device designed to absorb or disperse potentially dangerous energy created through dynamic loading.

Load Releasing Hitch (LRH) A configuration of cordage and/or webbing designed to allow controlled elongation under load. Often used together with a Tandem Prusik Belay system.

Load Watch A person designated to maintain direct visual contact with a person being moved by a rope system.

Lock Off The means of securing (hands-free) a specific descent control device within a rope rescue system to prevent further movement of the load to which it is attached.

Lockout/Tagout A method for keeping equipment from being set in motion and endangering workers. A disconnect switch, circuit breaker, valve, or other energy-isolating mechanism to hold equipment in a safe position. A lock is attached in accordance with U.S. Federal Regulations, so that equipment cannot be energized. This is usually performed in combination with a tagout procedure in which a warning tag is applied to the lockout device to alert personnel to the danger.

Long-Spine Immobilizer A body-length device used to immobilize the spine and body (from head to toe) in areas without size and/or space restrictions.

Loop One element of a knot created by a configuration of cordage or webbing having a shape, order, or path of motion that is circular or curved over on itself.

Low Point Anchor An anchor point situated at or below the level of an opening or structure over or through which the rope system is to be passed.

Lower Explosive Limit (LEL) The lowest concentration of a product that will explode or burn when it contacts a source of ignition of sufficient temperature.

Lower Flammable Limit (LFL) See Lower Explosive Limit (LEL)

Lowering To let, bring, or move down to a lower level.

Major Axis (Of a carabiner) the axis parallel with the spine, along which the carabiner is meant to be loaded.

Material Safety Data Sheets (MSDS) A document that contains information regarding the chemical composition, physical and chemical properties, health and safety hazards, emergency response, and waste disposal of the material as required by 29 CFR 1910.1200.

Mechanical Advantage (M/A) A force created through mechanical means including, but not limited to, a system of levers, gearing, or ropes and pulleys. It usually creates an output force greater than the input force and expressed in terms of a ratio of output force to input force.

Minor Axis (Of a carabiner) the axis which generally runs between the spine and the gate.

Munter Hitch A type of running knot that slips around a carabiner to create friction against itself. It is commonly used in belaying.

Needs Assessment A report that analyzes the technical rescue needs of a specific response agency including manpower and equipment.

National Fire Protection Association (NFPA) An international voluntary membership organization to promote improved fire protection and prevention, establish safeguards against loss of life and property by fire. The NFPA develops and publishes national voluntary consensus standards (e.g., NFPA 1983, *Fire Service Life Safety Rope and System Components*).

Non-Entry Rescue The removal of persons from a specific confined space not requiring entry of rescue personnel into the space.

OATH A crude means of communication involving the use of a series of tugs on a rope at one or the other ends: One tug means "okay," two tugs means "advance line," three tugs means "take up slack," and four tugs means "help."

Occupational Safety and Health Administration (OSHA) Component of the United states Department of Labor, an agency with safety and health regulatory and enforcement authorities for most United States industries, business and states.

Offset Belay The manual means of creating friction on a rope by wrapping it around two persons' waists while they face each other, slightly offset, and in an "S" configuration.

Off-site Rescue Team A rescue team located off-site but responsible for rescue within the confines of a given facility such as a plant or mill.

One Person Load 300 lb. (136 kg).

Open-circuit SCBA A type of breathing apparatus that vents the wearer's exhalations to the surrounding atmosphere.

Operations Level The National Fire Protection Association (1670—Standard on Operation and Training for Technical Rescue Incidents) term that describes a response agency with the operational capability of hazard recognition, equipment use, and techniques necessary to safely and effectively support, and participate in, a technical rescue incident. This level can involve search, rescue, and recovery operations, but usually operations are carried out under the supervision of technician- level personnel.

P Method A theoretical means of determining the forces applied to, and the mechanical advantage of, a hauling system.

Packaging Providing a stabilized patient appropriate protection from the environment and optimal comfort while allowing access for medical interventions during transport.

Performance Evaluation A criterion-based examination of a skill, based on specified requirements.

Permissible Exposure Limit (PEL) The concentration of a toxin that most people could safely be exposed to for 8 hours.

Permit Space See Permit-required Confined Space

Permit-required Confined Space By OSHA definition, a confined space that also has one or more of the following characteristics: contains or has a potential to contain a hazardous a hazardous atmosphere, contains a material that has the potential for engulfing an entrant, has an internal configuration such that an entrant could be trapped or asphyxiated by inwardly converging walls or by a floor that slopes downward and tapers to a smaller cross-section, or contains (or has the potential to contain) any other recognized serious safety or health hazard. NOTE: Unlike OSHA, the National Fire Protection Association (NFPA) standards 1670 - Technical Rescue Operations and Training and 1006 - Professional Qualifications for Rescue Technicians, use one definition (similar to OSHA's Permit-required Confined Space definition) to refer to all Confined Spaces. There is no differentiation made between *Confined Spaces* and *Permit-required Confined Spaces,* since these standards only address rescue from spaces assumed to contain additional hazards.

Personal Protective Equipment (PPE) Equipment provided to shield or isolate a person from the chemical, physical, and thermal hazards that may be encountered at a specific emergency incident. Adequate personal protective equipment should protect the respiratory system, skin, eyes, face, hands, feet, head, body, and hearing.

Personal Use An NFPA term referring to a designation of auxiliary equipment system components intended for the sole use of the rescuer for personal escape or self-rescue, or for the sole use of the rescuer in gaining access to victim. Designed for one-person loads only.

Pick-off Techniques for removing persons from an isolated area by accessing them with rope, attaching them to the rescuer's system, and rappelling or being lowered to a safe area with the victim attached.

Piggyback System The attachment of a rope/pulley mechanical advantage system to a separate rope or rope system to increase haul capability.

Portable Anchor An assembly or equipment component designed to provide an anchor system that can be moved or transported for rope rescue operations. Examples include ladder A-frame, tripod, and quadpod.

Positive Pressure A type of fresh-air breathing apparatus where air within the mask assembly is maintained at a slightly higher pressure than the atmosphere outside the mask. This creates an outward flow of air should a slight leak occur in the seal of the mask.

Preplan A written plan of action developed in anticipation of a potential emergency incident and based on specific conditions and resources.

Primary Anchor The anchor point within an anchor system intended to support most of the load or potential load.

Primary Entrant concerning a confined space entry, the first person to make entry into the space for a given purpose.

Primary Survey concerning a sick or injured person, the initial assessment by medical personnel to determine immediately life- threatening conditions.

Prusik Hitch A type of friction knot used to grab a rope when placed under load.

Prusik Minding Pulley A pulley whose sideplate configuration is designed to hold a Prusik Hitch in an "open" configuration while the rope to which it is attached is pulled through in a specific direction. This is particularly useful in conjunction with hauling operations where a Tandem Prusik Belay system is used.

Rappel To perform a controlled descent of a fixed line by use of a descent control device.

Rappel Master The person in charge of a rappel operation who is responsible for checking the system and the rappeller's rigging and connections before starting the descent. The Rappel Master is also generally responsible for communication of any necessary operating commands.

Ratchet Cam A rope grab device used within a hauling system to hold a load in a static position when activated. Often used to hold the load in place while some type of system reset occurs.

Ratchetman The person designated to manage the ratchet cam within a rope rescue system when such management is necessary.

Recovery 1. Activities and programs designed to return the entity to an acceptable condition, and 2. removal operation of low urgency where there is no chance of rescuing the victim(s) alive.

Rescue Those activities directed at locating endangered persons at an emergency incident, removing those persons from danger, treating the injured, and providing for transport to an appropriate health care facility.

Rescue Coverage Referring to the conditions surrounding the provision of rescue capability to a given response area.

Rescue Team The group of individuals assigned to perform rescue activities.

Rigging The assembly of rope and hardware to form anchoring and associated rope rescue systems.

Rigging Plate A piece of auxiliary equipment designed as a gathering point for various other rescue system components. Usually employed in the creation of load-distributing and load- sharing anchor systems.

Rope Grab Device An NFPA term used to describe an auxiliary equipment system component, a device used to grasp a life safety rope for the purpose of supporting loads, and can be used in ascending a fixed line.

Round Turn A full wrap of a rope around an object so that both ends emerge from the same side.

Safety Knot A type of knot (usually an Overhand or Barrel hitch) used to secure the loose end(s) of the principle knot to prevent it from coming untied accidentally.

Safety Line Belay One type of belay system independent of the primary rope system that incorporates a line attached to a separately anchored belay device. This type of belay system works effectively to provide a back up for both a failure of the primary rope system or loss of control by operators.

Safety Margin (Safety Factor) The ratio between the maximum load expected on a rope or rope system component and its breaking strength. The larger the ratio, the greater the safety factor.

Superfund Amendments and Reauthorization Act (SARA) Created to establish federal statutes for right-to-know standards and emergency response to hazardous materials incidents. It re-authorized the federal superfund program and mandated states to implement equivalent regulations/requirements.

Screw Link A type of metal connector with a threaded screw-type metal gate used for securing rope system components together. These connectors maintain their integrity only after the threaded female gate has been fully secured to the male threaded body of the link.

Secondary Anchor The anchor point within certain anchor systems intended to act as a backup to the primary anchor in case of its failure.

Secondary Entrant concerning a confined space entry, the person(s) designated to make entry subsequent to the primary entrant.

Secondary Survey concerning a sick or injured person, the thorough assessment by medical personnel to determine the type and extent of all injuries and other adverse medical conditions.

Secure To make firm or tight, to fasten.

Self Contained Breathing Apparatus (SCBA) A positive-pressure fresh-air breathing apparatus whose air supply is contained on a backpack assembly as part of the unit, certified by the national Institute for Occupational Safety and Health (NIOSH) and the Mine Safety and Health Administration (MSHA), or the appropriate approval agency for use in atmospheres that are immediately dangerous to life or health (IDLH).

Self-rescue The ability to carry out the method by which a person will escape should they become trapped. Often used in the context of confined space rescue and includes self-actuated methods (such as climbing a ladder or crawling through a horizontal manway opening) as well as those methods externally applied and operated (such as a hauling system attached to the entrant and operated by the rescue team).

Shock 1. The acute loss of capillary blood perfusion that results from a loss of pressure within the cardiovascular system, or 2. Dynamic loading of a system or object.

Shock Load (Impact load) Dynamic loading of a system often due to a fall or failure of a system or system component.

Shock Absorber See Load Limiter

Short Spine Immobilizer A short device used to temporarily immobilize the spine (from head to pelvic area) in areas where full spine immobilizers cannot be used due to size and/or space restrictions.

Side Load The loading of a carabiner along its minor axis.

Side Plate The structural members of a pulley forming the walls housing the sheave. Rescue pulleys are usually of a "swing-side" type allowing the side plates to be opened for attachment to a rope anywhere along its length.

Simple M/A A rope mechanical advantage system containing the following: 1. A single rope, 2. One or more moving pulleys (or similar devices), all traveling at the same speed and in the same direction, attached directly or indirectly to the load, and 3. in the case of mechanical advantage systems greater than 2:1, one or more stationary pulleys or similar devices.

Size-up The process of gathering information relative to the incident to include but not limited to weather, resource capabilities and limitations and, most critically, evaluating potential hazards to the rescuer(s) and patient(s).

Sked Litter A brand of flexible litter manufactured by Skedco, Inc.

Soft Ascender The use of cordage to create a hitch for grabbing and/or ascending rope.

Software A category of rope system components that is not hardware. In this category are rope and webbing.

Span of Control A term within the Incident Management System indicating the number of persons, sectors, groups, or divisions one person can effectively supervise. Although variable, this number is generally considered to be between three and seven with five being the optimum.

Spider Strap A type of pre-fabricated lashing device often used in conjunction with long-spine immobilizers. These devices have a webbing configuration that somewhat resembles the body and legs of a spider.

Spinal Immobilization To fix the position of the entire spine as with a splint or cast.

Spinal Precautions Care taken to prevent additional injury to a potentially traumatized spine.

Spineboard See Long-spine Immobilizer.

Society of Professional Rope Access Technicians (SPRAT) A membership-based agency instituted for the development of voluntary standards relative to work practices requiring rope and rope systems for access.

Stabilize 1) To make stable or steadfast, 2) To maintain the stability of by means of a stabilizer, or 3) To keep from fluctuating, fix the level of.

Standardized Operational Guidelines (SOGs) Also known as Standard Operating Procedures (SOPs), they serve to act as a guide to standardized operations within a particular agency relative to specific events. These guidelines are generally written in a broad fashion to allow easy application without restricting the use of independent judgement.

Static Kernmantle Rope A low-stretch kernmantle rope intended for use where potential for falls is limited and rope system control is vital.

Station The demonstration area where different evolutions will be performed.

Stokes Basket See Basket Litter.

Stopper Knot A type of knot secured in the loose end of a line to prevent its slipping through a system or system component.

Supplied Air Respirator (SAR) Positive pressure fresh-air breathing apparatus supplied by either an airline hose or breathing air cylinders connected to the respirator by a short airline (or pigtail). When used for rescue in hazardous atmospheres, a secondary source of air supply is required.

System A group of interacting, interrelated, or interdependent elements forming a complex whole.

Tag Line Line attached to litter or other object to pull away from obstacles that might cause the object to hang up.

Tandem Prusik Belay (TPB) A belay system usually constructed with two loops of accessory cord attached to the belay line with triple-wrap Prusik hitches at the distal end and attached to a load releasing hitch and/or anchor system at its proximal end (may include additional equipment such as pulleys). The hitches are intended to bind on the belay rope in case of failure of the primary rope system.

Technician Level A National Fire Protection Association (1670—Standard on Operation and Training for Technical Rescue Incidents) term that describes a response agency with the capability of hazard recognition, equipment use, and techniques necessary to safely and effectively coordinate, perform, and supervise a technical rescue incident. This level can involve search, rescue, and recovery operations.

Third Man Rescue A type of pick-off rescue performed by a rescuer who rappels or is lowered to a person who has no other means of safe egress. The victim is then attached to the rescuer via appropriate rigging and is transferred to a safe area by means of a rappelling or lowering operation.

Trauma Damage to the body caused by violent external means.

Traveling Pulley A pulley within a rope/pulley mechanical advantage system that moves when the system is operated. These type of pulleys create mechanical advantage within the system.

Turnaround The suspension of normal operation for a unit or plant so that required maintenance may be performed. Also known as "shut-down," "outage," etc.

Two Person Load 600 lbs. (272 kg).

Utility Belt A specific brand of adjustable-length anchor strap manufactured by The Roco Corporation.

Webbing Woven material in the form of a long strip. It can be of flat or tubular weave.

Z-Rig Common name given to a specific type of 3:1 hauling system. The name is derived from the shape the rope path makes as it travels through the system.

Index